Health Care: A Women-Centered Approach

Health Care: A Women-Centered Approach

Edited by Tim Grayson

hayle medical

New York

Hayle Medical,
750 Third Avenue, 9th Floor,
New York, NY 10017, USA

Visit us on the World Wide Web at:
www.haylemedical.com

ISBN: 978-1-63241-628-5

Printed in China.

Cataloging-in-Publication Data

Health care : a women-centered approach / edited by Tim Grayson.
p. cm.
Includes bibliographical references and index.
ISBN 978-1-63241-628-5
1. Women's health services. 2. Medical care. 3. Health facilities.
4. Health services administration. I. Grayson, Tim.
RA564.85 .H43 2019
610.82--dc23

Table of Contents

Preface

The main aim of this book is to educate learners and enhance their research focus by presenting diverse topics covering this vast field. This is an advanced book which compiles significant studies by distinguished experts in the area of analysis. This book addresses successive solutions to the challenges arising in the area of application, along with it; the book provides scope for future developments.

Health care is concerned with the maintenance and improvement of health. Its main goals are to ensure good quality of life, to provide high quality medical resources and assistance to those needing them, to cure diseases and to extend life expectancy. Women's health is often influenced by factors such as poverty, gender differences, family responsibilities and employment. Breast cancer, lung cancer and cervical cancer are some of the most common chronic diseases in women. Other common health conditions in women include anemia, dementia, osteoporosis and depression. This book studies, analyzes and upholds the pillars of women's health and its utmost significance in modern times. Different approaches, evaluations, methodologies and advanced studies on health care have been included herein. This book is a collective contribution of a renowned group of international experts.

It was a great honour to edit this book, though there were challenges, as it involved a lot of communication and networking between me and the editorial team. However, the end result was this all-inclusive book covering diverse themes in the field.

Finally, it is important to acknowledge the efforts of the contributors for their excellent chapters, through which a wide variety of issues have been addressed. I would also like to thank my colleagues for their valuable feedback during the making of this book.

Editor

A Comparison of 25 µg with 50 µg Misoprostol for Cervical Ripening and Induction of Labor

Francis Olayemi Adebayo*, Olatunde Onafowokan and Nathaniel Adewole

Department of Obstetrics and Gynecology, University of Abuja Teaching Hospital, Abuja-FCT, Nigeria

***Corresponding author:** Francis Olayemi Adebayo, Department of Obstetrics and Gynecology, University of Abuja Teaching Hospital, Abuja-FCT, Nigeria, E-mail: preciousdavis67@yahoo.com

Abstract

Background: Misoprostol is increasingly being accepted as a standard agent for cervical ripening and induction of labor. The lowest effective dose is still not known.

Materials and Methods: This was an open label clinical trial of one hundred and eighty four women with obstetrics or medical indications for induction of labor at University of Abuja Teaching Hospital, Abuja. Women were grouped to receive either 25 µg or 50 µg of intravaginal misoprostol. The main outcome measure was induction-vaginal delivery interval while the secondary outcome measures were requirements for oxytocin augmentation, mode of delivery, frequency of tachsystole/hyperstimulation, as well as feto-maternal outcomes. Data was analyzed using SPSS version 21.0. Chi-square test was used to compare categorical variables. Mann-Whitney test was used to analyze continuous variables of the two treatment groups. P-value of less than 0.05 was accepted as indicating statistical significance.

Results: Mean induction delivery interval was 13.8 ± 5.9 and 14.0 ± 5.7 hours (P=0.842) with the 25 µg and 50 µg misoprostol respectively. The delivery rate within 24 hours of 66.3% (61/92,) in 25 µg group was lower than 67.4% (62/92) recorded in the 50 µg group but the difference was not statistically significant (P=0.156). The rates of caesarean section and operative vaginal delivery were similar in both groups. There were no significant difference in maternal side effects and neonatal outcomes among the women in the two groups.

Conclusion: There were no statistically significant differences in the effectiveness and safety of either of the dose regimen over the other. The choice may therefore be guided by the physician's experience, availability and/or departmental protocol.

Keywords: Misoprostol; Labor; Pregnancy; Delivery; Cervical ripening

Introduction

Situations arise in obstetrics where it becomes necessary to end a pregnancy in the interest of the mother and/or baby. Thus, induction of labor (IOL) has merit as a therapeutic option when the benefit of expeditious delivery outweighs the risks of continuing the pregnancy. The benefits of cervical ripening and induction of labor therefore must be weighed against the potential maternal and fetal risks associated with this procedure [1-3]. Induction of labor usually involves not a single intervention but a complex set of interventions with a tendency of posing challenges for both the obstetrician and mother [4,5].

The search for an ideal agent, timing and dosage interval to convert an unfavorable cervix to one receptive to delivery is an ongoing process [6]. The ideal induction agent would be one that is efficient, cost effective, easy to store, non-invasive, without side effects, and whose effects on mother and fetus can be readily monitored [7].

The well documented effectiveness of misoprostol in several gynecological and obstetric applications has resulted in enthusiasm for its use. The purpose of induction of labor is to achieve vaginal delivery by stimulating uterine contractions before the spontaneous onset of labor. However, it does appears challenging to a obstetricians when the cervix is not favorable [8,9]. There is paucity of data about the use of preformed 25 µg intravaginal misoprostol for cervical ripening and labor induction in West African Sub-region especially in Nigeria.

With the availability of the 25 µg preparation, it may become objectively feasible to compare the effectiveness and efficacy of the 25 µg with 50 µg in cervical ripening and induction of labor. This study was designed to compare the efficacy and safety of 25 µg and 50 µg intravaginal misoprostol tablets for cervical ripening and induction of labor when administered at an interval of 6 hours.

Materials and Methods

This was a clinical trial of one hundred and eighty four women with obstetrics or medical indications for induction of labor at University of Abuja Teaching Hospital, Abuja. Women were randomized to receive either 25 µg or 50 µg of intravaginal misoprostol. The study population comprised of all eligible pregnant women admitted for induction of labour at term with unfavorable cervix during the study period.

Included were all pregnant women who had given consent and with; singleton cephalic presenting pregnancy at term with no contraindication for vaginal delivery. Other inclusion criteria were prerequisite reactive Cardiotocograph (CTG) and, intact membrane with unfavorable cervix for induction (Bishop's score of ≤ 5).

Patients who refused consent to participate were excluded alongside those with singleton fetus with weight greater or equal to 4 kg and multiple gestation. Other exclusion criteria were patient with ruptured membrane, unsatisfactory CTG and contraindication to vaginal delivery.

Enrolled patients were randomly allocated to one of the two therapeutic regimens of 25 µg or 50 µg misoprostol tablets. Randomization was performed using computer-generated list by means of sequentially numbered, opaque, sealed envelopes indicating their medication. One group of patients received 25 µg misoprostol and the other group 50 µg misoprostol (two 25 µg misoprostol).

The sample size on each arm of the dosing regimen was calculated using the formula [10]:

Sample size, N=2M

M=required minimum sample size for each study arm

$M=(Z\alpha+Z\beta)^2\{H0(1-H0)+H1(1-H1)\}/(H1-H0)^2$

Where; $Z\alpha$=percentage of normal distribution corresponding to the required significant level of 5%

=1.96

$Z\beta$=point of normal distribution corresponding to the statistical power of 90%

=1.28

H0=Response in the first group (From previous study)39=0.97

H1=Expected response in the second group=0.82

Thus $N=(1.96+1.28)^2\ \{0.97(1-0.97)+0.82(1-0.82)\}/(0.97-0.82)^2$

N=82.4

Therefore, the minimum sample size in each group was 83.

Adding 10% attrition rate to the value obtained above, each trial group was allocated 92 patients. The total sample size was 184 pregnant women for both arms.

Data were analyzed using Statistical Package for Social Science (SPSS version 21) categorical variables using Chi square test. P-value of less than 0.05 was accepted as indicating statistical significance. Comparison of means was done using a Student's t-test. Mann-Whitney U test and Fisher's exact test was also employed as found appropriate. The ethical clearance was obtained from the Research Ethics Committee of the University of Abuja Teaching Hospital and signed consent for participation was obtained for all the patients.

Results

A total of 1318 deliveries were recorded during the period of study and out of which 189 were assessed for eligibility. One hundred and eighty four met inclusion criteria and were enrolled into the study. Five women did not meet the inclusion criteria and were excluded. There were neither opt out cases nor incidence of protocol violations. All 184 enrolled were available for final analysis. Patient population was divided into two groups; group A received 25 µg misoprostol per vaginally and group B received 50 µg. Thus, the rate of cervical ripening and induction of labor was 14.3%.

Table 1 shows maternal demographic profile of the women included in the study. Both groups were comparable with respect to maternal age, parity, mean gestational age at the time of induction and Bishop's score at commencement of cervical ripening and labor induction. The mean age of patients in the 25 µg group was 29.28 ± 4.71, while the mean age in the 50 µ 29.39 ± 4.00, P=0.85; Nulliparity (47.8% *vs.* 45.7%, P=0.09) and multiparity (52.2% *vs.* 54.3%) respectively for 25 µg and 50 µg were not statistically different. The mean gestational age (40.30 ± 1.92 *vs.* 39.54 ± 4.50, P=0.14); and initial Bishop's scores (3.84 ± 0.97 *vs.* 3.88 ± 1.06, P=0.37) were similar respectively for 25 µg and 50 µg groups.

	25 µg Misoprostol	50 µg Misoprostol	P-value
Characteristic	n=92 (%)		
Age[a] (Years) (Mean ± SD)	29.28 ± 4.71	29.39 ± 4.00	0.85
Parity[b]			
Nulliparous	44 (47.8)	42 (45.7)	0.09
Multiparous	48 (52.2)	50 (54.3)	-
Gestational age (Weeks) (Mean ± SD)[c]	40.30 ± 1.92	39.54 ± 4.50	0.14
Initial Bishop Score (Mean ± SD)[c]	3.84 ± 0.97	3.88 ± 1.06	0.37

Table 1: Maternal characteristics of the study groups [[a]Mann-Whitney U test; [b]Chi square; [c]Student's t-test].

The indications for cervical ripening and induction of labor were similarly distributed in both groups. Postdate is the single most frequent indication constituting more than 50% in both groups of the study (Table 2).

Indication for labor induction[b]	25 µg Misoprostol	50 µg Misoprostol	P-value
	n=92 (%)		
Post date	60 (65.1)	46 (50.0)	0.28
Hypertensive disorder of pregnancy	20 (21.8)	26 (28.2)	0.43
IUFD	3 (3.3)	1 (1.1)	0.32
IUGR	1 (1.1)	3 (3.3)	0.32
Others	8 (8.7)	16 (17.4)	0.12

Table 2: Indications for induction [[b]Chi square].

Majority of women in both groups delivered vaginally (86.9% in 25 µg group and 88% in the 50 µg group). The 25 µg misoprostol group had a lower delivery rate with a single dose compared with the 50 µg group (32.6% and 39.1% respectively). However, 25 µg group had more deliveries than 50 µg group with increasing number of misoprostol doses (39.1% *vs.* 34.8%, and 17.4% *vs.* 16.3% for 2 doses and 3 doses respectively). The need for oxytocin augmentation among participants was higher in the 25 µg group (20.4%) than in 50 µg group (17.4%). This was however not statistically significant (P=0.64) (Table 3).

Variables	25 μg Misoprostol n=92 (%)	50 μg Misoprostol	P-value
Number of Misoprostol doses[b]			
1	30 (32.6)	36 (39.1)	0.53
2	36 (39.1)	32 (34.8)	0.68
3	16 (17.4)	15(16.3)	0.87
4	10 (10.9)	9(9.8)	0.83
Induction vaginal delivery interval[a]	13.8 ± 5.9	14.0 ± 5.7	0.84
<12 hrs (n,%)[b]	28 (30.4)	32 (34.8)	0.78
12- < 24 hrs (n,%)[b]	38 (41.3)	40 (43.4)	0.81
≥ 24 hrs (n,%)[b]	14 (15.2)	9 (9.8)	0.32
Oxytocin augmentation[b]	19 (20.6)	16 (17.4)	0.64

Table 3: Intrapartum variables [[a]Mann-whitney U test; [b]Chi square test].

There was no difference between the two groups with regard to the proportion of patients who had a successful induction. Eighty percent of patients allocated to 25 μg group and 76.1% of those in 50 μg group had spontaneous vaginal delivery while 6.5% and 11.9% of participants had instrumental vaginal delivery in 25 μg and 50 μg respectively (Tables 4 and 5).

Delivery[b]	25 μg Misoprostol n=92 (%)	50 μg Misoprostol	P-value
Spontaneous vaginal delivery	74 (80.4)	70 (76.1)	0.8
Instrumental vaginal delivery	6 (6.5)	11 (11.9)	0.25
Caesarean section	12 (13.1)	10 (10.9)	0.69
Others (Laparotomy)[c]	-	1 (1.1)	0.32

Table 4: Outcome of induction of labor [[b]Chi-square test; [c]Fisher's Exact test].

Indication	25 μg Misoprostol n=12 (%)	50 μg Misoprostol n=10 (%)	P-value
Fetal distress[b]	7 (7.6)	5 (5.4)	0.82
Non progress of labor[c]	3 (3.3)	1 (1.1)	0.32
Others[c]	2 (2.2)	4 (4.3)	0.42

Table 5: Indications for caesarean delivery [[b]Chi square; [c]Fisher's Exact test].

The incidence of caesarean section was similar in the two groups, twelve women (13.0%) in the 25 μg group and ten women (10.9%) in the 50 μg required emergency caesarean delivery for one reason or the other (P=0.82). No differences were noted in the overall incidence of caesarean section.

As highlighted in Tables 6 and 7, there was no significant difference in the secondary outcomes variable such as neonatal outcomes and intrapartum complications. No significant differences were found in both groups regarding intrapartum stillbirth, Apgar scores of less than 7 at 5 minutes and the number of neonates admitted to the Special Care Baby Unit.

The only recorded still birth in the 50 μg group was a consequence of ruptured uterus. The 50 μg misoprostol group recorded the highest number of cases with abnormal uterine contractions (2.2%) compared with misoprostol 25 μg group (1.1%).

Outcome	25 μg Misoprostol n=89 (92-3 IUFD) (%)	50 μg Misoprostol n=91 (92-1 IUFD) (%)	P-value
Foetal outcome			
Alive[b]	89 (96.7)	90 (97.8)	0.96
Dead[d]	-	1 (1.1)	0.32
Apgar score < 7			
At 1 min[b]	7 (7.6)	7 (7.6)	0.97
At 5 min[d]	5 (5.4)	2 (2.2)	0.25
SCBU admission[d]	5 (5.4)	3 (3.3)	0.47

Table 6: Fetal outcome [[b]Chi square; [d]Fisher's Exact test].

Complication[d]	25 μg Misoprostol n=2 (%)	50 μg Misoprostol n=7 (%)	P-value
Uterine contraction abnormalities	1 (1.1)	0.567	0.567
Uterine tachysystole	1 (1.1)	0.75	0.75
Uterine hyperstimulation syndrome	-	0.32	0.32
Ruptured uterus	-	0.32	0.32
Postpartum hemorrhage	-	2 (2.2)	0.16
Perineal laceration	-	2 (2.2)	0.16

Table 7: Intrapartum complications [[d]Fisher's Exact test].

With regards to potential adverse effects, no patient in any group had nausea, vomiting, diarrhea and fever in the study population. No case of hypertonus was recorded. Fetal distress requiring surgical intervention occurred in 12 patients. In each of these patients, management was initially conservative using nasal oxygen, adequate hydration and nursing on the left side. Caesarean sections were done when these measures failed to correct the adverse fetal cardiac activity. Uterine abnormalities were observed in both regimens; one case each while a case of uterine tachysystole was seen in 50 μg group. However, the observations were not significant statistically (P=0.57).

One multigravida in the 50 μg group had uterine rupture accounting for 0.54% of patients in the whole study. It was later discovered that she had a previous termination of pregnancy that was associated with complications. Two women in the 50 μg group developed postpartum hemorrhage compared to none in the 25 μg group (P=0.16). No maternal death was recorded in the study. All results tended to be more favorable in 25 μg group, but did not reach statistical significance.

Discussion

Misoprostol is increasingly being used for cervical ripening and induction of labour more than ever before. This was also observed in this study where there was an increase in rate from 13% recorded previously to 14.3% in the same institution [11]. The explanation for this could be attributed mainly to a rise in patients acceptability of induction of labour with misoprostol compared to 'painful' oxytocin. It is also lower to that of more developed nations like UK, United States and Canada. (18% UK, 20% US and 19% Canada) [12].

The women in the study were homogenous in terms of age, gestational age and parity in both groups. The most common indication for cervical ripening and induction of labour was postdate, accounting for 57.6%, followed by preeclampsia, accounting for 13.0%. This is similar to that obtained in a prospective study of labour induction [5] The same commonest indication was recorded in Korle Bu, Ghana [7], however, the second indication was sickle cell disease as against preeclampsia in Nigeria. These trends may be due to the fact that there are more postdated pregnancy now than before, probably due to better dating of gestational age and earlier booking.

The results of this study indicate that 25 μg of intravaginal misoprostol every 6 hours was as efficacious as 50 μg for cervical ripening and labor induction. There was no statistical significant difference between the two misoprostol regimens in terms of clinical efficacy. Although the study found that induction delivery interval was similar among the two groups, other investigators [13-18] had demonstrated that it was shorter in the 50 μg group. In a meta-analysis comparing 25 μg with 50 μg misoprostol, the induction vaginal delivery interval was nearly five hours shorter in the 50 μg group [19]. This difference as against meta-analysis may be due to small sample size and non-blinding of the study.

The proportion of women delivering within the first twelve hours and next twelve hours of induction were similar among the groups, which is consistent with the finding by other investigators [14,17]. This is contrast to the finding of Meydanli et al. [19] and Elhassan et al. [17] Meydanli reported that more women delivered between 12-24 hours in the 25 μg group while El-hassan reported that fewer delivered vaginally in the 25 μg group. The explanation for the differences may be in the methodology. Both researchers used compounded misoprostol prepared by different methods.

There was no difference in the overall caesarean section delivery rates unlike increase in caesarean section rate in the 50 μg group reported by Has et al. [14] Elhassan et al. [17] showed an increase in caesarean section rate in 25 μg group. In this study, there was no significant difference in occurrence of uterine contraction abnormalities among regimens, although some researchers have demonstrated an increase incidence of uterine contraction abnormalities in the 50 μg groups [13-15]. The higher incidence of hyper stimulation in Diro et al. [13] study is possibly due to higher dose of misoprostol received by most women. Although not statistically significant, the incidence of haemorrhage due to perinear laceration was more in the 50 μg group in this study. However, both El-hassan and El-sherbiny et al. [15] reported significantly increased incidence of atonic postpartum hemorrhage in 50 μg group.

Even though higher dose misoprostol (50 μg) enhance cervical ripening and labor during induction in a more efficient way than lower dose (25 μg), concern persist with respect to intrapartum fetal wellbeing. The price for using a higher misoprostol dosage to achieve higher delivery rate is increased risk of hyper stimulation syndrome, abnormal fetal heart rate, meconium staining liquor and perinatal mortality and morbidity from asphyxia. In this study, though not statistically significant, the 50 μg misoprostol group accounted for a high number of cases with abnormal uterine contraction (1.1% *vs.* 2.2%, Fisher exact test=0.375). However, the caesarean section for suspected fetal distress was not significant for both groups (7.6% *vs.* 5.4%, P=0.821). This may be due to early detection of abnormal fetal heart rate and early corrections.

The concern about safety of misoprostol is not limited to the fetus alone but extends to the mother. There was a case of uterine rupture in the 50 μg misoprostol group. Statistical analysis comparing this effect showed no significant difference. Even though the use of misoprostol for cervical ripening and induction of labor has been associated with uterine rupture, most reviews found no difference with other conventional methods.

Attempting an explanation for the aforementioned side effects in misoprostol use and taken into account other reports, it appears that the increase in clinically relevant adverse effects may be dose dependent rather than misoprostol related. The relationship between previous uterine evacuation and posterior uterine ruptured has previously been documented [20-22] as in this study. However, it is not strong evidence to exclude such patients from misoprostol use.

Conclusion

It appears that 25 μg of intravaginal misoprostol is as safe as 50 μg for cervical ripening and induction of labor. The choice may therefore be guided by the physician's experiences, availability and/or departmental protocol. It may also appeared safe to suggest that WHO recommendation on the use of low dose 25 μg misoprostol be applicable to our pregnant population provided strict selection criteria are upheld.

References

1. Girija S, Manjunath AP (2011) A randomised controlled trial comparing low dose vaginal misoprostol and dinoprostone gel for labour induction. J Obstet Gynaecol Ind pp: 153-160.
2. American College of Obstetrician and Gynaecology (2009) Clinical management guidelines for Obstetrician-Gynaecologist. Induction of labour. ACOG Practice Bulletin, Washington DC.
3. Caughey AB, Sundaram V, Kaimal AJ (2012) Maternal and neonatal outcomes of elective induction of labour. AHRQ Evidence Report, US.
4. Dodal JM, Crowther CA, Robinson JS (2006) Oral Misoprostol for induction of labour. BMJ 332: 509-513.
5. Ekele BA, Oyetunji JA (2002) Induction of labour at Usmanu Danfodiyo University Teaching Hospital, Sokoto. Trop J Obstet Gynaecol 19: 74-77.
6. Bano K, Mahjabeen, Bhutta ZS (2009) Oral misoprostol for induction of labour at term Pak J Surg 14: 38-41.
7. Kwawukume EY, Ayertey RP (2002) The use of misoprostol for induction of labour in a low resource setting. Trop J Obstet Gynaecol 19: 78-81.

8. Bahar AR, Archibong EI, Zaki ZMS (2003) Induction of labour using low and high dose regimens of prostaglandin E2 vaginal tablets. East Afr Med J 80: 51-55.
9. Appiah GE, Hofmeyr GJ, Moodley J (2005) Misoprostol in Obstetrics and Gynaecology-benefits and risks. SAJOG 11: 9-10.
10. Campell MJ, Machin DC (1990) Comparison of proportion. In: Medical Statistics, a common sense approach. John Wiley & Sons Ltd. West Sussex, England p: 148.
11. Onafowokan O, Kailani S, Offiong RA (2006) Outcome of labour induced with Misoprostol. Trop J Obstet Gynaecol 23: 1.
12. Lovold A, Stanton C (2008) Use of oxytocin and misoprostol for induction or augmentation of labour in low resource settings. A report of a working meeting POPPHI Project, PATH, Washington DC.
13. Diro M, Adra A, Gilles JM, Nassar A (2002) A double blind randomised trial of two dose regimens of misoprostol for cervical ripening and labour induction. Obstet Gynaecol 99: 145-151.
14. Has R, Batukan C, Ermis H (2002) Comparison of 25 and 50 mcg vaginally administered misoprostol for preinduction of cervical ripening and labour induction. Gynaecol Obstet Invest 53: 16-21.
15. El-Sherbiny MT, El-Gharieb IH, Gewely HA (2001) Vaginal misoprostol for induction of labour: 25 vs. 50 μg dose regimen. Int J Gynaecol Obstet 72: 25-30.
16. Elhassan EM, Mirghani OA, Adam I (2005) Cervical ripening and labour induction with 25 mcg vs. 50 mcg of misoprostol. Inter J Gynaecol Obstet 90: 234-235.
17. Farah LI, Ramous LS, Rosa C (1997) Randomised trial of two doses of the prostaglandin E1 analog misoprostol for labour induction. Am J Obstet Gynaecol 177: 364-371.
18. Adeniji AA, Odukogbe AA, Olayemi A, Oladokun O, Adenij AO, et al. (2014) Randomization of two dosing regimens of vaginal misoprostol for cervical ripening and labour induction in a low resource setting. Niger J Clin Pract pp: 287-291.
19. Meydanli MM, Caliskan E, Burak F (2003) Labour induction post-term with 25 micrograms vs. 50 micrograms of intravaginal misoprostol. Int J Gynaecol Obstet 81: 249-255.
20. Lalos O, Lundstrom P, Probst FP (1997) Spontaneous rupture of the uterus in the third trimester with a living fetus expelled into the abdominal cavity. Acta Obstet Gynaecol Scand 56: 153-156.
21. Hawe JA, Olah KS (1997) Posterior uterine rupture in a patient with a lower segment caesarean section scar complicating prostaglandin induction of labour. Br J Obstet Gynaecol 104: 857-858.
22. Chew SI, Choo HT (1982) Spontaneous uterine rupture through perforation scar of previous curettage. Singapore Med J 23: 283-285.

Effect of Complete Antenatal Care on Birth Weight of Children in India: Evidence from National Family Health Survey (NFHS) Data

Sanjay Jayawant Rode*

Department of Economics, S.K. Somaiya College, Mumbai University, India

***Corresponding author:** Sanjay Jayawant Rode, Assistant Professor, Department of Economics, S.K. Somaiya College, Mumbai University, India, E-mail: sanjayjrode@gmail.com

Abstract

Prenatal care consists of counseling, medical care and supplementary nutrition. As per WHO guidelines are concerned then all the pregnant women are expected to visit four times to health care staff, hospitals and get the counseling, medical care and supplementary food. We have used National Family Health Survey (NFHS)-1, 2, and 3 data and analyzed such data in STATA@10 software. We found that, lower access to health care facilities; education and poverty, religion and caste background do not support the pregnant women to have minimum four required prenatal visits. The multi-nominal logic regression result shows that poor, illiterate, lower age group, Scheduled caste and Tribe pregnant women do not get the minimum required prenatal care. Such variables are positively correlated and statistically significant with low birth weight babies in India. India has high infant, child mortality, malnutrition and morbidity. Adequate prenatal visits by all pregnant women will certainly reduce the incidence of mortality, illness and malnutrition in country. Government must broadcast prenatal related programs on television and radio. Government must open up more sub centers in villages and in urban areas. Government must promote private clinics/hospitals to provide prenatal care especially to poor pregnant women. Such efforts will certainly improve health status of women and children and reduce the prevalence of child malnutrition, morbidity and mortality in India.

Keywords: Nutrition; Breastfeeding; Healthcare; Malnutrition; Pregnancy; Antenatal care

Introduction

Developing countries have high incidence of neonatal, infant, child mortality and malnutrition [1]. Governments, international organizations and non-government organizations have taken number of steps over the period of time to reduce infant, child mortality and malnutrition and maternal mortality. In India, incidence of child malnutrition and mortality is not declining and still it is observed as very high. High malnutrition among children affects physical and intellectual growth. They become less educated and un-productive adults in the long term. Malnutrition in the long run effects on total productivity, economic growth of country. In order to reduce the low birth weight babies, neonatal, infant mortality and malnutrition, prenatal care is one of the best instruments [2]. The study also indicates that adequate use of prenatal care increases birth weight, holding other factors constant [3]. The maternal health production function explains that early onset of prenatal care and having a minimum number of prenatal care visits is important for improvement in health of mother as well as unborn child.

The prenatal care as per World Health Organization (WHO) consists of four visits by pregnant women to health care facility and health specialists. The four antenatal care ensures adequate nutrition, vitamin intake, proper vaccination, exercise, negative behavioral modification and institutional delivery. Pregnancy constitutes one of the most sensitive period of a women's life, both physically and mentally [4]. Good care during pregnancy is important for the health of mother and the development of the unborn baby. During pregnancy, healthy behaviors as well as care and parenting skills, medicines are required. Antenatal care is an umbrella term used to describe the medical procedures and care that are carried out during pregnancy. In promoting antenatal care, it is essential that the effectiveness of this service leaves no room for doubt [5]. Prenatal care is a key strategy for achieving public health goals, primary healthcare objectives, and the Millennium Development Goals [6].

During four antenatal visits, the health care facility and skilled health staff certainly plans delivery, understand danger signs during pregnancy through various physical tests and modify unhealthy behaviors and advice healthy diets. The health staff get chance to work for normal delivery. In the literature, it is well documented that those women received four antenatal care have lower rates of maternal and infant mortality as well as good pregnancy outcome. A proper utilization of prenatal care is co-related to high birth weight of babies and gestational age. The preterm deliveries and low birth weight babies contribute neonatal and infant mortality [6,7]. In the literature, it is stated that children of mothers did not receive prenatal care are twice as likely to die during infancy as children of mothers who received prenatal care. Despite the evidence that prenatal care is associated with desirable birth outcomes, it is not an easy step to conclude cost effectiveness. Although, the incidence of low and very low birth weights, premature labor, transfers to acute-care facilities, and early death was significantly greater for those women who had no prenatal care, the combined impact on total cost of care is not large in an absolute sense [8]. The major objective of this paper is to study the impact of prenatal care on birth weight of babies in India [9-13].

Data and Methodology

We collected secondary data from three National Family Health Surveys. The NFHS-1 (1992-1993), NFHS-2 (1998-1999) and NFHS-3

(2005-2006) data is collected in different states in India. International Institute for Population Science provides the state-wise health data with different health indicators. We studied the prenatal care related data from three surveys. We classified and analyzed the prenatal care data in spss@20 and stata@10.

The pregnant woman had either no antenatal visit or they have multiple antenatal visits. We classified the total antenatal visits of each woman in different states and socio-economic characteristics. For the regression, the number of visits took as dependent variable and women's socio-economic and demographic factors are considered as independent variables. We have used multinomial logit regression model to find the co-relation of dependent variable with independent variable.

Economic Model

We have developed economic model for prenatal care in India. The prenatal visits are categorized as follows:

PV=(NV, OV, TWV, THV, FMV)

The prenatal visits to health care facility and health specialist by pregnant women is categorized as No Visit (NV), One Visit (OV), Two Visits (TWV), Three Visits (THV) and Four or More (FMV) visits. All the pregnant women are expected to visit to health care facility and health care specialist. But due to socio-economic, demographic factors, the pregnant women either do not visit or visit less number of times to health care facility. The variables such as religion, caste, education and place of residence are considered as follows. The education of the women is considered into following categories:

E=(P, S, HS, C)

Education of pregnant women is considered as primary, secondary, high school and college.

R=(H, M, C, S, O)

Religion of pregnant women is categorized as Hindu, Muslim, Christian, Sikh and Others.

Wq=(PST, PER, MLE, RER, RST)

Wealth quintiles of pregnant women are classified as poorest (PST), poorer (PER), middle (MLE), richer (RER), richest (RST).

C=(SC, ST, OBC, O)

Caste background of pregnant women is categorized as Scheduled Caste (SC), Scheduled Tribe (ST), Other Back ward Class (OBC) and Other (O) caste. We have used above variables to examine the prenatal care among pregnant women in selected states in India.

The WHO Recommendations for Prenatal Care

The World Health Organization recommends (WHO) 9 at least four antenatal visits to health care facility during pregnancy of each women. We have used such standards for this study. The first visit is recommended before the end of the first trimester or before 12 weeks of pregnancy. The first visit to health care facility is expected to take 30-40 minutes. In this visit, pregnant woman's medical and obstetric history is collected, certain physical examinations are done and some advice is given to avoid certain risks during pregnancy. The second visit is recommended during the 2nd trimester or 24-26 weeks.

It takes around 20 minutes. Blood test measurement, uterine height and some tests for urinary infection are performed in this period. The third visit should take place around the 32nd week and it is supposed to take place for 20 minutes. Routine check-up and any necessary test are recommended in this period. If the 2nd visit is missed then all test of 2nd visit should be performed during 3rd visit. The period of third visit should comprise as 32 weeks. The fourth or final visit should take place between 36 and 38 weeks. At this time, the fetus's condition will be checked and if any abnormality found then the mother is advised to go to an obstetrician.

Health Care during Prenatal Visits

During four visits, variety of enquiries, testes, check-ups are conducted and advices are given to pregnant women and relatives. Usually the first contact of women to the health care staff takes place to confirm pregnancy. Suppose the pregnancy is confirmed then antenatal care should start immediately. Antenatal care (ANC) services are considered to be the key element in the primary health care delivery system of a country, which aims for a healthy society.

Over the past 60 years, the maternal health situation in the country has been staggering despite several changes in a rapidly evolving socioeconomic environment. The roles and responsibilities of primary care physicians have also been revised continuously in this context. Under their leadership, different cadres of health workers have been appointed to address the problem [10]. Therefore this study is making an attempt to understand the antenatal care among pregnant women and information provided about antenatal care to pregnant women.

Access and Visits of Prenatal Care in India

The prenatal access is very low among pregnant women in India. The doctors, nurses and midwives are the main providers of antenatal care. But they do not know potential barriers to utilization of antenatal care services. There are many barriers in utilization of prenatal care. Health care staff must be sensitive to women's socio-economic situation and their cultural and traditional beliefs and their communication skills. We have computed the total antenatal visits of each pregnant woman to health care facilities in India (Table 1).

Survey	Area	No ANC	Three ANC visits	Four and above ANC
NFHS-1	Rural	40.97	38.81	20.22
	Urban	17.19	33.29	49.52
NFHS-2	Rural	36.36	39.05	24.59
	Urban	11.55	29.91	58.54
NFHS-3	Rural	19.67	41.29	39.05
	Urban	8.94	25.49	65.57

Table 1: The prenatal visits by pregnant women in India (%).

Above table shows that in NFHS-1, around 40.97% women never received ante-natal care in rural area. The coverage of antenatal care is very low due to location of health care facilities. But in urban area, women without antenatal care are only 17.19% in NFHS-1. In NFHS-2, 36.36% women never received any antenatal care in rural area. In this survey, small increase in prenatal care is observed. It may be because of awareness of health care and development of transportation and communication technology.

In the urban area, 11.55% pregnant women never received any antenatal care at all. In the NFHS-3 survey, 19.67% pregnant women have not received antenatal care. In urban area, health care access is more. Therefore, only 8.94% of pregnant women have not received antenatal care. The coverage of antenatal care is higher in urban area as compare to rural area in India. It is simply because health facilities in rural area are located far away. The pregnant women cannot travel long distance for antenatal care.

In urban area, health care facilities are not far away. Therefore, access and utilization of antenatal care is more. We have also measured the outcome of the prenatal care. The study has pointed out the birth weight and that a delays in antenatal care. The study states that delay in obtaining prenatal care or receiving no prenatal care have been associated with increased frequencies of low birth weight and other adverse pregnancy outcomes [11].

We have studied the relationship of different socio-economic factors with the antenatal care of pregnant women. We have studied the prenatal care among pregnant women in relation to standard of living index. The standard of living index consists of holding various assets by the family members of pregnant women. The score of different assets is given as standard of living index (Table 2).

	No ANC		Three ANC		Four ANC	
SLI	Rural	Urban	Rural	Urban	Rural	Urban
Low	49.9	29.6	38.1	21.65	24	7.1
Medium	44.9	55.61	50.6	53.67	51.8	43.86
High	5.23	14.8	11.4	24.68	24.3	49.04

Table 2: Prenatal visits according to standard of living Index in NFHS-2 (%).

The table shows that half of pregnant women from rural area with low standard of living index had not received antenatal check-ups. Poverty is the main reason of not getting the four antenatal care. But only 5.23% pregnant women from high standard of living index had not received antenatal care. In urban area, 55.61% pregnant women with medium standard of living index have not received any antenatal care. Half of pregnant women from rural area with medium standard of living index have received three antenatal cares. In urban area, 53.67% of pregnant women have received the three antenatal care. As far as four antenatal cares are concerned then 51.75% pregnant women of medium standard of living index have received four antenatal cares. In urban area, 49.04% of pregnant women of high standard of living index have received four antenatal cares. It means that women of higher socioeconomic status are more likely to receive early and adequate prenatal care, compared to those of a lower socio-economic status. In fact, continuity of care during pregnancy is influenced by financial resources and social support. Above data and results also show that poor pregnant women from rural area have either no or few visits of antenatal care. We have also studied the coverage of prenatal care as per the wealth quintile of households of pregnant women in India. The results are presented in the following table (Table 3).

	No ANC		Three ANC		Four ANC	
Wealth quintile	Rural	Urban	Rural	Urban	Rural	Urban
Poorest	42	13.17	28.6	4.43	10	0.94
Poorer	30.6	19.49	27.8	11.29	16.6	2.97
Middle	19.2	27.73	24	21.79	26	10.64
Richer	7.09	27.89	15	36	27.2	27.46
Richest	1.18	11.71	4.69	26.49	20.2	57.98

Table 3: Prenatal visits according to wealth quintile in NFHS-3 (%).

It is found that 41.97% pregnant women of poorest quintile of rural area have not visited for any antenatal care. In urban area, 27.89% of pregnant women of richer quintile have not visited for prenatal care. It means they have missed all four tests which are performed during pregnancy. In poorest quintile, the 28.59% pregnant women have received three antenatal cares. Only 4.69% pregnant women of richest quintile in rural area have received three antenatal cares. In the urban area of country, 4.43% pregnant women of poorest quintile have received three antenatal cares as far as NFHS-3 data is concerned. Only 10.03% pregnant women of poorest quintile have received four antenatal cares in rural area. Such coverage of four antenatal cares is very low among poor women.

The 20.22% pregnant women of richest quintile in rural area have received four antenatal cares. The 2.97% pregnant women of poorer quintile of urban area have received four antenatal cares. The 57.98% women of richest quintile of urban area have received four antenatal check-ups. We have also considered the age related factor of pregnant women for antenatal care in India. One key medical and health issue of adolescent reproduction is its association with poor pregnancy outcomes for the mother and child. The study 12 has compared to women of more mature age, pregnancy and childbearing during the teen years have been observed to present much higher risks of low birth weight, neonatal mortality, infant mortality and pregnancy-related medical complication. This study is more practical and significant for birth outcome (Table 4).

		NFHS-1			NFHS-2			NFHS-3		
Age group	Region	No ANC	Three ANC visits	Four and above ANC	No ANC	Three ANC visits	Four and above ANC	No ANC	Three ANC visits	Four and above ANC
	R	38.82	39.7	21.48	37.02	41.22	21.76	22.76	49.15	28.09
	U	35.89	39.89	24.23	12.41	42.11	45.49	11.19	36.06	52.75
15-19	T	37.21	39.8	22.99	32.83	41.37	25.8	19.74	45.74	34.52

	R	37.11	38.65	24.24	34.1	40.28	25.62	19.44	44.81	35.75
	U	31.42	38.16	30.43	10.62	31.53	57.85	8.17	28.12	63.71
20-24	T	33.83	38.36	27.8	28.09	38.04	33.86	15.27	38.64	46.09
	R	40.52	35.51	23.97	38.66	36.97	24.36	22.83	40.36	36.81
	U	32.68	34.35	32.97	10.52	26.22	63.26	7.74	24.06	68.2
25-29	T	35.9	34.82	29.28	30.47	33.84	35.68	16.31	33.32	50.37
	R	48.64	31.54	19.82	46.58	34.19	19.23	27.95	39.4	32.64
	U	40.2	30.41	29.39	12.51	28.94	58.55	8.65	22.35	69
30-34	T	43.7	30.88	25.42	36.84	32.69	30.47	19.59	32.02	48.39
	R	56.98	28.76	14.27	52.72	31.97	15.3	37.51	36.14	26.35
	U	49.02	29.92	21.06	18.63	27.94	53.43	13.1	25.27	61.63
35-39	T	52.43	29.42	18.15	44.32	30.98	24.7	28.38	32.08	39.54
	R	58.94	28.14	12.93	58.1	29.89	12.01	44.82	37.63	17.56
	U	54.09	28.12	17.79	19.4	38.81	41.79	22.09	27.13	50.78
40-44	T	56.25	28.13	15.62	52	31.29	16.71	37.97	34.46	27.57
	R	68.6	23.67	7.73	59.79	28.87	11.34	58.14	25.58	16.28
	U	65.29	22.73	11.98	33.33	55.56	11.11	36.17	27.66	36.17
45-49	T	66.82	23.16	10.02	57.55	31.13	11.32	53.42	26.03	20.55

Table 4: Age of women and prenatal visits (%).

In NFHS-1, 65.29% pregnant women of 45-49 age groups have not received any antenatal care. In NFHS-2, nearly 57.55% pregnant women of 45-49 age groups have not received any antenatal care. In NFHS-3, 53.42% of same age group has not received any antenatal care. It means pregnant women without antenatal care are declining but it is declining at very lower rate. In NFHS-1, nearly 38.81% women of 15-19 age groups have received up to three antenatal care. In NFHS-2, 39.05% women of 15-19 age groups have received up to three antenatal care. In NFHS-3, 41.29% women of same age group have received up to three antenatal care. NFHS-1 data shows that, 32.97% pregnant women of 25-29 age groups have received four and above antenatal care.

The NFHS-2 shows that, 35.68% pregnant women of 25-29 age groups have received four and above antenatal care. In NFHS-3, 50.37% pregnant women of 25-29 age group have received three and above antenatal care. It means the antenatal care is increasing among pregnant women in India over the period of time. But there is need of more coverage of prenatal care. Health care staff must take more efforts for providing universal antenatal care in urban and rural area. Most of the time, health care staff is not available in hospitals for antenatal care. The four antenatal visits by pregnant women are also depends on the educational attainment. Highly educated women have more antenatal care as compare to illiterate and less educated women (Table 5).

Education	Region	NFHS-1			NFHS-2			NFHS-3		
		No ANC	Three ANC visits	Four and above ANC	No ANC	Three ANC visits	Four and above ANC	No ANC	Three ANC visits	Four and above ANC
Illiterate	R	52.97	33.99	13.05	44.65	38.36	16.98	26.32	50	23.68
	U	50.04	35	14.96	22.58	29.03	48.39	30	30	40
	T	51.37	34.54	14.09	41.05	36.84	22.11	27.08	45.83	27.08
Primary	R	25.27	43.39	31.34	18.99	42.95	38.06	14.69	39.87	45.44
	U	21.56	43.08	35.36	5.34	27.91	66.75	4.6	23.77	71.62

	T	23.11	43.21	33.68	14.25	37.72	48.03	10.02	32.42	57.56
Secondary	R	12.56	36.77	50.67	19.36	37.41	43.22	10.12	36.03	53.85
	U	8.95	32.89	58.16	3.86	20.89	75.25	3.14	17.78	79.08
	T	10.22	34.25	55.52	12.48	30.08	57.43	6.39	26.27	67.34
High Secondary	R	3.09	19.75	77.16	5.74	24.36	69.89	2.19	18.88	78.93
	U	1.46	13.17	85.36	0.77	12.66	86.57	0.7	8.21	91.09
	T	1.72	14.22	84.06	2.55	16.85	80.59	1.03	10.58	88.39

Table 5: Women's education and prenatal visits (%).

In NFHS-1, only 14.09% illiterate pregnant women have received four or more antenatal care. In NFHS-2, it has increased up to 22.11%. In NFHS-3, 27.08% pregnant women have received four and above antenatal care. Illiterate women do not know much about minimum required antenatal care during pregnancy. Most of the time, they avoid the prenatal cares. In NFHS-1, 33.68% pregnant women have received four and above antenatal care but they are primary studied. In NFHS-2, 48.03% primary studied pregnant women have received four and above antenatal care.

In NFHS-3, 57.56% pregnant women have received four and above antenatal care. Nearly 55.52% secondary studied pregnant women have received four and above antenatal care. In NFHS-2, the prenatal coverage among pregnant women has increased. In this survey, 57.43% pregnant women have received four and above antenatal care. In NFHS-3, 67.34% secondary studied women have received four and above antenatal care. The 84.06% higher secondary studied pregnant women have received three and above antenatal care in NFHS-1.

In NFHS-2, 80.59% pregnant women have received four and above antenatal care. As far as NFHS-3 is concerned then 88.39% pregnant women have received four and above antenatal care and they are higher secondary studied. It means with increase in education, the antenatal care is also increases. The religious factors are also important in use of prenatal care by pregnant women (Table 6).

Religion	Region	NFHS-1			NFHS-2			NFHS-3		
		No ANC	Three ANC visits	Four and above ANC	No ANC	Three ANC visits	Four and above ANC	No ANC	Three ANC visits	Four and above ANC
Hindu	R	42.21	36.04	21.75	39.6	38.57	21.83	22.05	43.38	34.57
	U	35.72	35.33	28.95	11.45	30.01	58.54	7.56	24.24	68.19
	T	38.49	35.64	25.87	32.83	36.51	30.65	16.53	36.1	47.37
Muslim	R	45.46	34.84	19.7	42.44	33.07	24.49	28.89	39.7	31.41
	U	38.13	35.21	26.66	15.87	33.52	50.62	14.28	29.62	56.1
	T	41.01	35.06	23.93	33.25	33.22	33.53	21.81	34.81	43.38
Christian	R	40.32	28.68	31	30.11	39.34	30.56	36.99	34.31	28.7
	U	31.8	27.55	40.66	2.83	25.85	71.32	9.13	30.02	60.84
	T	35.37	28.02	36.61	22.34	35.5	42.16	26.84	32.74	40.42
Sikh	R	14.83	55.51	29.66	28.95	35.52	35.52	12.71	30.63	56.67
	U	12.36	51.11	36.53	8.86	12.66	78.48	0.64	9.62	89.74
	T	13.42	52.99	33.59	23.37	29.17	47.45	9.75	25.47	64.78
Other	R	54.23	25.71	20.06	42.13	41.7	16.17	28.57	38.22	33.2
	U	41.54	28.09	30.37	5.88	29.41	64.71	3.7	17.28	79.01
	T	46.73	27.12	26.15	33.99	38.94	27.06	19	30.17	50.83

Table 6: Prenatal visits and religion (%).

In Hindu religion, only 25.87% pregnant women have received four and above antenatal care in NFHS-1. But in same survey, 23.93% women of Muslim religion have received four and more antenatal care. In NFHS-2, only 30.65% women of Hindu religion have four and more antenatal care. They must have more access to health care facilities.

But utilization of antenatal care is very low. The 47.45% pregnant women of Sikh religion have four and more antenatal care. In NFHS-3, 64.78% pregnant women of Sikh religion have received four and more antenatal care.

In NFHS-1 and 2, pregnant women from Hindu religion have received consistently lower access to antenatal care in India (Table 7).

Ethnicity	Region	NFHS-1 No ANC	NFHS-1 Three ANC visits	NFHS-1 Four and above ANC	NFHS-2 No ANC	NFHS-2 Three ANC visits	NFHS-2 Four and above ANC	NFHS-3 No ANC	NFHS-3 Three ANC visits	NFHS-3 Four and above ANC
	R	45.16	37.77	17.07	42.12	39.09	18.78	25.04	45.98	28.97
	U	40.97	38.81	20.22	15.97	38.88	45.15	10.45	33.25	56.3
Scheduled Caste	T	42.82	38.35	18.83	36.36	39.05	24.59	19.67	41.29	39.05
	R	54.77	31.29	13.94	45.07	40.55	14.38	34.96	42.43	22.61
	U	50.69	31.74	17.57	11.58	33.12	55.31	11.42	34.02	54.56
Scheduled Tribe	T	52.59	31.53	15.88	40.09	39.45	20.46	29.6	40.52	29.88
	R	38.52	36.4	25.08	39.74	35.65	24.61	24.84	42.48	32.68
	U	31.61	35.07	33.32	12.84	28.53	58.63	12.35	26.23	61.42
Other Backward Classes	T	34.44	35.62	29.94	33.52	34	32.48	20.08	36.29	43.63

Table 7: Prenatal visits and ethnicity (%).

In NFHS-1, around 42.82% pregnant women of Scheduled Caste background have not received any antenatal care. The 36.36% female of Schedule Caste have not received antenatal care in NFHS-2. In NFHS-3, 19.67% women have not received any antenatal care. The number of women may have low birth weight babies, neonatal and infant mortality. In NFHS-1, nearly half of pregnant women of Scheduled Tribe (50.69%) have not received any antenatal care in India. The awareness and access of prenatal is very low among such women. In NFHS-2, 40.09% women of Scheduled Tribe have not received any antenatal care. In NFHS-3, 29.60% pregnant women of Scheduled Tribe have not received any antenatal care. The access to prenatal is increasing but it is increasing at very rate. As far as Other Backward Caste is concerned, then 34.44% pregnant women have not received any antenatal care. In NFHS-2, 33.52% pregnant women have not received any antenatal care. In NFHS-3, 20.08% pregnant women have not received any antenatal care of this caste. It means pregnant women with different ethnic background; the access to prenatal care is increasing but it is increasing at very slow rate in India.

The Multi-nominal Logit Regression Results

We have used multinomial logit regression model 13 to understand the different socio-economic and demographic factors responsible for antenatal care among pregnant women in India. The regression model is defined as follows.

$$Pr\left(y_i = j\right) = \frac{Exp\left(X_i B_j\right)}{1 + \sum_j{}^J exp\left(X_i B_j\right)}$$

$$Pr\left(y_i = 0\right) = \frac{1}{1 + \sum_j{}^J exp\left(X_i B_j\right)},$$

Where for the ith women, y_i is the observed outcome and X_j is a vector of explanatory variable. The parameters B_j are estimated by maximum likelihood. The positive and negative parameters are compared with the reference category of pregnant women those had four prenatal cares. The results are presented in the following table (Table 8).

NFHS-1	Rural				Urban			
	No ANC		Three ANC		No ANC		Three ANC	
Variables	Co-efficient	Z-test	Co-efficient	Z-test	Co-efficient	Z-test	Co-efficient	Z-test
13-14	-3.67** (1.15)	10.14	-0.45 (0.63)	0.52	-2.03** (0.64)	10.04	-0.18 (0.51)	0.12
15-19	-0.0915	16.51	-0.17 (0.15)	1.23	-0.0564	15.03	-0.01 (0.13)	0.01
20-24	-0.042	17.83	-0.14 (0.10)	1.92	-0.0272	17.75	-0.04 (0.08)	0.21

25-29	-0.0196	14.78	-0.12 (0.07)	2.34	-0.0138	15.16	-0.04 (0.65)	0.52
30-34	-0.18** (0.06)	8.81	-0.09 (0.06)	2.14	-0.14** (0.04)	9	-0.04 (0.04)	0.75
35-39	-0.10*** (0.05)	3.79	-0.06 (0.05)	1.29	-0.06*** (0.04)	2.75	-0.01 (0.04)	0.1
40-44	-0.09** (0.04)	4.17	-0.05 (0.04)	1.28	-0.07*** (0.03)	3.63	0.02 (0.00)	0.47
Illiterate	-0.17 (0.39)	0.19	-0.74*** (0.38)	3.7	-0.14 (0.34)	0.16	-0.2574	5.55
Primary	-0.636	16.23	-1.23** (0.38)	10.19	-0.544	21.45	-1.28** (0.33)	14.92
Secondary	-0.9438	37.42	-0.627	18.28	-2.60 (0.34)	56.38	-0.594	29.53
High secondary	-1.8792	41.28	-0.9143	28.7	-1.616	98.4	-0.9588	68.15
Hindu	0.21* (0.05)	13.46	0.09 (0.05)	2.54	0.12** (0.04)	6.94	0.06 (0.04)	1.97
Muslim	0.16** (0.09)	3.33	-0.0208	9.83	0.08 (0.08)	1.14	-0.0217	18.45
Christian	-0.1274	56.88	0.24* (0.09)	7.18	-0.95* (0.11	64.27	0.21** (-0.07)	7.54
Sikh	0.25** (0.14)	3.06	-0.26*** (0.14)	3.1	0.28** (0.12)	4.87	-0.12 (0.11)	1.13
Scheduled caste	0.08*** (0.05)	2.55	0.09** (0.05)	3.13	0.13** (0.04)	7.59	0.14** (0.04)	10.3
Scheduled tribe	0.79* (0.06)	151.57	0.45* (0.06)	48.29	0.92* (0.06)	242.71	0.52* (0.05)	78.96
Lbw	-0.0264	685.66	-0.0036	648.76	-0.0168	1063.29	-0.0034	1029.89
	2.56* (0.49)	26.88	2.13* (0.49)	18.49	2.18* (0.41)	27.07	1.81* (0.41)	18.88
	-2log likelihood=3169.19		Chi^2=7194.97		-2log likelihood=3169.19		Chi^2=7194.97	
	Sig=0.00		Cox and Snell=0.23		Sig=0.00		Cox and Snell=0.23	
Intercept	Nagelkerke=0.26		McFadden=0.12		Nagelkerke=0.26		McFadden=0.12	

Table 8: Multi-nominal regression results of prenatal visits with NFHS-1 [@*significant at 1%, **significant at 5%, *** significant at 10%].

The pregnant women without antenatal care in NFHS-1 are positively co-related with women of Hindi, Muslim and Sikh religion. The pregnant women of Christian religion have negative relationship with no antenatal care. The women of Christian community visit to health care facilities. Therefore such women have complete antenatal care. But there is possibility that the other women may not have antenatal check-ups. Therefore the no antenatal visits are positively co-related with women of Hindi, Muslim and Sikh religion. The pregnant women of scheduled tribe caste have no antenatal care. The relationship with no antenatal care is statistically significant and positively co-related. The health care facilities are located far away. The pregnant women do not have access to such facilities. They do not have knowledge about required antenatal care during pregnancy. As far as age of the pregnant women is concerned then no antenatal care is negatively co-related to all age group categories. It is clear that antenatal care is not provided on the basis of age. Any age category pregnant women can get the complete antenatal care in all health care facilities. Therefore, based on the age group of pregnant women, there is no difference in antenatal care. That is the reason where no antenatal care is negatively co-related and statistically significant. The pregnant women with primary, secondary and higher secondary school have negative co-relationship with no antenatal care. Any woman with more than primary education has more antenatal visits.

Therefore, it is negatively co-related and statistically significant. The lower weight babies have negative co-relationship with no antenatal care. The women of Muslim and Sikh religion do not have adequate prenatal care. No antenatal care is negatively co-related with women of Muslim and Sikh religion. The women of Christian religion have three antenatal care visits. It is statistically significant and positively co-related. The women of the scheduled caste and tribe have positive co-relationship with three antenatal care. The women of scheduled caste and tribe are economically poor. They do not have knowledge of required antenatal care. An access to health care facilities is also low. Due to high opportunity cost of time, they do not visit health care facilities and get the four antenatal cares. Therefore it is positively co-related and statistically significant. The illiterate, primary, secondary and higher secondary educated women have negative co-relationship with three antenatal care. There is no difference in three antenatal cares as far as education of women is concerned. The three antenatal cares is negatively co-related and statistically significant with low birth weight babies. During pregnancy, the women have not visited four times to health care facilities. Therefore, the women delivered low birth weight babies. In order to have healthy child, at least four antenatal visits are required by each pregnant woman. But it is negatively co-related and statistically significant.

In the urban area of county, no antenatal care is positively correlated to women of Hindu religion. The women of Hindu religion have not visited for antenatal care to hospitals in urban area. That is why it could be negatively co-related and statistically significant. The pregnant women of Christian religion have negatively co-relationship with no antenatal care. They have knowledge of minimum required prenatal care. Therefore, they visit to health care facilities and health specialist. That is why the relationship is negatively co-related and statistically significant. The women of Sikh religion in urban area have negative co-relationship with no antenatal care. The women of scheduled caste and tribe have positive co-relationship with antenatal care. This is mainly because the women from such community are poor and they have less educational achievement and knowledge. They have also less knowledge of health care facilities and required antenatal care during pregnancy.

Therefore, it is positively co-related and statistically significant. The women of all age groups have negative co-relationship with antenatal care. There is no any discrimination in prenatal care on the basis of age of pregnant women. Any pregnant women can get the prenatal care in each health care facility. Therefore, it is statistically significant and negatively co-related with no antenatal care. The women with primary, secondary and higher secondary are negatively co-related with no antenatal care. The pregnant women with primary and secondary education can visit health care facility for prenatal care. Therefore they can have more than one antenatal care but certainly they do not have zero antenatal care. The low birth weight is negatively co-related with the no antenatal care (Table 9).

	Rural				Urban			
	No ANC visits		Three ANC visits		No ANC visits		Three ANC visits	
Variables	Co-efficient	Z test	Co-efficient	Z test	Co-efficient	Z test	Co-efficient	Z test
15-19	0.77*** (0.44)	3.08	-0.28 (0.41)	0.48	-1.32 (1.24)	1.14	-0.90 (1.14)	0.63
20-24	-0.4452	6.44	-0.00 (0.40)	0	-1.26 (1.23)	1.04	-1.19 (1.13)	1.1
25-29	-0.4961	8.49	-0.22 (0.40)	0.3	-1.28 (1.29)	1.08	-1.37 (1.13)	1.44
30-34	-0.4662	7.05	-0.30 (0.40)	0.55	-1.09 (1.23)	0.98	-1.19 (1.14)	1.1
35-39	-0.91** (0.42)	4.6	-0.23 (0.40)	0.32	-0.82 (1.24)	0.43	-1.26 (1.14)	1.22
40-44	-0.96 (0.45)	1.02	0.08 (0.43)	0.03	-0.84 (1.29)	0.42	-0.84 (1.17)	0.5
Illiterate	0.35 (0.82)	0.18	-0.33 (0.79)	0.18	-0.77 (0.49)	2.46	-0.89** (0.44)	4.1
Primary	-0.148	494.93	-0.0465	294.54	-0.176	262.67	-0.0574	128.01
Secondary	-0.224	494.93	-0.063	454.57	-0.2665	240.25	-0.088	185.97
Higher secondary	-	-	-	-	-15.79 (74422.58)	0	-16.94 (4617.35	0
Hindu	-0.3052	14.33	-0.41*** (0.21)	3.96	0.75 (0.59)	1.6	0.43 (0.36)	1.42
Muslim	-0.61** (0.29)	4.33	-1.09 (0.21)	0.25	0.83 (0.60)	1.88	-0.50 (0.37)	1.8
Christian	-0.56*** (0.29)	3.61	-0.16 (0.21)	0.59	-0.25 (0.65)	0.15	0.29 (0.37)	0.62
Sikh	-2.92** (1.05)	7.74	-1.27** (0.34)	13.41	0.36 (0.67)	0.28	-0.61 (0.44	1.92
Buddhist	-0.8164	8.96	-0.294	10.76	0.54 (0.82)	0.44	0.37 (0.46)	0.65
Jain	-1.84*** (1.05)	3.05	-0.7752	8.9	1.03 (0.97)	1.12	-0.47 (0.65)	0.52
Jewish	-16.22 (0.00)	1.03	-16.29 (677.75)	0	-13.07 (0.00)	0	-15.37 (654.35)	0
No religion	-17.66 (39.64)	0	-0.45 (1.03)	0.19	-1.97*** (1.12)	3.07	0.85 (0.77)	1.21
Scheduled caste	1.36 (0.22)	38.43	1.16* (0.13)	76.23	-1.30** (0.60)	4.72	-0.5457	4.36
Scheduled tribe	1.44 (0.23)	37.41	1.15* (0.14)	64.55	-0.29 (0.31)	0.88	-0.42 (0.26)	2.57
Other backward caste	1.44 (0.20)	48.55	0.85* (0.12)	45.26	-0.8201	5.46	-1.41** (0.51)	7.57
None of above	0.79 (0.21)	14.32	0.61* (0.12)	23.52	-0.9735	7.7	-1.45** (0.51)	8.03
Lbw	1.43 (0.06)	512.08	0.71* (0.02)	609.62	-0.3042	403.98	-0.336	469.51
Intercept	-6.17 (0.60)	105.3	-1.6121	52.01	-2.40 (1.47)	2.64	2.86 (1.29)	4.9
	-2log likelihood=1319.30		McFadden=0.11		-2log likelihood=2458.70		McFadden=0.181	

	Sig=0.00	Chi^2=727.84	Sig=0.00	Chi^2=2516.13
	Nagelkerke=0.24	Cox and Snell=0.21	Nagelkerke=0.338	Cox and Snell=0.285

Table 9: The regression results for antennal care in NFHS-2 [@*significant at 1%, **significant at 5%, ***significant at 10%].

Age of the women is positively co-related to no antenatal visits. In India, girls get marry at early age. After marriage, women conceive too early. They do not have knowledge of contraceptives. The antenatal care is not observed among the young women. During pregnancy, they do not visit to health care facilities. Therefore, the antenatal care among different age groups is negatively co-related to no antenatal visits. They do not visit regularly to health care facilities. Therefore, no antenatal visits by pregnant women in all age groups are statistically significant and negatively co-related. The women with primary and secondary education have negative relationship with no antenatal visits. Women are not discriminated on the basis of education. They easily get the antenatal care in public or private health care facilities.

Therefore, primary and secondary education of pregnant women is negatively co-related with no antenatal visits. The religion of pregnant women of Hindu, Muslim, Christian, Sikh, Buddhist, Jain and no religion is negatively co-related to no antenatal visits. The antenatal care is not discriminated on the basis of religion of women in India. All pregnant women of different religion have equal access to health care facilities. Therefore, it is negatively co-related and statistically significant. The women of scheduled caste, tribe, Other Backward Class (OBC) and none of above religion have negative co-relationship with no antenatal visits. The women of any caste background have negative co-relationship with prenatal care. The women of scheduled caste, tribe and other backward caste are poor. They do not have knowledge of minimum required antenatal care. They do not visit to health care facilities.

Therefore, no antenatal visits are negatively co-related and statistically significant. The lower birth weight of children is positively co-related to no antenatal visits. The pregnant women during pregnancies do not get antenatal care. It results into lower birth weight of children. The antenatal cares during pregnancies involve variety of methods such as counseling of food, breastfeeding, medicines. Therefore, every pregnant woman is expected to get four antenatal visits to avoid the lower birth weight babies, morbidity and mortality.

As far as three antenatal cares are concerned then they are negatively co-related with primary and secondary education of pregnant women. The pregnant women do not find any problem for getting up to three antenatal visits. The women of Hindu, Sikh, Buddhist and Jain have negative relationship with three antenatal visits. These women do not get the three antenatal visits and the visits are negatively co-related and statistically significant. The women of scheduled caste, tribe, other back ward caste and none of the above religion are positively co-related with three antenatal care in NFHS-2. The lower birth weight is positively co-related to three antenatal visits. It is clear that below three antenatal care leads to lower birth weight among children in NFHS-2 data. Therefore, every pregnant woman must have the four antenatal visits. We have also studied the prenatal care to pregnant women and its access with NFHS-3 data (Table 10).

	Rural				**Urban**			
	NO ANC visits		**Three ANC visits**		**NO ANC visits**		**Three ANC visits**	
Variables	**Co-efficient**	**Z test**	**Co-efficient**	**Z test**	**Co-efficient**	**Z test**	**Co-efficient**	**Z test**
15-19	-0.28 (0.25)	1.31	0.76** (0.26)	8.39	-0.3388	3.08	0.28 (0.41)	0.48
20-24	-0.60** (0.24)	6.28	0.50** (0.25)	3.85	-01.06** (0.42)	6.44	-0.00 (0.40)	0
25-29	-0.55 (0.24)	5.31	0.34 (0.25)	1.76	-1.21** (0.42)	8.49	-0.22 (0.40)	0.3
30-34	-0.39** (0.24)	2.72	0.36 (0.25)	1.95	-01.11** (0.41)	7.05	-0.30 (0.40)	0.55
35-39	-0.15 (0.25)	0.4	0.26 (0.26)	1.74	-0.91 (0.42)	4.6	-0.23 (0.40)	0.32
40-44	-0.20 (0.27)	0.6	0.66** (0.28)	5.47	-0.46 (0.45)	1.02	-0.08 (0.43)	0.03
Illiterate	-0.52 (0.50)	1.07	-0.09 (0.43)	0.05	-0.35 (0.50)	0.18	-0.33 (0.79)	0.18
Primary	-0.0695	735.4	-0.028	290.12	-0.148	494.93	-0.0465	294.54
Secondary	-0.1044	693.35	-0.0352	346.23	-0.224	494.44	-0.063	454.57
Hindu	-0.49** (0.15)	9.77	-0.11 (0.14)	0.66	-01.09** (0.28)	14.33	-0.41 (0.21)	3.96
Muslim	-0.28** (0.16)	2.86	0.03 (0.15)	0.04	-0.61 (0.29)	4.33	-0.10 (0.21)	0.25
Christian	0.26*** (0.13)	2.62	0.03 (0.15)	0.04	-0.56*** (0.13)	3.61	-0.16 (0.21)	0.59

Sikh	-0.2684	29.19	-0.51** (0.18)	7.83	-3.066	7.74	-0.4318	13.41
Buddhist	-0.15 (0.24)	0.4	-0.06 (0.21)	0.08	-01.57 (0.52)	8.96	-0.294	10.76
Jain	-19.25 0.00)	1.04	0.23 (01.16)	0.04	-1.84 (1.05)	3.05	-1.52** (0.51)	8.9
No religion	-0.60 (0.83)	0.52	-0.48 (0.89)	0.29	-17.66 (3964.58)	0	-0.45 (1.03)	0.19
Scheduled caste	1.25* (0.12)	108.15	0.73* (0.09)	63.62	1.36* (0.22)	38.43	1.16* (0.13)	76.23
Scheduled tribe	1.50* (0.12)	153.75	0.93* (0.09)	97.42	1.44* (0.12)	37.41	1.15* (0.14)	64.55
Other backward class	1.22 (0.11)	117.67	0.62* (0.08)	53.12	1.44 (0.23)	48.55	0.85* (0.12)	45.26
None of above	0.91 (0.11)	65.87	0.44* (0.08)	26.99	0.79 (0.21)	14.32	0.61* (0.12)	23.52
Lbw	1.09 (0.2)	1589.15	0.59* (0.01)	0.01	1.43 (0.3)	512.08	0.71* (0.02)	609.62
	-1.8909	288.82	-03.46 (0.31)	124.48	-2.03709	105.3	-1.6121	52.01
	-2log likelihood=5589.66		McFadden=0.14		-2log likelihood=4145.46		Chi2-=3895.45	McFadden=0.159
Intercept	Nagelkerke=0.295		Chi2-=6738.67		Nagelkerke=0.289		Cox and Snell=0.235	

Table 10: The antenatal visits and its determinants in NFHS-3 [@*significant at 1%, **significant at 5%, ***significant at 10%].

In NFHS-3, not received any antenatal check-ups are negatively co-related to age group of 20-24 and 30-34. The pregnant women's primary, secondary education is negatively co-related to no antenatal check-ups. The religion of pregnant women such as Hindu, Muslim and Sikh is negatively co-related with no antenatal check-ups but it is positively co-related to pregnant women of Christian community. As far as pregnant women's caste is concerned then scheduled caste, tribes have positive co-relation with no antenatal check-ups. It is statistically significant and positively co-related with no antenatal care.

As far as three antenatal visits are concerned then they are negatively co-related to 15-19, 20-24 and 40-44 age group. In this age group, pregnant women have not received antenatal care. They must get four antenatal cares to avoid the low birth weight babies. The three antenatal visits are negatively co-related to primary and secondary education. Basically all pregnant women should get the antenatal care irrespective of their education. The Prenatal care relates to any event or condition that occurs or exists in the embryo or the mother during the period between conception and delivery of the infant [14].

The study does not differentiate on the basis of education of women and nature of antenatal care. The pregnant women of Sikh community have negative co-relationship with three antenatal care. The women of scheduled tribes and scheduled caste, other backward caste and none of above caste have negative relationship with below three antenatal visits. The below three antenatal visits are also negatively co-related to low birth weight babies. In rural areas, the pregnant women must get the four antenatal care in order to avoid infant, child mortality, morbidity and malnutrition.

In the urban area, no antenatal check-ups are negatively co-related with pregnant women of Muslim religion. These women of Muslim religion visit health care facilities more frequently in urban areas. Therefore, the prenatal visits are negatively co-related and statistically significant. The pregnant women of Sikh community have three antenatal visits and it is statistically significant and positively co-related. They do not complete required four antenatal cares. The women of scheduled caste and scheduled tribe have up to three antenatal visits. They do not complete all four antenatal care. They are poor and do not have health care knowledge as well as access to health care in urban area. The health care facilities are overcrowded and each visit has high opportunity cost of time. That is why minimum antenatal visits are not completed. An illiterate, primary, secondary, higher secondary studied women have negative co-relationship with three antenatal care. The three antenatal visits are negatively co-related with the educational background of women. The three antenatal visits are negatively co-related with low birth weight of babies. The low birth weight babies in NFHS-3 do not have three antenatal visits during pregnancy of women. The low birth weight could occur below three antenatal cares. Therefore pregnant women should have four antenatal visits in order to eliminate low birth weight babies in India.

Policy Implication and Conclusion

There are number of studies linked to prenatal care and birth weight of babies. Adequate utilization of prenatal health care services positively associated with improved maternal and neonatal, infant and mortality, morbidity and other health outcomes. The full prenatal care is expected to have impact on the development of the fetus and infant as well as mothers health. This can only be achieved through early antenatal visits and regular attendance of antenatal clinic. The trend of maternal mortality in developing countries has been increasing and various international organizations have reported that an important factor related to maternal and infant mortality has been linked to lack of antenatal care [15]. This study is important as an impact factor of birth weight to low birth weight, mortality and morbidity. Therefore, the prenatal care is significant determinant of birth weight, mortality and morbidity in India. The high stunting, wasting and underweight among children are observed in urban and rural area. All the pregnant women in urban and rural areas must get four antenatal cares. The four antenatal cares are expected to reduce the prenatal complexities and improve the birth weight of babies through counseling medical check-ups, medicines, balanced diet and breastfeeding awareness. But the women with low educational status are less likely to visit to health care facilities for the antenatal care. They do not have knowledge of minimum four antenatal visits and what tasks are performed in four visits. They do not visit hospitals and health care experts because they do not find pregnancy is a health problem.

The pregnant women of Hindu, Muslim, Sikh religion do not visit health care facilities for prenatal care. The women of scheduled caste and tribe are less likely to visit to health care facilities for antenatal care. The hospitals are located far away in rural areas. The opportunity cost of using health care facilities is very high. Due to high waiting cost, medicines and transport cost, the poor women do not visit frequently to health care facilities. Therefore the poor women skip the number of prenatal visits. It is found that the pregnant women of the poorer wealth quintiles often skip the number of antenatal visits than the pregnant women of richest wealth quintiles. The richer class women have more economic resources and they can visit to health care facilities. The poor women are daily wage earners or depend on family members for health care. In order to visit to health care facility, they required to take leave from work or ask the family members to accompany them. The direct cost of prenatal care is high for poor pregnant women. We have used multi-nominal logic model to examine the socio-economic and demographic factors with prenatal care. We found positive co-relationship with age, educational status, religion and caste of pregnant women. In order to reduce the incidence of malnutrition among children and mothers, government must establish more health centers in urban and rural area. Government must fill the vacancies of doctors on urgent basis which are lying since many years. Central and state governments must spend more money on health care facilities. Government must prepare the prenatal care related programs and must broadcast on the radio and television. It will provide more awareness about prenatal care among pregnant women in rural and urban area. In urban areas, more hospitals are required as per the density of population.

All the prenatal care related policies are required on urgent basis to tackle the lower coverage of prenatal care. We estimated that the full coverage of prenatal care will be possible after 2034 in rural area and 2040 in urban area. The health care staff must promote healthy practices during delivery period of each pregnant woman. Most of the pregnant women have fear of caesarean deliveries than normal deliveries. They avoid visiting health care facilities during such period. The present speed of antenatal care and it coverage is very low. There are number of socio-economic, demographic, psychosocial and behavioral factors are also responsible for the low coverage of antenatal care. All these factors are associated with reductions in mean birth weight and with increases in the odds of low birth weight. Smoking, drinking and using drugs during pregnancy all had very strong, adverse effects on outcomes, even after we controlled for other psychosocial, socio-economic and demographic factors [16].

For Indian sample, this study is not much useful because pregnant women do not take drugs and smoke. Poor perinatal outcomes impact individual families, society, and an overburdened health-care system. Because of technological advances in medicine, babies born too early are surviving. If longer gestation periods and higher birth weights could be achieved through improved models of prenatal care and education, a significant beneficial impact on birth outcomes could be achieved. With the growing trend toward evidence-based practice, nurses not only have a strong voice but also have a responsibility to change perceptions regarding the need to adopt research evidence into nursing practice. The patients receiving medical and/or nursing care in a group format is not a new concept. Group medical appointments have evolved in the management of patients with chronic diseases, such as diabetes, hypertension, and chronic obstructive pulmonary disease. The group care format is one alternative to the traditional delivery of medical care [17]. The study shows that despite various efforts by the Government of India, utilization of antenatal care (ANC) services continue to be low among women from rural areas particularly those belonging to the Scheduled Tribes [18]. Therefore, central government must focus on tribal women for complete antenatal care. It will reduce the malnutrition, morbidity and mortality among children.

The study suggested that the utilization of maternal health services is a complex phenomenon and it is influenced by several factors [19]. Antenatal care may play an indirect role in reducing maternal mortality by encouraging women to deliver with assistance of a skilled birth attendant or in a health facility [20]. The study highlights the need for coordinated effort from government and stakeholders to improve women's education, as well as strengthen community participation. Furthermore, the study recommended the need to scale up the quality of ANC and family planning services backed by improved and equitable access, availability and quality of skilled delivery care services [21]. Awareness and perception creation towards skilled maternity service utilization need to be enhanced. Facilities and transport services should be more accessible as pointed out by this study [22]. To ensure safe motherhood initiative, government should pay special attention to reduce inequality in seeking skilled delivery assistance [23]. The study shows that women's autonomy was significantly associated with the maternal health care utilization by skilled attendants [24].

The study emphasized that the use of institutional delivery services was very low even among antenatal care attendees. Targeted programmatic efforts are necessary to increase skilled attendant-assisted births, with the ultimate goal of reducing maternal mortality [25]. Addressing the underlying determinants for the inequities and bridging the quality gaps in maternal and new born services with due emphasis on respectful care for migrant women need tailored intervention and prioritization [26]. The long term sustainable policies for universal prenatal care are an urgent requirement to reduce mortalities, improve birth weights and reduce morbidities in India. Present study will certainly help to create awareness, understand present coverage, future challenges and policies for universal pre-natal care among pregnant women in India.

Important Notes

- Government of India along with International Institute for Population Science (IIPS) conducted National Family Health Survey (NFHS) three times in India. First NFHS was conducted in 1992-1993 period. The second NFHS survey was conducted in 1998-99. The third NFHS was conducted in 2005-06 in India. We have used same data for this analysis.
- We have considered four antenatal visits to health care facility by each pregnant woman as per World Health Organization (WHO) standards and guidelines.

References

1. Adam W (2000) Socio-economic inequalities in child mortality: Comparisons across nine developing countries. Bulletin of the World Heal Organ 78: 19-29.

2. Bibha S, Teijlingen ER, Porter M, Simkhada P (2008) Factors affecting the utilization of antenatal care in developing countries: Systematic review of the literature. J Advan Nurs 61: 244-260.
3. Awiti JO (2014) A multilevel analysis of prenatal care and birth weight in Kenya. Health Econ Rev 4: 33.
4. Ashraf G, Mirzaei F, Dokht FA (2011) Relationship between prenatal care and the outcome of pregnancy in low-risk pregnancies. Open J Obstet Gynecol 1: 109-112.
5. Marilyn M (1996) Is antenatal care effective in reducing maternal morbidity and mortality? Health pol and plan 11: 1-15.
6. Shayesteh H, Tehrani FR, Simbar M, Farzadfar F (2016) Factors influencing the use of prenatal care: A systematic review. J Midwife Reprod Heal 4: 544-557.
7. Akanda AS (2010) Relationship between prenatal care and infant mortality: Evidence from Bangladesh demographic and health survey. South Asian J Popul Health 3: 191-202.
8. Henderson JW (1994) The cost effectiveness of prenatal care. Health Care Financ Rev 15: 21-32.
9. WHO (2016) WHO recommendations on antenatal care for a positive pregnancy experience. WHO Press, Geneva, Switzerland.
10. Roy MP, Mohan U, Singh SK, Singh VK, Srivastava AK (2013) Determinants of utilization of antenatal care services in rural Lucknow, India. J Family Med Prim Care 2: 55-59.
11. William J, Gilbert GE, Davis L, Sturgill V (2003) Delayed prenatal care and the risk of low birth weight delivery. J Comm Health 28: 199-208.
12. Yeboah MK (2012) Social support and access to prenatal health services: A study of pregnant teenagers in Cape Coast, Ghana. J Sci and Tech 32: 68-78.
13. Greene W (2003) Econometric Analysis (5th edn.) Pearson Education Private Ltd, Indian Branch, Delhi, India.
14. Falah MA (2015) Females' satisfaction and perception about prenatal care services at primary health care centres. Int J Sci Res 5: 620-627.
15. Olayinka A, Joel A, Bukola D (2012) Factors influencing utilization of antenatal care services among pregnant women in Ife Central Lga, Osun State Nigeria. Adv in Appli Sci Res 3: 1309-1315.
16. Nancy ER, Teitler JO (2003) Effects of psychosocial risk factors and prenatal interventions on birth weight: Evidence from New Jersey's health start program. Persp Sexual Reprod Health 35: 130-137.
17. Thielen K (2012) Exploring the group prenatal care model: A critical review of the literature. J Perinat Educ 21: 209-218.
18. Tulsi A, Sahu D, Nair S, Saha KB, Sharma RK (2016) Factors associated with utilization of antenatal care services among tribal women: A study of selected States. Indian J Med Res 144: 58-66.
19. Jat TR, Ng N, Sebastian M (2011) Factors affecting the use of maternal health services in Madhya Pradesh state of India: A multilevel analysis. Int J Equity Health 5: 10-21.
20. Regassa N (2011) Antenatal and postnatal care service utilization in southern Ethiopia: A population-based study. Afr Health Sci 11: 390-397.
21. Fekadu M, Regassa N (2014) Skilled delivery care service utilization in Ethiopia: analysis of rural-urban differentials based on national demographic and health survey (DHS) data. Afr Health Sci 14: 974-984.
22. Girmaye M, Berhan Y (2016) Skilled antenatal care service utilization and its association with the characteristics of women's health development team in Yeky District, South-West Ethiopia: A multilevel analysis. Ethiop J Health Sci 26: 369-380.
23. Kamal SM, Hassan CH, Kabir MA (2015) Inequality of the use of skilled birth assistance among rural women in Bangladesh: facts and factors. Asia Pac J Public Health 27: 1321-1332.
24. Kc S, Neupane S (2016) Women's autonomy and skilled attendance during pregnancy and delivery in Nepal. Matern Child Health J 20: 1222-1229.
25. Cotter K, Hawken M, Temmerman M (2006) Low use of skilled attendants' delivery services in rural Kenya. J Health Popul Nutr 24: 467-471.
26. Mirkuzie AH (2014) Exploring inequities in skilled care at birth among migrant population in a metropolitan city Addis Ababa, Ethiopia: A qualitative study. Int J Equity Health 25: 110-115.

Awareness of Anemia and Associated Factors among Pregnant Women Attending Antenatal Care, South Ethiopia

Duko B, Tadesse B*, Gebre M and Teshome T

Faculty of Health Sciences, College of Medicine and Health Sciences, Hawassa University, Ethiopia

***Corresponding author:** Bruktawit Tadesse, Faculty of Health Sciences, College of Medicine and Health Sciences, Hawassa University, Ethiopia, E-mail: tblessedwaza@gmail.com

Abstract

Background: Anemia affects around half a billion women of reproductive age worldwide, women; especially pregnant women are at high risk of contracting anemia. The aim of this study was to asses' awareness of anemia among pregnant women and identifies associated factors with the level of awareness.

Methods: Institutional based cross-sectional study was conducted from April to June 2016 at Yrga Cheffe health center, South Ethiopia. Data were gathered using structured questionnaire. Simple random sampling technique was used to select participants. Sample frame was prepared from secondary data at antenatal care service unit. SPSS version 20 was used to analyze the data.

Results: Among 244 study participants about 94.3% (230) pregnant women were responsive and only 44.3% (102) of the women have comprehensive awareness of anemia. Awareness of anemia was significantly associated with number of ANC visit {AOR=7.407, CI=95% [3.247-16.895]}, occupational status {AOR=1.970, CI=95% [1.092-3.555]} and educational status {AOR=6.141, CI=95% [2.781-13.562]} of respondents.

Conclusion: Promoting the benefits of early and frequent ANC, enhancing the quality of ANC and counseling on the ad knowledge of women on anemia are essential elements for improving the awareness of anemia.

Keywords: Awareness; Anemia; Antenatal care; South Ethiopia; Regression analysis

Introduction

Awareness refers to "the state or level of consciousness where sense data can be confirmed by observer," or can be defined more broadly and simply as "knowledge or perception of a situation or fact [1,2]." According to the World Health Organization "anemia is a condition in which the number of RBCS or their oxygen-carrying capacity is insufficient to meet physiologic needs, which vary by age, sex, altitude, smoking, and pregnancy status [3]". It affects half a billion women of reproductive age worldwide that is 30.2% of non-pregnant and 41.8% of pregnant women aged 15-49 years [3]. The commonest type of anemia is IDA which is controlled by nutritional intake of Fe rich foods and taking IF supplementation [4], meanwhile women have less awareness about their health [5].

"Knowledge is the springboard for action [6]." It is believed that improving awareness motivates behavioral change and it is possible that limited knowledge about anemia interferes with ANC attendance, IF supplements use, dietary practices, and the use of anti-helminthes medicine [6].

That is why one of the most effective steps to reduce the prevalence of anemia during pregnancy is health promotion, which is the process of enabling people to improve their health through providing information, health education, and skill training [7]. Generally, anemia is serious public health problem with global prevalence of 48.8%, in Africa 40.7% for total population and 69% and 65.8% for global and African pregnant women respectively [3]. As Ethiopia is one of the low-income countries with poor health status and rapid population growth with 4.1 fertility rate [8], and has one of the highest rates of maternal mortality in Africa [9].

The prevalence of anemia in Ethiopian among women of 15-49 age group is 17% [10], southeast Ethiopia is 27.9% [11] Lack of awareness is the major retarding factor to reach millennium development goal [9], as the awareness of anemia among pregnant women is only 72% [12]. Anemia was found to be severe public health problem in Ethiopia that is greater than 40% of pregnant women were anemic [3]. Although identifying gap and creating awareness is essential for controlling anemia, to the best of our knowledge, studies have not been conducted to assess the level of awareness on anemia among pregnant women in Yrga Cheffe town, Ethiopia.

Methods

Study setting and population

The study was conducted among pregnant women attending ANC service at Yrga Cheffe health center. Yrga Cheffe is located in Gedeo zone, SNNPR, approximately 395 Km south of Addis Ababa, and 125 Km away from regional capital Hawassa. About 773 pregnant women attended ANC service at the health center during study period. All pregnant women who visited the health institution for ANC follow up where included on the study, while pregnant women who were critically and mentally ill were excluded. The study was carried out from April 2016 to June 2016.

Study design and sampling method

A total of 244 pregnant women were enrolled in this study, with 5.7% non- response rate. Sample size was estimated using the general formula for single population proportion, with the following assumptions: Awareness of anemia (P) of 72% and using the 95% Confidence level and 5% marginal error. This gave us 310; since, the total population is 773, we used correction formula to find the sample size. 10% is added for non-response rate, this gives the total sample size of 244.

Simple random sampling technique was used. Sample was collected from pregnant who were attending ANC service at Yrga Cheffe health center regardless of gestational age and number of ANC visit. The sample frame for participants was prepared from patient record at ANC service of Yrga Cheffe health center.

Data collection

Data was gathered by using structured and pretested questionnaire which asked questions on anaemia and associated factors. It had five parts, these were socio demographic, life style and maternal related factors, awareness of anaemia and its adverse effects, risk and cause, sign and symptom, and prevention and treatment of anaemia were asked.

Pregnant women those who score mean (average) and above are considered as aware about anemia. Respondents who were aware of anemia and know at least one of its major causes, symptoms and consequences during pregnancy were considered to have comprehensive knowledge.

The mean awareness of the term anemia, risk, cause, prevention and treatment were 6.8 as comprehensive awareness. The questionnaire was prepared in English and translated to Amharic and highly reliable in the study (Cronbach's α=0.94).

Data management and analysis: At the end of each day the questionnaire was checked for clear, correct and complete answer of each question, and data was carefully entered into SPSS version 20 and, checked for completeness throughout the study. Pre-test was done on 5% of sample size, (12) at Hawassa University Referral Hospital, which was no included in the samples and some corrections was made prior to applying on the study. Data was coded in order to avoid missing and entered in to SPSS version 20.0 for analysis of descriptive data.

Frequency distributions, proportions both bivariate and multivariable logistic regression analysis with 95% CI was used to see the association between each independent variables and awareness of anemia.

Finally those variables which showed statistical significance at P<0.05 and 95% CI in the final model was reported as associated with awareness of anemia. The substantial difference about awareness of anemia was computed and the data is summarized in tables, charts and figure.

Results

Socio demography characteristics

The mean age of the respondents was 24.48 (± SD=4.339) years. More than half 62.6% (144) of the pregnant women was within the age range of 15-25 years followed by 47.4% range of 25 to 34 years. Many of them were married, 96.5% (222). Majority of the pregnant women were house wives 51.7% (119), urban residents 58.7% (135) and has primary education 41.3% (95).

The majorities of the participants were Gedeo 56.1% (129) in ethnicity followed by Amhara 17.8% (41) and Gurage 11.3% (26). The majority 58.7% (135) of the study participants were protestant Christian followers. Extreme poverty is highly prevalent as 44.8% (103) of pregnant have monthly income less than 750 ETB with mean of mean 1336.11 (Table 1).

Parameter		Frequency	Percentage (%)
	15-25	144	62.6
	26-36	81	35.21
Age group	34-44	5	2.1
	Protestant	135	58.7
	Orthodox	83	36.1
	Muslim	9	3.9
Religion	Other*	3	1.3
	Gedeo	129	56.1
	Amhara	41	17.8
	Gurage	26	11.3
	Oromo	26	11.3
Ethnicity	Other**	8	3.47
	Illiterate	62	27
	Primary	95	41.3
	Secondary	58	25.2
Education	College/university	15	6.5
	House wife	119	51.7
	Labor	12	5.2
	Farmer	21	9.1
	Government worker	32	13.9
	Merchant	35	15.2
Occupation	Other***	11	4.8
	Married	222	96.5
	Single	8	3.5
Marital status	≤ 750 ETB	103	44.78
	751-1200 ETB	41	17.826
Income****	≥ 1201 ETB	86	37.39
Other*: Catholic, Adventist, Other**: Wolayta, Other***: Student, Income****			

Table 1: Distributions of socio demographic characteristics of study subject at Yrga-Cheffe health center, SNNP, Ethiopia, 2016.

Maternal related factors

More than three fourth, 80% (184), of respondents had followed ANC service only twice and less. About Two-thirds, 66% (152), of the participants were multi gravidas, and 51.37% (75) of respondents delivered at health institutions. Less than one fourth of 15.75% (23), 14.86% (22) respondents had still birth and abortion respectively (Table 2).

Parameter		Frequency	Percentage (%)
ANC visit	01-Feb	184	80
	03-May	32	13
	06-Oct	14	6.1
Place of delivery	Health facility	75	51.37
	Home	71	48.63
Still birth	Yes	23	15.75
	No	123	84.24
Abortion	Yes	22	14.86
	No	126	85.13

Table 2: Distributions of maternal related factors of study subject at Yrga- Cheffe health center, SNNP, Ethiopia, 2016.

Life style related factors

Source health information: More than three fourth, 76.5% (176), of respondents got health information from health professional, 12.2% (28) from TV and radio, while only 12.3% (26) from friend.

Dietary intake: Consumption of Dark green vegetable is highly consumed among pregnant 95% (218), followed by, meat 94.3% (217) and kocho (false banana), 92.6% (213) (Table 3).

Parameter	Frequency	Percentage (%)
Consumption of kocho	213	92.6
Consumption of dark green leafy vegetables	218	51.3
Consumption of fruits	134	58.3
Consumption of meat	217	94.3
Consumption of milk	74	32.2
Consumption legumes	205	89.1

Table 3: Distributions of dietary intakes of study subject at Yrga-Cheffe health center, SNNP, Ethiopia, 2016.

Awareness of anemia among the pregnant women

Regarding the awareness of Anemia, 44.3% (102) of the women were aware of the term anemia, and 55.7% (128) of them has poor comprehensive awareness of anemia; with the highest being in the age group 15-25 with a 40.97% (59).

Only 26.5% (61) of respondents were aware of some adverse outcome of anemia during pregnancy to both maternal and child health. Only 26.5% (61) of respondents were aware of some negative consequences of anemia during pregnancy to both the mother and child (Table 4).

Character	Frequency	Percentage (%)
Awareness about anemia	102	44.3
Knowledge about outcome of anemia during pregnancy	61	26.5
Maternal death	53	23
Still birth	16	7
Infant mortality	28	12.2
Premature delivery	17	7.4
Impaired development	9	3.9
Increased BP	7	3
Other (like bleeding)	1	0.4

Table 4: Distributions of awareness of anemia and its adverse outcomes of study subject at Yrga-Cheffe health center, SNNP, Ethiopia, 2016.

Awareness of pregnant women about risk factors of anemia

The majorities of the participants were aware of sign and symptom of anemia, 67.18% (86), than cause and risk of anemia, 42.18% (54), and 39.84% (51) respectively (Figure 1).

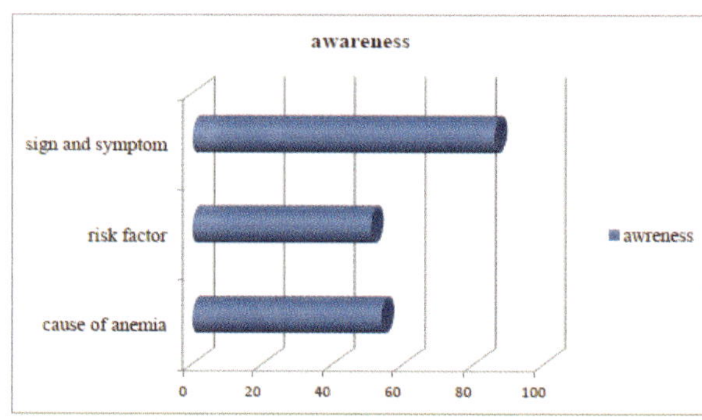

Figure 1: Distributions of awareness about risk/cause and sign/ symptom of anemia of study subject at Yrga-Cheffe health center, SNNP, Ethiopia, 2016.

Awareness of pregnant women about prevention and treatment of anemia

Among all study participants, more than three fourth, 89 (87.3%), of respondents had awareness about prevention of anemia.

Similarly, more than half of the respondents had an awareness about iron/foliate tablet and its usage 68.6% (70) major sources of iron reach food 59.4% (60), importance of birth spacing towards prevention of anemia 66.6% (68), and treatments of anemia 78.2% (79) (Table 5).

Parameter		Frequency	Percentage (%)
Knowledge about the prevention of anemia	Yes	89	87.3
	No	13	12.7
Awareness about Iron/ foliate tabs	Yes	70	68.6
	No	32	31.4
Knowledge about the use of Iron/foliate tabs	Drugs used to prevent infection	6	8.6
	Supplements used to prevent anemia	60	85.7
	Treatment of morning sickness	4	5.7
Awareness about Fe rich foods	Yes	60	59.4
	No	41	40.6
Awareness about major sources of Iron rich foods	Liver	44	73.3
	Red meat	16	26.7
	chicken	7	11.7
	Fruits	18	30
	Green leafy vegetables	27	45
	Honey	1	0.4
Awareness about birth spacing	Yes	68	66.6
	No	34	33.3
Inter pregnancy gap	≤ 6 months	6	8.7
	1-2 years	10	14.5
	3-4 years	35	50.7
	≤ 5 years	18	26.1
Knowledge about treatment of anemia	Yes	79	78.2
	No	129	56.1
Knowledge about method of treatments of anemia	Provision of Iron/ foliate tab	71	88.8
	Blood transfusion	26	32.5
	Treating malaria	12	15
	Deworming	12	15
	Other*	4	5

Other*: Drinking juice.

Table 5: Distributions of awareness about risk/cause and sign/symptom of anemia of study subject at Yrga-Cheffe health center, SNNP, Ethiopia, 2016.

Comprehensive awareness of pregnant women about anemia

From total of 230 study participants, only 44.3% (102) were aware of anemia (Figure 2).

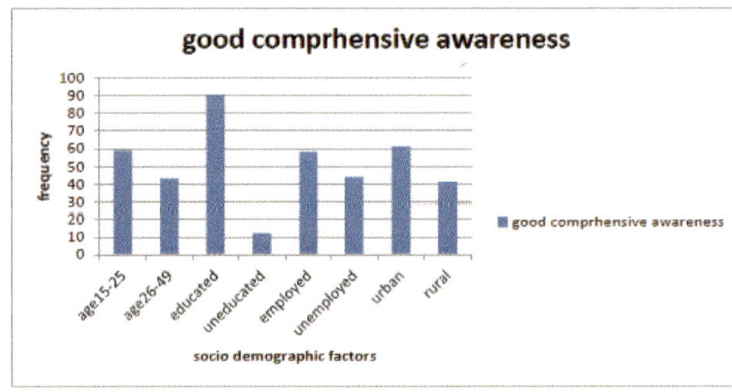

Figure 2: Distributions of comprehensive awareness of anemia among pregnant women who ware on ANC service at Yrga-Cheffe health center, SNNP, Ethiopia, 2016.

Association of dependent and independent variables

Comprehensive knowledge of anemia was measured using a mean awareness index constructed based on multiple indicators (Table 6).

Parameter		No Awareness n=128	Awareness n=102	COR (95% CI)	AOR (95% CI)
		No (%)	No (%)		
Educational status	Illiterate	50 (80.6%)	12 (19.3%)	4.8 [2.4-9.7]	6.14 [2.78-13.56]
	Literate	78 (46.4%)	90 (53.6%)		
Occupation	Unemployed	75 (63%)	44 (37%)	1.9 [1.1-3.16]	1.97 [1.09-3.55]
	Employed	53 (47.7%)	58 (52.2%)		
Access to health service	<15 Km	107 (52.4%)	97 (47.5%)	0.26 [0.09-0.72]	-
	≥ 15 Km	21 (80.8%)	5 (19.2%)		
Educational status of husband	Illiterate	13 (86.7%)	2 (13.3%)	5.65 [1.24-25.65]	-
	Literate	115 (53.5%)	100 (46.5%)		
Number of ANC visit	01-Feb	117 (63.9%)	66 (36.1%)	5.8 [2.8-12.15]	7.4 [3.25-16.9]
	≥ 3	11 (23.4%)	36 (76.6%)		

*Significant association (p<0.05), COR-Crudes Odds Ratio, AOR-Adjusted Odds Ratio, CI-Confidence Interval.

Table 6: Association of the overall awareness of anemia and associated factors among pregnant women on ANC follow-up at Yrga-Cheffe Health center.

Ethical Consideration

Ethical clearance and approval for the study was obtained from the ethical committee of Hawassa University, college of health science school of nursing and midwifery. Permission was also been obtained from Head of Yirga Cheffe health center and ANC unit. Privacy, confidentiality and anonymity had been guarded. Scientific objectivity of the study was maintained with honesty and impartiality. Thus, oral and written consent was obtained from all the respondents after explaining the purpose of the study, risks and benefits to the subject, confidentiality of records, right to refuse and terminate participation on study at any time of study.

Conclusion

The awareness of anemia among pregnant women attending ANC service at Yrga Cheffe Health Center is generally low, as pregnant women have less than average awareness about anemia. Pregnant women who are uneducated, unemployed and have only one ANC visit had a low awareness of anemia. Awareness creation on the consequences of anemia during pregnancy should be given to women in child bearing age in general and pregnant women in particular.

Recommendation

Promoting the benefits of early and frequent ANC, enhancing the quality of ANC counseling and promoting the knowledge of women on anemia are essential elements for improving the awareness of anemia. Therefore, Yrga Cheffe health center and health office have to consider incorporating health extension workers and social workers in order to improve strong involvement in the dissemination of health information.

Limitation

We didn't get validated and standard data collection tool. Therefore, they data were collected by a questionnaire which was prepared by researchers. This might affect outcome of the study.

Acknowledgment

We would like to thank staff members of Yrga Cheffe health center, particularly the antenatal care unit, for their cooperation during data collection. We are grateful to the study participants. This study was financially supported by Hawassa University.

References

1. World Health Organization (2011) Global nutrition targets 2025: Anemia policy brief.
2. Anthony SF (2015) Harrison principle of internal medicine, 19th edition, McGraw-Hill Education, 625-650.
3. Hussain T, Shu LY (2010) Awareness of iron deficiency anemia among women of reproductive age in Hubei province, China. Asian J Med Sci 1: 12-13.
4. Mbule MA, Byaruhanga YB, Kabahenda M, Lubowa A (2013) Determinants of anaemia among pregnant women in rural Uganda. Rural Remote Health 13: 2259.
5. World Health Organization (2014) Global Nutrition Targets 2025: Policy brief series.
6. Ethiopia mini demographic and health survey 2014 (2014) Central statistical agency, Addis Ababa, Ethiopia 41-53.
7. Ethiopia demographic and health survey 2011 (2012) Central statistical agency, Addis Ababa, Ethiopia.
8. Kefiyalew F, Zemene E, Asres Y, Gedefaw L (2014) Anemia among pregnant women in Southeast Ethiopia: Prevalence, severity and associated risk factors. BMC Res Notes 7: 771.
9. Gebremedhin S, Samuel A, Mamo G, Assefa T (2014) Coverage, compliance and factors associated with utilization of iron supplementation during pregnancy in eight rural districts of Ethiopia: A cross-sectional study. BMC Public Health 14: 607.
10. Pareek P, Hafeez A (2015) A study on anemia related knowledge among adolescent girls. Int J Food Sci Nutr 4: 273-276.
11. Kakade NR, Kakade SN (2012) A study to assess knowledge of mothers of fewer than five children regarding nutritional anemia from Karad urban area. Int J Sci Res 3: 1007-1009.
12. Fredanna ADM, Judy CD (2012) Assessment of anemia knowledge, attitudes and behaviors among pregnant women in Sierra Leone. Health Educator 44: 9-16.

Criteria Based Clinical Audit of Cesarean Section in a General Hospital in West Tigray, Ethiopia

Solomon Gebre[1*], **Ataklti Negasi**[2] **and Assefa Hailu**[3]

[1]*Mearg General Hospital, Emergency Surgical Department, Dansha, West Tigray, Ethiopia*

[2]*Mygaba Primary Health Unit, Emergency Surgical Department, Mygaba, West Tigray, Ethiopia*

[3]*Freweyni Primary Hospital, Emergency Surgical Department, Freweyni, Eastern Tigray, Ethiopia*

***Corresponding author:** Solomon Gebre, Mearg General Hospital, Emergency Surgical Department, Dansha, West Tigray, Ethiopia, E-mail: solomongebre300@gmail.com

Abstract

Improving the quality of obstetric care is an urgent priority in low income countries, where maternal and perinatal morbidity and mortality remain high. Clinical audit is a tool to improve quality of care. Specifically clinical audit in MNCH is a tool to reduce maternal and perinatal morbidity and mortality. Cesarean section is among "five auditable" MNCH scenarios according 2012 women lung foundation. This study is a one year retrospective cross-sectional study among 99 women who delivered by cesarean section from July 2016-June 2017 in Mearg general hospital in West Tigray, Ethiopia. The aim of this survey was to investigate cesarean section rate (CSR) and indications of cesarean section to improve quality of obstetric care by reducing unnecessary cesarean sections. In the study period 99 women delivered by cesarean section among 749 institutional deliveries which gives an institutional cesarean section rate of 13.2%. Medical records were retrieved for 81 mothers. The most common indications for cesarean section were cephalopelvic disproportion (CPD) in 19 women (23.5%), antepartum hemorrhage in 11 (13.6%) and obstructed labor in 10 (12.3%). Majority of the cesarean sections 75(88.9%) were done under spinal anesthesia. Seven (8.6%) mothers had no justified indication for cesarean section according to criteria based audit. From the total 99 cesarean sections there was one (1.0%) maternal death. There was significant number of cesarean sections done with medically unjustified indications but comparatively low with the country and global figure. The three common indications for CS in this study were CPD, APH, and obstructed labor. A huge percentage of lost medical files was observed. Keeping medical records is the safest, simplest and cheapest way to analyze cesarean section indications, to reduce unjustified/unnecessary cesarean sections.

Keywords: Cesarean section rate; Clinical audit; Obstetric care; Delivery

Abbreviations: APH: Antepartum Hemorrhage; CEmOC: Comprehensive Emergency Obstetric Care; CP: Contracted Pelvis; CPD: Cephalo Pelvic Disproportion; CS: Cesarean Section; CSR: Cesarean Section Rate; LUSCS: Lower Uterine Segment Cesarean Section; MNCH: Maternal, Neonatal and Child Health; NRFS: Non Reassuring Fetal Status; OL: Obstructed Labor; VBAC: Vaginal Birth after Cesarean Section

Introduction

Cesarean section (CS) is one of the ten signal functions of comprehensive emergency obstetric and neonatal care (CEmONC) that includes seven basic emergency obstetric care (parenteral antibiotics, anticonvulsants, uterotonic agents, manual removal of placenta, manual vacuum aspiration, basic neonatal resuscitation and assisted vaginal delivery) and blood transfusion, anesthesia and cesarean section [1]. The term clinical audit has been defined as "in depth analysis of clinical performance of health care over a specified period of time" [2]. There are three main approaches to obstetric audit namely audit of deaths (maternal or perinatal), audit of severe morbidity (or near-miss), and audit of clinical practice. Audit is based on criteria (or standards) of care which can be either implicit or explicit (e.g., criterion based audit) [3].

Improving the quality of obstetric care is an urgent priority in low income countries, where maternal and neonatal morbidity and mortality remain high [4]. Cesarean section can be a life-saving intervention for mother and baby when it is clearly indicated or vaginal birth is contraindicated, unnecessary cesarean section poses avoidable risks to the mother and her child, increased morbidity and mortality and may impact negatively on a woman's future reproductive health.

Birth by caesarean section also places extra demands on maternity services and provision of resources or needlessly raising cost [5-7]. The national population based cesarean delivery rate in Ethiopia is 0.6% with variation between the regions from 0.2% to 9% and the overall institutional rate was 18%, which varied between 46% in the private for profit sector and 15% in the public sector. Currently about 20 million cesarean section (CS) deliveries occur each year worldwide [8,9].

Average global CSR is 19% of all births, ranging from 6-27%. Regions with high rates of CS include Latin America, North America and the Caribbean's (30-40%), followed by Europe (25%), Asia (19%) and Africa (7.3%). The international healthcare community has considered the ideal rate for caesarean sections to be between 10% and 15%, but not less than 5%. Since then, caesarean sections have become increasingly common in both high and low income countries. Medically justified caesarean section can effectively prevent maternal and perinatal mortality and morbidity.

However, there is no evidence showing the benefits of caesarean delivery for women or infants who do not require the procedure [10-12].

Methods

Study design and population

This cross sectional study was performed from July 2016 to June 2017. All mothers who delivered by CS in the study period are included except those mothers' of whom medical records were lost or without information.

Data collection and audit process

For these criteria based audit mothers' medical records were thoroughly reviewed by the auditing team using structured data collection abstraction. The checklist contained questions about background characteristics, time and date of admission, parity, cervical dilatation at the time decision for CS, partograph, type of anesthesia, status of membrane rupture, oxytocin augmentation, and indications for CS, maternal and perinatal outcome.

The list with criteria for absolute indications for CS (Table 1) was used to assess whether the indication for CS was in accordance with these audit criteria.

Absolute Indications	Remark
Absolute CPD	In the presence of adequate contractions failure to progress of labor e.g., contracted pelvis (CP) or malpresentations
APH	with active bleeding that endangers maternal or fetal live
Obstructed labor	Action line is crossed, a membrane is ruptured and presences of signs of imminent Uterine rupture.
Two previous CS scar	-
Single non LUSCS	Classical or low vertical CS
NRFS	Persistent bradycardia FHB<100 BPM or persistent tachycardia FHB>180 BPM despite intrauterine resuscitations
Cord prolapse	pulsating cord and instrumental vaginal delivery was not feasible or failed
Malpresentation	transverse lie, footling breech, hand prolapse, shoulder, brow, face (persistent mento-posterior/mento-transverse)
Failed induction	Despite adequate contractions or maximum dose of uterotonic agent achieved for at least 6-8 hours and no adequate progress of labor
Failed VBAC	After TOL in mothers previously give birth via CS after fulfill prerequisites of trial of vaginal delivery and failure to progress labor
Twin pregnancy	First baby non vertex or failure to progress of labor

Table 1: Criteria based audit and absolute indications for CS used for this survey.

Operational Definitions

Despite several existing CS classification systems, based on obstetric characteristics or on indications, a universally accepted list of absolute indications with clear criteria for CS does not exist.

Justified indication

Acceptable partogram

This is the basis for everything. If the partogram is not good enough for action to be taken it is clearly unacceptable.

Documentation

If there is no documentation on cesarean section indication the cesarean section is said to be unjustified.

Strong contractions

There must be either a clear maternal or fetal indication or both. "Big baby" is never an acceptable indication! If the partogram indicates obstructed labor or mechanic dystocia there must be sufficient contractions documented and insufficient progress (crossing of action line) in spite of membranes ruptured. Insufficient (too weak) contractions imply dynamic dystocia, which is different from obstructed labor. This is never in itself a justification for cesarean section unless oxytocin augmentation has been initiated.

Correct management

Membrane rupture

Cesarean section in case of poor progress of labor with intact membranes is never justified if there is no maternal indication of cesarean section. Rupture of membranes should be followed by oxytocin augmentation if contractions do not follow after rupture of membranes. If membranes were ruptured ("ARM") by health worker, indicate the hour of this procedure.

Augmentations

Oxytocin infusion must be given with caution, particularly in multiparas women. A cesarean section is never justified in cases with insufficient (weak) contractions unless augmentation (stimulation with oxytocin) has been tried. Indicate also the hour when oxytocin infusion was started.

Data Analysis

Data analysis was performed with SPSS version 22. All results are reported as numbers (n) and frequencies (%) (Tables 2 and 3).

Variables	Clinical characteristics	N	Percentage (%)
Date and time delivery	Yes	80	98.8
	No	1	1.2
Parity	0	25	30.9
	01-Apr	45	55.6
	>5	10	12.3
	Unknown	1	1.2
Previous CS scar	One scar	6	7.4
	Two scar	1	1.2
	No scar	74	91.4
Rupture membrane	Yes	38	46.9
	No	33	40.7
	Unknown	10	12.3
Strong contraction	Yes	41	50.6
	No	20	24.7
	Unknown	20	24.7
Induction/ Augmentation	Yes	19	23.5
	No	58	71.6
	Unknown	4	4.9
Cervical dilation	0-3 cm	26	32.1
	4-9 cm	32	39.5
	Full	7	8.6
	Unknown	16	19.8
Type of anaesthesia	Spinal	72	88.9
	GA	6	7.4
	Unknown	3	3.7
Maternal outcome	Alive	80	98.8
	Died	1	1.2
Perinatal outcome	Alive	81	97.6
	Still birth	2	2.4
Justified indication	Yes	74	91.4
	No	7	8.6
Correct management	Yes	75	92.6
	No	6	7.4
Acceptable parthograph	Yes	37	45.7
	No	9	11.1
	Not applicable	35	43.2

Table 2: Clinical characteristics (n=81).

Indications	N	Percentage (%)
CPD	19	23.5
Obstructed labor	10	12.3
APH	11	13.6
Failed induction	9	11.1
Others	9	11.1
NRFS	8	9.9
Failed VBAC	6	7.4
Breech	5	6.2
Twin	2	2.5
Cord prolapse	2	2.5
Total	81	100

Table 3: Indications for CS.

Results

In the study period 99 women delivered by cesarean section among 749 institutional deliveries which gives an institutional cesarean section rate of 13.2%. Medical records were retrieved for 81 mothers. The most common indications for cesarean section were cephalopelvic disproportion (CPD) in 19 women (23.5%), antepartum hemorrhage in 11 (13.6%) and obstructed labor in 10 (12.3%). Majority of the cesarean sections 75 (88.9%) were done under spinal anesthesia. Seven (8.6%) mothers had no justified medical indication for cesarean section according to criteria based audit. From the total 99 cesarean sections there was one (1.0%) maternal death and from the audited 81 cesarean section there were two (2.4%) perinatal deaths (Figures 1 and 2).

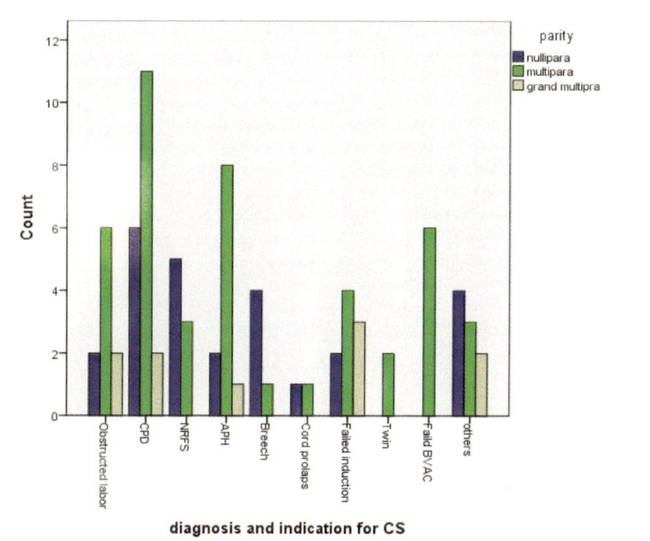

Figure 1: Indications of cesarean section by parity.

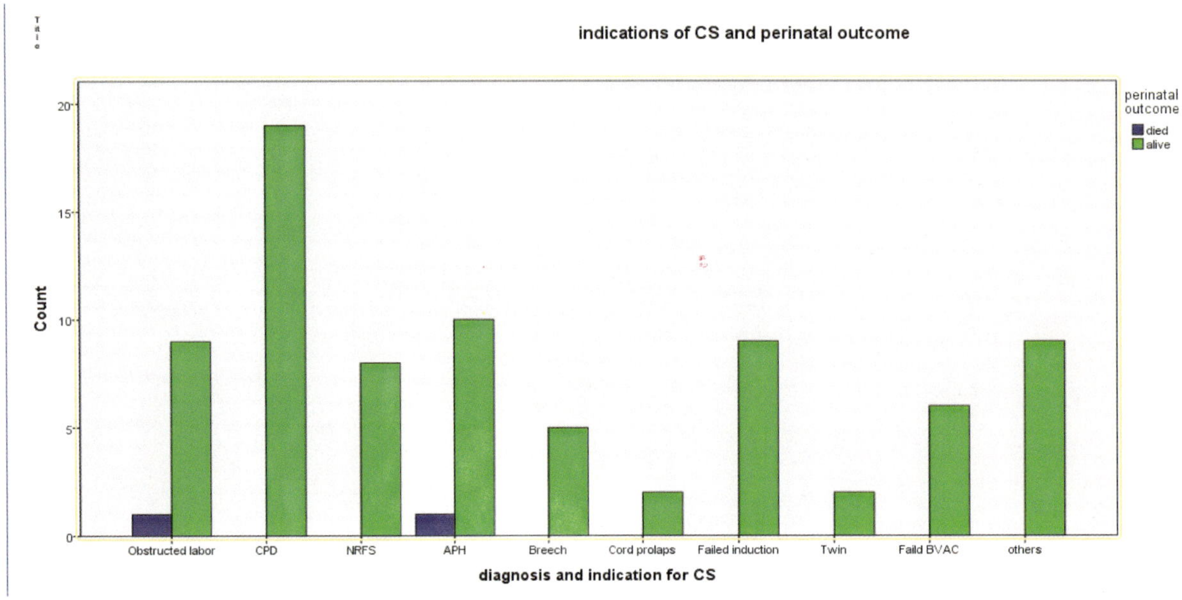

Figure 2: Indications for caesarean section and perinatal outcomes.

Discussions

Although CSR is rising globally but in fact there is no single evidence that increasing population based CSR above 10% reduces maternal and perinatal morbidity and mortality according to the ecological study from 159 countries [13]. This study revealed 13.4% institutional based CSR; this finding did not include those mothers who delivered elsewhere outside the hospital in the catchment area (Home, health post, health center and primary hospital deliveries). According the EDHS 2016 institutional delivery rate is 26.2% [14], so it is possible to imagine what will be the overall population based CSR, which is too far below the WHO recommended rate. The CSR in this survey is comparable with the study in Adigrat hospital (14.3) [15], but below the national figure (18%) [8], and the study shown in Addis Ababa (19.2%), Mizan Aman hospital southwest Ethiopia (21.1%), Jimma university specialized teaching hospital (28.1%), Attat hospital Gurage zone (27.6%), Harar East Ethiopia (34.3%) both in public (26.6%) and private (58.7%).

This discrepancy might be due to differences in the study area and most of the above study was conducted in specialized referral teaching hospitals [16-20]. Our survey finding was also far below the global figure, North America (32.3%), Oceania (31.1%), Europe (25%), Asia (19.2%) but above the African rate of CS (7.3%) [21]. CPD (25.3%) was the leading indication for cesarean section in this survey which is comparable with other studies from Ethiopia (Adigrat, Jimma specialized hospital and Atta hospital) [15,18,19] and other African countries like northern Namibia, Nigeria [22,23].

This could be explained by high rate of childhood malnutrition in low income countries which leads to contracted pelvis but needs further investigation, but study in Tikur Anbessa showed that the leading indication for CS were repeated CS (32.4%) as compared to our study 7.4% which might be explained by high primary CS rates [24]. A study performed by Medecins sans Frontieres in some Sub-Saharan African countries showed obstructed labor (31%) was the commonest indication for CS. which comparatively higher than (12.3%) the finding on this study but in modern obstetrics having obstructed labor is completely obsolete [25]. In this study there were seven (8.6%) CS done without justified medical indication according the criteria based audit which is similar with report from Addis Ababa (6.9%) [16] but lower than the report from Tanzania (19.5%), global survey by WHO (14.2%) and china (69%). This might be due to clinicians/physicians' clinical decision making skills difference [5,26]. Majority of CS procedures were performed under spinal anesthesia 75 (88.9%) which is with accordance WHO guideline recommendation and study done in Adigrat hospital Northern Ethiopia (94.1%) [15].

Conclusion

The institutional CSR in this survey were within the WHO population based CSR recommended limit but still there was significant number of cesarean sections done with medically unjustified indications but comparatively low with the country and global figure. The three common indications for CS in this study were CPD, APH, and obstructed labor and there were high medical records lost observed. Improving the quality of obstetric and perinatal care is an urgent priority worldwide and criteria base clinical audits can play key role in this process by critical analysis of current medical practice and identification of substandard care factors. Keeping medical records is the safest, simplest and cheapest way to analyze cesarean section indications, to reduce unjustified/ unnecessary cesarean sections.

Recommendation

This is an eye opening survey or clinical audit finding on CS which can be baseline for other studies or clinical audit across the region as well at country level. Even though the number of CS done for unjustified medical indications are comparatively low to the studies done worldwide, but still the hospital needs clear indication protocol to minimize unnecessary obstetric surgeries, thereby it is possible to reduce needlessly short and long term maternal and perinatal complications as well cost expenditures.

We observe there were unexpectedly high rate of patient's card lost in the study area/Mearg general hospital, and the hospital management body should establish strong system that kept medical records safe.

Acknowledgement

First and foremost our deepest gratitude extends to Van Jos Roosmalen (Professor), who was on our side from inception of this survey up to this level, without your support this study would not have been completed. Your wisdom and knowledgeable commitment inspired and motivate us up to the highest standard. We would like to thank the auditing team (Saddam Abdurrahman (MD), Ato Kidane Gebresilasie, Ato Hafte Kefil, Ato Efrem Gizaw and Ato Major Teklay) for their efforts, support and contribution. Finally, special and profound thanks to all Mearg general hospital senior management team who allowed us to conduct this survey.

Ethical Clearance

Ethical clearance was collected from Mearg general hospital senior management committee after the research proposal was reviewed. Confidentiality was maintained throughout the study.

Funding Issue

There was no funding for this study from any governmental or private organization.

References

1. WHO, UNFPA, UNICEF, AMDD (2009) Monitoring emergency obstetric care. Sexual and Reproductive Health. Geneva.
2. Wylie BJ, Mirza FG (2008) Cesarean delivery in the developing world. Clinics in Perinatology 35: 571-582.
3. Lewis G (2003) Beyond the numbers: Reviewing maternal deaths and complications to make pregnancy safer. Geneva, Switzerland.
4. Graham W, Wagaarachi P, Penney G, Binns MC, Antwi KY, et al. (2000) Criteria for clinical audit of the quality of hospital based obstetric care in developing countries. Reproductive Health 78: 5.
5. Souza JP, Gulmezoglu A, Lumbiganon P, Laopaiboon M, Carroli G, et al. (2010) Caesarean section without medical indications is associated with an increased risk of adverse short-term maternal outcomes: The 2004-2008 WHO global survey on maternal and perinatal health. BMC Medicine 8: 71.
6. Villar J, Carroli G, Zavaleta N, Donner A, Wojdyla D, et al. (2007) Maternal and neonatal individual risks and benefits associated with caesarean delivery: Multicentre prospective study. BMJ 335: 1025.
7. Ronsmans C, Holtz S, Stanton C (2006) Socio-economic differentials in caesarean rates in developing countries: A retrospective analysis. Lancet 368: 1516-1523.
8. Fesseha N (2011) A national review of cesarean delivery in Ethiopia. Int J Gynecol Obstets 115: 106-111.
9. Betran AP, Merialdi M, Lauer JA, Bing-Shun W, Thomas J, et al. (2007) Rates of caesarean section: analysis of global, regional and national estimates. Paediatr Perinat Epidemiol 21: 98-113.
10. Dumont A, Bernis L, Bouvier-Colle MH, Breart G (2001) Caesarean section rate for maternal indication in Sub-Saharan Africa: A systematic review. Lancet 358: 13281333.
11. WHO UNFPA, UNDPA, World Bank (2015) WHO Statement on caesarean section rates. Department of reproductive health and research world health organization, Geneva.
12. NICE (2002) Principles for best practice in clinical audit. Abingdon, United Kingdom Radcliffe Medical Press.
13. Zhang J, Mikolajczyk R, Torloni MR, Gülmezoglu AM, Betran AP (2016) Association between rates of caesarean section and maternal and neonatal mortality in the 21st century: A worldwide population-based ecological study with longitudinal data. BJOG 123: 745-753.
14. Ethiopian health and demographic survey (2016) Central Statistical Agency, Addis Ababa, Ethiopia.
15. Kahsay S, Berhe G, Gebremariam A, Birhane B (2015) Determinants of caesarean deliveries and its major indications in Adigrat Hospital, Northern Ethiopia: A case control study. Epidemiology (sunnyvale) 5: 192.
16. Bayou YT, Mashalla YJS, Tshweneagae G (2016) Patterns of caesarean-section delivery in Addis Ababa, Ethiopia. Afr J Prm Health Care Fam Med 8: a953.
17. Gutema AS (2014) Caesarean section and associated factors at Mizan Aman General Hospital Southwest Ethiopia. J Gynecol Obstet 2: 37-41.
18. Taye A, Yuya M (2015) One year retrospective analysis of prevalence of caesarean section in Jimma University Specialized Hospital, South Western Ethiopia. J Preg Child Health 2: 172.
19. Moges A, Adem B, Akessa G (2015) Prevalence and outcome of caesarean section in Attat Hospital, Gurage Zone, SNNPR, Ethiopia. Arch Med 7: 1-6.
20. Tsega F, Mengistie B, Dessie Y, Mengesha MM (2015) Prevalence of cesarean section in urban health facilities and associated factors in Eastern Ethiopia: Hospital based cross sectional study. J Preg Child Health 2: 169.
21. Betran AP, Ye J, Moller AB, Zhang J, Gulmezoglu AM, et al. (2016) The increasing trend in caesarean section rates: Global, regional and national estimates: 1990-2014. PLoS One 11: e0148343.
22. Dillen TM, Petrova V, Roosmalen JV (2007) Caesarean section in a semi-rural hospital in Northern Namibia. BMC Pregnancy and Childbirth 8: 2.
23. Geidam AD, Audu BM, Kawuwa BM, Jessy YO (2009) Rising trends and indications of cesarean sections at university of Miaduguri teaching hospital Nigeria. Annals of African Medicine 8: 127-132.
24. Tadesse E, Adane M, Abiyou M (1996) Caesarean section deliveries at Tikur Anbessa Teaching Hospital, Ethiopia. East Afr Med J 73: 619-622.
25. Chu K, Cortier H, Maldonado F, Mashant T, Ford N, et al. (2012) Cesarean section rates and indications in Sub-Saharan Africa: A Multi-country study from Medecins sans Frontieres. PLoS ONE 7: e44484.
26. Heemelaar S, Mode P, Kidano H, Roosmalen J, Stekeleburg J (2016) Criteria-based audit of caesarean section in a referral hospital in rural Tanzania. Trop Med Int Health 21: 525-534.

Domestic Violence among Women in Jeddah

Fageeh WMK*

Department of Obstetrics and Gynecology, Faculty of Medicine, King Abdulaziz University Hospital, Kingdom of Saudi Arabia

***Corresponding author:** Fageeh WMK, Department of Obstetrics and Gynecology, King Abdulaziz University Hospital, Jeddah 21589, Kingdom of Saudi Arabia, E-mail: fageeh.wafa@gmail.com

Abstract

Objective: This study aimed to determine the prevalence of domestic violence and the common health problems reported by abused women.

Methods: This cross-sectional survey was conducted between December 15, 2011 and May 30, 2012 on female residents of Jeddah who presented to King Abdulaziz University Hospital, King Abdulaziz Oncology Medical Center, or King Fahd General Hospital.

Results: A total of 203 women were recruited. The lifetime prevalence of domestic violence was 34.0%. Emotional abuse was the most common form of abuse (31.3%); physical and sexual abuses were reported in 21.6% and 4.8% of the participants, respectively. Only 1% of Saudi victims of domestic violence planned to seek help from social services.

Conclusion: Although domestic violence is a common problem among women in Jeddah, only a negligible proportion of women plan to seek help. Policy makers should therefore improve social support services to encourage and cater for the needs of abused women.

Keywords: Domestic violence; Emotional abuse; Physical abuse; Sexual abuse; Women

Introduction

Domestic violence (DV) is defined by the World Health Organization [1] as "the range of sexually, psychologically, and physically coercive acts used against adult and adolescent women by current or former male intimate partners." It represents a unique aspect of the wider set of problems faced by women in most societies worldwide.

Much qualitative evidence and analysis demonstrate that DV has a deleterious effect on the physical and mental health of women [2]. An estimated 35% of women visit emergency departments as a result of DV, and abused women are reported to have a 50-70% increase in gynecological, central nervous system, and chronic stress-related problems compared with non-abused women [3]. Gynecological problems may include sexually transmitted diseases, fibroids, pelvic pain, vaginal bleeding, or infection. Chronic stress-related problems that have been reported include functional gastrointestinal disorders, appetite loss, and colds [3]. There are also reports, including those of a meta-analysis of 14 studies, that women exposed to abuse during pregnancy had an increased risk of miscarriage, abortion, and stillbirth [4,5].

Population-based data on the prevalence and effects of DV are limited in Arab countries and are only available from few countries in the region. The prevalence of DV in Arab countries ranges between 23 and 35%, similar to internationally reported data [6,7]. In a conservative country such as Saudi Arabia, there are no official reports on the prevalence of DV, and only a few hospital-based studies [8,9] have focused on the prevalence and health consequences of DV. In a study conducted among married women in Al-Ahsa, Saudi Arabia [9], the prevalence of lifetime DV was 39.3% (35.9% for mental, 17.9% for physical, and 6.9% for sexual violence). To the best of our knowledge, no population- or hospital-based study has been conducted in Jeddah to assess the prevalence of DV among women. In this paper, we explore DV in women who lived in Jeddah, with the aim of estimating its prevalence and the common health problems reported by abused women.

Methods

Participants

This was a cross-sectional survey conducted from December 15th, 2011 to March 30th, 2012 at King Abdulaziz University Hospital, King Abdulaziz Oncology Medical Center, and King Fahd General Hospital, which are three leading tertiary care hospitals in the western region of Saudi Arabia.

The target population included a convenience outpatient and inpatient sample of women (patients, caregivers, and visitors) aged 15-70 years who were willing to participate in this study. We could not include participants from women's gathering groups because our approach was hampered by resistance from the administration owing to the relatively sensitive nature of our theme.

A total of 2301 women were included from the outpatient and inpatient departments of the above-mentioned hospitals. Of these, 2072 respondents completed the full interview, representing an overall response rate of 90.0%. Of the total number of non-responders (n=229), 10.0% provided partial or incomplete information. A follow-up study of non-responders was not performed, as the survey was conducted in a public place.

A psychologist and a professional health assistant explained the purpose of the research to all the women who consented to participate in the survey. The women were then asked to fill a 50 item questionnaire that comprised questions to identify ever exposure to DV. Special assistance was provided to the illiterate and in cases where further explanation was required. All questionnaires were collected immediately after they were filled.

Instrument

We used a questionnaire that was available in English and Arabic. The questionnaire was developed by selecting items from two validated questionnaires: the NorVold Domestic Abuse Questionnaire [10] and the Kansas Marital Satisfaction Scale [11].

Items assessed

Violence

The questionnaire was composed of five sections:

- Eleven items on the personal data of the women
- Twenty-five items on violence, namely two items for general violence, ten items for physical violence, six items for psychological or emotional violence, and seven items for sexual violence
- Five items that explored the respondents' options to ask for help
- Five items that assessed the damaging effect of DV on the victims
- Four items that evaluated sexual dysfunction and three items that scored the level of happiness, extracted from the Kansas Marital Satisfaction Scale [12].

For the purpose of this study, physical violence was defined as having ever been pushed, beaten, slapped, kicked, hit with a fist or object, pulled by the hair, dragged, burned, or threatened or attacked with a knife or gun by a spouse or family member.

Psychological abuse was defined as having ever been threatened by a spouse or family member, prevented from visiting or calling family members and friends, or insulted. Sexual violence was defined as having ever been forced by a spouse or family member to have unwanted sexual intercourse.

Marital satisfaction

Marital satisfaction was categorized into the following: extremely dissatisfied, very dissatisfied, somewhat dissatisfied, mixed feelings, somewhat satisfied, very satisfied, and extremely satisfied.

Health problems

Closed-ended questions on general well-being, including body self-image and perception of self and others, were asked to document health problems experienced by the participants.

Statistical analysis

The data were analyzed using the Statistical Package for the Social Sciences (SPSS IBM Inc., New York, US), version 18. The independent t-test was used for equal variance and Welch's t-test for unequal variance. The chi-square test was used to determine the relationship between variables. Differences were considered statistically significant at a p-value of <0.05. Results are expressed as mean ± standard deviation (SD) and frequency (%).

The Biomedical Ethics Research Committee of King Abdulaziz University provided ethical review and approval for the survey, including voluntary recruitment, rigorous confidentiality provisions, and written informed consent.

Results

General characteristics of the study population

A total of 2301 women were recruited. The mean ± SD age of the women was 34.4 ± 10.9 years. Of the 2301 women, 2235 (97.1%) were Muslim, whereas 23 (1.0%) were Christian; 43 women did not specify their religion. Saudi women constituted 58.3% (n=1342) of the sample.

Among the participants, 1516 (65.9%) were married, 606 (26.3%) were divorced, 58 (2.5%) were widowed, and 34 (1.5%) were separated; 87 (3.8%) did not specify their marital status. Most of the participants came from big families where the mean number of siblings was 7.1 ± 3.4.

Abuse

Emotional abuse

The prevalence of abuse (physical, emotional, and sexual) was 34.0%. Emotional or psychological abuse was the most common form of abuse, which was reported by 720 women (31.3%).

Nearly one in five women (n=492, 21.4%) reported divorce threats from their husbands, 340 (14.8%) reported being prevented from visiting or calling their families, 264 (11.5%) reported their husbands had threatened to marry another wife, 183 (8.0%) received threats of getting thrown out of their homes, and 163 (7.1%) had money withheld from them (Table 1).

Emotional abuse	Yes	No	Total	No respons e
Did your husband ever threaten you with divorce?	492 (21.4)	1792 (77.9)	2284 (99.3)	17 (0.7)
Did your husband ever threaten to throw you out of your home?	183 (8.0)	2103 (91.4)	2286 (99.3)	15 (0.7)
Did your husband ever threaten to marry another woman?	264 (11.5)	2013 (87.5)	2277 (99.0)	24 (1.0)
Did your husband ever withhold money from you?	163 (7.1)	2119 (92.1)	2282 (99.2)	19 (0.8)
Did your husband ever prevent you from visiting or calling your family?	340 (14.8)	1952 (84.8)	2292 (99.6)	9 (0.4)

Table 1: Frequency of responses to questions that assessed emotional abuse (Data presented as frequency (percent).

Physical abuse

A total of 290 women (12.6%) reported physical abuse. Almost one in ten women reported ever experiencing physical violence in the form of beating (n=237, 10.3%), hitting with the fist (n=222, 9.6%), or slapping (n=194, 8.4%).

Of the 2301 women, 88 (3.8%) reported serious injury that required medical intervention or hospital care; 46 (2%) were threatened with a knife or gun.

One hundred and thirty-six women (5.9%) reported severe beating during childhood (Table 2).

Physical abuse	Yes	No	Total	No response
Did your husband ever throw an object at you?	93 (4.0)	2073 (90.1)	2166 (94.1)	135 (5.9)
Did your husband ever slap you?	194 (8.4)	1983 (86.2)	2177 (94.6)	124 (5.4)
Did your husband ever push or grab you?	237 (10.3)	2045 (88.9)	2282 (99.2)	19 (0.8)
Did your husband ever hit you with a fist?	222 (9.6)	2062 (89.6)	2284 (99.3)	17 (0.7)
Did your husband ever kick or bite you?	87 (3.8)	2199 (95.6)	2286 (99.3)	15 (0.7)
Did your husband ever choke or beat you up?	88 (3.8)	2203 (95.7)	2291 (99.6)	10 (0.4)
Did your husband ever use a knife or gun to threaten you?	46 (2.0)	2242 (97.4)	2288 (99.4)	13 (0.6)
Did your husband ever cause you injury that required medical intervention?	88 (3.8)	2205 (95.8)	2293 (99.7)	8 (0.3)
Were you ever a victim of severe beating during childhood?	136 (5.9)	2051 (89.1)	2187 (95.0)	114 (5.0)

Table 2: Frequency of responses to questions that assessed physical abuse (Data are presented as frequency (percent)).

Sexual abuse

One hundred and eleven women (4.8%) reported being sexually abused by a family member. Sixty-six women (2.9%) reported sexual penetration during childhood, and 68 women (3.0%) reported ever experiencing forceful anal intercourse.

Forty-four women (1.9%) reported that their husbands kicked them during intercourse (Table 3).

Sexual abuse	Yes	No	Total
Did your husband ever beat you during intercourse?	44 (1.9)	2225 (96.7)	2269 (98.6)
Did your husband ever rape you?	68 (3.0)	2206 (95.9)	2274 (98.8)
Did your husband ever force you to have anal intercourse?	68 (3.0)	2227 (96.8)	2295 (99.7)
Were you a victim of child abuse?	182 (7.9)	2013 (87.5)	2195 (95.4)
Were you a victim of sexual abuse?	111 (4.8)	2077 (90.3)	2188 (95.1)
Were you fondled?	6 (0.2)	66 (2.6)	130 (5.2)

Table 3: Frequency of responses to questions that assessed sexual abuse (Data are presented as frequency (percent)).

Health problems reported by abused women

The frequency of health problems was higher in abused than non-abused women (Table 4).

These included loss of trust in others (P<0.0001), irritable colon or gastric ulcer (P<0.0001), hopelessness (P<0.0001), body self-hatred (P<0.0001), and food addiction (P<0.0001) (Table 4).

	Non-abused		Abused		Total		P-value
Variables	Yes	No	Yes	No	Abused	Non-abused	
Loss of trust in others	290 (20.2)	1144 (79.8)	227 (31.2)	500 (68.8)	517 (23.9)	1644 (76.1)	< 0.0001
Body self-hatred	80 (5.6)	1349 (94.4)	82 (11.3)	644 (88.7)	135 (7.5)	1993 (92.5)	< 0.0001
Food addiction	102 (7.1)	1330 (92.9)	119 (16.4)	607 (83.6)	221 (10.2)	1937 (89.8)	< 0.0001
Irritable colon or gastric ulcer	219 (15.4)	1202 (84.6)	209 (28.8)	517 (71.2)	428 (19.9)	1719 (80.1)	< 0.0001

Table 4: Most common medical and mental problems reported by abused and non-abused women (Data are presented as frequency (percent)).

Marital and sexual satisfaction

The proportion of women who were unsatisfied with their marriages was higher in the abused than non-abused group (P≤0.0001 for emotional, physical, and sexual abuse).

One thousand eighty-three women (52.3%) reported they did not enjoy sex with their spouses; 746 women (54.7%) in the non-abused group did not enjoy intercourse as compared with 337 women (47.7%) in the abused group (P=0.003). Two hundred twenty-nine (10.0%) women declined to respond to the question on sexual satisfaction (Table 5).

	Physically abused*		Sexually abused*		Emotionally abused*		Ever abused*	
Satisfaction scale	No	Yes	No	Yes	No	Yes	No	Yes
Extremely dissatisfied	24 (1.3)	19 (7.1)	34 (1.6)	9 (8.2)	17 (1.1)	26 (3.9)	16 (1.1)	27 (3.7)
Very dissatisfied	25 (1.3)	14 (5.2)	32 (1.6)	7 (6.4)	15 (1.0)	24 (3.6)	15 (1.0)	24 (3.3)
Somewhat dissatisfied	29 (1.5)	22 (8.2)	40 (1.9)	11(10.0)	14 (0.9)	37 (5.5)	11 (0.8)	40 (5.4)
Mixed	236 (12.4)	76 (28.3)	279 (13.5)	33 (30.0)	180 (12)	132 (19.6)	170 (11.8)	142 (19.3)
Somewhat satisfied	627 (33.0)	68 (25.3)	676 (32.8)	19 (17.3)	456 (30.5)	239 (35.5)	436 (30.3)	259 (35.3)
Very satisfied	655 (34.4)	45 (16.7)	681 (33.0)	19 (17.3)	557 (37.2)	143 (21.2)	537 (37.4)	163 (22.2)
Extremely satisfied	306 (16.1)	25 (9.3)	319 (15.5)	12 (10.9)	258 (17.2)	73 (10.8)	252 (17.5)	79 (10.8)

Table 5: Marital satisfaction scale showing how satisfied the women were with their marriages (Data are presented as frequency (percent)) (*P ≤ 0.0001).

Help-seeking action

A very small proportion of the women sought help from their families (n=72, 3.1%) or husbands' families (n=73, 3.2%). Only 56 women (2.4%) responded that they planned to see a psychiatrist; 24 women (1.0%) planned to contact social services.

Discussion

The definition of women abuse varies in different cultures. In fact, the various methods that are used to measure violence can cause wide variations in its assessment, leading to great difficulties in estimating its prevalence. In a conservative society such as Saudi Arabia where male authority is predominant, it is a quite difficult and complicated task to assess abuse against women.

According to some data [13], there is a growing body of evidence pointing to the range of negative health consequences of DV, and women are reportedly victims of violent deaths, which are either a direct (through homicide) or indirect (through suicide) result of DV. In this study, we attempted to explore violence against women living in Jeddah.

Our analysis showed that the lifetime prevalence of DV was 34.0%, which falls within the 23-35% range of prevalence rates for Arab countries [6,7]. Conversely, the prevalence reported in the current study is relatively lower when compared with results from studies conducted in other regions of Saudi Arabia. Afifi et al. [9] reported that the lifetime prevalence of DV among women in the Eastern Province of Saudi Arabia was 39.3%, and Tashkandi and Rahseed [8] reported that the lifetime prevalence of abuse in women who attended primary health centers in Medina was 57.7%. The lower percentage observed in the current study could be explained by the heterogeneous nature of our population, which consisted of women from various cultural backgrounds.

Emotional abuse was the most frequent form of abuse (31.3%) in our study; 12.6% of the participants reported physical abuse, whereas 4.8% reported sexual abuse. Other authors [7,9,14,15] have also cited emotional abuse to be the most common form of abuse, which we believe might be because all forms of abuse have an emotional component. In one report from Sari, Iran [16], it was found that the prevalence of physical, emotional, and sexual abuse was 73.5%, 92.2%, and 49.6%, respectively. In another report from the United States [14], the authors found that up to 97.2% of the women in their study were emotionally abused. Sexual abuse was also the least common form of abuse, reported in 16.5% of the women.

Domestic violence is known to affect women's health and well-being seriously [17-20]. In the current study, loss of trust, body self-hatred, food addiction, and irritable bowel syndrome or gastric ulcers were significantly more common among abused women. This finding might be related to the fact that psychological or emotional abuse, which was the most common form of abuse in our study, is positively related to negative health perceptions [21]. Furthermore, our finding of poor sexual fulfilment, which was more common among abused women, is not surprising because sexual health requires a positive and respectful approach to sexuality and sexual relationships, as well as the possibility of having pleasurable sex experiences, free of coercion, and violence [22].

Many women in our study declined to make comments on their spouses or marital fulfilment; however, the level of marital satisfaction was high in the respondent group. Most women (79.9%) were satisfied to extremely satisfy although over half of them (52.3%) reported they did not enjoy sex with their husbands. In Saudi Arabia, interpretations of the local culture and traditions, as well as social peer pressure, have been reported to have a negative impact on women's well-being [23]. As a result, women tend to tolerate their husbands and thus feel they are satisfied with their marital lives, or they decline to talk about their spouses for fear that it is socially improper to do so. More so, because sex is generally a subject of taboo in Saudi Arabia like in many Arab countries [24,25], most women tend to ignore the importance of sexual satisfaction in marriage or judge that it is not important.

We found that only 1% of DV victims planned to seek help from social services. Few participants left their contact numbers with the prospect that we could help them gain access to social services since personal efforts were unsuccessful, and the limited available services were only accessible to local citizens. It is plausible that some women do not report cases of DV because social services are underdeveloped in Saudi Arabia or because of the poor perception of social services by the local population [25]. In addition, Arab women are in general expected to balance their needs and well-being against loyalty to their spouses and preservation of family reputation [26]. Besides, fear of retaliation by the spouse has also been reported to be more common among Arab women, whose concerns are not only limited to increasing violence, but also to being separated from their children, a technique that is commonly applied by violent spouses [7]. However, this may be more of a cultural than a religious issue, as Prophet Muhammad (10 A.H.) in his last sermon said: "Do treat your women well and be kind to them for they are your partners and committed helpers."

Approximately 90% of countries have ratified international conventions specifically banning discriminations against women, including the Convention on the Elimination of All Forms of Discrimination against Women [27] and the Declaration on the Elimination of Violence against Women [28]. In Africa, human rights groups such as the Protocol to the African Charter on Human and People's Rights on the Rights of Women in Africa [29] stipulates that "States Parties shall prohibit and condemn all forms of harmful practices which negatively affect the human rights of women and which are contrary to recognized international standards. States Parties shall take all necessary legislative and other measures to eliminate such practices."

This study has several limitations. First, because women were recruited from hospitals, the results may not be representative of the local population in Jeddah. Second, the use of close-ended questions in the questionnaire probably introduced bias since women with no opinion were constrained to respond. Third, we could not obtain information from some participants due to barriers associated with fear of breach of privacy, tensions about limited confidentiality, and frustration linked to feelings of unsafety after releasing information to strangers. Fourth, our use of questionnaires implied that we relied on the participants' honesty and memories thereby increasing the risk of bias during data analysis. Finally, the interpretation of happiness and satisfaction is purely subjective and cannot be accurately assessed.

However, our study highlights the magnitude of DV among women who were interviewed at three of the largest hospitals in Jeddah. We recommend that social service policy makers make their facilities available to victims of DV by encouraging women to disclose their abuse, changing the perception of social services in our society, and providing victims of abuse with mandatory prevention, counselling, and support. Furthermore, the role of care managers (specially trained nurses) should be explored in abused women needing medical attention. A previous model that incorporated care managers to support general practitioners and specialists in managing patients showed that patients were more satisfied with health care services due to their strong partnership with care managers who collaborated effectively with physicians [30].

Conclusions

Domestic violence affects 34.0% of women attending the outpatient and inpatient clinics of three of the main tertiary hospitals in Jeddah. Mental and medical disorders are more frequent among victims of DV. Furthermore, only a small proportion of abused women seeks or plans to seek help either from family members or social security services. Policy makers should, therefore, improve the social support services to encourage and cater for the needs of abused women. It is necessary for health policy decision-makers to set rules and regulations to carefully assess this problem, which can be done by improving the level of awareness about violence against women and developing social support services to cater for the needs of abused women. In addition, health care providers should consider developing a valid and culturally appropriate violence screening method in pregnant women to enable health professional's screen and estimate suffering, and hence provide victims of DV with adequate care and support.

Funding

This work did not receive any specific grant from any funding agency in the public, commercial, or non-profit sector.

Acknowledgments

The author wishes to thank Mr. Kalvin Balucanag for his help in analyzing the data. The author would like to thank the staff at King Abdulaziz University Hospital, King Abdulaziz Oncology Medical Center, and King Fahd General Hospital for their help in collecting data.

Declaration of Interest

As the sole author, Wafa M.K. Fageeh wrote and approved the manuscript for submission. She warrants that this article is her original work and it has not received prior publication nor is it under consideration for publication elsewhere.

Competing Interests

The author has no competing interests.

References

1. World Health Organization (1997) WHO/WHD. Violence against women: A priority health issue, Geneva: World Health Organization.
2. Guth AA, Pachter LH (2000) Domestic violence and the trauma surgeon. Am J Surg 9: 134-140.
3. Campbell J, Jones AS, Dienemann J, Kub J, Schollenberger J, et al. (2002) Intimate partner violence and physical health consequences. Arch Int Med 162: 1157-1163.
4. Murphy CC, Schei B, Myhr TL, Du Mont J (2001) Abuse: a risk factor for low birth weight? A systemic review and meta-analysis. CM AJ 64: 1567-1572.
5. Yoshikawa K, Agrawal NR, Poudel KC, Jimba M (2012) A lifetime experience of violence and adverse reproductive outcomes: findings from population surveys in India. Biosci Trends 6: 115-121.
6. Boy A, Kulczycki A (2001) What we know about intimate partner violence in the Middle East and North Africa. Violence Against Women 14: 53-70.
7. Usta J, Farver JA, Pashayan N (2009) Domestic violence: the Lebanese experience. Public Health 121: 208-219.

8. Tashkandi A, Rasheed FP (2009) Wife abuse: a hidden problem. A study among Saudi women attending PHC centres. East Mediterr Health J 15: 1242-1253.
9. Afifi ZE, Al-Muhaideb NS, Hadish NF, Ismail FI, Al-Qeamy FM (2011) Domestic violence and its impact on married women's health in Eastern Saudi Arabia. Saudi Med J 32: 612-620.
10. Swahnberg IM, Wijma B (2003) The NorVold Abuse Questionnaire (NorAQ): validation of new measures of emotional, physical, and sexual abuse, and abuse in the health care system among women. Eur J Public Health 13: 361.
11. Kotelchuck M (2006) Pregnancy risk assessment monitoring system (PRAMS) possible new roles for a national MCH data system. Public Health Rep 121: 6-10.
12. Crane DR, Middle KC, Bean RA (2000) Establishing criterion scores for the kansas marital satisfaction. Am J Fam Ther 28: 53-60.
13. Garcia-Moreno C, Watts C (2011) Violence against women: an urgent public health priority. Bulletin of the World Health Organization. Bull World Health Organ 89: 2-2.
14. Grossman SF, Lundy M (2007) Domestic violence across race and ethnicity: implications for social work practice and policy. Violence Against Women 13: 1029-1052.
15. Hegarty KL, O'Doherty LJ, Chondros P (2013) Type and severity of intimate partner violence on women's health and service use: Findings from a primary care trial of women afraid of their partners. J Interpers Violence 28: 273-294.
16. Ghahhari S, Mazdarani S, Khalilian A (2008) Spouse abuse in Sari-Iran. Iran J Psychiatry Behav Sci 2: 31-35.
17. Rachana C, Suraiya K, Hisham AS, Abdulaziz AM, Hai A (2002) Prevalence and complications of physical violence during pregnancy. Eur J Obstet Gynecol Reprod Biol 103: 26-29.
18. Ellsberg M, Heise L, Watts CH, Moreno CG (2005) Researching violence against women a practical guide for researchers and activists. Washington DC: World Health Organization, PATH.
19. Ellsberg M, Jansen HA, Heise L (2008) WHO multi-country study on women's health and domestic violence against women study team. Intimate partner violence and women's physical and mental health in the WHO multi-country study on women's health and domestic violence: an observational study. Lancet 371: 1165-1172.
20. Mohammadi G, Amiraliakbari S, Ramezankhani A (2011) Poor reproductive health among a group of socially damaged Middle Eastern women: a cross-sectional study. Int J Womens Health 3: 399-403.
21. Straight E, Harper F, Arias I (2003) The impact of partner psychological abuse on health behaviors and health status in college women. J Interperl Violence 18: 1034-1054.
22. World Health Organization. Sexual and reproductive health: gender and human rights.
23. Mobaraki AE, Soderfeldt B (2006) Gender inequity in Saudi Arabia and its role in public health. East Mediterr Health J. 16: 113-118.
24. Lootah W (2009) Top secret: Sexual guidance for married couples. 4th ed. Dubai: Dubai distribution office, United Arab Emirates.
25. Alzahrani A (2011) Women's sexual health in Saudi Arabia: A focused ethnographic study. Yorkshire: University of Sheffield.
26. Yahia MMH, Sadan E (2008) Issues in intervention with battered women in collectivist societies. J Marital Fam Ther 34: 1-13.
27. Convention on the Elimination of All Forms of Discrimination against Women. (2010). New York: UN GAOR.
28. http://www.ohchr.org/english/law/eliminationvaw.htm
29. http://www.gtz.de/de/dokumente/en-fgm-maputoprotocol.pdf
30. Ciccone MM, Aquilino A, Cortese F, Scicchitano P, Sassara M, et al. (2010) Feasibility and effectiveness of a disease and care management model in the primary health care system for patients with heart failure and diabetes (Project Leonardo). Vasc Health Risk Manag 6: 297-305.

Anxiolytic Benefits of Exercise Classes for Mothers

Currie J*

Health and Physical Education, University of Technology Sydney, Australia

***Corresponding author:** Currie J, Health and Physical Education, University of Technology Sydney, Australia, E-mail: Janet.Currie@uts.edu.au

Abstract

Objective: The importance of women accessing physical activity has been shown in the literature as being even more critical for wellbeing following birth of a child. As there is scant research available specifically purporting the mental health benefits of exercise classes, this paper examines the anxiolytic or anxiety-reducing benefits gained from involvement in a 3-month, twice-weekly group low-impact exercise class program for a group of mothers (n=21).

Method: Quantitative data were obtained by measuring acute pre and post-changes (or pre and post-60 minutes interval for the exercise group and a non-exercising control) in the level of state anxiety (i.e. how you feel 'right now'), through the Spielberger et al. State Anxiety Inventory (STAI).

Results: The mean state anxiety levels experienced pre and post-activity showed a significant change (decrease) in exercising mothers as compared to non–exercising mothers at both Week 1 (Measurement A) and at 12–weeks (Measurement B) ($p<0.05$).

Conclusion: Mothers are able to experience a decrease in acute anxiety following participation in exercise classes. Further strategies that allow for enhanced access and the continuation of care of children or relatives by others while the mother takes time out for health promoting exercise for leisure will need to be developed.

Keywords: Mothers; Anxiety; Exercise classes; Stress; Women's fitness; State anxiety inventory; Anxiolytic

Introduction

Individual health includes maintaining a sense of balance between the physical, emotional/mental, social and spiritual aspects of our wellbeing. These areas are interrelated and interdependent [1]. As the pace of life in Western society continues to accelerate, gaining access to quality leisure becomes even more important from a health point-of-view [2,3]. More recently, research recommends leisure pastimes as being a means of coping with such daily stress. Not only has exercise been clinically proven to improve mood or lower depressive and anxiety states, recent research has demonstrated that exercise might also help us to engage in more positive things, thereby improving our overall lifestyle and perceived satisfaction with quality of life [4-7].

Even perceiving one's self as being physically active compared with peers has been concluded as an important factor related to health status and predicted mortality. For example, in Zahrt and Crum's major study, individuals who perceived themselves as less active than others were up to 71% more likely to die in the follow–up period than those who perceived themselves as more active, even after accounting for the effects of actual physical activity levels and other known determinants of mortality [8]. Therefore, it's not surprising participation in exercise is often recommended for enhancing wellbeing [9-12]. Mothers have been identified as a group that could significantly benefit from physical activity interventions for enhancing social and emotional wellbeing, particularly stress levels [12,13]. However, mothers perceive more barriers to accessing exercising than women without children do [13-15].

The combination of little control and attempting to be on–call meeting the relentless demands of caring may account for the stressfulness of these roles [15]. One of the major shocks for mothers after the birth of a child is that their own needs for time, space and nurture have suddenly become secondary to the baby's needs [16]. In a vicious circle, women also involved in outside employment often experience "role overload" which is associated with negative health outcomes including elevated levels of stress, depression, and anxiety [17,18]. Lack of time is also the principal and most prevalent reason given for an inactive lifestyle [9,13,19]. With many mothers reporting high levels of stress and constraints in managing their busy lifestyles, the importance of them being able to access active leisure becomes even more critical for maintaining individual health and wellbeing [18,19].

A paradox exists in that while mothers value the role of physical activity as part of their wellbeing, they report on finding it difficult to access or find suitable formats [18,20]. One active leisure activity that has been proposed as a potentially more convenient and accessible option for mothers is exercise classes [9,12,18]. Its perceived benefits may vary across age groups, but overall women state perceived enjoyment from the 'feel good' aspects involved from their exercise class participation [21]. However, there is scant evidence-based research that has been published on the benefits of exercise class participation for women. Most reports are typically anecdotal in nature, or promoted through the mass media [22,23]. Health care providers prefer recommending the most reliable and evidence-based forms of exercise available. Likewise, participants themselves would benefit from understanding the mental health efficacy associated with a particular activity. With fitness classes and gym being the second most commonly participated recreation activity undertaken by women in Australia after walking, it is surprising that so little research has been undertaken regarding its perceived benefits as a potential leisure activity [24,25]. Therefore, the purpose of this study was to discover whether participation in exercise classes is reported by mothers as positively impacting on stress levels.

Method

Research design

As the study aimed to examine any potential anxiolytic or anxiety–reducing phenomenon associated with exercise class participation, a group of exercising mothers and a non–exercising control group both completed inventories intending to evaluate reported measures of individual anxiety levels. A quasi–experimental research design was implemented using non-randomised group pretest–posttest results, with 'treatment' consisting of a 12-week, low impact group exercise class program. STAI Measurements were examined pre and post-activity at Week 1 and Week 12 to assess consistency and also note any possible changes due to cumulative adaptation.

Sample

A sample of convenience of exercising mothers (n=21) volunteered to take part while the non-exercising control group of mothers (n=21) were recruited from those mothers who were attending local health centers with their child. Hence the self–volunteering mothers in the exercise group may have been more motivated to be involved in exercise and lowering their stress compared with the control group of mothers. All women in the sample lived in the same metropolitan region of Sydney, NSW, Australia. The mean age of the exercise group was 37.3 years and the non-exercise group 29.2 years. The exercising mothers had a mean number of 2.2 children each, and the non-exercisers 1.4 children each. The mean age of the exercising mothers' children was 10.4 years the non-exercising group's children only 3.6 years of age. So, while on average the exercising mothers had more children to care for, a younger child could be considered more demanding in terms of the amount of care required [26]. Thirteen of the exercising mothers were involved in outside employment compared with only three in the non-exercising group. Respondents had to meet the inclusion criteria of being a mother of one or more children, identify as well, and living in the Warringah area of Sydney, Australia. Only mothers who did not withdraw from the study or miss a session were included in the results. The control group contained 21 mothers who did not engage in any exercise for the duration of the 12 week program.

Exercise treatment

The exercise classes included 60-minute, moderate intensity, Low–Impact aerobics or group exercise classes conducted twice a week, for 12 weeks in a local community hall. 'Low-impact' means that at least one foot is always landed and weight-bearing on the ground at any one time, so the class involves mainly stepping or walking movements with no running or jumping. The format consisted of a gradual warm-up, rhythmic movements or steps conducted in the upright or standing position, muscle conditioning exercises conducted on the floor such as leg raises, abdominal exercises, followed with a final cool down and stretching phase.

Procedures

Results were obtained by administering the State Anxiety Inventory Form Y-1 (STAI) to the two groups of women [27].

The two groups being assessed were:

- **Exercise Group**-those who participated in a regular twice-weekly exercise program and completed all sessions for twelve weeks (n=21); and
- **Non-Exercise Group**-those who did not participate in an exercise program (n=21).

The STAI is a 20–item inventory or survey measurement tool able to be self-administered to reliably detect any changes in a person's level of state or acute anxiety, for how stressed s/he is feeling, 'right now'. State anxiety is the intensity of any unpleasant emotional state of how we may be experiencing or responding to stressors at a given point in time, characterised by the degree an individual perceives any feelings of tension, apprehension, nervousness or worry. Each Likert-scale response (1-20) attracts a score of 1-4, with 20 points the lowest and 80 points the maximum possible. A decrease in the STAI post-activity indicates a reduction on anxiety. Therefore, it is the negative change that is able to indicate whether an activity is anxiolytic or not.

The STAI is the most commonly used instrument in exercise studies for measuring anxiety levels and has been documented as a reliable, valid and sensitive indicator of changes in state anxiety [28]. It was explained to respondents that the inventory required them to report how they felt 'right now…at this moment'. Each member of the two groups in the sample answered the STAI questionnaire before and after an activity of one hour's duration. For example, members of the exercise group were given the inventory to answer before commencing the exercise class, and then immediately afterwards for the researcher to notice the difference in scores and therefore define the respondent's acute response/change. Members of the non–exercise group, however, were given the inventory to answer immediately before and after a non-exercise related activity such as household work. An important factor which does reflect positively on the equivalence of the two groups is the 'baseline' STAI scores of the two groups of mothers as they entered the program. The mean STAI scores of the recorded at Week 1 were:

- Exercise Group: 35.38
- Non-Exercise Group: 36.05.

The first occasion that the STAI was administered is illustrated in the results as 'Measurement A'. The inventory was distributed again after a 12-week period to members of each group to gauge consistency in responses. This is illustrated in the results as 'Measurement B'.

Data Analysis

To test the significance of the changes in mean STAI scores for the two groups of mothers, pre to post activity at the two intervals (Measurements A and B), an independent one-tailed t-test was selected [29]. All data were analyzed using the t-test for independent samples of group from SPSS [30]. For the purposes of this study, a confidence interval of 0.05 was used. The next section presents the results of the inventory measurements of anxiety levels pre and post activity.

Findings

The aim of this study is to report on the perceived stress–relieving benefits reported by mothers who have been able to carve time out to participate in exercise classes compared with a group who participated in non-exercise activities. The quantitative results are concerned with any changes in the mothers' STAI inventory scores post–activity compared with pre–activity. The average changes in STAI scores for the exercise groups were -5.76 and -8.00 Measurements A and B respectively. However, the average changes for the non-exercise group were +4.81 and +2.52 for Measurements A and B (at Week 1 and 12), respectively. A decrease in anxiety is indicated by a negative figure whereas a positive figure indicates an increase in anxiety. Therefore, the greatest decrement in anxiety pre-post activity was present in the exercise group for Measurements A and B, with the exercise group as a whole achieving decreases in STAI scores of -121 and -168, for Measurements A and B. In contrast, the non–exercise participants increased their STAI scores by a total of 101 and 53, for Measurements A and B respectively.

The results were tested to see if they were significant using a 95% confidence interval, and confirmed the hypothesis that mothers who participate in exercise programs experience a significant decrease in stress after exercising compared with mothers who don't exercise. The t-test used was to test the significant difference in scores before and after (exercise/non–exercise) between the two independent groups of mothers. The t values for Measurements A and B were -4.27 and -4.68 respectively. The mean change of -5.7619 (exercising group, 21 cases) compared with 4.8095 (non–exercising group, 21 cases) for Measurement A at .05 level of confidence (for a one tailed t–test) was significant. The mean change of -8.000 (exercising group, 21 cases) compared with 2.5238 (non–exercising group, 21 cases) was also significant for Measurement B, at .05 level of confidence (for a one tailed t–test). The decrease in anxiety post–exercise session was also significant at the 0.0025% confidence level. Therefore, both measurements A and B showed a significant change in exercising mothers as compared to non–exercising mothers ($p<0.05$). The factors influencing these results will now be examined.

Discussion

The reported subjective decrease in stress associated with the class participation may be associated with the general anxiolytic nature of exercise per se [31-34]. According to Johnsgard, exercise can produce a very significant tranquillising effect, which usually lasts for two hours [35]. This may be due to release of endorphins or a simple decrease experienced in overall tension and improved mood [12,35]. If the classes were of too high an intensity, or not well received, the exercise may have led to increases in anxiety, tension and fatigue, suggesting that moderate intensity, continuous aerobic activity may be best [6]. Bahrke and Morgan found that less intensive non–exercise activities such as meditation and quiet rest can also achieve reductions in state anxiety [32]. However, these methods may not be as practical or readily achievable and convenient for the mother, unless she has individual childcare organised and a quiet space available. Non–exercise activities also don't provide the fitness–related benefits of exercise, such as increased cardiovascular capacity, or improvements in strength or muscle tone.

The exercising group's positive experiences regarding reported decreased stress, as reflected in their STAI, may have been moderated *via* the stress-reducing mechanism of social support [35-38]. Access to social support is associated with psychological wellbeing and a lower probability of physical illness, however, social isolation is associated with psychological distress and postnatal depression [39,40]. The non-exercising mothers may have felt more anxious if they considered themselves to be isolated in a negative way at home. These buffering effects may occur only when the kinds of support available match the needs elicited by the stress a person is experiencing. For instance, the exercisers may have felt less stressed due to the availability of childcare and having a break. However, perhaps the class wouldn't have been so anxiolytic if participants found the other mothers unfriendly or the instructor and atmosphere unwelcoming.

The various modes of social support available to the exercising group of mothers in this study able to impact positively on wellbeing included [41]:

- **Esteem support:** Includes mothers talking to each other and ventilating feelings;
- **Status support:** Other mothers sharing a common bond.
- **Informational support:** Exchanging and sourcing information and ideas.
- **Instrumental support:** Provision of free childminding and parking.
- **Social companionship.**
- **Motivational support.**

A greater proportion (18 out of 21) of the mothers in the non–exercising (control) group were involved in unpaid, full–time home duties. Unpaid work includes household work (such as cleaning, washing, home maintenance), caring for family members, and volunteer community work. Almost half of the exercising mothers were involved in part– or full–time outside paid employment, and the rest in full–time home duties. The fact that a greater proportion of the mothers in the non–exercising group were involved in 'unpaid' work or perhaps feeling somehow more constrained by this feature [42], may have negatively influenced their STAI results. The non–exercising group may not have been able to relieve their anxiety as effectively the exercisers because they felt more trapped in their role on the occasions the STAI was completed. There are many reasons for lower rates of physical activity experienced by women [43]. However, it is mainly due to them reporting having less time and ironically, feeling too tired due to greater responsibilities for housework and childcare [19].

Limitations to interpretation of the findings

There are numerous limitations to interpreting the study's findings. Perhaps the largest limitation is the fact that the exercise group volunteered to exercise, rather than being randomly assigned to exercise/non–exercise. However, this may be attributed to the local community, low–cost nature of the exercise setting used for the study and its sample of convenience. The Spielberger et al. STAI purports to measure the level of state anxiety in an individual, that is, how anxious a person feels 'right now, at this moment' [27]. It is therefore situation–specific and sensitive to changes in the level of tension, nervousness, worry and anxiety present in a person over time. However, it does rely on the respondent's honesty and integrity. Respondents have to select only one answer or position on the Likert Scale out of the four possibilities available for each question, and they may not like to 'pigeon hole' or label themselves in this way.

Although the STAI can act like a temperature gauge in noting if a person is either relatively relaxed or highly stressed, it cannot provide the reasons why a person feels that way. Therefore, people can feel stressed for different reasons, but this won't be detected or included in the STAI score results. The STAI utilised in this study may have been insensitive to monitoring particular aspects or the magnitude of the respondents' stress experience. The mothers may have found certain questions inappropriate to their own individual situation, or that more applicable categories able to capture how they were feeling were absent from the inventory. Some symptoms that were experienced by the mothers in this study may not be highlighted or available on the anxiety inventory. If a symptom seems commonplace to the mother, for example feeling tired, it may also be considered as normal and therefore not defined as illness or stress. Some of the mothers who may have been 'rushed' or 'tense and jittery' on the day of the measurement may have been so used to feeling these symptoms that they believed they were part of feeling normal as a mother and their score was lower due to under-representation or desensitisation. Consequently, these symptoms may have been played down in their own anxiety inventory results. While the employment status of respondents did not change during the study, mothers considering themselves to be unemployed or those experiencing factors considered beyond their own control, may have had their high stress levels under-represented. Respondents may have also answered some questions according to what is culturally acceptable for a 'good mother' to be like.

If a mother is too 'jittery' (Question 13, STAI), 'frightened' (Question 9, STAI) or 'indecisive' (Question 14, STAI), then this may indicate weakness. Individuals with higher self-esteem may have been more truthful in their responses. State levels of anxiety are influenced by a person's trait or stable individual differences in anxiety proneness plus their interpretation of the situation they are experiencing; is it considered threatening, dangerous or worrying, for example. Those mothers with a normally low degree of trait or general personality-type level of anxiety might have recorded lower state responses to the STAI. It is of concern that STAI measurements may be biased by having high mean trait levels existing within a sample. Future research might incorporate the impact of individual levels of trait and state anxiety, motivation, self-efficacy, resilience, responses to class-specific influences such as music, and the effect of socio-economic factors on results. Due to the small numbers involved and local nature of the investigation, the findings aren't generalizable. However, they do help point to initial, quantifiable evidence suggesting that exercise classes may be of specific mental health benefit for mothers, helping inform and offer efficacy to program recommendations. All respondents taking part identified as 'well' and not experiencing illness or disease, however it was not discovered if any mother's responses at the time of completing the inventory was influenced by medication or an undisclosed mental condition. Accessing a meaningful, fulfilling and positive leisure lifestyle for one's self is an important component of health promotion and maintenance of wellness. The basic characteristics of this leisure experience may include enjoyment, relaxation, intrinsic motivation, commitment, control, challenge and freedom of choice. The aerobics classes in this study could be thought of as a leisure experience if the mothers thought of them as pleasurable, self-determined, yet enjoyable, and an area where they felt competent and in control. This would not be possible if the instructor's style was too autocratic, if they did not design the program to meet the needs of the clientele, or if the women felt driven to attend through obligation, rather than pure motivation.

Leisure experiences such as the classes, involving intrinsic motivation of a self-determining nature can result in psychological benefits. Further research is warranted to discover the particular anxiolytic mechanism within the exercise class, such as the music, the time out, the availability of childcare, or aspects of the exercise process itself [41]. It has also not been discovered within the limits of this study if the exercising mothers delegated tasks more often than the non-exercising mothers. This aspect would be worthy of greater investigation in combination with leisure lifestyles. Resistance by mothers in the form of task delegation or rationalization has to ensure that they can participate effectively in leisure activities [19,44]. Otherwise mothers may feel too bombarded with work when they return from leisure, or may feel too busy or constrained by housework to be able to afford the time off [43]. Ignoring stress symptoms, or not being able to utilize a coping strategy such as exercise can unfortunately create more distress in the long term [18]. Due to the ethic of care associated with 'good' mothering or possible guilt, some working mothers (both paid or unpaid) may be less willing to take time out to exercise for leisure [45]. Women can find it difficult to plan leisure in advance with any degree of certainty due their caring and housework responsibilities. This pressurizes them into being constantly available and on call to care for others. Some even feel unwilling to relinquish their child-minding duties in order to access leisure time for self, or feel guilty when doing so [19]. As mothers face many barriers to spend leisure time outside the home, much so-called free time for leisure is spent on activities centered around the home or with children present [13]. Health is about helping individuals develop a critical awareness of their situation and enabling them to master their environment to achieve self-determination. When the mothers take time-out to exercise, they can become 'master' of their own environment for a change, even if only for an hour at a time. This is in direct conflict with the view of Condon [46] who stated that women can never fully escape the influence of the socially constructed gender roles that "restrict their freedom of thought, will and action".

Ethical Approval

All procedures performed in the study involving human participants were in accordance with the institution's ethical standards for the National Statement on Ethical Conduct in Human Research issued by the National Health & Medical Research Council of Australia.

Conclusion

The mothers participating in the exercise program achieved significant decreases in acute anxiety compared with those mothers who did not exercise. This conclusion supports the findings of previous qualitative studies [12,19]. As a population group however, most mothers potentially miss out on these benefits [20,43]. Mothers usually have limited opportunities for leisure. This may form a barrier to them receiving the consistent mental health benefits that active leisure has to contribute [19,47]. Women have identified that physical activity is an important aspect of them maintaining wellness after the birth of a child [15,19]. A sense of freedom and control is critical for actual leisure involvement and also for mental health. The anxiolytic benefits gained from participation in exercise classes can assist mothers in managing the stresses of everyday life. Further strategies that allow for enhanced access and the continuation of care of children or relatives by others while the mother takes time out for health promoting exercise for leisure will need to be developed. Taking time out to exercise with childcare available allows a mother to experience a separate space free the usual burdens associated with her role, decrease stress, and promote wellbeing.

Informed Consent

Informed consent was obtained from all individual participants included in the study.

References

1. Donatelle RJ (2015) Health: The Basics (11th edn). Pearson, Harlow, Essex, UK.
2. Hamilton Smith E (1991) The Construction of Leisure, in BL Driver, PJ Brown, GL Peterson (Eds), Benefits of Leisure. Venture Publishing, Pennsylvania pp: 445-450 .
3. Mannell RC (2007) Leisure, Health and Well–Being. World Leis J 49: 114-128.
4. Stathopoulou G, Powers MB, Berry AC, Smits JA, Otto MW (2006) Exercise interventions for mental health: A quantitative and qualitative review. Clin Psych: Sci & Prac 13: 179-193.
5. Strohle A (2009) Physical activity, exercise, depression and anxiety disorders. J Neural Trans 116: 777.
6. Steptoe A, Cox S (1988) Acute effects of aerobic exercise on mood. Health Psych 7: 329.
7. Young KC, Machell KA, Kashdan TB, Westwater ML (2018) The cascade of positive events: Does exercise on a given day increase the frequency of additional positive events? Pers & Ind Diff 120: 299-303.
8. Zahrt OH, Crum AJ (2017) Perceived physical activity and mortality: Evidence from three nationally representative US samples. Health Psychol 36: 1017.
9. Hayosh T (2017) Engagement is serious leisure as practice for coping with the stress of daily life. World Leis J 59: 206-217.
10. Mannell RC, Salmoni AW, Martin L (2002) Older adults caring for older adults: Physically active leisure lifestyles as a coping resource for the health of caregivers. Soc & Leis 25: 397-420.
11. Elavsky S, McAuley E, Motl RW, Konopack JF, Morquez DX, et al. (2005) Physical activity enhances long–term quality of life in older adults: Efficacy, esteem, and affective influences. Ann of Behav Med 30: 138-145.
12. Currie J (2018) Radical leisure: How mothers gain well-being and control through participation in exercise classes. Common Ground Research Networks, Champaign, IL.
13. Verhoef MJ, Love EJ (1994) Women and exercise participation: The mixed blessings of motherhood. Health Care Women Int 15: 297-306.
14. Welch N, McNaughton S, Hunter W, Hume C, Crawford D (2009) Is the perception of time pressure a barrier to healthy eating and physical activity among women? Pub Health Nut 12: 888-895.
15. Currie J (2008) Conditions affecting perceived coping for new mothers: Analysis of a pilot study, Sydney, Australia. Int J Ment Health Prom 10: 34-41.
16. O'Brien W, Lloyd K, Riot C (2017) Exploring the emotional geography of the leisure time physical activity space with mothers of young children. Leis Stud 36: 220-230.
17. Luecken LJ, Suarez EC, Kuhn CM, Barefoot JC, Blumenthal JA, et al. (1997) Stress in employed women: Impact of marital status and children at home on neurohormone output and home strain. Psychosom Med 59: 352-359.
18. Shivakumar G, Brandon AR, Snell PG, Santiago–Munoz P, Johnson NL, et al. (2011) Antenatal depression: A rationale for studying exercise. Depr & Anx 28: 234-242.
19. Currie J (2004) Motherhood, stress and the exercise experience: Freedom or constraint? Leis Stud 23: 225-242.
20. Currie J (2009) Managing Motherhood: Strategies used by new mothers to maintain perceptions of wellness. Health Care Women Int 30: 653-668.
21. Currie JL (2013) Perceived Benefits of Women's Participation in Exercise Classes. Int J Sport & Soc 3: 1-7.
22. Carroll W (2017) Benefits of group exercise: My Body + Soul.
23. Veling J (2017) The Benefits of Group Fitness Classes: Active. http://www.active.com/fitness/articles/the-benefits-of-group-fitness-classes
24. Australian Bureau of Statistics (ABS) (2012) 4156.0-Sports and physical recreation: A statistical overview, Australia, 2012.
25. Choi PYL, Van Horn JD, Picker DE, Roberts HI (1993) Mood changes in women after an aerobics class: A preliminary study. Health Care for Women Int 14: 167-177.
26. Kimmel J, Connelly R (2007) Mothers' time choices: caregiving, leisure, home production, and paid work. J Hum Res 42: 643-681.
27. Spielberger CD, Gorsuch RC, Lushene RE (1983) Manual for the State-Trait Anxiety Inventory STAI (Form Y): ("Self-Evaluation Questionnaire"). Consulting Psychologists Press, Palo Alto, California.
28. Marteau TM, Bekker H (1992) The development of a six–item short–form of the Spielberger State–Trait Anxiety Inventory (STAI) Brit J Clin Psych 31: 301–306.
29. Croucher JA, Oliver E (1979) Statistics: An introduction. McGraw–Hill, Sydney.
30. Norussis MJ (1993) SPSS Inc.SPSS for Windows: Base System User's Guide. SPSS Incorporated, Chicago.
31. Anderson E, Shivakumar G (2013) Effects of Exercise and Physical Activity on Anxiety. Front Psych 4: 27.
32. Bahrke MS, Morgan WP (1978) Anxiety reduction following exercise and meditation. Cog Ther Res 2: 323-333.
33. Salmon P (2001) Effects of physical exercise on anxiety, depression and sensitivity to stress: A unifying theory. Clinical Psychology Review 21: 33-61.
34. Carmeli E (2013) Physical activity reduces stress and anxiety. Aging Sci 2: e108.
35. Johnsgard KW (1989) The exercise prescription for depression and anxiety. Plenum Press, New York.
36. Leach J (2015) Improving mental health through social support: Building positive and empowering relationships. Jessica Kingsley Publishers, London.
37. Lloyd K, Little DE (2010) Self–determination theory as a framework for understanding women's psychological well–being outcomes from leisure–time physical activity. Leis Sci 32: 369-385.
38. Oakley A (1992) Social support and motherhood: The natural history of a research project. Blackwell, Cambridge, Massachusetts.
39. Lawson JS, Callaghan A (1991) Recreating the village: The development of groups to improve social relationships among mothers of newborn infants in Australia. Aust J Pub Health 15: 64-66.
40. Leigh B, Milgrom J (2008) Risk factors for antenatal depression, postnatal depression and parenting stress. BMC Psychiatry 8: 24.
41. Cohen S, Syme SL (1985) Issues in the study and application of social support, in S Cohen & SL Syme (Eds), Social Support and Health. Academic Press, Florida pp: 3-22.
42. Wanamaker NJ, Bird GW (1990) Coping with stress in dual career marriages. Int J Sociol Fam 20: 199-211.
43. Brown WJ, Mishra G, Lee C, Bauman A (2000) Leisure time physical activity in Australian women: relationship with well being and symptoms. Res Quart Ex Sport, 71: 206-216.
44. Iso-Ahola SE, Weissinger E (1984) Leisure and well–being: Is there a connection? Parks & Rec 19: 40-44.
45. Wearing B (1990) Beyond the ideology of motherhood: Leisure as resistance. J Sociol 26: 36-58.
46. Condon EH (1992) Nursing and the caring metaphor: Gender and political influences on an ethic of care. Nursing Outlook 1: 69-84.
47. Warburton DE, Nicol CW, Bedi SS (2006) Health benefits of physical activity: The evidence. Canad Med Assoc J 174: 801-809.

7

Evaluation of the *in vitro* Human Skin Percutaneous Absorption of Progesterone in Versabase® Using the Franz Skin Finite Dose Model

August S Bassani, Daniel Banov and Maria Carvalho*

Professional Compounding Centers of America (PCCA), Houston, TX, USA

***Corresponding author:** Carvalho M, Manager of PCCA Science, Professional Compounding Centers of America (PCCA), R&DELTA, Houston, TX, USA, USA, E-mail: mcarvalho@pccarx.com

Abstract

Women may benefit from hormone replacement therapy to alleviate undesirable menopausal symptoms such as hot flashes, disruption of sleep and fatigue. Transdermal hormone replacement therapy consists in the delivery of hormones through the skin and into the blood stream, avoiding gastrointestinal drug absorption difficulties and the first pass effect. Transdermal compounded medications may be customized to meet the individual needs of women by changing the hormones used, the respective concentrations and the medicine's formulation. Two compounded medications were prepared for progesterone 50 mg/g, as follows: Progesterone in VersaBase® Cream and progesterone in VersaBase® Cream Gel. The purpose of this study is to determine the *in vitro* human skin percutaneous absorption of progesterone for both test formulations. The Franz Skin Finite Dose Model was the methodology used to evaluate the total absorption, the rate of absorption and the skin content of progesterone applied to the outer surface of *ex vivo* skin. This model has proven to be a valuable tool for the study of percutaneous absorption of topically applied drugs and to accurately predict *in vivo* permeation kinetics. The skin samples were obtained within 24 h to 48 h of death from three adult Caucasian donors and a total of 17 Franz diffusion chambers were prepared for testing. Results are presented as the mean ± standard error per parameter, for each test formulation. The rate of percutaneous absorption, presented as mean flux, was similar for the two test formulations and characterized by 2 peaks at approximately 6 hours and 28 hours after dose application, followed by a decline in flux over time. The total absorption and the skin content of progesterone were also similar: 21.6% and 21.8% of the applied doses for the test formulations 1 and 2, respectively. Although *in vitro*, these results suggest that progesterone in VersaBase® is likely to be delivered through the skin and into the general circulation for systemic effects. Practitioners may then consider transdermal progesterone as a viable route of drug administration for menopausal women.

Keywords: Skin absorption; Progesterone; Hormone replacement therapy; Menopause; Pharmacokinetics

Introduction

Progesterone is a sex hormone naturally produced by a women's body mainly to regulate the menstrual cycle. There are several conditions in which the levels of progesterone are decreased and women may choose to supplement the body's natural production of progesterone by taking hormone replacement therapy (HRT) [1]. Menopausal women, for instance, benefit from HRT to relieve the undesirable menopausal symptoms such as hot flashes, disruption of sleep and fatigue [2,3]. A drug delivery system routinely used for the administration of hormones is the transdermal drug delivery, in which hormones are delivered through the skin and into the general circulation for systemic effects, avoiding gastrointestinal drug absorption difficulties and the first pass effect.

The percutaneous absorption is non-invasive and provides extended therapy with a single topical application. Transdermal HRT may be customized to meet the individual needs of patients by changing the hormones used, the respective concentrations and the medicine's formulation [4]. Customized HRT formulations may be prepared by compounding pharmacists in accordance to the patient's specific hormone needs [1]. Progesterone administered transdermally is perceived as beneficial over conventional menopausal therapy due to the successful relief of symptoms and individuality of treatment [3,5].

The skin is a major barrier to drug absorption and thus not all drugs are suitable candidates for transdermal delivery. Skin permeation depends on the physical and chemical properties of the drugs, such as: molecular weight, solubility, partition coefficient and dissociation constant [4].

Progesterone is suitable for transdermal delivery provided that it is formulated in an adequate carrier vehicle that facilitates the percutaneous absorption. VersaBase® Cream and VersaBase® Gel, two compounding proprietary bases by Professional Compounding Centers of America (PCCA; Houston, Texas), were the carrier vehicles selected to evaluate the percutaneous absorption of progesterone. VersaBase® Cream is a topical cream base that simulates the natural moisturizing barrier of the skin through its emulsion system whereas VersaBase® Gel is a topical gel base that is resiliency to low pH and has good compatibility with polar solvents [6].

Progesterone USP micronized 50 mg/g was incorporated in VersaBase® Cream and in a mixture of VersaBase® Cream and VersaBase® Gel (95:5). The human skin percutaneous absorption of the test formulations was evaluated *in vitro* using the Franz Skin Finite Dose Model.

Methodology

The Franz Skin Finite Dose Model was the methodology selected to characterize the percutaneous absorption of progesterone into and through the skin by evaluating the total absorption, the rate of absorption and the skin content of progesterone applied to the outer surface of the skin. This model has proven to be a valuable tool for the study of percutaneous absorption and determination of the pharmacokinetics of topically applied drugs.

It consists in using *ex vivo* human trunk skin mounted on specially designed Franz diffusion chambers which provide an intimate contact between the dermal layers of the skin and the receptor solutions, parallel to the *in vivo* contact between the underlying tissues of the skin and the blood stream. Furthermore, these chambers allow the skin to be maintained at a temperature and humidity that match normal *in vivo* conditions. Because of these characteristics, the Franz Skin Finite Dose Model has proven to accurately predict *in vivo* percutaneous absorption kinetics [7].

Preparation of skin samples and Franz diffusion chambers

The percutaneous absorption of progesterone was measured using *ex vivo* human trunk skin samples, without obvious signs of disease, obtained within 24 h to 48 h of death from three adult Caucasian donors. The skin samples were dermatomed, prepared for cryopreservation, sealed in a water-impermeable plastic bag and stored at approximately -70°C until the day of the experiment.

Prior to use, the skin samples were thawed in water at approximately 37°C and rinsed in tap water to remove any adherent blood or other material from the surface. The skin samples from each donor were then cut into small sections to fit on the nominal 1.0 cm^2 chamber compartment.

The receptor solution compartment was filled to capacity with a reservoir solution of phosphate-buffered isotonic saline (PBS), pH 7.4 ± 0.1, and the chamber chimney left open to ambient laboratory conditions. All Franz diffusion chambers were mounted on a diffusion apparatus in which the bathing solution was stirred magnetically at approximately 600 RPM and the skin surface temperature was maintained at 32.0°C ± 1.0°C.

The integrity of each skin section was evaluated by testing its permeability to titrated water prior to the experiment. Following a brief equilibrium period of 30 minutes to 1 hour, $3H_2O$ (NEN, Boston, MA, sp. Act. ~0.5 µCi/mL) was layered across the top of the skin with a dropper so that the entire exposed surface was covered (approximately 200 µL to 500 µL).

After 5 minutes, the $3H_2O$ aqueous layer was removed and after 30 minutes, the receptor solution was collected and analyzed for radioactive content by liquid scintillation counting. The skin samples were considered acceptable when absorption of $3H_2O$ was less than 1.56 µL-equ/cm^2.

Preparation of test formulations

Two test formulations were prepared, in duplicate, containing the active pharmaceutical ingredient (API) Progesterone USP, PCCA Special Micronized (particle size average<10 microns) 50 mg/g and the wetting agent Pentylene Glycol 10%. The test formulation 1 was incorporated in VersaBase® Cream and the test formulation 2 was incorporated in a mixture of VersaBase® Cream and VersaBase® Gel (95:5), named below as VersaBase® Cream-Gel. The test formulations were prepared at PCCA and shipped to PRACS Institute, Ltd. (Fargo, North Dakota, USA) for *in vitro* testing.

Dosing application and diffusion

The receptor solution was replaced with a solution of phosphate-buffered isotonic saline (PBS) with 0.1% Volpo and placed bathing the inner surface of the skin sections in order to measure the rate of appearance of progesterone. The chamber chimney was removed from the diffusion cell to allow full access to the epidermal surface of the skin. Each test formulation was applied to the skin sections of the three donors, in triplicate, using a positive displacement pipette set to deliver a finite dose of 5 µL formulation/cm^2/skin section, and it was spread across the surface with the Teflon tip of the pipette.

Due to the limited number of skin sections by one donor that passed the integrity test, the test formulation 1 was replicate twice instead. As a result, there were a total of 8 Franz diffusion chambers for the test formulation 1 and 9 Franz diffusion chambers for the test formulation 2. One non-dosed chamber was included in the study to serve as blank control.

The percutaneous absorption of progesterone was evaluated over a period of 48 hours. At pre-selected times after dose application (4, 8, 12, 24, 32 and 48 hours), the receptor solution was removed entirely and replaced with new solution; an aliquot of the receptor solution was saved for posterior analytical assay testing.

After the collection of the last aliquot at 48 hours, the skin surface was washed twice with equal parts of methanol and water in order to collect unabsorbed test formulation from the surface of the skin. Subsequently, the skin section was removed from the chamber, tape stripped to remove the stratum corneum and separated into epidermis and dermis for evaluation of the skin content of progesterone.

Analytical assay testing

The quantification of progesterone from the aliquots was performed by the analytical method High Performance Liquid Chromatography with Ultraviolet Detection (HPLC/UV). A volume of 10 µL of each aliquot was injected in the HPLC/UV, which was conducted on a Hewlett-Packard 1100 Series system with an Agilent 1100 Series LC and a diode array detector at a wavelength of 245 ηm (5 ηm) to 480 ηm (50 ηm). The solvent system consisted of 85% methanol (solvent A) and 15% water (solvent B), which was run through a Phenomenex Luna C18 column (100 mm × 4.6 mm; 3 µ) at a flow rate of 0.5 µL/min, the column temperature was maintained at 40°C.

Results and Discussion

To characterize the percutaneous absorption of progesterone, the following parameters were determined for each Franz diffusion chamber: rate of absorption, total absorption, skin content (epidermis and dermis) and surface wash. The absorption of progesterone refers to the percutaneous diffusion of the drug through the skin whereas the skin content refers to the distribution of the drug into the skin. Results are presented as the mean ± standard error (SE) per parameter, for each test formulation. Statistical significance was determined using p-values obtained from a student's t-test. A p-value of <0.05 is considered statistically significant.

The rate of percutaneous absorption of progesterone was determined by dividing the amount of progesterone collected in the receptor solutions during a specified time interval, over the 48-hour study period, for all 17 Franz diffusion chambers. This is a time-averaged parameter presented as flux (μg/cm²/h) and reported at midpoint of sample collection. The mean flux profile of percutaneous absorption for progesterone in both test formulations is shown in Table 1 and Figure 1.

Mid-Time (hr)	Progesterone in VersaBase® Cream	Progesterone in VersaBase® Cream-Gel
2	0.094 ± 0.024	0.099 ± 0.015
6	0.156 ± 0.021	0.192 ± 0.020
10	0.150 ± 0.012	0.158 ± 0.017
18	0.104 ± 0.010	0.101 ± 0.017
28	0.12 ± 0.011	0.229 ± 0.127
40	0.092 ± 0.018	0.101 ± 0.032

Table 1: Mean flux (ug/cm²/hr ± SE) of percutaneous absorption of progesterone in VersaBase® Cream and in VersaBase® Cream-Gel over 48 hours (across donor summary). Time is shown as midpoint of sample collection.

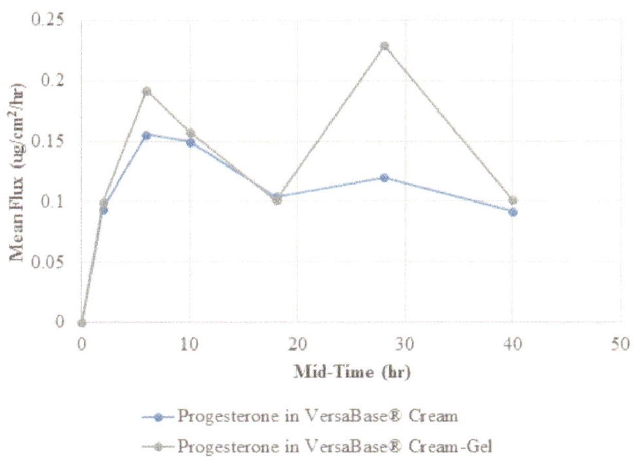

Figure 1: Mean flux profile of percutaneous absorption for progesterone in two test formulations.

The two test formulations exhibit similar penetration profiles, characterized by a rise in absorption to a peak at approximately 6 hours after dose application, followed by a slow decline in flux over time. A secondary peak is present for both formulations at approximately 28 hours after dose application, though progesterone in VersaBase® Cream-Gel exhibits a much higher peak (Figure 1), possibly due to a depot of some of the applied dose in the epidermis.

The total absorption of progesterone corresponds to the amount of progesterone (μg) collected in the receptor solutions over the 48-hour study period, for all 17 Franz diffusion chambers. The mean total absorption of progesterone in VersaBase® Cream was 5.285 μg ± 0.682, which corresponds to 2.1% of the applied dose; whereas the mean total absorption of progesterone in VersaBase® Cream-Gel was 6.470 μg ± 1.814, which corresponds to 2.6% of the applied dose, as displayed in Table 2.

Parameter	Progesterone in VersaBase® Cream (%)	Progesterone in VersaBase® Cream-Gel (%)
Total absorption	2.114 ± 0.273	2.588 ± 0.726
Epidermis	18.376 ± 10.098	18.696 ± 3.500
Dermis	1.088 ± 0.284	0.520 ± 0.095
Surface wash	67.145 ± 13.663	68.436 ± 4.036

Table 2: Total absorption, skin content (epidermis and dermis) and surface wash (mean ± SE) of progesterone in VersaBase® Cream and in VersaBase® Cream-Gel as percent of applied dose over 48 hours (across donor summary).

The two formulations were found to be statistically similar with regards to the total absorption of progesterone since the p-value obtained was 0.574 (>0.05). These results show that the bioavailability of transdermal progesterone may not be high but it is important to consider that the skin samples used referred to the torso, which is thicker and less irrigated than other body parts commonly used in transdermal therapy, such as the inner wrists. Furthermore, the test formulations were applied to 1.0 cm² skin samples, which is a very small area in comparison to the *in vivo* potential areas of exposure.

The skin content of progesterone corresponds to the amount of progesterone (μg) recovered from the epidermis and the dermis layers of the skin sections following the 48 hours post-dose application, for all 17 Franz diffusion chambers. For the progesterone in VersaBase® Cream, the mean distribution content of progesterone in the epidermis was 45.939 μg ± 25.244 (18.4%) and in the dermis was 2.721 μg ± 0.710 (1.1%).

For the progesterone in VersaBase® Cream-Gel, the mean distribution content of progesterone in the epidermis was 46.739 μg ± 8.750 (18.7%) and in the dermis was 1.301 μg ± 0.237 (0.5%) (Table 2). When combining the total absorption and the skin content of progesterone, it is concluded that 21.6% (test formulation 1) and 21.8% (test formulation 2) of the applied doses permeated the skin.

The surface wash of progesterone corresponds to the amount of progesterone (μg) recovered from the surface of the skin sections following the 48 hours post-dose application, for all 17 Franz diffusion chambers. The mean surface wash of progesterone in VersaBase® Cream was 167.861 μg ± 34.158, which corresponds to 67.1% of the applied dose; whereas the mean surface wash of progesterone in VersaBase® Cream-Gel was 171.090 μg ± 10.090, which corresponds to 90.2% of the applied dose (Table 2).

Despite the vast majority of the applied dose for both test formulations was found to be either on the epidermal layer of the skin or remaining on the surface of the skin, as demonstrated above, progesterone was able to penetrate through and into the skin. These *in vitro* results may be used in practice to predict the *in vivo* rate and extent of percutaneous absorption for progesterone. Future clinical studies are needed though to establish a correlation between the *in vitro* results and the *in vivo* conditions. However, there is already clinical evidence regarding the efficacy of multiple hormones, including progesterone 100 mg/mL, in VersaBase® applied to postmenopausal women. According to the pilot study by Glaser et al., both saliva and blood testing proved the systemic absorption of hormones following topical application of a combination cream to the mucous membranes of the labia and vagina [8]. These *in vitro* and *in vivo* studies are important evidence to support the use of transdermal progesterone in HRT.

The total recovery of progesterone, calculated as a sum of all parameters (total absorption, skin content and surface wash), was 88.7% for the test formulation 1 and 90.2% for the test formulation 2. Although the mass accountability of the applied dose was high, a total recovery of progesterone was not achieved potentially due to the limitations of the study. For instance, due to adsorption of progesterone to the Franz diffusion chamber, binding of progesterone to skin tissue proteins, concentration of progesterone in the test formulations lower than labeled, instability of progesterone or incomplete extraction of progesterone for analytical assay testing.

Albeit the widespread use of the Franz Skin Finite Dose Model, there are additional limitations that should be considered when studying the percutaneous absorption of drugs. Inadequate study protocols generate inadequate data; the experimental conditions must be carefully designed taking into account the formulation tested and the physicochemical characteristics of the drug [9]. Preferably, the study protocols should be validated to reduce data variability and to enhance reproducibility [10].

Animal skin is often employed in these studies due to the limited availability of human skin excised from cadavers or obtained from plastic surgeries; these samples do not always correlate to the human skin absorption as a result of differences in thickness, follicular structure and vascular anatomy, among others [9]. When human skin is used, variables such as the anatomical site, the skin hydration and the age of the person also affect the skin absorption [11]. Another limitation to consider is the number of the samples used to obtain significant results; it is not always possible to employ as many samples as required for statistical power. Furthermore, *in vitro* evaluations cannot fully reproduce the complexity of biological systems; when extrapolated, the study results should be considered only a prediction of the *in vivo* skin absorption [9].

Conclusions

Women may benefit from transdermal progesterone to alleviate undesirable menopausal symptoms. The Franz Skin Finite Dose Model has demonstrated that progesterone does penetrate through and into *ex vivo* skin, following topical application of both test formulations. Although *in vitro*, these results suggest that progesterone in VersaBase® is likely to be delivered through the skin and into the general circulation for systemic effects. Practitioners may then consider transdermal progesterone as a viable route of drug administration for menopausal women.

Financial Disclosure

The authors are affiliated with Professional Compounding Centers of America (PCCA), the manufacturer of VersaBase® and the sponsor of the study.

Acknowledgements

The authors would like to acknowledge Paul A Lehman (QPS, LLC, Newark, Delaware, USA; formerly PRACS Institute, Ltd., Fargo, North Dakota, USA) for conducting this study.

References

1. Newton S (2007) The history of progesterone. Int J Pharm Compd 11: 274-277.
2. Kuntz R (2005) Natural progesterone handout. Int J Pharm Compd 9: 281-282.
3. Stephenson K, Neuenschwander P, Kurdowska A, Pinson B, Price C (2008) Transdermal progesterone: Effects on menopausal symptoms and on thrombotic, anticoagulant, and inflammatory factors in postmenopausal women. Int J Pharm Compd 12: 295-304.
4. Allen L (2011) Transdermals: The skin as part of a drug delivery system. Int J Pharm Compd 15: 308-315.
5. Spark M, Dunn R, Houlahan K (2009) Women's perspective on progesterone: A qualitative study conducted in Australia. Int J Pharm Compd 13: 345-349.
6. http://www.pccarx.com/pcca-products/pcca-exclusives/bases
7. Franz TJ, Lehman PA, Raney SG (2009) Use of excised human skin to assess the bioequivalence of topical products. Skin Pharmacol Physiol 22: 276-286.
8. Glaser RL, Zava DT, Wurtzbacher D (2008) Pilot study: Absorption and efficacy of multiple hormones delivered in a single cream applied to the mucous membranes of the labia and vagina. Gynecol Obstet Invest 66: 111-118.
9. Ruela ALM, Perissinato AG, Lino S, Mudrik ME, Pereira GR (2016) Evaluation of skin absorption of drugs from topical and transdermal formulations. Braz J Pharm Sci 52: 3.
10. Ng SF, Rouse JJ, Sanderson FD, Meidan V, Eccleston GM (2010) Validation of a static franz diffusion cell system for *in vitro* permeation studies. AAPS PharmSciTech 11: 1432-1441.
11. Bartosova L, Bajgar J (2012) Transdermal drug delivery *in vitro* using diffusion cells. Curr Med Chem 19: 4671-4677.

8

Disordered Eating Attitudes and Behaviors: Gender Differences in Adolescence and Young Adulthood

Massaldjieva R Ivanova*, Desislava Bakova, Maria Semerdjieva, Bianka Torniova, Boris Tilov and Ekaterina Raikova

Department of Health Care Management, Medical University of Plovdiv, Bulgaria

***Corresponding author:** Massaldjieva RI, Associate Professor in Psychology, Department of Health Care Management, Medical University of Plovdiv, Bulgaria, E-mail: rada_ivanova@yahoo.fr

Abstract

Introduction: Dieting, obsessive weight control practices, fears of fatness, negative body image, food and weight preoccupation and other distorted attitudes and behaviors are proven risk factors with a serious potential to facilitate the development of anorexia and bulimia nervosa and the so called "atypical ED". They are not enough studied in Bulgaria. The purpose of this study was to assess the prevalence and the gender differences in disordered eating attitudes and behaviors in adolescents and young adults from Bulgaria.

Methods: We studied two age groups – 886 (80.7%) adolescents from 14 to 19 years and 212 (19.3%) young adults from 20 to 40 years, 402 male and 696 female. The respondents were Bulgarian high school students, undergraduate university students and volunteers from the general population with higher education. All participants anonymously completed the Eating attitudes and behaviors questionnaire (EABQ); Bulgarian version of the SCOFF, The Eating Disorder Diagnostic Scale (EDDS) and gave information about their age, gender, height and weight, the lowest body weight during the last three months; the frequency of measuring the body weight. We calculated three composite EDDS sub-scores.

Results: The boys and girls total and composite questionnaires scores differed significantly. There were no significant gender differences in young adults, except for EABQ total score. The mean ranks in the adolescent group showed that the female subjects reported more disordered eating behavior and risky attitudes compared with the males. In both age groups, the total SCOFF and EABQ scores and the composite scores of EDDS correlated significantly and proportionally (Spearman's correlation, $p<0.01$). The mean results from EABQ showed more distorted eating attitudes and behaviors in the groups above the SCOFF "Yes" risk threshold, the EABQ scores of males and females from the groups at risk and from the non-risk groups differed significantly ($p<0.05$).

Conclusion: More than one fifth (22.5%) of the girls examined are at risk for ED development and have significantly lower BMI values than boys. The risk in adult women and in males from both age groups is smaller. EABQ showed good discriminative capacities.

Keywords: Disordered eating attitudes; Healthy adolescents; Healthy young adults; Gender differences; Bulgaria

Introduction

Eating disorders (ED) anorexia nervosa, bulimia nervosa and binge eating disorder are one of the leading causes of disability among young women [1]. Adolescence and early adulthood are the periods of life with a highest incidence of ED and gender, together with age is a very important predictor of the risk for developing an ED [1-4]. The ED treatment is difficult and time consuming. Anorexics tend to deny the seriousness of their problems and have a high suicidal risk and mortality rate up to 15% from long-term studies [5].

Patients with bulimia nervosa are often distressed and ashamed by the loss of control over eating. They frequently experience depression and anxiety symptoms and are vulnerable to self-injuries. Many of the so-called "atypical ED" is also severe and long lasting [6]. ED and the eating behavior in men are not as frequently studied as in women. Nevertheless some authors report an increasing ED risk in males [7-11].

Restrictive or binge eating, purgative behavior, excessive exercising, limited or excessive drinking, body checking or body avoidance, physical symptoms-weight loss, menstrual cycle impairments, reduced libido, fatigue; and body image disturbances are common characteristics of ED [12].

Distorted eating attitudes and behaviors have been proven as risk factors for ED. Dieting and other obsessive weight control practices, fears of fatness and negative body image, intensive food and weight preoccupation are forms of eating impairment with a great potential to facilitate the development of anorexia and bulimia nervosa [13,14].

Disordered eating attitudes and behaviors have a significant impact on the health and their scientific study could enrich the knowledge of the ED risk. Development of effective preventive programs depends on the early determination of the groups at risk. Reliable data about the pathologic attitudes towards the body and the body weight are scarce in Bulgaria [15].

The purpose of this study was to examine the prevalence and the gender differences in disordered eating attitudes and behaviors in adolescents and young adults from Bulgaria.

Methods

The study was carried out in two big South Bulgarian cities between September 2014 and June 2016. Participants were 1098 volunteers, 402 male and 696 female, aged 14-40 years. Initially, the sample included 1232 respondents, but 136 were excluded because of the positive response to the question whether they have ever sought psychiatric help.

We recruited high school students, from four schools; undergraduate university students, from three universities and volunteers from the general population with higher education, all of Bulgarian origin and Caucasian.

The sample was divided in two age groups – 886 (80.7%) adolescents from 14 to 19 years and 212 (19.3%) young adults from 20 to 40 years.

The number of women was greater in both age groups. Demographic characteristic are presented in Table 1.

	Gender				Age		BMI			
	Males		Females							
Age Group	n	%	n	%	Mean	SD	Min	Max	Mean	SD
Adolescents	356	40.2	530	59.8	16.45	SD=1.522	12.5	33.14	20.74	2.88
Young adults	46	21.7	166	78.3	25.39	SD=5.634	15.15	38.06	22.77	4.2

Table 1: Demographic characteristics.

All participants anonymously completed three self-report scales, under the supervision of one researcher. The subjects answered as well questions about their age, gender, height and weight, the lowest body weight during the last three months; the frequency of measuring the body weight. The respondents gave verbal consent for inclusion in the study.

Study Measures

The Eating attitudes and behaviors questionnaire (EABQ)

It is a new questionnaire, developed by a multidisciplinary team to assess disordered eating attitudes and behaviors. The team included physicians, specialists in social medicine and nutrition; psychologists, general practitioners and health care professionals.

The set of items of EABQ was generated on the basis of the core features of eating disorders, included in the diagnostic criteria of DSM5 and ICD10, as well as risky eating attitudes and behaviors, discussed in the literature [16-20].

EABQ consists of 25 items (Likert scale: 1-always; 2- frequently; 3-sometimes; 4-no, never), describing eating and weight concerns and preoccupations; fears and other feelings, related to body image, self-evaluation and food consumption; dietary restraints and behaviors, linked to restrictions of food intake, eating rules, purging and other compensatory activities.

The bigger total score means less risky eating attitudes and behaviors. A pilot study was conducted with the first EABQ version. It included students and staff of the Medical University in Plovdiv and the feedback received was discussed by our project team, then the final version of the questionnaire was made.

A four-factor structure of EABQ was found by Principal Component Analysis, oblimin rotation. The content of the items, loading on each of the factors extracted permitted us to give them the following labels: "Body shape and weight concerns" 9 items, "Personal control over eating and calories intake" 6 items, Dieting 6 items" and "Preoccupation with food and binge eating" 4 items [21].

Bulgarian version of the SCOFF

SCOFF is an eating disorder screening questionnaire [22] comprising essential characteristics of anorexia and bulimia nervosa [23].

This questionnaire includes 5 questions with dichotomous "Yes" or "no" answers. They are related to "food dominance in life", "beliefs about fatness", significant weight loss in a 3-month period and worries about the control over eating and self-induced vomiting.

With SCOFF coding in our study the bigger the total scores, the smaller the risk of eating disorders.

The Eating Disorder Diagnostic Scale (EDDS)

A diagnostic scale for anorexia, bulimia and binge eating disorder in accordance with DSM-IV criteria for eating disorders.

It is a 22 items questionnaire with different response scales-Likert scale for four items; Yes-no answers for nine items; frequency reporting for seven items and two write-in responses [24].

EDDS was developed to provide diagnoses of ED. We used it mainly to assess the psychometric qualities of our EABQ questionnaire. For the statistical analyses we calculated three composite sub-scores from:

- The items, assessing eating attitudes with a Likert-scale (the bigger score means higher eating disorder risk)
- The Yes-no items, concerning eating behaviors (the bigger score means smaller eating disorder risk)
- The items, assessing eating behavior by a frequency reporting (the bigger score means bigger frequency of disordered eating behavior)

This procedure allowed us to compare the results from our questionnaire and from the SCOFF with the results from EDDS, related to disordered eating attitudes and behaviors.

We received permission to translate and to use The SCOFF (from the author) and EDDS (from The American Psychological Association).

Statistical Analysis

Our data were analyzed with the Statistical Package for Social Sciences (SPSS 16.0) statistical software. Normality of the data was assessed by skewness, kurtosis and Kolmogorov-Smirnov test. We used descriptive statistics-means and percentages to calculate age and gender group characteristics.

Comparisons between the groups were made by the Mann-Whitney U test. Spearman Rank Order coefficient was used to test for possible associations among the variables tested. By single item analysis we interpreted the SCOFF results and respondents answers to questions related to risky behaviors. Chronbach Alpha was calculated for the results from the three questionnaires. Statistical significance was set at $p<0.05$ (two-tailed analyses).

Body mass index-BMI, was calculated on the base of self-reported height and weight (BMI=weight (kg)/height (m)^2.

Results

Descriptive statistics (min, max, means and SD) for the measures, used in our study are shown in Table 2. We found significant age differences (Mann-Whitney test) for the total results from SCOFF ($p=0.003$) as well as for the composite sub-scores from EDDS items, assessing eating attitudes ($p=0.024$).

Scales	Min	Max	Mean	SD
SCOFF				
Adolescents	5	10	8.72	1.2
Young adults	6	10	9	1.07
EABQ				
Adolescents	27	98	80.94	11.38
Young adults	40	97	80.38	10.66
EDDS eating attitudes				
Adolescents	0	24	8.04	6.89
Young adults	0	21	7.66	6.05
EDDS presence of disordered eating behavior				
Adolescents	6	12	10.37	1.6
Young adults	7	12	10.72	1.27
EDDS frequency of disordered eating behavior				
Adolescents	0	77	8.7	10.74
Young adults	0	55	7.36	8.63

Table 2: Descriptive statistics (total and composite scores) for SCOFF, EABQ and EDDS.

The total SCOFF and EABQ scores and the composite scores of EDDS correlated moderately and significantly (Spearman's correlation, $p<0.01$), in both age groups (Tables 3 and 4). The positive and negative relationships found were directly proportional.

Scales	SCOFF	EABQ	EDDS (1)	EDDS (2)	EDDS (3)
SCOFF	-	r=0.600**	r=-0.523**	r=0.380**	r=-0.440**
EABQ	r=0.600**	-	r=-0.694**	r=0.368**	r=-0.526**
EDDS eating attitudes (1)	r=-0.523**	r=-0.694**	-	r=-0.271**	r=0.403**
EDDS presence of disordered eating behavior (2)	r=0.380**	r=0.368**	r=-0.271**	-	r=-0.423**
EDDS frequency of disordered eating behavior (3)	r=-0.440**	r=-0.526**	r=0.403**	r=-0.423**	-

Table 3: Spearman's correlations between the total scores from SCOFF, EABQ and EDDS in adolescents [**Correlation is significant at the 0.01 level (2-tailed)].

Scales	SCOFF	EABQ	EDDS (1)	EDDS (2)	EDDS (3)
SCOFF	-	r=0.491**	r=-0.497**	r=0.314**	r=-0.358**
EABQ	r=0.491**	-	r=-0.673**	r=0.384**	r=-0.497**
EDDS eating attitudes (1)	r=-0.497**	r=-0.673**	-	r=-0.312**	r=0.532**
EDDS presence of disordered eating behavior (2)	r=0.314**	r=0.384**	r=-0.312**	-	r=-0.461**
EDDS frequency of disordered eating behavior (3)	r=-0.358**	r=-0.497**	r=0.532**	r=-0.461**	-

Table 4: Spearman's correlations between the total scores from SCOFF, EABQ and EDDS in young adults [**Correlation is significant at the 0.01 level (2-tailed)].

The scales results of the males and females in the total sample differed significantly except for EDDS presence of disordered eating behavior.

When we analyzed the gender differences of the scales results in the age groups, we found that scores differed significantly in adolescents, but not in young adults, except for EABQ total score (Table 5).

The mean ranks in the adolescent group showed that the female subjects reported more disordered eating behavior and risky attitudes compared with the male.

Scales	M rank		U	p
	Men	Women		
SCOFF: Total sample	636.95	485.31	97680.5	P<0.001
Adolescents	524.33	374.47	59555.5	P<0.001
Young adults	110.52	105.39	3633	P=0.595
EABQ: Total sample	641.88	446.13	76953.5	P<0.001
Adolescents	516.2	347.06	48884	P<0.001
Young adults	119.93	98.37	2797	P=0.033
EDDS eating attitudes				
Total sample	395.1	628	77854	P<0.001
Adolescents	309.42	522.38	46873.5	P<0.001
Young adults	95.23	109.62	3299.5	P=0.158
EDDS presence of disordered eating behavior				
Total sample	552.07	518.8	122506	P=0.079
Adolescents	454.13	413.01	79934	P<0.05
Young adults	98.4	103.03	3393	P=0.628
EDDS frequency of disordered eating behavior				
Total sample	477.34	562.8	109831	P<0.001
Adolescents	383.65	457.08	72636	P<0.001
Young adults	90.83	108.27	3052.5	P=0.083

Table 5: Gender differences in the total and composite scores from SCOFF, EABQ and EDDS [Mann-Whitney test].

We found age differences in the answers to three SCOFF items 1,4 and 5: A significantly higher percentage of adolescent boys and girls, compared with the young adults reported self-induced vomiting (7.1% *vs.* 2.8%; χ^2=5.365, df=1, p=0.021); "thinking oneself fat, when others say being too thin"; (40.0% *vs.* 28.8%; χ^2=9.225, df=1, p=0.002); and food dominance into life (29.5% *vs.* 20.3%; χ^2=0.241, df=1, p=0.007). In the adolescents group there were significant gender differences in the SCOFF positive answers to two of the five items 2 and 4.

The prevalence of female subjects who answered "Yes" to the items related to worries about the control over eating and to feeling oneself fat was significantly higher than that of males (respectively 32.4% *vs.* 12.5%; χ^2=45.149, df=1, p<0.001 and 55.8% *vs.* 16.5%; χ^2=1.358, df=1, p<0.001).

In the group of adult the results showed a bigger prevalence in male subjects, who reported significant weight loss in a 3 month period (34.8% *vs.* 20.5%; χ2=4.087, df=1, p=0.043).

We found a higher prevalence of women, feeling themselves fat (32.5% *vs.* 15.2%; χ^2=5.268, df=1, p=0.022). The frequencies of the total scores from EABQ in the adolescent and adult gender groups are shown on Figure 1.

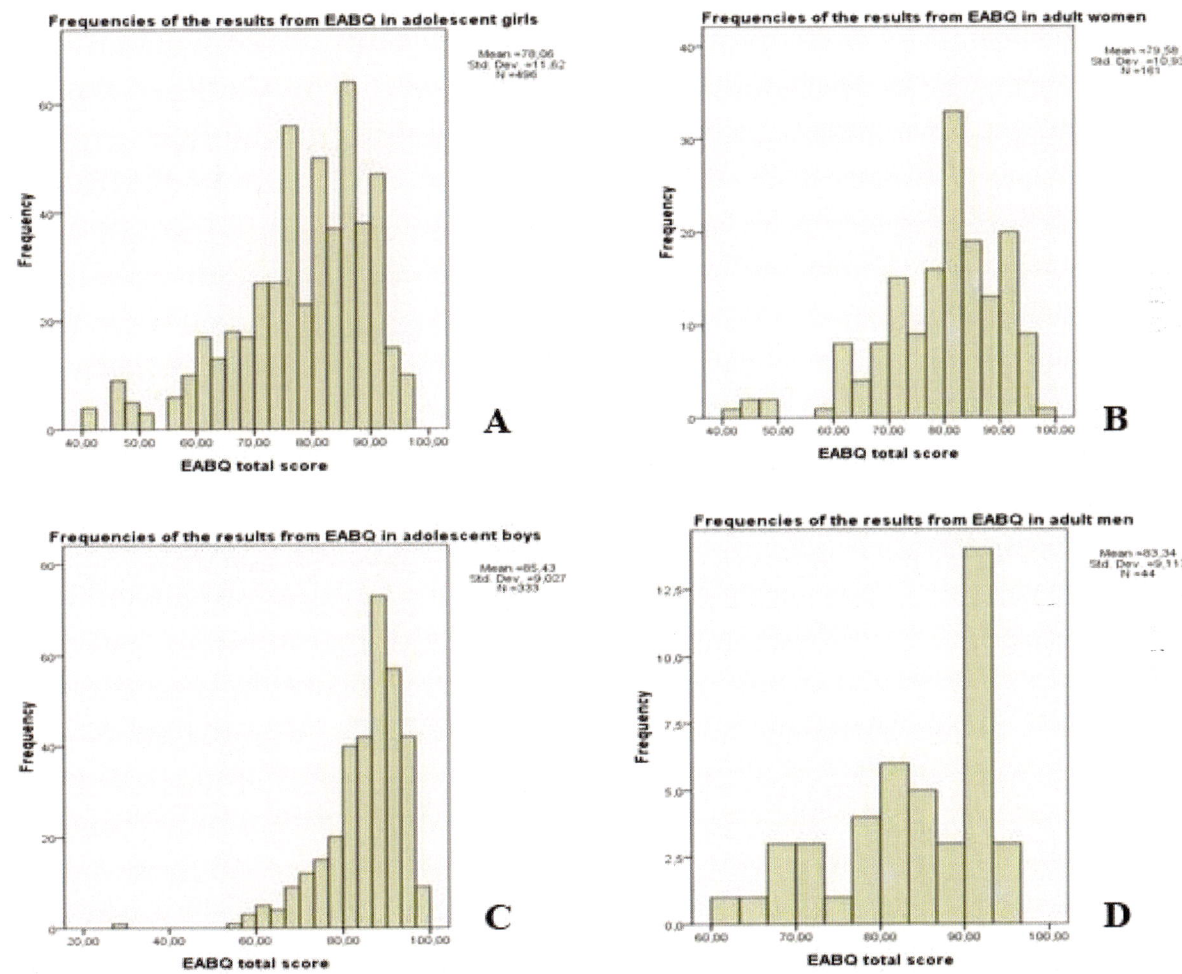

Figure 1: A. Frequencies of the results from EABQ in adolescent girls; B. Frequencies of the results from EABQ in adult women; C. Frequencies of the results from EABQ in adolescent boys; D. Frequencies of the results from EABQ in adult men [Note: EABQ - The Eating attitudes and behaviors questionnaire].

To assess the concurrent validity of EABQ we compared the mean ranks of the male and female respondents in the age groups with SCOFF "Yes" score equal to 2 and less than 2.

Two positive answers to SCOFF items are a sensitive cutoff used to classify the groups at risk for anorexia and bulimia [22,23,25].

The results are presented in Table 6. The EABQ total scores of males and females, adolescents and young adults, from the groups at risk and from the non-risk groups differed significantly (p<0.05).

The mean results from EABQ showed more distorted eating attitudes and behaviors (smaller values) in the groups above the SCOFF "Yes" risk threshold.

The small number of men in early adulthood (n=2) is a limitation of this analysis (Table 6).

Variables	SCOFF "Yes" groups	Frequency SCOFF "Yes" N	%	Mean	SD	M rank	U
Adolescent girls	SCOFF "Yes" ≤2	402	77.50%	81.49	8.61	280.09	
	SCOFF "Yes">2	116	22.50%	65.93	12.9	114.29	6444.00*
Adolescent boys	SCOFF "Yes" ≤ 2	322	90.70%	86.44	8.28	176.5	
	SCOFF "Yes">2	33	9.30%	75.32	9.85	69.44	1656.50*
Women in early adulthood	SCOFF "Yes" ≤ 2	139	87.40%	80.81	10.44	82.92	
	SCOFF "Yes">2	20	12.60%	69.83	11.09	36.56	487.00*
Men in early adulthood	SCOFF "Yes" ≤ 2	43	95.60%	84.41	8.48	22.85	
	SCOFF "Yes">2	2	4.40%	69	1.41	4.5	6.00*

Table 6: Means and mean ranks of EABQ in gender groups, based on the SCOFF "Yes" cutoff=2 [Mann-Whitney test; *P<0.05].

The results concerning the frequency of measuring the body weight in school boys and girls were as follows: 33.1% check their weight once every few months; 26.5% once a month; 19.4% once a week; 12.1% several times a week; 6.6% every day and 1.8% several times a day. In the adult group 41.5% once every few months; 25.0% once a month; 20.3% once a week; 8.0% several times a week; 3.8% every day and 1.4% several times a day. The sum of the percentages in the adolescents who frequently check their weight (more frequently than once a week) was greater than that of the adults, but there were no significant differences between the age groups χ^2=8.527, df=5, p=0.129. As to gender female respondents checked their weight more frequently than male in both age group, the difference not reaching statistical significance (χ^2=10.450, df=5, p=0.063 for adolescents and χ^2=6.838, df=5, p=0.233 for the adults) (Table 7).

Scale	BMI	M rank Men	U	M rank Women	U
SCOFF	BMI ≤ 17.5	212.93		395.95	
	BMI>17.5	195.52	3708.5	330.16	16978.5*
EABQ	BMI ≤ 17.5	247.75		457.28	
	BMI>17.5	184.1	2335.0*	308.28	10310.5*
EDDS eating attitudes	BMI ≤ 17.5	164.41		222.25	
	BMI>17.5	197.88	3364	353.11	13523.5*
EDDS presence of disordered eating behavior	BMI ≤ 17.5	197.08		331.31	
	BMI>17.5	191.72	3528.5	330.41	19.811.5
EDDS frequency of disordered eating behavior	BMI ≤ 17.5	141.68		269.92	
	BMI >17.5	195.29	2623.5*	339.13	17003.5*

Table 7: Mean ranks in disordered attitudes and behaviors in underweight males and females, compared with these with BMI>17.5 [Mann-Whitney test; *P<0.05].

Significant gender differences were found for BMI in both age groups (Mann-Whitney test, p<0.01), with smaller mean rank values (389.24 in adolescents; 99.49 in adults) for females. The mean ranks for males were 501.17 in adolescents and 129.36 in adults. A larger number of female subjects 73 (10.7%) 63 adolescents and 10 adults, than male 22 (5.6%) 21 adolescents and 1 adult, were underweight (BMI=17.5) [18]; Pearson χ^2=4,196, df=1, p=0,041. Sixty six (7.59%) school boys and girls were overweight (BMI ≥ 25) [26]. The prevalence of overweight adults was 48 (22.75%). We compared the scales mean ranks in the underweight women and in these with BMI>17.5 and the results showed significant differences (p<0.05) between them, except for EDDS presence of disordered eating behavior. There were significant differences only for EABQ and for EDDS frequency of disordered eating behavior in men with BMI under the norms and those with BMI>17.5 (Table 7).

The analysis of the BMI influence on the scales results in the age groups was not appropriate, because of the small number of underweight adult subjects. Values of the mean ranks in the groups based on BMI showed that the higher weight increases the likelihood of disordered eating attitudes and behaviors.

We analyzed the reliability of the questionnaires scores, received in our study. The internal consistency of EABQ, SCOFF and the results from the EDDS composite scores are presented in Table 8.

Scale		Cronbach's Alpha	No. of items
SCOFF	Adolescents	0.479	5
	Young adults	0.425	
EABQ	Adolescents	0.883	25
	Young adults	0.877	
EDDS	Adolescents	0.592	22
	Young adults	0.546	

Table 8: Cronbach's Alpha for EABQ, SCOFF and EDDS results.

Discussion

The adolescence is a developmental period focusing the interest of scientists as a "time of risk" [27]. It is characterized by different changes and some of them, such as the changes of self-perception, could be a basis for problematic and distorted attitudes and behaviors. Reports confirm that the adolescents are at the highest risk for ED [8,25,28].

Simultaneously, it was proven that the female gender increase the vulnerability to different forms of disordered eating [1-2,4]. Thin-ideal internalization and body dissatisfaction, largely influenced by the exposure to media images, as well as dieting and elevated body weight are risk factors with considerable effects on the onset or worsening of ED [1].

In a large sample of healthy Bulgarian adolescents and young adults, we used self-report scales with questions about respondents height and weight, the lowest body weight during the last three months; the frequency of weight measuring and risky eating attitudes and practices. The questionnaires of those subjects who have sought psychiatric help were not included in the processing of the results. Our first aim was to examine the prevalence of distorted attitudes and behaviors in these two groups representing the young urban Bulgarian population. As a second purpose of this cross-sectional study we planned to analyze the gender differences in risky for clinically significant disorders eating attitudes and practices.

The results revealed that one fifth (20.5%) of the adolescent subjects frequently checked their weight from several times a week to several times a day. This frequency was lower in the adults (13.2%), but the difference was not significant. The urge on controlling body weight was stronger in female groups of both age samples, without statistical significance of this difference. In a large female teenage sample (12-18 years) Jones et al. [29] found that 38% reported feeling overweigh and 47% felt unhappy about their weight. Our findings show lower significance of the weight, expressed in the frequency of its measurement. At the same time we found higher percentages of girls (55.8%) who reported feeling fat, than in the Jones et al. [29] sample.

In 154 young women from Greece, of normal body weight, 6.2% were measuring their body weight on a daily basis [30]. Our results are similar 6.6% of the adolescents and 3.8% of the young adults checked their weight every day. This similarity may be associated with common cultural traits of the Balkan region. The SCOFF frequencies showed significantly higher percentage of adolescents than young adults with self-induced vomiting, thoughts and fears of fatness and food dominance into life.

SCOFF "Yes" answers of female adolescents to questions about worries related to control over eating and to feeling oneself fat was significantly higher than those of males. One finding that leads towards the conclusion that disordered eating behavior is not primarily a female problem is the significantly bigger prevalence of males from the adult group, who reported significant weight loss in a 3-month period, although generally women adolescents are at higher risk of disordered eating. In the adult age group the females showed significantly higher prevalence of answers revealing fears of fatness, compared with adult men.

The analyses on the basis of BMI in our study gave significantly lower BMI values in females from both age groups; the same was true with respect to abnormally low weight (BMI=17.5). In the above cited study of Jones et al. [29] of adolescent girls, BMI was positively related with drive for thinness, body dissatisfaction, dieting, binge eating and bulimia. In our study the underweight women (with BMI=17.5) showed lower risk of disordered eating (better total and composite scores from SCOFF, EABQ and EDDS, except for EDDS presence of disordered eating behavior), i.e. the higher the weight in adolescence, the bigger the risk of eating pathology. This result probably reflects the pursuit of body thinness in healthy young women. It would be interesting to compare this finding in a clinical sample with similar demographic features [30].

We found significant proportional correlations between the scores from the three self-report scales, $p<0.01$, in the age groups, which confirms the acceptable psychometric features of our eating attitudes and behaviors questionnaire. In the same direction is the significant difference of EABQ total result between males and females from the groups with SCOFF "Yes" under and above the cutoff of 2, giving information about the individuals at risk for ED.

In the second half of the 20th century in the Western countries a belief was established, that the thin body shape, as a guaranty for beauty and success, can be obtained through dieting, exercises and other practices [31] some of them increasing the risk of ED. This phenomenon is not enough studied in Bulgaria. The analyses of our SCOFF results confirmed that the prevalence of self-induced vomiting, fears of fatness and food dominance is significantly higher in adolescence and that the adolescent girls have significantly more worries about the control over eating and feeling to be fat compared with the boys. This, together with the highest percentages of SCOFF "Yes" score in girls confirm other countries data [25,32-34] about the biggest risk of eating pathology in female adolescent. We found as well that young women are more at risk than young men.

The internal consistency of SCOFF results in our study was similar to that of other authors [25]. EABQ results showed acceptable reliability (Cronbach Alpha>0.8). The explanation of Cronbach Alpha values greater than 0.5 for the composite score of EDDS could be the small number of items in the group of items we used.

Conclusion

The main objective of our study was to collect and to analyze data about the distorted eating attitudes and behaviors in Bulgarian high school and undergraduate university students and volunteers from the general population up to 40 years.

The results showed that more than one fifth (22.5%) of the girls examined are at risk for ED development and have significantly lower BMI values than boys. The risk in adult women and in males from both age groups is smaller.

The scores of the questionnaire that we developed as a screening tool for distorted eating attitudes and behaviors (EABQ) correlated significantly with the other measures of this study (SCOFF and EDDS) and had discriminative capacity for the groups at risk for ED. Its internal consistency was assessed by Cronbach Alpha, which was greater than 0.8.

Our study results confirmed the Western countries tendency for a biggest risk of eating pathology in adolescent girls that have to be the main target group for prevention programs and practices.

Acknowledgements

This research was supported by a grant in the framework of University Research Scientist Projects of Medical University in Plovdiv, Bulgaria, 2014-2016.

References

1. Moore RH, Bulik CM (2007) Risk factors for eating disorders. Am Psychol 62: 181-198.
2. Jacobi C, Hayward C, Zwaan M, Kraemer HC, Agras WS (2004) Coming to terms with risk factors for eating disorders: Application of risk terminology and suggestions for a general taxonomy. Psychol Bull 130: 19-65.
3. O'Dea JA, Abraham S (1999) Onset of disordered eating attitudes and behaviours in early adolescence: Interplay of pubertal status, gender, weight and age. Adolescence 34: 671-679.
4. Touchette E, Henegar A, Godart NT, Pryor L, Falissard B, et al. (2011) Subclinical eating disorders and their comorbidity with mood and anxiety disorders in adolescent girls. Psychiatry Research 185: 185-192.
5. Shader M (1994) Manual of psychiatric therapeutics. Little, Brown and Co., Boston.
6. Fairburn CG, Harrison PJ (2003) Eating disorders. Lancet 361: 407-416.
7. Herzog DB, Norman DK, Gordon C, Pepose M (1984) Sexual conflict and eating disorders in 27 males. Am J Psychiatry 141: 989-990.
8. King MB (1990) Eating disorders in general practice. JR Soc Med 83: 229-232.
9. Pope HG, Katz DL, Hudson JI (1993) Anorexia nervosa and "reverse anorexia" among 108 male bodybuilders. Comprehensive Psychiatry 34: 406-409.
10. Moore RH, Silberstein LR, Rodin J (1986) Toward an understanding of risk factors for bulimia. Am Psychol 41: 246-263.
11. Thiel A, Gottfried H, Hesse FW (1993) Subclinical eating disorders in male athletes. A study of the low weight category in rowers and wrestlers. Acta Psychiatr Scand 88: 259-265.
12. Treasure J, Claudino AM, Zucker N (2010) Eating disorders. Lancet 375: 583-593.
13. Currie A, Crosland J (2009) Responding to eating disorders in sport-UK guidelines. Nutr Food Sci 39: 619-626.
14. Yannakoulia M, Matalas AL, Yiannakouris N, Papoutsakis C, Passos M, et al. (2004) Disordered eating attitudes: an emerging health problem among Mediterranean adolescents. Eat Weight Disord 9: 126-133.
15. Boyadjieva S, Steinhausen HC (1996) The eating attitudes test and the eating disorders inventory in four bulgarian clinical and nonclinical samples. Int J Eating Disorders 19: 93-98.
16. Tsai LY, Ghaziuddin M (2014) DSM-5 ASD moves forward into the past. J Autism Dev Disord 44: 321-330.
17. Bulik CM, Reba L, Riz AM, Kjennerud T (2005) Anorexia nervosa: Definition, epidemiology, and cycle of risk. Int J Eating Disorders 37: S2-S9.
18. International classification of diseases (ICD 10) (1998) National center for complex human investigation, Sofia.
19. Dahlmann B (2009) Adolescent eating disorders: Definitions, symptomatology, epidemiology and comorbidity. Child Adolesc Psychiatr Clin N Am 18: 31-47.
20. Sepulveda AR, Carrobles JA, Gandarillas AM (2008) Gender, school and academic year differences among Spanish university students at high-risk for developing an eating disorder: an epidemiologic study. BMC Public Health 8: 1.
21. Massaldjieva R, Bakova D, Semerdjieva M, Tilov B, Raikova E, et al. (2016) The hidden picture: Unhealthy eating attitudes and behaviours in a non-clinical population from Bulgaria. CBU International conference proceedings. Prague pp: 693-699.
22. Morgan JF, Reid F, Lacey JH (1999) The SCOFF questionnaire: Assessment of a new screening tool for eating disorders. BMJ 319: 1467-1468.
23. Garcia FD, Grigioni S, Chelali S, Meyrignac G, Thibaut F, et al. (2010) Validation of the French version of SCOFF questionnaire for screening of eating disorders among adults. World J Biological Psychiatry 11: 888-893.
24. Stice E, Telch CF, Rizvi SL (2000) Development and validation of the eating disorder diagnostic scale: A brief self-report measure of anorexia, bulimia, and binge-eating disorder. Psychol Assess 12: 123-131.
25. Sans P, Campos JA, Morgan JF (2007) The SCOFF-c: Psychometric properties of the Catalan version in a Spanish adolescent sample. J psychosomatic Research 64: 81-86.
26. https://www.cdc.gov/obesity/downloads/bmiforpactitioners.pdf
27. Eccles JD, Midgley C, Wigfield A, Buchanan C, Reuman D, et al. (1993) Development during adolescence: The impact of stage-environment fit on young adolescents' experiences in schools and in families. Am Psychol 48: 90-101.
28. Pastore DR, Fisher M, Friedman SB (1996) Abnormalities in weight status, eating attitudes, and eating behaviors among urban high school students. J Adolesc Health 18: 312-319.
29. Jones JM, Bennett S, Olmsted MP, Lawson ML, Rodin G (2001) Disordered eating attitudes and behaviours in teenaged girls: A school-based study. CMAJ 165: 547-552.
30. Michou M, Costarelli V (2011) Disordered eating attitudes in relation to anxiety level, self-esteem and body image in female basketball players. J Exerc Sci Fit 9: 109-115.
31. Levine M, Smolak L, Hayden H (1994) The relation of sociocultural factors to eating attitudes and behaviours among middle school girls. J Early Adolescence 14: 471-490.
32. Croll J, Sztainer D, Story M, Ireland M (2002) Prevalence and risk and protective factors related to disordered eating behaviors among adolescents: relationship to gender and ethnicity. J Adolescent Health 2: 166-175.
33. Maor NR, Sayag S, Dahan R, Hermoni D (2006) Eating attitudes among adolescents. Isr Med Assoc J8: 627-629.
34. Rosen JC, Gross J, Vara L (1987) Psychological adjustment of adolescents attempting to lose or gain weight. J Consulting Clin Psychol 55: 742-747.

"Everything Happened So Quickly" Living Through Events Immediately Before and After Initial Breast Cancer Diagnosis: An Exploratory Study of the Experiences of a Group of Women in Cape Town, South Africa

Krishnavelh Kathleen Nadasen*

Department of Anthropology and Sociology, University of the Western Cape, Bellville, South Africa

***Corresponding author:** Krishnavelh Kathleen Nadasen, Lecturer, University of the Western Cape, Robert Sobukwe Rd, Bellville, Cape Town, 7535, South Africa, E-mail: knadasen@uwc.ac.za

Abstract

This article provides information on an aspect of the author's research on colored women's experiences of breast cancer and deals specifically with events immediately before and after the initial diagnosis. The experiences of this group of South African women have remained largely undocumented. Individual in-depth interviews were conducted with 30 colored women. Qualitative data were collected and analyzed using thematic content analysis. The main themes that emerged relate to the discovery of the lump, reaction time, response to diagnosis, the question of whether a lumpectomy or a mastectomy should be conducted, counseling and family reactions. The findings show, inter alia, that these women are not accorded sufficient time to deal with the magnitude of the diagnosis and that access to appropriate counseling is insufficient. This study has implications for health professionals and for women in general and suggests further areas of investigation within the field of breast cancer research.

Keywords: Breast cancer; Colored women; Health; Mastectomy

Introduction

The World Health Organization [1] reported that breast cancer continues to remain a common and fatal disease affecting more than 1.2 million women each year around the world. Furthermore, 58% of deaths caused by breast cancer occur in the developing countries [1].

The Cancer Association of South Africa [2] notes that breast cancer is the most prevalent type of cancer among South African women and the lifetime risk of developing breast cancer is 1:33 and this figure is increasing steadily each year. The seriousness of this disease is clearly evident when compared to the prevalence of other types of cancer found among women. In the case of cervical cancer, the lifetime risk for South African women is one in 42 and for uterine cancer it is one in 160 [2]. The prevalence of colorectal cancer is one in 182 South African women and for esophageal cancer it is one in 239 [2].

According to CANSA [2], 6224 cases of breast cancer were diagnosed nationally in South Africa in 2009 with colored women having a one in 22 lifetime risk of developing this disease. It is reported that in the Western Cape alone, 1500 cases of breast cancer are diagnosed annually but, because the cancer registry is voluntary, the cases are underreported and the actual figures are not known [3].

The majority of South Africans are black/African (80.2%) while the colored community is a minority group nationally (8.8%); however, the colored community dominates in the Western Cape (54%), with women making up more than half of this population group [4].

This group is largely working class but is affected by high levels of unemployment. The areas in which these women reside are predominantly mono-racial and are also plagued by high levels of community violence, gang activity [5], drug and alcohol abuse and economic marginalization [6].

Relatively little is known about the experiences of colored women with breast cancer in the Western Cape and it appears that their specific experiences have not been directly documented before. The research presented here is part of a larger exploratory study which examines colored women's experiences of breast cancer. The intention of the study was to gather preliminary data in order to supplement gaps in the literature on the experiences of this particular group of breast cancer survivors.

A review of the literature reveals that there has been a proliferation of studies on breast cancer in recent years and most have been done from either a psychosocial or clinical perspective or in terms of body image, identity and sexuality [7-12]. There has also been an increase in studies on survivorship, coping strategies and partner relationships [13-17].

It appears that these studies were conducted after the women underwent surgery and very little has been written about women's lived experiences before and after the initial diagnosis.

Where studies have included some of these experiences, they were peripheral to the main research question. The intention of this article is therefore to document colored women's concerns and reactions just before and after the initial diagnosis. These existential events, according to Landmark and Wahl [18], are also fundamental in recuperation and survival.

Methods

A snowball sampling method was utilized to recruit women for this study [19]. The initial participant, who is from the designated population group, was recruited during a breast awareness campaign in Cape Town, South Africa. Using the snowball method, 29 women who are survivors of breast cancer were subsequently contacted and interviewed. The inclusion criteria for the present study were that the woman be diagnosed with breast cancer within the previous five years and that she is from the designated population group.

The timeline for diagnosis of five years ensures a more vivid recollection of the individual's experiences. Informed consent was obtained from all the participants. The University's Ethics Committee approved the consent forms. Participation was voluntary and no monetary compensation was exchanged for participation. Twenty five of the 30 interviews took place in the homes of the participants while the others were conducted at a place convenient to the respondent.

The grounded theory method, which uses observation and data, guided this study. Besides race, other demographic information was obtained from the participants and a 60-minute face-to-face interview was conducted with each woman. The interview schedule consisted of open-ended questions relating to the participants' initial fears, concerns and reactions. The interviews were audio-recorded and transcribed verbatim. Fictitious names were used to guarantee confidentiality and anonymity. The transcripts were analyzed using the inductive approach [20] and themes that emerged during the interviews were identified. An open coding process was utilized to identify varying and recurring sections in the transcripts [21].

The codes were then grouped into six themes and thematic content analysis was applied to the data [20]. The themes that emerged are: the discovery of the lump, the response to diagnosis, the reaction time, the decision between a lumpectomy and a mastectomy, counseling, and informing the family and the family's reaction. Each theme is discussed later in this article under the section on the research findings.

The qualitative nature of this study allowed the participants' own experiences to be prioritized and for their voices to be heard and included in the findings and discussion [22]. The value of this methodology is also noted by the breast cancer researcher, [23] who states that few studies directly quote or include women's perspectives and experiences in relation to their illness.

In addition, Kasper [24] emphasized the imperative to understand breast cancer from the standpoint of women themselves. For Landmark and Wahl [18], it is important to capture the wholeness of women's experiences while Frank's [25] view is that health narratives provide a voice for people living with ill health and allows meaningful insight into their existential experiences with their illness. The current study therefore uses the participant's voices extensively in an attempt to capture and communicate their experiences.

Characteristics of the Participants

Thirty (30) colored women participated in this study and they ranged in age from 17 to 81 years old. The mean age (M) is 49 years and the standard deviation (SD) is 13.1 years. Table 1 below provides selected demographic and medical information of the participants. The women are from varying socioeconomic backgrounds with 21% having had tertiary training, 66% having completed high school and 13% have a primary school level of education. Less than half of the respondents (40%) are in full-time employment.

The majority (54%) of the women are married, 13% are divorced, 13% are single and 20% are widowed. While 57% of the respondents reported a family history of breast cancer, only 21% reported undergoing regular mammograms. Prior to diagnosis, the majority (63%) of the women had not been for a mammogram while 16% were considered too young to go through the procedure.

Participants (N=30)	
Age range	17-81 years of age (Mean: 49; SD: 13.1)
Marital status	
Married	54%
Divorced	13%
Widowed	20%
Single	13%
Education	
Primary school	13%
High school	66%
Tertiary	21%
Employment status	
Full-time	40%
Self-employed	14%
Unemployed	30%
Pensioners	16%
Family history of breast cancer	57%
Mammogram prior to diagnosis	
Regular	21%
Never underwent	63%
Too young	16%
Surgery and treatment received	
Lumpectomy	26%
Mastectomy	74%
Chemotherapy/radiation	100%

Table 1: Demographics and medical history of participants.

Findings

The six themes which relate to the lived experiences of these women are discussed in the sections to follow:

Discovery of the lump

The women spoke at length about the detection of the lump and the action they took thereafter. More than half of the participants (63%) had not had regular mammograms before the appearance of the lump. Therefore, it is not surprising that the majority of the women discovered or felt the lump themselves, that is, by means of self - detection. Most commonly, the women felt the lump while they were in the shower or dressing or while lying in bed. Some individuals noticed a lump as small as a "frozen pea" which they were not concerned about initially, however, they now feel that this was a big mistake. One participant stated that she had had a lump for about a year. Initially it was small and gave no problems but later it increased in size to that of an egg and it was only at that point that she decided to consult a doctor. In order to make sure that there is in fact a lump in the breast, women often asked their family members or friends to feel the breast and confirm its presence.

One participant, who went for regular mammogram screening, thought she would not develop breast cancer because the mammogram would detect any abnormality before it could become a problem. However, she noticed a lump and, after the diagnosis, it was found that the lump was malignant. This person stated "I followed the rules and yet it still happened".

The younger women who had pain in their breasts told their mothers. The mothers initially thought that the pain was part of a young woman's normal development. Only when the pain became unbearable and, as one individual explained, the lump was "as hard as a rock and stretching my skin, that I was taken to the doctor" (Shireen 17). Laura (27) stated that she had had the lump for ten years before her breast began to swell and her "nipples were oozing". She thought she was pregnant and went to the local clinic.

The women who do regular self-examinations were surprised that the lumps appeared so suddenly. For example, Mary (60) stated that she had always had lumpy beasts and was advised by the doctor not to be concerned. But, one lump she detected was "different, harder" although there was "no pain." Mary stated that this was "a wake-up call" for her.

Janice (46) mentioned that she felt the lump while she was showering. "It was a strange lump, it was never there before and suddenly I spot something unusual. There was no pain, no infection, no oozing, just a big round lump". Kathy (47) stated "One day you feel nothing and the next day there is this lump in your breast. It appears like a thief in the night".

Two of the participants initially felt that they could have hurt themselves in physical activity. Judy (48) stated that the lump felt like a ball and she thought she had strained herself with her housekeeping chores. Maxie (37) thought she had "pulled a muscle" and she said "there was no pain just a bit of discomfort". Both of these women felt there was no need to go to the doctor immediately.

For some of the participants the lumps were discovered by accident. Sue (50) stated that she had unintentionally placed her hand over her breast while lying in bed. She felt an unusual small lump and she had that diagnosed by a doctor. Pat (81) said that her diagnosis was "an act of God as I did not feel a lump, I did not have a lump. I went to the hospital for a bone scan but the machines were faulty. I went for a mammogram instead and a small lump was discovered by the nipple". Joy (68) stated that she did not really know how to examine her breasts and she discovered the lump by accident when she was putting on her bra.

Participants with a family history of breast cancer were more vigilant and regularly examined themselves, but some had doubts about the process. Jane (32), whose mother died of breast cancer, endeavored to be aware of her health in this regard and therefore examined herself after each menses. She mentioned, "After the last cycle the right breast didn't feel normal. There was a bump in the right one and nothing in the left. This made me suspicious. Knowing full well what my mother went through, I consulted the doctor immediately. I thought I was being overcautious".

Another participant, Nancy (48), stated that she discovered a lump in her breast when she was 36 years old. She consulted the doctor who prescribed anti-inflammatory medication and she subsequently did not feel the lump nor was there any pain. A mammogram was never recommended. Nancy was concerned because her grandmother had breast cancer. She was sent for a mammogram when she was 46 and she was diagnosed with breast cancer. Nancy wonders if she could have been spared the experience if the mammogram was done earlier.

One participant was pregnant when she discovered fluid being emitted from the nipple. She stated, "I thought it was part of the pregnancy. The liquid contained traces of blood. I could not go for a mammogram because the appointment coincided with the day I gave birth to my baby. I went a month later and three lumps were discovered at the tip of the nipple" (Sybil 34).

Reaction time

There seems to be no uniformity in the way the participants reacted when they discovered an irregularity in their breast.

According to Evelyn (67), she had the lump for several months but, because it was small and gave no problems at first, she did not react immediately. Mary (54) stated, "When I felt the lump there was no urgency. It was a week after I discovered the lump that I went to the day hospital". For Judy (48) "The lump was not a gradual thing. One day it was there. I carried it for two long weeks before I decided to see the doctor".

Maxi (35) was not concerned at first but, upon examination at the clinic, the nursing sister advised her to consult her doctor immediately. She said:

I had to take my baby for a check-up and casually asked the doctor to examine my breasts. He advised me to go for a mammogram. It was only two weeks later that I actually went for the mammogram. Everything was more important than me going for the x-rays. My needs were secondary.

Laura (27) stated "My breasts were swollen and I thought I was pregnant then. I had oozing nipples. I went to hospital, was given medication but it started again a few weeks later. I knew the lump was in my breast since I was 16. I never took note of it. At the hospital, they said it was not dangerous. I felt sick and was coughing. I thought it was TB. I knew something was wrong but did not know what it was. The swelling continued and I decided that something is definitely wrong. I went to the local clinic and that was when arrangements were made for the mammogram".

Noelle (57) explained that it took her "about two weeks eventually when I finally went to the clinic. I definitely did not think it was too serious and breast cancer did not even cross my mind".

According to Linda (46) "In 2012, I felt the lump and went to a specialist. A biopsy was done and it came out clean. Nevertheless the specialist advised me to have it removed. I did not take notice of his advice. I thought why remove it if there is no cancer or pain. So I just left it because we are women and in many situations we do not consider ourselves as the most important person in our lives, so I just put it aside. Whenever I went to my *General practitioner,* I would tell him to examine my breast. He never advised me to have a mammogram. He said if it is not painful then it's ok. It was only in May 2013 that I was finally diagnosed with breast cancer".

On the other hand, Wendy (48) mentioned that she was actually reprimanded by the radiologist who said, "Why do you women wait so long before coming for a mammogram?"

The researcher noted that those with a family history of breast cancer reacted almost immediately and went for the necessary tests.

Response to diagnosis

There were varied reactions to being diagnosed with breast cancer. Some of the participants thought this was the end for them. Evelyn (67) stated, "Yes, when I was diagnosed I did feel as though this was the end, that I will not live long. I sobbed".

Joy (68) said "I was shocked. It came as a blow to me, like cold water in your face. I did not expect that. The news did not sink in at that time, it is only when I got home did I *realize* that it was cancer. For me, cancer is death. I thought I was going to die. I became emotional. I felt sorry for myself and I did not know what is goin*g to happen. I was living alone*".

Nancy (48) was concerned about how she would handle "the fear ... death... I was probably in denial but more scared. I thought it would have spread to the other organs. I spent four days in my room. I did not want to see or talk to anyone because I felt I had to work through this". Sue (50) associated cancer with death and said, "You always hear about the one that died, not the one that survived."

A few of the participants were in a state of confusion and did not want to believe the diagnosis. Betty (48) explained, "At first I thought this can't be, it is not real. I was in denial" Shireen (17) stated, "At the news I did not really feel anything. No shock or anything. I did not know what cancer was at that time" Janice (46), on the other hand, hoped that the diagnosis was incorrect. She said, "Initially, deep down I expected them to tell me that they are wrong. It is just something that needs to come out or it's just a non-cancerous lump. It happened so fast, you really need to absorb it".

Some of the participants were more pragmatic in their reaction. Mary (54) said, "I was not concerned about myself. I was worried about the children. Each in their own stage in their life and had different concerns about losing a mother. After losing a father, this was like a wake-up call for them".

Sue (50) stated that she was anxious when she heard the news but her concerns were more for her children. She said, "I was scared and worried about my family. Perhaps it is a women's thing. You have your own little fears but you worry about how they feel, how will they cope".

For Sybil (34) the news did not register immediately because she had just given birth. She stated, "I felt very confused but I had to confront and deal with this thing. I felt get it done and over with because my children needed me".

Maxi (35) noted that she was not anxious. For her "something happened, get it over and done and move on... that was always my attitude".

Jane (32) said, "Things go through your mind. If I am sick, who is going to care for my child? I thought, rather leave that, I must think of the positive. I am not going to let him grow up without a mother. He is going to see me. He is going to know me". The views expressed above are similar to the findings of Gonzalez and Davis [26] who noted that the women they interviewed were also fearful and anxious about not being able to care for their children.

A few of the women were not ready for such devastating news. Bernie (60) said, "When I received the results I was not prepared. I felt nothing, I can't explain. I was alone. My family asked if they could go with me. I said no, thinking there is nothing wrong".

Judy (48) explained, "I was with my husband when the cancer was confirmed. I was devastated. I thought, why me*?* Why did God do this to me?"

Participants with a family history of breast cancer were more accepting of the diagnosis. Laura (27) said, "I was not actually scared because breast cancer is in my family. My aunt has breast cancer and she is still living after being diagnosed five years ago".

Doreen (46) felt positive, as she explained "No, I wasn't really scared because I said I am going to pass through this because if others can then I can. My grandmother had breast cancer and she died of a heart attack at 87. I thought of positive things. I did not think that I am going to die."

Wendy (60) did not associate breast cancer with death even though she had lost a sister through breast cancer. She said, "Reading about breast cancer put my mind at ease because the information stated that breast cancer could be beaten".

Mastectomy or lumpectomy?

The majority of the women were asked to decide whether they wanted a mastectomy or a lumpectomy and 74% of the women had a mastectomy and 26% had a lumpectomy. In three instances the women were told that the cancer was at an advanced stage and the only option was a mastectomy.

Sybil (34) stated, "The doctors said they had to work fast as the cancer was in stage 2 and it was in the milk ducts. If they were to remove half then the cancer may still be behind that. I was fine with their decision".

Janice (46) said, "The doctor mentioned that the cancer was at stage 3 and because the lump inside was so huge, it was the size of a tennis ball, the entire breast had to be removed".

Some of the participants did not have the mastectomy immediately.

Enid (67) stated, "At the hospital I had to undergo several tests to make sure that the cancer had not spread. Thank goodness the cancer was only in the breast. I had to first go on chemotherapy to shrink the lump. I was on chemo for seven months and only after that I had the mastectomy".

In some instances the choice between a mastectomy and a lumpectomy was a difficult one and a few of the women had to consult with significant others before making the final decision. Betty (48) explained that the doctor wanted to operate almost immediately but she wanted to go home and speak to her family before making the final decision. She stated, "They did not really know what to say as this was the first in the family. My sister who works at the hospital advised that it would be better to remove the breast. I had to decide what was best for me. I went back and had the mastectomy". Judy (48) was accompanied by her husband when she consulted with the surgeon. She stated,

"The more I said that I wanted a lumpectomy, the more my husband said cut it off...cut it off! Well I was glad in the end. My husband took the final decision. He told me later that a colleague of his had a lumpectomy and after a while she had to have the breast removed. He wanted to prevent this from happening to me. I was happy about the decision ".

On the other hand, Berny (60) made a personal decision and opted for a mastectomy because the cancer was at stage 2. Her husband questioned her decision and enquired whether that was the only available option. She explained, "I told my husband that it is my body and I do not want the cancer to spread so I am going for the mastectomy. I was happy with my decision".

One participant made her decision based on information she found on the Internet. Through her search Rita (42) came to the decision that, even if the lump was removed, the chance of the cancer recurring is never completely ruled out. Rita stated, "I did not want to go through a second operation, so I decided to remove everything".

Another participant stated that because she had medical insurance she opted for a lumpectomy. With medical insurance she was able to undergo the other treatments, i.e., chemotherapy and radiation, as well as taking expensive medication. It is interesting to note that this participant later mentioned, "If I must have it over again I would rather have a mastectomy because I have lots of swelling due to the radiation and I had another operation to have the nodes removed" (Doreen, 46). Doreen was also fearful of the fact that the cancer may recur.

Shireen (17) described her experience as follows: "The doctors decided that a lumpectomy was best for me. I did not really care. All I wanted at that point was for the lump and the pain to be removed. The pain was so severe the painkillers did not help".

Some of the women faced another dilemma. After receiving chemotherapy they were notified that the lump was completely destroyed but they still had to have a mastectomy. Nancy (48) stated, "The doctor said, based on what was found initially and to make doubly sure that there is no cancer, it has to be a mastectomy. Considering all the facts I wanted the mastectomy".

Two of the participants had a bi-lateral mastectomy. Maxi (35) initially had a lumpectomy but, a few years later, it was discovered that there was "a tumour in the operated breast and fresh one in the other. After having chemo to shrink the tumours both breasts were removed." While Maxi did not have a choice, Sue (50), on the other hand, had a mastectomy and, two years later, wanted to have a reconstruction. She decided to have the remaining breast removed and, according to her, "It was a major decision, I thought I was crazy. I had another mastectomy and the surgeon constructed both. I am happy with my decision *today*" In their study, Grimes and Hou [27] also noted that their participants wanted both breasts removed even though it was not necessary. But, unlike Sue whose decision was based on body image, Grimes and Hou indicate that the participants in their study took the decision because they were afraid of a recurrence of the cancer. Both Maxi and Sue said that they were satisfied with their decision, albeit for different reasons.

Counseling

The participants revealed that they did not receive any professional counselling after being diagnosed. The majority stated that they did not have sufficient knowledge about the cancer and what was going to happen. The women said that some sort of professional counselling would have been preferable after the diagnosis because they were fearful and anxious about the events that were to follow. Shireen (17) stated, "If I had more information it would have been helpful and would have put me at ease to a certain extent." Two of the women, Judy (48) and Janice (46), saw social workers. However, Judy explained "I thought I am really going to die. The doctor sent me to the social worker to discuss all my problems. I told her I cannot do this on my own. Although my family is there they cannot get into your head. The social worker explained the anxiety attacks that I was experiencing and she put me on some drugs. She advised that I must just talk and the person listening to me must put themselves in my shoes. I did not know what to do and the advice did not help".

For Janice the events around her diagnosis happened very quickly. The day she obtained her results she was also sent to the social worker. She said "The social worker mentioned that they are there for the cancer patients. Anytime if there are questions or if you need to chat, they were there to help. But this did not help me at all".

Informing the family and the family's reaction

After receiving confirmation of the cancer the women had to face the arduous task of informing their families. Hilton, Emslie, Hunt, Chapple and Ziebland [28] note that informing one's family of the cancer appears to be the most difficult part of the process. According to Evelyn (67), "My family was upset but they said it was for my own good. They all accept now, even my husband. He was not with me when I received the news". Betty (48), who is single, stated, "My family encouraged me to be positive". Doreen (46) mentioned, "My husband was more upset he just said he couldn't take it". Because Shireen (17) was still young she felt that it was very traumatic for her parents. They lost a relative through cancer and Shireen said, "They knew what cancer was all about and they were afraid that I was going to go the same way". Mary (54), who is a widow, found it difficult to inform her children. She stated:

Because of my concern for my children, I thought, I must rise above this. They must not really see my fear. My eldest son was in prison. He was the last to know because I had to get permission to visit him. I found it extremely difficult to tell my daughter so I had to ask a friend to come and share this with her. My middle son had a girlfriend who was a nurse so she knew what it entailed and she tried to reassure them. But my children reacted badly, especially my daughter who was very fearful and very concerned. She thought she was going to lose me. Being 14 years old I just reassured her. I had to be strong for her.

Maxi (35) stated: The day I received the news I phoned my husband and told him that it was cancer and that my breasts will have to be removed. I shed a few tears. He did not cry. He said this is going to be a long journey for us. Both of us agreed that our sons needed to know. I wanted to assure them it was not a death sentence because I was positive I was not going to die. When we spoke to them that evening my eldest son wanted to know if I was going to die, that is like a given. I said I believe I am not going to die because I believe in a higher power. They were at peace but I cannot say how they were feeling or if there were unasked questions for them but they were scared.

Sue (50) found a measure of relief because her husband was with her when she received the news but she stated, "Telling the children was not easy. They did not ask anything, they were nervous. The death issue was scary". Pat (81) said that her children were very shocked when they found out that she had to deal with this at this point in her life as she had always been strong and healthy. Laura (27) explained her situation at the time of diagnosis as follows:

I was alone when I got the news. My family was not actually with me throughout this whole thing. Just before I went for the operation, I met this wonderful guy. He is still with me now. He is the one that made everything so much easier and he is still there for me. If you got someone like that in your life then it is important... You must have someone to care so much about you... otherwise you won't be able to do it.

Rita (42) stated that her daughter thought it was a "death sentence. She was very afraid". Janice (46) said, When I came home-I have a disabled daughter, she does not communicate as normal but she understands us – as I walked in, she looked at my face and I broke down. She wanted to know why I was crying. I also did not want to hide it from her. I was very open. When I told her she was just devastated... She understands everything and she felt she was going to lose her mum. I do most of the things for her. She is in a wheelchair. My eldest daughter was not in. My husband is not very emotional and not supportive. That night he went to tell my daughter. They had a few words in the room and he broke down at that point. I think that was the only part of the journey that he cried a bit.

Jane (32), whose mother died of breast cancer, stated, I came home and had to explain to my dad and brother. My dad has been through this with my mother. It is not news that you want to give to your family. My dad did not expect it. I did not tell him why I went to the doctor in the first place... just wanted to do it on my own. I thought it was a precaution. My dad and brother were shocked. He said we will pray that it is a positive outcome and that we must be strong. He assured me. It's not news you want to bring to your father... The thing that happened to his wife is happening to his daughter. I told my fiancé the same night. He was not happy and was very quiet. The reactions are all different. He did not want anything to happen to me.... don't want to lose me. He said all those things and that he will stand by me... he did not run away.

Nancy (48) described her experiences when telling her family as follows, I am a divorcee and I depend a lot on my brother and his wife. When I told them they broke-down, they sobbed. I asked them to support me and that they have to be strong for me, especially my brother. My daughter just walked out of the room. She did not want to hear anything. Because I breast fed her for about three years... people say you don't get breast cancer if you have breast fed... that's a lot of crap. She walked out of the room. I was unable to console her.

According to Rene (46), her husband was with her all the time but did not say anything. She said, Men do not show emotions but it was very emotional for me and our children. They knew what was happening. We sat together and explained everything. My daughter was very emotional. I think everyone was emotional but she showed it more being a woman. I feared more for her than for me because she is a woman, she could be the next victim here.

Discussion

During the interviews the participants spoke at length about their experiences. Each part of their journey has its own significance and elicited different emotions and related to different issues.

The majority of the women in this study discovered the lump themselves. This finding correlates with a previous study which reported that "a vast majority of breast cancers are found by women themselves" [29]. Thind, Diamant, Hoq and Maly [30] also note that it is more common for women to detect their breast cancer themselves and this is especially common among women who have no medical insurance or who do not have regular access to health care prior to diagnosis. Some of the women discovered the lump accidentally while others discovered it through regular self-examination.

Once a lump is detected, most of the women go through a period of denial, anxiety and fear and do not really know what to do or they hope that the lump will disappear. Because no pain was experienced in majority of the cases, the respondents felt that there was no urgency in having the lump tested. It is interesting to note that some of the participants ask family members or close friends to confirm what they had initially felt in the breast. None of the women mentioned the role their husbands played in discovering the lump. It seems that, initially, some of the women avoided involving their husbands and went for the medical examination alone. This is in contrast to a WHO [31] report which describes the experience of a housewife from New Delhi who found a lump in her breast and wanted to see a doctor about it. She told her husband immediately and he accompanied her to the hospital. A possible explanation could be socio-cultural differences but a few of the women in this study also mentioned that their husbands had their own issues like unemployment and alcoholism. Perhaps further research could shed more light on this.

In line with women's gendered nurturing role, some felt that their health was not a priority and that the needs of their families took precedence and they thus delayed a medical examination. While it is undeniable that the needs of the family are important, it nevertheless seems likely that the underlying factor for stalling was fear and anxiety that the lump could be cancerous. These women therefore find themselves in a precarious position in that they are afraid of what a medical examination will reveal and they therefore avoid the examination which exacerbates their anxiety and/or the spread of the cancer. In retrospect, some of the participants stated that once a lump is detected it is better to have it examined as quickly as possible. For example, Shireen (32) stated:

If you are feeling a lump, it is better to go and find out what it is than sitting and taking all the medications that your friends tell you to take. Rather go and find out than walking around worrying about it. The anxiety of worrying about it can bring the cancer on. So it is better to have yourself checked than living with this fear.

Myrick [32] also confirms that many women are reluctant to have a mammogram because they fear the results. In some senses, these women were also afraid of the Foucauldian clinical gaze and initially felt that the body and especially the breasts are "private". The majority of the women therefore did not go for an immediate examination. Those with a family history of breast cancer reacted immediately and had the necessary tests done. The older women waited after the discovery of the lump for a few months, others for a week or two, before seeking medical attention. Some of the participants felt that other things were more important and needed immediate attention. Some of the women felt that, because the lump was relatively small and there was no pain, there was no reason to take immediate action.

A few of the participants also admitted that the possibility that the lump could be cancerous never crossed their minds. The younger women seemed to have experienced the lump or swelling of the breast for much longer periods and they depended on their mothers for guidance but no immediate action was taken. From the narratives of the participants the belief that if there is no pain then there is no cancer is evident. One woman reported that her GP never advised her to have a mammogram and he reiterated that if there was no pain then there was no need to be concerned. A year later she was diagnosed with breast cancer. In one particular instance, the participant was reprimanded by the radiologist for not being vigilant and for waiting so long before having a mammogram.

In instances where the women had been for a check-up and/or a biopsy and the results were negative for cancer, or when some of the participants were told that a mammogram was not necessary, the women trusted these results and advice. They were of the view that no further steps were necessary or that there was no urgency to have the lump tested again. These participants stressed the need to have a second and even a third opinion, especially in cases where there is a family history of breast cancer. It seems that the advice "no pain no cancer" is iatrogenic and misleading because most of these women reported no pain and yet were diagnosed with breast cancer. According to the biomedical perspective of health, patients put their trust in the doctors and expect the best advice from them and, for some women, when the doctor's advice did not live up to expectations a sense of doubt and anger developed.

Nancy (48) stated, "2012, 27 March was the worst day of my life. I was told I had breast cancer". According to Sue (50), "Waiting for the results was a traumatic experience for me". The initial reactions to the diagnosis are shock, anxiety, disbelief, numbness, denial, confusion and some respondents hoped that the diagnosis was incorrect. Upon hearing the words "breast cancer" some of the respondents immediately thought about death while others thought about their children. Some of the women also expressed relief that the cancer was only in the breast and had not spread to other organs. It is interesting to note that, at this point, none of the women expressed any concern for their spouses. Their immediate thoughts were for themselves and/or their children. Women with a family history of breast cancer were not as devastated as the other women because they were more prepared and aware that one could survive breast cancer. Prior knowledge about breast cancer also had a mediating effect in that some women read that breast cancer could be beaten and it is not necessarily a "death sentence".

The majority of the participants had a mastectomy and most were given a choice between a lumpectomy and a mastectomy. Three of the women had no option because the cancer was at an advanced stage. Some women were unable to make an immediate decision and consulted members of their families. In these instances, the women felt comforted by the fact that, although the decision was entirely theirs, they could consult with their families. In a few instances there were disagreements between the participants and their spouses but the women were satisfied with the final decision. It is interesting to note that the final decision between a lumpectomy and a mastectomy was based on family knowledge, experience of cancer, family history of breast cancer and information found on the Internet. Some of the women felt that because this was happening to their bodies they wanted complete ownership of the final decision and they saw no need for confirmation from their spouses. While some of the women had the operation almost immediately, others had to undergo chemotherapy in order to shrink the lump. This leads to additional trauma because of the effects of chemotherapy, especially hair loss and the impact of this on a woman's femininity. A few of the respondents also underwent several tests to determine if the cancer had spread to other organs.

The decision between a lumpectomy and mastectomy, in some instances, depended on the financial situation of the individuals. One respondent felt that because she had sufficient funds for continued medical treatment radical surgery could be obviated. It is interesting to note that only one woman's decision was based on body image and this was a factor which only arose sometime after the initial diagnosis.

At the time of diagnosis, none of the respondents mentioned any concerns about losing a breast and the implication of this for their femininity and sexuality. These issues were insignificant. The need to survive took precedence. Their immediate response was the fear that the cancer might spread to other organs. Nancy (42) stated, "When I received the diagnosis I told myself that I have a diseased organ and it must go. I did not want to live with the fear that the cancer may spread. That was my main concern". This finding is similar to a study by Fallowfield, Hall, Maguire and Baum [33] who found that the fear of losing a breast was not as bad as the fear of knowing that one has cancer. For the majority of the women in this study, it seems that the issues of body image, sexuality, identity or even femininity were stepsisters to survival and were not given any immediate consideration.

Twenty eight (28) of the participants attended a public academic hospital (as a direct consequence of not having any medical insurance) while two individuals were diagnosed at a private medical centre. In both of these instances the women did not have access to professional psychological counselling. At the public hospital some of the women were referred to social workers immediately after the diagnosis. Most of the women stated that they would have preferred more information from the doctors themselves about the procedures that were to follow rather than being sent to the social worker. According to Rottmann, Helmes and Vogel [34], early-stage breast cancer patients need information about the stage of the cancer and treatment options and they prefer verbal information from health care professionals. The results of the current study show that this was seriously lacking.

Janice (46) stated, "Everything happened so quickly, decisions had to be made there and then. One did not have time to let it all sink in and they sent me immediately to the social worker. I had to make a life-changing decision and I was not given time to think about it". The women felt that counselling from a psychologist would have been more helpful rather than from a social worker. Some respondents also felt that they should have been given more time to come to terms with the diagnosis and to inform their families before being sent to the social worker. At that point they were overwhelmed by the diagnosis and still in a state of shock and as Janice (46) mentioned "I am thinking I haven't even told my family yet and here I am with the social worker".

Furthermore, some of the women felt that they were being hurried and experienced a doctor-patient relationship which was dismissive and detached. Bitsika, Sharpley and Christie [35] stress that counseling interventions which take into account an individual's specific circumstances are more likely to succeed than a generalized approach. At the public facilities the women felt that because the doctors had many patients to attend to they were unable to reassure them when they needed it the most. The majority of the respondents clearly stressed the need for more information around breast cancer and the procedures and nearly all the women would have preferred professional counseling.

For most of the participants, attending a public facility and coming from impoverished backgrounds also meant that they had to use public transport. After hearing about the life threatening disease most women felt weak and extremely distressed and thoughts about using public transport in the future, especially after chemotherapy, surgery and other forms of treatment made them even more anxious.

Most of the women were concerned about informing their families. Being fearful for themselves, some of the women tried to put on a brave front and many stated that they had to be strong for their children and their family. Some of the children wanted to know if their mothers were going to die because of the cancer. Generally the women felt that they did not really know what was going through their children's minds but they were more anxious for their daughters, knowing that breast cancer could also affect them someday. In this study it seems that the daughters reacted more openly than the sons.

Without exception, the women did not want to keep the cancer a secret. They wanted their families to know what was happening. Many of the participants were generally reassured by the concern and support they received from their families. According to Rowland and Massie [36], social support is critical for all women at all stages of the process. However, some did not receive this support. Laura (27), for example, mentioned that it was a lonely journey for her as she did not receive the support she expected from her family. She stated, "You must have someone to care so much about you... otherwise you won't be able to do it". Janice (46) also mentioned that her husband was not very supportive and did not try to reassure her when she told him of the results. Some women stated that their husbands found it difficult to show their emotions. Although some women stated that their husbands were supportive at the initial stage, many were concerned about how their husbands would react after they underwent chemotherapy or after surgery. One respondent thought that when she informed her fiancé he would abandon her. Jane (32), being a single woman, had difficulties informing her father of the outcome of the tests. Jane explained that her father had been through the same situation with her mother and she wished that he did not have to be upset in this way again. It seems that, without exception, the women were fearful and concerned about the cancer but they had to put up a facade and appear strong for their families at the same time.

Implications of the Study

Several concerns and needs of the women came to the fore as the study progressed. These are the "no pain no cancer" advice given by medical personnel which left many women confused and angry when they were eventually diagnosed with breast cancer as well as instances where women felt they were misdiagnosed because they initially tested negative for breast cancer but later tested positive. They stressed that one should have a second and even a third opinion if possible but this is generally only possible for women on a medical aid. For the majority of the participants in this study, who are not on a medical aid, they depended on the initial diagnosis with little chance of a second opinion. Furthermore, almost all of the respondents would have preferred professional psychological counselling and more information on the procedures after the initial diagnosis.

They clearly felt that the social worker was not the person to see when confronted with breast cancer. With 63% of the women not having regular mammograms before diagnosis and the one in 22 chance of a woman developing breast cancer, the need for education and regular screening should be a sine qua non for women above a certain age. All the women stressed the need for regular self-examination and mammograms. As the majority of the women could not afford medical aid, the accessibility of medical and screening facilities is also a cause for concern.

While the findings from this research may have implications for the manner in which tests are conducted, or the manner in which medical personnel engage with patients, women also have a responsibility to maintain their health as best they can. The lessons derived through this study are that all lumps must be checked, no matter how small or inconsequential it may seem to be; one should listen instinctively to one's body as the presence of the lump is a sign that a serious problem may exist; women should have regular mammograms and that there should be breast awareness campaigns to educate and encourage women to have regular screening.

Study Limitations and Further Research

This study does have inherent limitations. For instance, the research presented here is based on interviews with individuals from a certain population group in South Africa. Only a group of 30 female coloured women from the Western Cape were interviewed. Being an exploratory study, it did not include the experiences of women who belong to other population groups and who may come from varying socio-economic backgrounds which may impact differently on their experiences of breast cancer. Neither did the research delve into how breast cancer impacted on the coloured women's femininity and the body image. The study was also confined to a particular area and, therefore, the findings cannot be generalised to represent the experiences of all breast cancer survivors in South Africa.

These limitations, however, provide a platform for further research in relation to breast cancer. For example, future researchers may consider how the marginalisation of coloured women impacts on their coping strategies. A cross-sectional study comparing the experiences of women from different cultural, racial and socio-economic backgrounds will also broaden the understanding of the experiences of breast cancer survivors in South Africa. It is necessary to ascertain to what extent South African women generally make use of mammography screening and to gauge the efficacy of the education around breast cancer and early detection.

In addition, a nuanced understanding of the notion of "femininity" in relation to breast cancer could ease the anxiety women experience when they have to have a breast or part of it removed. There is also a need to understand why women diagnosed with breast cancer are sent to social workers and not psychologists. The apparent lack of involvement of spouses and the impact of the wife's illness on the husband are important areas that require urgent attention also.

These studies may have further implications for policies around women's health with specific reference to breast health and breast cancer.

Conclusion

Although the experiences of the group of coloured South African women in the Western Cape who were interviewed may not differ widely from the experiences of other breast cancer survivors, it is nevertheless important to give these women recognition and a voice because of their marginalised status in the South African context. Many women commented on the cathartic nature of the interview and expressed surprise and gratitude that someone wanted to hear exactly what had happened to them during their cancer experience and this gave them a sense of recognition and validation.

The contributions of this study, besides documenting the experiences of a particular group of women in South Africa, are that:

(a) It highlights the importance of acknowledging the initial experiences of breast cancer survivors and the need for more time to process the diagnosis; (b) It emphasises the need for professional psychological counselling; (c) It suggests that access to health facilities, especially for mammogram screening, is crucial for women who do not have medical insurance and who have to depend on public transport; (d) It brought to the fore lessons that women must take note of in terms of their health; and (e) Being an exploratory study, it raises several pertinent issues which require further interrogation in order to adequately understand women's experiences in relation to breast cancer.

Self-reflection

As a woman listening to these survivors, the researcher became so immersed in the details of their experiences that for days and weeks after the interviews the researcher was acutely aware of subtle reactions and slight changes around her breast area and was constantly dogged by the question "Do I have breast cancer"? This feeling of over-identification is also noted by Johnson and Macleod Clark [37] who found that for some researchers dealing with sensitive topics, e.g. cancer, left them wondering if they too had this disease [38-40].

References

1. WHO (2015) Breast Cancer: Prevention and control.
2. CANSA (2015) Fact sheet on breast cancer in women.
3. Fokazi S (2011) Cancer victim talks of family's battle with illness. Cape Argus.
4. Statistics South Africa (2014) Mid-year Population Estimates.
5. Shields N, Nadasen K, Pierce L (2013) Community violence and psychological distress in South African and US children. Int Perspect Psychol: Research, Practice, Consultation 2: 286-300.
6. Daniels D, Quinton A (2010) Breaking with township Gangsterism: The struggle for place and voice. African Studies Quarterly 11: 45-57.
7. Avis NE, Crawford S, Manuel J (2004) Psychosocial problems among younger women with breast cancer. Psychooncology 13: 295-308.
8. Schulz U, Mohamed NE (2004) Turning the tide: benefit finding after cancer surgery. Soc Sci Med 59: 653-662.
9. Fallbjork U, Frejeus E, Rasmussen BH (2012) A preliminary study into women's experiences of undergoing reconstructive surgery after breast cancer. Eur J Oncology 16: 220-226.
10. Rasmussen DM, Hansen HP, Elverdam B (2010) How cancer survivors experience their changed body encountering others. Eur J Oncol Nurs 14: 154-159.
11. Manganiello A, Hoga LA, Reberte LM, Miranda CM, Rocha CA (2011) Sexuality and quality of life of breast cancer patients post mastectomy. Eur J Oncol Nurs 15: 167-172.
12. Kaiser K (2008) The meaning of the survivor identity for women with breast cancer. Soc Sci Med 67: 79-87.
13. Schetter CD, Feinstein LG, Taylor SE, Falke RL (1992) Patterns of coping with cancer. Health Psychol 11: 79-87.
14. Stanton AL, Snider PR (1993) Coping with a breast cancer diagnosis: A prospective study. Health Psychol 12: 16-23.
15. Lethborg CE, Kissane D, Burns WI (2003) "It's Not the Easy Part." The experiences of significant others of women with early stage breast cancer at treatment completion. Soc Work Health Care 37: 63-85.
16. Coggin C, Shaw-Perry M (2006) Breast cancer survivorship: Expressed needs of black women. J Psychosoc Oncol 24: 107-122.
17. Manne SL, Norton TR, Ostroff JS, Winkel G, Fox K, et al. (2007) Protective buffering and psychological distress among couples coping with breast cancer: The moderating role of relationship satisfaction. J Family Psychol 21: 380-388.
18. Landmark BT, Wahl A (2002) Living with newly diagnosed breast cancer: A qualitative study of 10 women with newly diagnosed breast cancer. J Adv Nurs 40: 112-121.
19. Neuman WL (1994) Social research methods, qualitative and quantitative approaches. Boston: Allyn and Bacon.
20. Ezzy D (2002) Qualitative analysis, practice and innovation. Sydney: Allan and Unwin.
21. Henning E, Rensburg W, Smit B (2004) Finding your way in qualitative research. Pretoria: Van Schaik.
22. Ingrisch D (1995) Conformity and resistance as women age. In: Arber S, Ginn J, Connecting Gender and Ageing: A Sociological Approach. London: Routledge pp: 151-165.
23. Bredin M (1999) Mastectomy, body image and therapeutic massage: A qualitative study of women's experience. J Adv Nurs 29: 1113-1120.
24. Kasper AS (1994) A feminist, qualitative methodology: A study of women with breast cancer. Qual Sociol 17: 263-281.
25. Frank AW (1998) Just listening: Narratives and deep illness. Family, Systems and Health 16: 197-212.
26. Gonzalez SJ, Davis C (2012) Understanding the unique experiences of undocumented Hispanic women who are living in poverty and coping with breast cancer. J Immigrant and Refugee Studies 10: 116-123.
27. Grimes TS, Hou S (2013) "A Breast ain't but a sandwich." Narratives of Ella, an African American social worker breast cancer survivor. Social Work in Public Health 28: 44-53.
28. Hilton S, Emslie C, Hunt K, Chapple A, Ziebland S (2009) Disclosing a cancer diagnosis to friends and family: A gendered analysis of young men's and women's experiences. Qual Health Res 19: 744-754.
29. Kearney AJ (2006) Increasing our understanding of breast self-examination: Women talk about cancer, the health care system, and being women. Qual Health Res 16: 802-820.
30. Thind A, Diamant A, Hoq L, Maly R (2009) Method of detection of breast cancer in low-income women. J Women's Health 18: 1807-1811.
31. http://www.searo.who.int/entity/noncomunicabledisease/advocacy/worldcancerday2014/en
32. Myrick S (2002) The patient perspective: Surviving breast cancer. The Breast Journal 8: 119-120.
33. Fallowfield LJ, Hall A, Maguire GP, Baum M (1990) Psychological outcomes of different treatment policies in women with early breast cancer outside a clinical trial. BMJ 301: 575-580.
34. Rottmann N, Helmes AW, Vogel BA (2010) Patients' needs and experiences at breast cancer diagnosis: How perceived threat influences the physician-patient interaction. J Psychosoc Oncol 28: 157-172.
35. Bitsika V, Sharpley CF, Christie DRH (2010) "What made me unhappy." Experiences of, and responses to, lifestyle changes in breast cancer patients. Br J Guidance Counselling 38: 179-189.
36. Rowland JH, Massie MJ (1998) Breast Cancer. In: Holland JC, Psycho-oncology. Oxford, New York pp: 380-401.
37. Johnson B, Clarke JM (2003) Collecting sensitive data: The impact on researchers. Qual Health Res 13: 421-434.
38. Fransch CJP (2010) "We would have no name": The porosity of locational and racial identities among the 'coloured" communities of Stellenbosch. African Studies 69: 403-422.
39. Isaacs-Martin W (2014) National and ethnic identities: Dual and extreme identities amongst the coloured population of Port Elizabeth, South Africa. Studies in ethnicity and nationalism, 14: 56-73.
40. Seekings J (2008) The continuing salience of race: Discrimination and diversity in South Africa. J Contemporary African Studies 26: 1-25.

10

Barriers of Maternal Health Seeking Behavior: A Bayesian Analysis

Pranti Dutta[1*] and Bodhisattva Sengupta[2]

[1]*Department of Biosciences and Bioengineering, Indian Institute of Technology, Guwahati, India*

[2]*Department of Humanities and Social Sciences, Indian Institute of Technology, Guwahati, India*

***Corresponding author:** Pranti Dutta, Research Consultant, Department of Biosciences and Bioengineering, Indian Institute of Technology, Guwahati, India, E-mail: prantidutta12@gmail.com

Abstract

Health outcomes depend on availability of and actual usage of formal institutional facilities. In this context, perhaps the most primary decision from a patient's point of view is to seek institutional care. The present study attempts to delineate main barriers of maternal health seeking behavior from select villages of Assam, an Indian state exhibiting highest MMR in spite of relative improvement in supply side scenario. Using multistage and snowball sample techniques, 169 interviewees are selected which include mothers who have children aged 0-24 months, subjects who are pregnant as well as members of families that have experience of maternal death. Data is analyzed with a Bayesian logistic regression model. Our analysis posits that non-availability of ambulance and female health providers; ignorance and hesitation; long queue at facilities, non-availability of supporting persons at home and heavy workload are main barriers to maternal health seeking behavior. Policy wise, the paper highlights the areas in which scarce public money should be spent.

Keywords: Maternal health; Maternal mortality; Pregnancy; Treatment

Introduction

Globally, about 830 women die in a day from pregnancy and childbirth related complications [1]. At the country level, India accounts for one-third of all global maternal deaths (ibid). At the national level, state of Assam has the dubious distinction of highest maternal mortality ratio of 300 per 1,00,000 live births (SRS, GOI 2013). Since 1997-98, Assam has always been one of the top (above the 3rd quartile) Indian states with MMR. The trend of Assam vis-a-vis India can be shown in the following graph (Figure 1), and a comparison with selected states of India is shown in Table 1.

This persistently high MMR cannot be explained solely in terms of supply side constraints. If one compares data from 2007 (facility health survey) vis-a-vis District Level Household Survey (DLHS)-IV (2012-2013), one can see that the number of facilities have increased across all the districts of Assam (Table 2A). District Level Household and Facility Survey (DLHS) IV (2012-2013) of Assam reveals that number of government health institutions have been increasing in 2014 compared to those reported existing in 2007, i.e. DLHS III (Table 2B).

Such expansion of formal facilities is incompatible with high (relative) MMR, and therefore we look into other explanations. One key variable is, of course, the demand side (e.g. utilization pattern). DLHS III shows that among currently married women aged 15-44 years, 35.3% of women had institutional delivery and 40.9% have safe delivery including either institutional delivery or home delivery attended by skilled health personnel. Further, 74.8% receive the minimum antenatal care during pregnancy. The same source reveals that about 60.2% of women of Assam had faced complications during pregnancy. However, only 45% of such women, who had reported at least one complication of pregnancy, sought treatment from the formal system.

This implies poor utilization of reproductive healthcare services and a low status of healthcare seeking behavior. Based on the observations, we propose the hypothesis that ceteris paribus, poor maternal outcomes result from inadequate utilization of facilities. Low utilization, in turn, is caused by significant barriers to Maternal Health Seeking Behaviour (MHSB) at the micro level. The paper seeks to explore such barriers in a systematic way. Understanding Maternal Health Seeking Behavior (MHSB) (or lack thereof) in Assam is crucial for improving the outcome of pregnancy and childbirth and thereby unlocking a key element of its development potential.

States/Years	Assam	Bihar	Kerala	Rajasthan	Tamil Nadu	Uttar Pradesh	West Bengal	India	Q1 (India)	Q3 (India)
1997-98	568	531	150	508	131	606	303	398	226.5	549.5
1999-01	398	400	149	501	167	539	218	327	192.5	450.5
2001-03	490	371	110	445	134	517	194	301	164	467.5
2004-06	480	312	95	388	111	440	141	254	126	414
2007-09	390	261	81	318	97	359	145	212	121	338.5

2010-12	328	219	66	255	90	292	117	178	103.5	273.5
2011-13	300	208	61	244	79	285	113	167	96	264.5

Table 1: Maternal mortality ratio in India in selected states (Per 1, 00,000 live births) [Source: Registrar General of India, Ministry of Home Affairs (SRS bulletins) Note: Q1 is the first quartile (25%); Q3 is the third quartile (75%)].

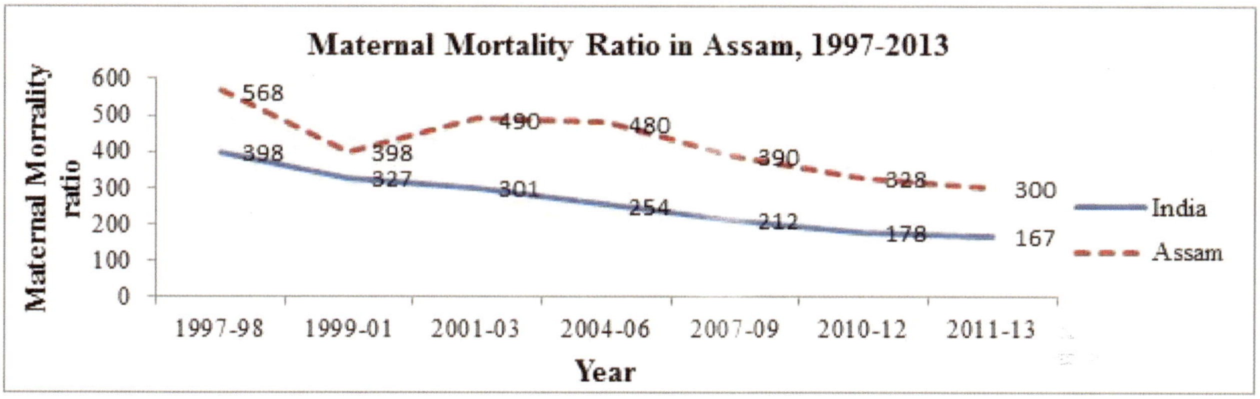

Figure 1: Maternal mortality ratio in Assam, 1997-2013 (Source: SRS reports).

PHC facilities	No. of PHC with facilities 07	No. of PHC with facilities 14
Medical officers	141	329
Lady Medical officers	29	119
ANM	146	359
Ambulance facility	60	175
Delivery services	63	186
Referral services	124	216

Table 2A: Availability of maternal care facilities at PHC in Assam between 2007 to 2014.

Health Institutions	DLHS IV	DLHS III
Community Health Center	214	83
Primary Health Center	375	195
Sub center	857	714

Table 2B: Number of health institutions in Assam as per DLHS III and DLHS IV.

Note that, such attempts have been made in different country or socio-economic contexts. For instance, Fenta et al. [2] suggests that maternal age, educational level, partner's attitudes towards health seeking care from doctors including the ignorance and lack of awareness about danger signs during pregnancy are major contributors to non-usage of maternal care services. Osubor et al. [3] showed that, in Nigeria, agents are more likely to prefer Traditional Birth Attendants (TBAs) due to greater accessibility, lower cost and more convenience. Further, local beliefs, perceptions, and knowledge of community members about maternal health problems also played an important role in MHSB. Koenig et al. [4] have examined MHSB in Bangladesh and identified that medical cost and socio-economic disparities are major factors. Tasnim et al. [5] in Bangladesh found that high cost, non-availability of drugs and beds, ignorance about complications, cultural norms and attitudes of health providers are major reasons for not availing health care services.

Jayaraman et al. [6] have revealed in Rwanda that the households with a female head and women with higher-order birth are less likely to access health care facilities. Further, supply side factors like availability, cost and quality of medical care also play an important role. Chomat et al. [7] in Guatemala have found poor utilization of maternal care services are caused by socioeconomic disparities, ethnic and linguistic differences, personal experience with health institutions and health providers, influence of husband and other family members. Benova et al. [8] has stressed that economic resourcefulness (household asset ownership, access to agricultural production and household consumption), and socio-cultural resourcefulness (woman years of education, literacy, male head of household occupational category, identity documents among members of the household) are positively associated with MHSB.

A limited number of similar studies are available for India. Navaneetham et al. [9] carried out their studies in Southern India (states of Andhra Pradesh, Kerala, Karnataka and Tamil Nadu). They showed that utilization pattern of maternal care varies due to variations in the implementation of maternal health care program and differences in availability and accessibility of the maternal services between the states as well. Agarwal et al. [10] examined the utilization pattern of maternal care in an urban slum in Delhi. Their results reflect that awareness and knowledge about maternity care and accessibility of modern maternity facilities have significant influence. Similarly, Mahapatro et al. [11] found that in Odisha, transportations and financial constraints, community perceptions and attitudes towards maternity care, influence of elderly person and other family members are the major barriers and determinants of maternal seeking behavior. Bhattacherjee et al. [12] found that in tea gardens of Darjeeling district of West Bengal, ignorance and distance to health care institutions are main reasons for non-utilization of health care services. Srivastava et al. [13] showed that in Rohilkhand Region of Uttar Pradesh that mother's education and husband's occupation are the strong predictors of utilization of maternal health care services. Likewise, Tiwari et al. [14] showed that accessibility and availability of maternal care services increased the utilization of healthcare facilities in Madhya Pradesh.

A few case studies regarding utilization of reproductive healthcare are available in the context of Assam, or North East India in general. For instances, Khound et al. [15] in Jorhat district of Assam found that socio-economic barriers (such as: lack of awareness, financial constraint, does not think it as necessary) are the major factors in decreasing the utilization of these services. Another study was done by Mazumder et al. [16] among the Karbis of Guwahati city revealed that mother's education is positively related to awareness of antenatal care and place of delivery. Yet, to the best of our knowledge, very little attention has been given to figure out determinants of barriers of MHSB in Assam (or anywhere in North East India) in a comprehensive manner. Studies carried out by Khound (op. cit) and Mazumder (op. cit) are case studies with limited scope. The current paper provides broader perspectives and hence has more precise policy prescriptions. Based on Mackin et al. [17], we considered the following variables to be significant barriers to MHSB (Table 3).

Category	Barriers	Measures	Variables
Geographical	Distance and physical access	Far from home	FH
		Bad roads	BR
Organizational	Quality care	Doctors not responsive	DnR
		Non availability of ambulance	NAmb
		Non availability of Female health provide	NFhP
Cultural	Knowledge and perceptions	Husband restriction	HR
		Hesitation	Hesi
		Ignorance	Ign
Socio-economic	Social structure and economic cost	Cost of drugs	CoD
		Cost of transportation	CoT
		Long queue	LQ
		Non availability of person at home	NPaH
		Heavy workload	HW
		Income level	Y
		Age of marriage	AoM
		Land ownership	LO
		Literacy	Lit

Table 3: Framework for maternal health seeking behavior.

Our study finds that non-availability of female health providers and ambulance reduces the probability of maternal health seeking care. In addition, ignorance, hesitation, long queues at formal facility, non-availability of persons at home to taking care of pregnant women as well as heavy workloads are barriers to MHSB. The rest of the paper is organized as follows. Section 2 discusses methodology of data collection and statistical analysis. Section 3 focuses on maternal healthcare in sample areas and presents the result and interpretation of statistical analysis. Section 4 and 5 provides the interpretation and discussion of our results. Section 6 concludes the whole paper and offers some policy implications.

Methodology

Selection of the study areas and data collection

Since secondary data (for example, DLHS IV data regarding utilization pattern in Assam) is non-existent, we carried a primary survey in order to get more insight about barriers to MHSB.

The survey was carried out in eight villages of four districts of Assam that are identified by multi-stage sampling. By using stratified sampling methods, all districts under four Administrative Divisions of Assam have been arranged as highest to lowest based on maternal mortality ratio (MMR) for the period of April 2013 and March 2014. This helps us to identify four districts with highest MMR. From each district, we have selected that Block Primary Health Centres (BPHC), which have reported the highest maternal death. Finally, as per reference with the Medical Officer (MO) from selected BPHC, two villages from each BPHC (total 8 villages) are selected purposively for carrying out the survey. The details are in Table 4.

District	Maternal Mortality Rate in Districts	Name of BPHC	Maternal Death at BPHC	Name of Village
Kamrup	230.1539	Chhaygaon	7	Muhimari, Patgaon
Dibrugarh	413.3103	Barbaruah	86	Janzimukh, Lepetkatta TE
Sonitpur	297.3435	Biswanath Chariali	14	Kadamani, Sakumato TE
Cachar	516.6315	Sonai	10	Motinagar, Silcoorie TE

Table 4: Selected districts and villages of Assam based on highest maternal mortality ratio reported in the period of 2013-2014.

Employing snowball sample techniques, we interviewed the following from each sample village

- Currently pregnant women
- Mothers who have children aged 0-24 months
- Members of a family that has experienced of maternal deaths.

We interviewed 169 subjects. The survey period was September 2014 to February 2015 with the reference period of 365 days preceding the date of the survey. The objective of the questionnaire was to obtain information on maternal health status and in-depth information on maternal deaths cases; socio-demographic characteristics of subjects; reproductive history as well as their attitude towards reproductive health and utilization of the maternal services from the health system. Our primary focuses being the socio-economic and cultural.

Maternal Healthcare in Surveyed Area

Maternal health outcome

It is clear from the Table 5 that along with the maternal deaths cases, there are reported cases of high-risk pregnancy and other complications during pregnancy. High-risk pregnancy is associated with conditions like preterm labour, preeclampsia, edema and problems with uterus and placenta. Complicated pregnancy refers to problem such as severe lower abdominal pain, vision problem, severe nausea, swelling of body etc. during pregnancy.

Maternal Outcome	No.	(%)
Maternal deaths	17	10.1
High risk pregnancy	29	17.2
Complications	27	16
Normal pregnancy	96	56.8
Total pregnancy	169	100

Table 5: Maternal health outcome at study villages (Source: Field data 2014-2015).

Socio-economic characteristics

Table 6 provides the detailed profile of the socio-economic and demographic characteristics of the respondents.

Socio-economic variables	No.	Percentage (%)	Socio-economic variables	No.	Percentage (%)
Age at Marriage			Family structure		
>18	28	16.6	Nuclear family	101	59.8
19-29	121	71.6	Joint family	68	40.2
Above 30	20	11.8			
Literacy			Housing condition		
Illiterate	88	52.1	Kutcha	139	82.3
Literate	61	36.1	Pucca	20	11.8
Only sign	20	11.8	Semi-pucca	10	5.92
Birth order			Drinking water facilities		
1	66	39.1	Pump tube well	92	54.4
2 to 3	76	45	Well	38	22.5
4 to 5	22	13	Pipe water	30	17.8

6 to 7	5	2.96	Stream water	9	5.33
Haemoglobin level			Income level		
<7	29	17.2	Below average	110	65.1
7 to 9	67	39.6	Above average	59	34.9
10 to 12	73	43.2	Average income	39615. 38	

Table 6: Selected socio-economic variables (N=169) (Source: Field data 2014-2015).

Utilization of maternal health care services

Figure 2 depicts the selected maternal health care services in the studied areas. The coverage of full antenatal care (those women who completed their three trimesters of pregnancy till the date of survey) is only 57%. The figure also shows that the institutional delivery (women who delivered till the date of survey) in studied villages is less than 80 %. Further, the use of contraceptive methods among studied population is also found very low i.e. only 11%.

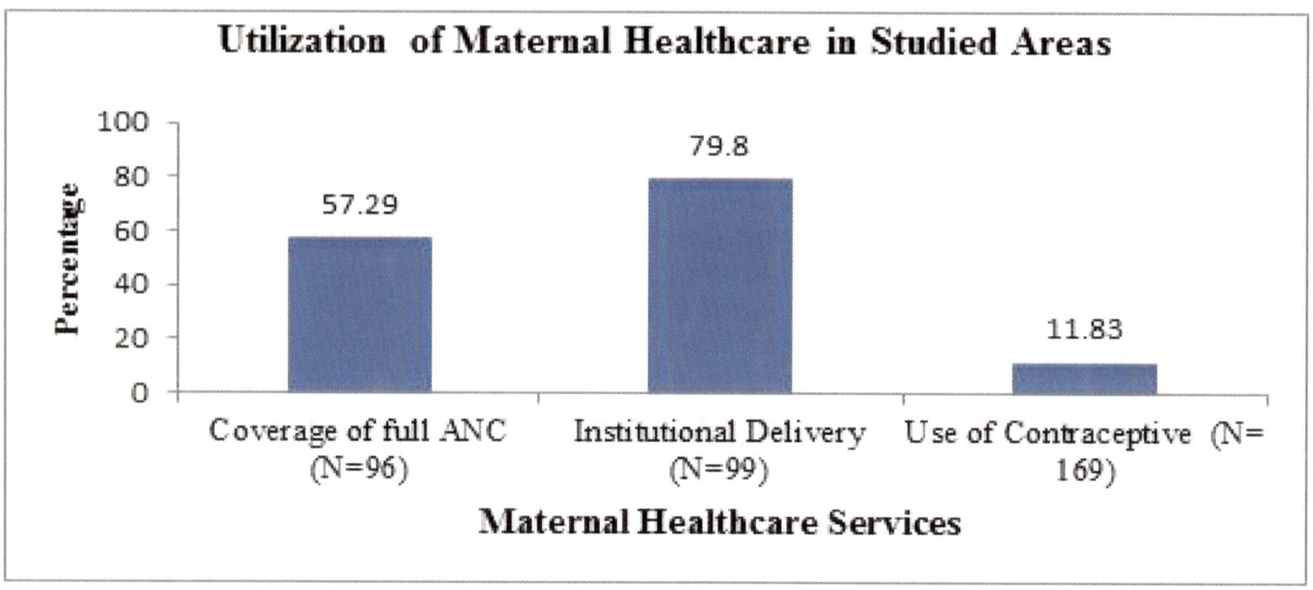

Figure 2: Utilization of maternal healthcare in studied areas (Sources: Field data 2014-2015).

Occupational profile

Occupational distribution is shown in Figure 3. This figure reflects that daily wage labour is the main source of the income of the larger sections of the sample households and very few are engaged in cultivation, own farming and business.

Apart from the socio-economic characteristics of the studied villages, interviews with pregnant women and health providers highlighted that although the pregnant women are familiar with the use of available facilities of sub-centre at the village level. On the other hand, they ignore referral advice provided by ANM's to seek medical help from nearby health institutions with better facilities.

Bayesian Logistic Regression

To assess the association of the outcome variable namely Not Seeking Care (NSC) with the selected independent variables one proceeds with standard logistic model:

$$\text{Logit (NSCi)} = \alpha + \beta 1 \text{ (GEOi)} + \beta 2 \text{ (ORGi)} + \beta 3 \text{ (CULi)} + \beta 4 \text{ (SOCECOi)} + \mu i \quad - (1)$$

In the left-hand side of the equation, NSCi denote the response of ith respondent regarding decision to seek care. It is a dummy variable such that NSC=1 implies "not seeking care" and zero otherwise. In the right-hand side of equation (1), α is the constant; β is the vector of coefficients and the independent variables are Geographical parameters (GEO), Organizational parameters (ORG), Cultural parameters (CUL) and Socio-economic parameters (SOCECO) which are coded as 1 for "if the factor causes problem in accessing health facilities" and zero otherwise. However, the parameters included in SOCECO land ownership, income level and age of marriage have continuous values (Table 7).

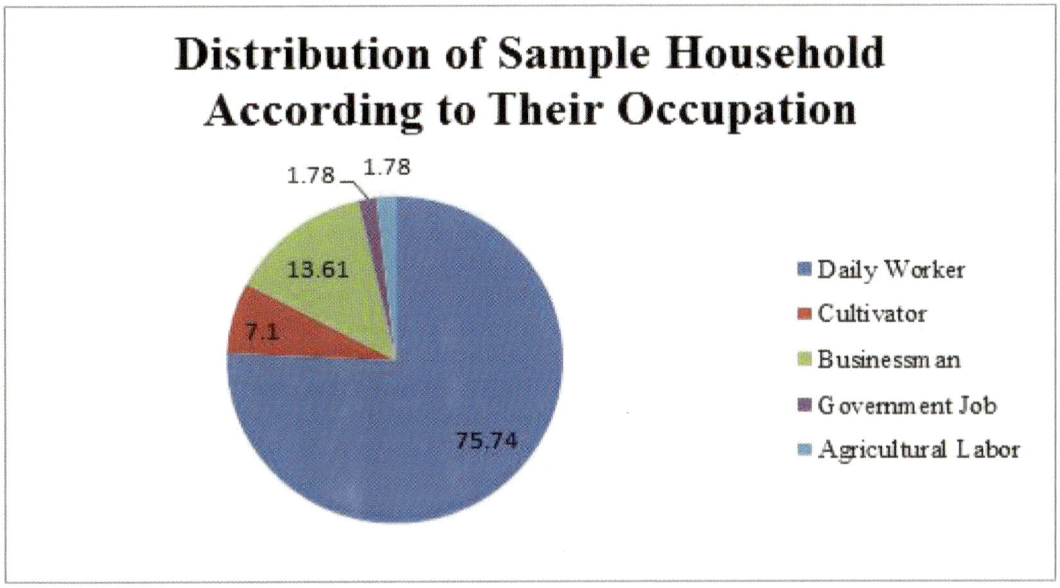

Figure 3: Distribution of sample household according to their occupation (Sources: Field data 2014-2015).

Measures	Variables	Mean	Std. Dev	Min	Max
Not seeking care	NSC	0.64497	0.47994	0	1
Far from home	FH	0.02959	0.16995	0	1
Bad roads	BR	0.00592	0.07692	0	1
Doctors not responsive	DnR	0.01183	0.10846	0	1
Non availability of ambulance	NAmb	0.02959	0.16995	0	1
Non availability of female health provides	NFhP	0.15385	0.36187	0	1
Husband restriction	HR	0.02959	0.16995	0	1
Hesitations	Hesi	0.05325	0.22521	0	1
Ignorance	Ign	0.0355	0.1856	0	1
Cost of drugs	CoD	0.11834	0.32397	0	1
Long queue	LQ	0.26627	0.44332	0	1
Non availability of person at home	NPaH	0.14201	0.3501	0	1
Heavy workload	HW	0.04734	0.21299	0	1
Literacy	Lit	0.39053	0.48932	0	1
Land ownership	LO	0.61462	1.09151	0	5.61
Income level	Y	39615.4	19011.9	10000	145000
Age of marriage	AoM	18	3.27872	12	28

Table 7: Descriptive statistics of the variables influencing maternal health seeking behavior.

Given the data set, a standard logistic regression cannot be estimated because of complete separation problem. The outcome variable separates a predictor variable or a combination of predictor variables completely. This result in very large standard errors the maximum likelihood estimate fails to converge [18-22]. In order to circumvent the problem, our analysis applies the Bayesian approach to logistic regression [20,22-24].

To estimate such model by using M-H Markov Chain Monte Carlo algorithm and credible intervals, we have used Jeffreys' (uninformative) prior. For the sampling process in the MCMC method, burn-in of 5,000 iterations with MCMC sample size of 12,000 and finally total 17,000 MCMC iterations were selected for the posterior inference, which is accurate and efficient with higher effective sample size (ESS) of all the parameters. Use of MCMC method produces some level of autocorrelation. To evaluate statistical efficiency of such methods, effective sample size is calculated, which is the number of effectively independent samples from the total number of posterior samples.

Low ESS relative to MCMC sample suggests convergence problem. In this analysis, due to low ESS, income level and age at marriage are excluded. The detail of the effective sample size table is presented in Table 8 in Appendix. The acceptance rate of the Metropolis-Hastings algorithm is 43% out of 12,000 MCMC sample size where average efficiency is 13%. We have used the 95% highest probability density (HPD) region for each parameter in the model.

ESS	Corr. time		Efficiency
Seeking care			
Far from home	2113.61	5.68	0.1761
Bad roads	2709.58	4.43	0.2258
Doctors not responsive	1941.9	6.18	0.1618
Non-Availability of ambulance	2158.74	5.56	0.1799
Non-Availability of female health provider	1357.69	8.84	0.1131
Husband restriction	2125.13	5.65	0.1771
Hesitation	1587.17	7.56	0.1323
Ignorance	1973.57	6.08	0.1645
Cost of drugs	1896.86	6.33	0.1581
Cost of transportation	1511.27	7.94	0.1259
Long queue	1123.91	10.68	0.0937
Non availability of person at home	1873.47	6.41	0.1561
Heavy workload	1729.66	6.94	0.1441
Land ownership	1313.51	9.14	0.1095
Literacy	787.4	15.24	0.0656

Table 8: Effective sample sizes of all variables.

Another important component of Bayesian inference is comparison of two models, say M1 and M2 which provides support for a model over another based on the Bayes' factor. The present analysis compares three models with three different prior distributions to find the one that best fits the data. In the first model (base l), we have considered normal prior with a fixed variance. Secondly, we compute the second model with uninformative prior and informative prior. For former one, we have used uninformative priors. To construct informative priors, we uses the information obtained for N~(μ, σ) from the former to replace the uninformative distributions N~(0, 1).

We add one final note regarding choice of variables to increase the parsimony of our model. It could be the case that many of the responses regarding different variables are not independent. If two variables are not independent, then we drop one of them.

We surmise that the following variables might be dependent:

- Far from home; Bad roads; Non-availability of ambulance; Cost of transportation.
- Unresponsive doctors, Non-availability of female health provider; Husband restriction; Hesitation; Ignorance
- Long queue; Non-availability of person at home; Heavy workload

Note that it could be the case that one group of variables (e.g. Organizational/Geographical) can have spillover effect on other group of explanatory variables (e.g. Cultural/Socioeconomic).

We performed Chi-square test for independence of variables.

Results are summarized in Tables 9-11. The results show that:

- Cost of transportation (as barrier of MHSB) is not independent to perception of roads and non-availability of ambulance are dependent. However, the latter two are independent (at least, the null could not be rejected). Therefore, we have dropped the variable Cost of Transportation, since its effect is likely to be captured in other two.
- Similarly, husband restriction is not independent to unresponsive doctors and non-availability of female health provider. Surprisingly, husband restriction is related to organizational factors, not hesitation

or ignorance. We have removed husband restriction and keep both organizational variables in our subsequent analysis.

- For the third group of variables, we could not reject the null of no independence. Hence, all of those are kept in subsequent analysis.

Variables	FH	BR	NAmb	CoT
Far from home (FH)	0	0.9	0.69	0
Bad roads (BR)	0.9	0	0.86	0.6
Non-availability of ambulance (NAmb)	0.7	0.9	0	0.3
Cost of transportation (CoT)	0	0.6	0	0

Table 9: Chi-squared (p-value): Variable group 1.

Variables	DnR	NAFhP	HR	Hesi	Ign
Doctors not responsive (DnR)	0	0.8	0	0.74	0.8
Non-availability Female health provider (NAFhP)	0.8	0	0	0.19	0.9
Husband restriction (HR)	0.01	0	0	0.59	0.7
Hesitation (Hesi)	0.74	0.19	0.6	0	0.6
Ignorance (Ign)	0.79	0.93	0.7	0.55	0

Table 10: Chi-Squared (p-value) test: variable group 2.

Variables	LQ	NAPaH	HW
Long queue (LQ)	0	0.23	0.9
Non-availability of person at home (NAPaH)	0.2	0	0.2
Heavy workload (HW)	0.9	0.24	0

Table 11: Chi-squared test (p-value) variable group 3.

Results

Table 12 provides the posterior probability distribution. The result shows that parameters of geographical determinants like far from home (distance), bad roads (road conditions); unresponsive doctors (organizational factor) and cost of drugs, land ownership and literacy (socio-economic determinants) have no significant effects on predicting the health seeking behavior. On the other hand, out of four categories of determinants, the HPD intervals of the factors of cultural determinants; parameters of organizational category such as non-availability of female health providers, non-availability of ambulance and variables of socio-economic determinants like long queue, non-availability of person at home and heavy workloads represent significant barriers to MHSB in the surveyed villages at Highest Posterior Density (HPD) of 95% credible interval for all parameters.

Categories	Measures	Posterior Means	Std. Dev.	MCSE	HPD (95% Cred. Interval)	
Geographical	FH	1.3669	2.6288	0.055	-3.604	6.777
	BR	0.1478	3.0012	0.058	-5.603	6.171
Organizational	DnR	1.7078	2.5192	0.0532	-3.188	6.531
	NAmb	3.6275	1.9804	0.0396	0.0696	7.856
	NFhP	4.9924	1.8831	0.046	1.3603	8.68
Cultural	Hesi	5.4343	1.6388	0.0355	2.3477	8.701
	Ign	5.494	1.6705	0.0388	2.438	8.833

Socio economic	CoD	2.3415	2.1767	0.0502	-1.562	6.869
	LQ	6.4431	1.5276	0.0361	3.5282	9.377
	NPaH	6.4397	1.4361	0.031	3.9396	9.366
	HW	5.5274	1.6628	0.0361	2.5754	8.961
	LO	-0.0406	0.3289	0.0092	-0.705	0.597
	Lit	-0.2451	0.8	0.025	-1.796	1.351

Table 12: Posterior distribution for binary logistic regression model in response to health seeking behavior in surveyed villages, (Not Seeking care=1, seeking care=0) (Base model) [Source: Authors' estimation based on field data (2014-2015); Note: The dependent variable is women choice between not seeking care and seeking care. Not seeking care is coded as 1, 0 otherwise. "C.I." means credible interval. Statistically significant factors have been highlighted].

Table 13 presents the results from the second model using the uninformative priors, and Table 14 presents results with informative priors. The HPD level of the both models show that the effects of organizational parameters such as non-availability of female health providers; cultural determinants like hesitation and ignorance; and socio-economic determinants like long queue, non-availability of person at home and heavy workloads remain significant in these models. However, road conditions (geographical factor) in model of uninformative priors and non-availability of ambulance facilities (organizational factors) are significant in model of informative priors. The difference in results in Tables 13 and 14 indicates that the prior information regarding the mean and standard deviation of the parameter has an impact on the estimates.

Categories	**Measures**	**Posterior Means**	**Std. Dev.**	**MCSE**	**HPD**	
					(95% Cred. Interval)	
Geographical	FH	-3.7332	2.078	0.0557	-7.912	0.2081
	BR	-7.3065	2.3921	0.0588	-11.88	-2.469
Organizational	DnR	-3.0179	2.0642	0.0661	-7.065	0.9737
	NAmb	0.142	1.608	0.0384	-2.848	3.4049
	NFhP	5.707	1.7233	0.0597	2.303	8.9809
Cultural	Hesi	2.9595	1.158	0.0264	0.7871	5.2609
	Ign	2.9975	1.1156	0.024	0.8452	5.2511
Socio-economic	CoD	0.1339	1.436	0.0406	-2.498	3.0767
	LQ	4.9284	1.1346	0.0316	2.9163	7.2242
	NPaH	4.2514	0.9917	0.0218	2.5328	6.3405
	HW	2.9993	1.119	0.0245	0.8938	5.274
	LO	-0.0611	0.2624	0.0074	-1.591	0.4498
	Lit	-0.4774	0.5857	0.0176	-1.591	0.6883

Table 13: Posterior distribution for binary logistic regression model with uninformative priors in response to health seeking behavior in surveyed villages (Not Seeking care=1, Seeking care=0) [Source: Authors' estimation based on field data (2014-15)].

Categories	**Measures**	**Posterior Means**	**Std. Dev.**	**MCSE**	**HPD**	
					(95% Cred. Interval)	
Geographical	FH	2.0207	2.667	0.0542	-2.777	7.657
	BR	0.0427	3.0411	0.0576	-6.205	5.666

Organizational	DnR	2.2889	2.5527	0.0551	-2.603	7.246
	NAmb	4.1578	2.1078	0.0437	0.1621	8.235
	NFhP	5.2331	1.9747	0.0441	1.4814	9.004
Cultural	Hesi	5.8137	1.7912	0.0392	2.5277	9.28
	Ign	5.7952	1.648	0.0345	2.955	9.303
Socio-economic	CoD	2.8301	2.3509	0.0515	-1.593	7.367
	LQ	6.7153	1.5714	0.0352	3.8688	9.863
	NPaH	6.7932	1.537	0.0356	4.1089	9.937
	HW	5.7867	1.6602	0.0357	2.9572	9.136
	LO	-0.1884	0.8004	0.0246	-1.776	1.359
	Lit	-0.1884	0.8004	0.0246	-1.776	1.359

Table 14: Posterior distribution for binary logistic regression model with informative priors in response to health seeking behavior in surveyed villages (Not Seeking care=1, seeking care=0) [Source: Authors' estimation based on field data (2014-2015)].

Computation of Bayes factor indicates that the uninformative prior model performs worse than other two models. The value log (BF) 4.98 provides strong evidence in favor of the informative priors' model. Thus, the informative priors model (Table 14) is the best fit among the three (Table 15).

Variables	DIC	log(ML)	log(BF)
Uninformative Priors	68.2116	-133.27	-99.5461
Informative Priors	27.9266	-28.743	4.98422
Base Model	31.3606	-33.727	-

Table 15: Bayes factor of the considered models [Note: Marginal likelihood (ML) is computed using Laplace-Metropolis approximation].

Analysis based on our sample thus demonstrates that non-availability of female health provider and ambulance facilities increase the probability of not seeking care for maternal health. Similarly, this probability tends to increase in presence of hesitation and ignorance (which is quite intuitive).Additionally, long queues in hospital, non-availability of person at home and heavy workload are significant barriers to MHSB.

Discussion

Barriers of maternal health seeking behavior

The result of posterior probabilities indicates that out of four broad categories of determining factors of MHSB, the parameters of geographical factor (distance and road conditions) have no significant effects on shaping MHSB among studied population. Previous studies such as Gleia et al. [25] and Chomat et al. [7] also have found similar results, suggesting that accessibility might not necessarily translate into increased utilization of services if these facilities are lacking of essential infrastructure.

In the context of organizational determinants, non-availability of female health providers has significant effects on discouraging person to seek maternal healthcare from health facilities. It may be the case that respondents are not comfortable to share their reproductive problem with male doctors. This observation is consistent with observation from Schepper et al. [26] Singh et al. [27] and Qureshi et al. [28]. Our study also indicates that non-availability of ambulance at the time of emergency is a critical factor. The respondents argued that they do not have financial resources to afford a vehicle in a short notice. Further, other than the delivery of a baby, ambulance services are not free for the patients. Frequently they use bicycle, but it is not convenient during last trimester or with newborn. This result of our study also found consistent with findings from the studies of Ruth et al. [29] and Munguambe et al. [30].

The parameters of cultural determinants namely hesitation and ignorance have a strong influence on MHSB. Such factors have a large impact on shaping wider health seeking behavior [9,31]. Ignorance and hesitations for maternal healthcare during pregnancy are common factors that develop due to cultural practice and beliefs [2,12,32].

Other factors such as long queue in hospital, non-availability of helping persons at home and heavy workloads are found to be significant. About 26 percent of respondents want to avoid standing in a long queue. Heavy household responsibilities prevent women from visiting health institutions for regular checkup. Pregnant women do not want to stay longer in health institutions after her delivery (required for minimum time frame is 48 hours after delivery), because of non-availability of attendants in the hospitals, cost of lodging and foods of attendants. Similar result has found in studies of Yiran et al. [33] and Simkhada et al. [34]. Our study has also identified that patients often do not find any person to accompany her to the hospitals at the time of emergency or for a regular check-up in the last month of her pregnancy: husbands are not available at home during daytime and neighbors are busy with their daily household activities.

Conclusions

The paper has discussed the factors influencing MHSB of the population in selected districts of Assam based on the primary data collected from field observations. The results indicate that the MHSB of an individual is influenced by

- Organizational factors such as non-availability of female health providers and ambulances.
- Cultural factors viz. ignorance, hesitations and
- Socio-economic factors such as long queue, non-availability of persons at home, heavy workloads.

To be sure, sometimes distinctions between the various factors are blurred, or point to some other problems. Long queue, for example, can be result of inadequate provision of medical facility compared to number of patients. Non availability of female health providers could be a problem with organization as well as a cultural factor. Cultural factors point to a social setting where the "value" of women is less as a person due to (already entrenched) patriarchal biases. Such patriarchal biases work through heavy workload which nobody is willing to share because the workload is a "woman's job and duty" at the same time.

As Millennium Development Goals (2000-2015) unraveled, one distinct pattern emerged. It is comparatively easy to make progress where a material change is required: for example, providing safe drinking water or reducing poverty. However, shortfalls do remain where the target includes a significant behavioral change. The same parallel can be drawn in case of our survey. Provision of adequate, low cost and quality healthcare, tracking and monitoring pregnant women throughout pregnancy, improvement in connectivity etc. although difficult, are not insurmountable hurdles for government. The main challenges are probably poverty coupled with women's "perceived" place within a patriarchal society.

Apart from regular awareness camps, a tentative prescription is substantial social insurance targeted to the patients. This may help to increase the value of women and prove beneficial in long run. However, Central Schemes like Janani Suraksha Yojana (JSY) are inadequate and ineffective to an extent. A report on assessment of JSY in Assam during 2007 revealed that the cash assistance under JSY to pregnant women is not sufficient to cover all the expenses for institutional delivery. Further, the report also suggested for improving the quality care at PHC and sub-centre to provide services to normal deliveries, making payment on time to JSY beneficiaries, proper arrangement for transport facilities (CORT) [35]. Moreover, to encourage people to seek medical help, ensuring availability of physical infrastructure and female health providers, community level awareness and maternal education are much needed. This will help the population to upgrade their knowledge and perception towards women reproductive health issues. Broad conclusions from the study can be strengthened with a survey which must be covering more districts and more participants [36-42].

References

1. WHO (2016) Maternal Mortality: Fact sheet. Geneva.
2. Fenta M (2005) Assessment of factors affecting utilization of maternal healthcare services in Ayssaita and Dubti Towns, AFAR Regional State, North East Ethopia. Thesis submitted to The School of Graduate Studies of Addis Ababa University pp: 1-95.
3. Osubor KM, Fatusi AO, Chiwuzie JC (2006) Maternal health-seeking behavior and associated factors in a rural Nigerian Community. Maternal and Child Health Journal 10: 159-169.
4. Koenig MA, Jamil K, Streatfield PK, Saha T, Ahmed AS, et al. (2007) Maternal health and care-seeking behavior in Bangladesh: Findings from a national survey. International Family Planning Perspectives 33: 75-82.
5. Tasnim S, Rahman A, Chowdhury S, Shahabuddin A (2009) Challenges for utilization of antenatal and delivery care services in urban setting of Bangladesh. South Asian Federation of Obstetrics and Gynecology 2: 44-47.
6. Jayaraman A, Chandrasekhar S, Gebreselassie T (2008) Factors affecting maternal health care seeking behavior in Rwanda. Demographic and Health Research (Working paper) 59: 1-25.
7. Chomat AM, Solomons NW, Montenegro G, Crowley C, Bermudez OI (2014) Maternal health and health-seeking behaviors among indigenous Mam mothers from Quetzaltenango, Guatemala. Revista Panamericana Salud Publica 35: 113-120.
8. Benova L, Campbell OM, Sholkamy H, Ploubidis GB (2014) Socio-economic factors associated with maternal health-seeking behaviours among women from poor households in rural Egypt. Int J Equity Health 13: 1-14.
9. Navaneethama K, Dharmalingamb A (2002) Utilization of maternal health care services in Southern India. Social Science & Medicine 55: 1849-1869.
10. Agarwal P, Singh M, Garg S (2007) Maternal health-care utilization among women in an urban slum in Delhi. Indian J Comm Med 32: 203-205.
11. Mahapatro M (2015) Equity in utilization of health care services: Perspective of pregnant women in southern Odisha, India. Indian Journal Medical Research 142: 183-189.
12. Bhattacherjee S, Datta S, Saha JB, Chakraborty M (2013) Maternal health care services utilization in tea gardens of Darjeeling, India. J Basic Clin Reprod Sci 2: 77-84.
13. Srivastava A, Mahmood S, Mishra P, Shrotriya V (2014) Correlates of maternal health care utilization in Rohilkhand region, India. AMHSR 4: 417-425.
14. Tiwari S, Nigam R, Waware RS, Chandorkar RK (2014) Health care seeking behavior and awareness of maternal and child health practices in a rural village of Madhya Pradesh. National J Community Med 5: 105-108.
15. Khound S (2016) Utilization of maternal and child health care service: A case study in Jorhat district. Imperial J Interdisciplinary Research 2: 329-331.
16. Mazumder MN (2016) Utilization of maternal health care services among the karbis of Guwahati City. Indian Journal of Research 5: 404-406.
17. Mackian S, Bedri N, Hermione L (2004) Up the garden path and over the edge: where might health-seeking behaviour take us? Health Policy and Planning 19: 137-146.
18. Hosmer D, Lemeshow S (2000) Applied Logistic Regression. John Wiley & Sons. Inc.: USA.
19. Heinze G, Schemper M (2002) A solution to the problem of separation in logistic regression. Statistics in Medicine 21: 2409-2419.
20. Allison P (2003) Convergence problems in logistic regression. In: Altman M, Gill J, McDonald MP (1st Edtn.) Numerical issues in statistical computing for the social scientist. John Wiley & Sons, Inc. New York pp: 219-233.
21. Zorn C (2005) A solution to separation in binary response models. Political Analysis 13: 157-170.

22. Abrahantes JC, Aerts M (2012) A Solution to separation for clustered binary data. Statistical Modelling 12: 3-27.
23. Gelman A, Carlin JB, Stern HS, Dunsun DB, Vehtari A, et al. (2014) Bayesian data analysis. Taylor & Francis Group, New York.
24. Rainey C (2014) Dealing with separation in logistic regression models. Working paper, University of Buffalo pp: 1-34.
25. Gleia DA, Goldman N, Rodriguez G (2003) Utilization of care during pregnancy in rural Guatemala: does obstetrical need matter? Social Science & Medicine 57: 2447-2463.
26. Scheppers E, Dongen E, Dekker J, Geertzen J, Dekker J (2005) Potential barriers to the use of health services among ethnic minorities: a review. Family Practice 23: 325-348.
27. Singh RK (2012) Lifestyle behavior affecting prevalence of anemia among women in EAG states, India. Population Association of America 2012 Annual Meeting Program. San Francisco, CA pp: 1-22.
28. Qureshi RN, Sheikh S, Khowaja AR, Zaidi S, Sawchuck D, et al. (2013) Health care seeking behaviours in pregnancy in rural Sindh, Pakistan: a qualitative study. Reproductive Health 13: 75-81.
29. Ruth J, Tesfay FH, Gebrehiwot TG (2016) Health extension workers' and mothers' attitudes to maternal health service utilization and acceptance in Adwa Woreda, Tigray region, Ethiopia. PLoS One 11: 1-15.
30. Munguambe K, Boene H, Vidler M, Bique C, Sawchuck D, et al. (2016) Barriers and facilitators to health care seeking behaviors in pregnancy in rural communities of southern Mozambique. Reproductive Health 13: 83-97.
31. Babalola S, Fatusi A (2009) Determinants of use of maternal health services in Nigeria: Looking beyond individual and household factors. BMC Preg Childbirth 9: 1-13.
32. Ramarajan A (2011) Social cultural and economic issues in SAMM. In: Ramarajan A. Severe acute maternal morbidity. Jaypee Brothers Medical Publishers Private Limited. New Delhi, India pp: 1-252.
33. Yiran GSA, Teye JK, Yiran GA (2015) Accessibility and utilization of maternal health services by migrant female head porters in Accra. J Int Migration Integration 16: 929-945.
34. Simkhada B, Porter MA, Teijlingen ER (2010) The role of mothers-in-law in antenatal care decision-making in Nepal: a qualitative study. BMC Pregnancy and Childbirth 10: 1-10.
35. Centre for Operations Research and Training (CORT) (2007) Assessment of Janani Suraksha Yojana in Assam. Vadodara: Race Course Circle.
36. Chamberlain J, Watt S, Mohide P, Muggah H, Trim K, et al. (2007) Women's perception of self-worth and access to health care. Int J Gynecol Obstet 98: 75-79.
37. Currie D, Wiesenberg S (2010) Promoting women's health-seeking behavior: Research and empowerment of women. Health Care for Women International 24: 880-899.
38. Godefay H, Byass P, Graham WJ, Kinsman J, Mulugeta A (2015) Risk factors for maternal mortality in rural Tigray, Northern Ethiopia: A case-control study. PLoS one 10: 1-12.
39. Goubar A, Ades AE, Angelis DD, McGarrigle CA, Mercer CH, et al. (2008) Estimates of human immunodeficiency virus prevalence and proportion diagnosed based on Bayesian multiparameter synthesis of surveillance data. J Royal Statistical Society 171: 541-580.
40. Spiegelhalter DJ, Jones MJ (2000) Bayesian methods in health technology assessment: a review. Health Technology Assessment 4: 38.
41. Ward H, Mertens T, Thomas C (1997) Health seeking behavior and the control of sexually transmitted disease. Health Policy and Planning 12: 19-28.
42. Wilmoth J (2009) The lifetime risk of maternal mortality: Concepts and measurement. Bulletin of the World Health Organization 87: 256-262.

An Awareness and Experiences of Pregnant Women towards Antenatal Weight Management at a Maternity Hospital in Najran City, KSA

Nasser Saeed Al-Qahtani*

Department of Family and Community Medicine, College of Medicine, Najran University, KSA, Saudi Arabia

Corresponding author: Nasser Saeed Alqahtani, Assistant Professor, Department of Family and Community Medicine, College of Medicine, Najran University, KSA, Saudi Arabia, E-mail: drnasser1000@hotmail.com

Abstract

Background: One of health priorities for women during pregnancy is the attainment of healthy weight both in the antenatal and postpartum periods. This study is aiming to evaluate pregnant women awareness and experiences towards the management of obesity and weight gain during pregnancy.

Method: This was a cross-sectional study (n=416) conducted over 3 months in 2017 of pregnant women attending antenatal clinics at a maternity hospital, Najran city, KSA. An interviewer administered, questionnaire was used.

Findings: Results were shown 58.7% of participants (n=244) had low awareness for management of obesity and weight gain during pregnancy, with the highest level of awareness regarding management objectives and strategies (77.2%), while the lowest level of awareness folic acid (44%). In addition, 90.4% (n=376) showed poor experience in counselling about obesity management in pregnancy. Four risk factors were shown to be important indicators of awareness and experience of participants with largest being an occupation (Adjusted OR=2.7, p=0.001), nationality (Adjusted OR=2.4, p=0.015), regular follow up (Adjusted OR=1.7, p=0.049) and education level (Adjusted OR=1.3, p=0.009).

Conclusion: Study findings are consistent with earlier findings indicating that low level of awareness for management of bodyweight during pregnancy in addition to bad experience in counselling about recommended guidelines for that may explain up to some extent why women are not being served appropriately regarding bodyweight and its health risks in the antenatal care.

Keywords: Pregnancy; Caesarean section; Family planning; Bariatric surgery; Nutrition

Introduction

Obesity has become a worldwide epidemic health condition with estimates suggesting that over 50% of women enter pregnancy with a BMI in excess of 25 kg/m^2 [1]. It is evident that a combination of poor dietary choices, an increase in sedentary time and reduction in physical activity are all contributors to the development of overweight and obesity. One of health priorities for women during the childbearing stage is to implement interventions (e.g. having a healthy diet and undertaking enough moderate-to-vigorous physical activity) that aim to support attainment of healthy weight both during the antenatal and postpartum periods. With this in mind, current research has reviewed 44 randomized controlled trials (7278 women) where interventions including diet, physical activity or both were evaluated for their influence on maternal weight during pregnancy.

Results indicate that all were significantly effective in reducing gestational weight gain (GWG) compared with the control group [2]. A recent systematic review of the literature evaluated the adequacy and effectiveness of the methodological designs implemented in dietary intervention trials for obesity in pregnancy. Thirteen randomized controlled trials were identified where reduced gestational weight gain was observed in nine studies and a number of studies demonstrated improved dietary behaviour in response to diet and/or lifestyle interventions [3].

During the year 2010-2011, a retrospective study conducted in Al-Khobar city, Eastern Saudi Arabia, recommended that health education sessions should be conducted to all females with particular attention to pregnant women regarding hazards associated with overweight, obesity and the different methods of its control, with special emphasis on lifestyle modification [4]. However, many national studies addressed the prevalence of overweight and obesity in pregnancy and estimated the accompanied complications. As far as the researcher explored no local study focusing on weight managing during pregnancy, therefore this study aim to examine that issue in order to fill the gap between the guidelines and real practice.

Objectives

General objective

To evaluate the awareness and explore experience of pregnant women at maternity hospital, Najran city, KSA, concerning the management of obesity and weight gain during pregnancy.

Specific objectives

- To measure the level of awareness of pregnant women regarding the goals and strategies in treating obesity and weight gain during pregnancy.
- To measure the level of awareness of pregnant women regarding the nutrition guidance in treating obesity and weight gain during pregnancy.
- To measure the level of awareness of pregnant women regarding the exercise guidance in treating obesity and weight gain during pregnancy.
- To measure the level of awareness of pregnant women regarding the folic acid guidance in treating obesity and weight gain during pregnancy.
- To explore the experiences of pregnant women about counseling in treating obesity and weight gain during pregnancy.
- To identify the relevant factors that might affect the awareness and experiences of pregnant women toward the managing of obesity and weight gain during pregnancy.

Methodology

This study is a cross-sectional, interviewer administered, questionnaire-based survey, conducts from June to August 2017 in Najran city, which is a city in south-western Saudi Arabia. It is the capital of Najran Province. Designated a new town; its population has risen to 569332 persons in 2016, 253868 of them are women, around 67.6% of them in 15-64 year age group and 58.8% are married [5]. The antenatal health services are provided through different sectors with high preference and overutilization to Maternity and Children's Hospital, Najran where we conduct our study. The study population is all pregnant women attended antenatal clinic (ANC), the sampling frame is all pregnant women attended ANC in Najran Maternity & Children's Hospital during the study period, which were able to communicate and granted permission to participate in the study.

We enrol all listed in ANC register as simple random sampling, while the sample size determined (n=416) in taking account a 5% allowable error value (margin of error), 95% confidence level in addition to the prevalence of obesity and overweight in pregnancy in similar studies around 52% [4,6-9]. Researcher develops the questionnaire that has been pretested before using. It consists of two parts, part one is focusing on demographics, medical and gestational variables, part two is focusing on awareness and experiences toward the management of obesity and weight gain during pregnancy. While dependent variable is awareness and experiences towards the management of obesity and weight gain during pregnancy, and independent variables are all the demographic, medical, gestational characteristics (age, nationality, educational status, occupation, medical/surgical/psychiatric illness, medications, parity, caesarean section, miscarriage, gestational age, risk categories, family planning, antenatal care, weight in (pre-pregnancy/3 months) and clinician action toward weight (pre-pregnancy/3 months), awareness about management of obesity and weight gain during pregnancy (goals and strategies, nutrition guidance, exercise guidance, folic acid guidance), experience towards management of obesity and weight gain during pregnancy (receiving counselling, discussion about weight gain during pregnancy and readiness for healthy change, advise about obesity and its associated health risks that can be improved with good lifestyle habits, assessment for obesity and its related health risks during pregnancy and assisting for management obesity and weight gain during pregnancy).

The questionnaires content and relevance have been tested and evaluated for their appropriateness; reliability and average time needed to administer the questionnaire by pre-test have been conducted on 24 of the study population who did not include in the main study. Where the internal consistency was tested using Kurder Richardson 20 (KR-20) due to the dichotomous nature of the answers scores (Yes/No or do not know). KR-20 for all domains ranged from 0.71 for folic acid guidance to 0.86 for management goals and strategies, the tool stability was tested using test-retest reliability as measured by intra-class correlation coefficients (ICC) which ranged from 0.87 for experience to 0.99 for management goals and strategies. Content validity evaluated on reviewing all scale items by three different experts, any conflicts were treated using discussion or voting, and any suggested modifications were done. Construct validity validated using the simplest method using simple correlation coefficient and all items were highly correlated with its overall score (convergent validity) and poorly correlated with other domains totals (discriminant validity), correlation coefficients ranged from 0.38 to 0.95.

The questions in the questionnaire were prepared in a structured way in English and then translated into Arabic and again back to English by language professionals in each language, to see its consistency. One day training has been given to data collectors, in a face-to-face delivery mode; an interviewer is physically present to ask the questionnaire questions and to facilitate the respondent in answering them. Then, corrections have been made accordingly before the actual data collection time. After data was collected, it was checked for their completeness, coded and fed to statistical software IBM SPSS version 20. The given graphs were constructed using Microsoft Excel software.

All statistical analysis was done using two-tailed tests and an alpha error of 0.05. A P-value $\leq$ 0.05 was considered to be statistically significant. Regarding scoring system, the correct answer was given a score of one point otherwise, zero score was given. The items discrete scores of dimension and the total score was calculated by summing the scores given for its responses.

All scores were transformed into score percentage as:

Score %=(The observed score/The maximum score) $\times$ 100

Then score percentage (%) was categorized into poor awareness if the participant had core percentage (%) <60% and good awareness if score percentage (%) $\geq$ 60%.

Descriptive statistics

Frequencies and percentage were used to describe the frequency of each category for categorical data. Mean with standard deviation was used to describe scale data. Chi-square test/Mont Carlo exact test and Fishers exact test were used to test for association between awareness level and sample characteristics if there were many small expected values. Multiple logistic regression analysis was used to identify which of the studied factors can determine the participant level of awareness and on adjusting all other factors.

Results

All participants (n=416) completed questionnaire interview, with response rate 100%. Descriptive analysis of participants data (N=416) reveals that most are Saudi and ranged in age from 20 to 35. The majority were free of disease with notice (n=10, 2.4%) had been bariatric surgery. For most, the current pregnancy was a first for 23.6% and 13.5% labelled them in high-risk pregnancy. More than a third had a history of caesarean section and miscarriage (socio-demographic characteristics of all the interview participants can be found in Appendix A, with medical and obstetric details in Appendix B) (Tables 1-3 and Figure 1).

Domains	Poor		Good	
	No	Percentage (%)	No	Percentage (%)
Total Awareness Score	244	58.70%	172	41.30%
Management goals and strategies	62	14.90%	354	85.10%
Nutrition guidance	281	67.50%	135	32.50%
Exercise guidance	131	31.50%	285	68.50%
Folic acid guidance	257	61.80%	159	38.20%
Experience Score	376	90.40%	40	9.60%
Poor: Score % <60%		Good: Score % ≥ 60%		

Table 1: Awareness and experience level for management of obesity and weight gain during pregnancy of pregnant women attending Maternity and Children Hospital in Najran city, KSA during 2017.

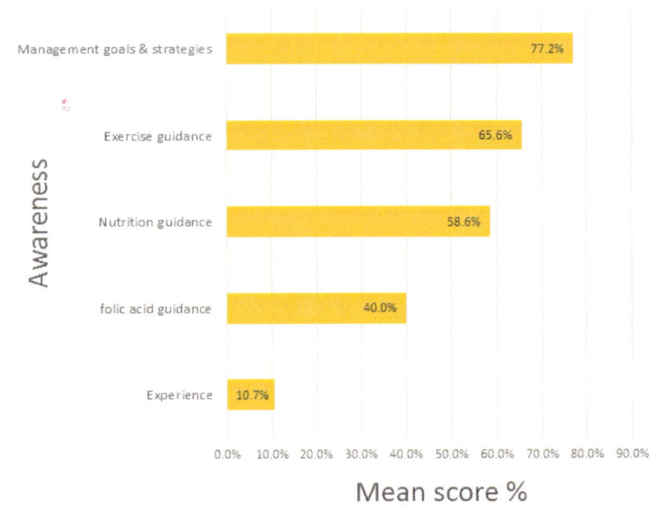

Figure 1: Average awareness and experience level for management of obesity and weight gain during pregnancy of pregnant women attending Maternity and Children Hospital in Najran city, KSA during 2017.

Variables		No	Percentage (%)
Antenatal care	Regular	324	77.90%
	Irregular	92	22.10%
Number of visits	1-4	161	38.70%
	5-11	255	61.30%
Health provider	One	177	42.50%
	Multiple	239	57.50%
Place of antenatal care	PHC	25	6.00%
	Maternity hospital	151	36.30%
	Private sector	2	0.50%
	Others	238	57.20%
Weight in pre-pregnancy/3 months	Normal	295	70.90%
	Abnormal	75	18.00%
	Don't know	46	11.10%
Clinician action towards weight (Pre-pregnancy/3 months)	Nothing	371	89.20%
	Reassurance	17	4.10%
	Counselling for weight loss	28	6.70%

Table 2: Antenatal care for pregnant women attending Maternity and Children Hospital in Najran city, KSA during 2017.

Variables		Yes		No		Don't know	
		No	%	No	%	No	%
Management goals and strategies	Do you think the obesity in pregnancy is a significant risk factor for adverse maternal and infant outcomes?	320	76.90%	34	8.20%	62	14.90%
	Do you think the pregnancy is opportunity for the promotion of healthy lifestyle behaviours?	338	81.30%	49	11.80%	29	7.00%
	Do you think that encourage is important factor for healthy lifestyle	394	94.70%	13	3.10%	9	2.20%
	Do you think that one of aims for management of obesity in pregnancy is loss of excess in preconception weight?	334	80.30%	30	7.20%	52	12.50%
	Do you think that one of aims for management of obesity in pregnancy is prevention the excess in gestational weight gain?	162	38.90%	183	44.00%	71	17.10%
	Do you know the recommended weight gain in obese pregnant women is 5-9 kg?	188	45.20%	55	13.20%	173	41.60%
	Do you think that providing counselling in nutrition & physical activity regarding obesity in pregnancy is recommended?	401	96.40%	5	1.20%	10	2.40%
	Do you think the drugs for obesity are not safe in pregnancy?	355	85.30%	22	5.30%	39	9.40%
	Do you think the obesity surgeries are not safe in pregnancy?	294	70.70%	25	6.00%	97	23.30%
	Do you think the herbal preparations for obesity are safe in pregnancy?	360	86.50%	24	5.80%	32	7.70%
	Do you think monitoring of weight throughout pregnancy and providing feedback on progress toward the goal are recommended?	385	92.50%	26	6.30%	5	1.20%
Nutrition guidance	Do you think that in first 3 months; a continuing same intake of total daily energy is recommended for obese pregnant?	86	20.70%	176	42.30%	154	37.00%
	Do you think that after first 3 months, an increasing daily calories by 400 calories is recommended for obese pregnant?	89	21.40%	82	19.70%	245	58.90%
	Do you think that keep balanced healthy food in pregnancy is recommended?	408	98.10%	6	1.40%	2	0.50%
	Do you think that consuming essential micronutrients -rich diets such as calcium, iron, folic acid and vitamin D in pregnancy is recommended?	392	94.20%	8	1.90%	16	3.80%
Exercise	Do you think that in the absence of either medical or obstetric complications the exercise is encouraged in pregnancy?	293	70.40%	93	22.40%	30	7.20%
	Do you think that physical activity for 30 minutes for most, if not all, days of the week is recommended?	307	73.80%	75	18.00%	34	8.20%
	Do you think that moderate intensity activities in pregnancy is recommended	219	52.60%	160	38.50%	37	8.90%
Folic acid guidance	Do you think that benefit of folic acid to prevent neural tube defect?	76	18.30%	46	11.10%	294	70.70%
	Do you think that obese pregnant at moderate risk of neural tube defect?	274	65.90%	10	2.40%	132	31.70%
	Do you think that take a higher dose (5 mg) of folic acid is recommended for obese pregnant?	107	25.70%	60	14.40%	249	59.90%
	Do you think that start to take a folic acid 3months before pregnancy is recommended?	193	46.40%	67	16.10%	156	37.50%
	Do you think that continue to take a folic acid throughout pregnancy is recommended for obese pregnant?	189	45.40%	91	21.90%	136	32.70%
Experience	I have been received counseling in the obesity and weight gain during pregnancy	69	16.60%	347	83.40%	0	0.00%
	I have been discussed about weight gain during pregnancy and readiness for healthy change	66	15.90%	350	84.10%	0	0.00%
	I have been advised about obesity and its associated health risks that can be improved with good lifestyle habits.	70	16.80%	346	83.20%	0	0.00%
	I have been assessed for obesity and its related health risks during pregnancy	55	13.20%	361	86.80%	0	0.00%

	I have been assisted for managing obesity and weight gain during pregnancy	31	7.50%	385	92.50%	0	0.00%

Table 3: Descriptive of dimensions of awareness and experience towards the management of obesity and weight gain during pregnancy of pregnant women attending Maternity and Children Hospital in Najran city, KSA during 2017.

In consideration of predictors of an awareness and experience regarding the management of obesity and weight gain during pregnancy, a multiple regression predicting an awareness and experience regarding the management of obesity and weight gain during pregnancy was conducted and statistics are provided in Table 4.

Predictor	S.E.	P	Adjusted OR	95% C.I for OR	
				Lower	Upper
Age	0.253	0.589	1.146	0.699	1.88
Nationality	0.351	0.015	2.354	1.183	4.685
Education level	0.114	0.009	1.348	1.078	1.685
Working	0.305	0.001	2.7	1.51	3.65
Medical history	0.838	0.072	4.511	0.873	23.306
Parity	0.197	0.134	1.343	0.913	1.976
Gestational age	0.167	0.94	1.1	0.711	1.62
High risk	0.331	0.864	1.2	0.494	1.808
Planned pregnancy	0.227	0.656	1.106	0.709	1.726
Regular ANC	0.273	0.049	1.7	1.1	2.71
Abnormal pre-pregnancy weight	0.169	0.8	1.044	0.749	1.453
Constant	1.805	0.581	0.369	-	-

Table 4: Results of multiple stepwise logistic regression for predictors of an awareness and experience regarding the managing of obesity and weight gain during pregnancy for pregnant women attending Maternity and Children Hospital in Najran city, KSA during 2017 [SE: Standard error; OR: Odds Ratio; C.I: Confidence interval].

Discussion

Many local studies estimated the prevalence of overweight and obesity, and found the overweight and obesity are common (>52%) among pregnant women in Saudi Arabia [4,6-9]. This study shows the most of the pregnant women have poor satisfaction level of awareness for management of obesity and weight gain during pregnancy in addition to bad experience in counselling about recommended guidelines for that (58.7% and 90.4% perceptively). These reasons (women awareness and counselling practicing) may explain up to some extent the dissociation between scientific guidelines and a real practice. Similar to international studies suggest that few women receive directed pre-conception health programs and interventions and research has found the reasons for this to be limited awareness of current pregnancy weight gain guidelines, belief that such counselling is ineffective, or awkwardness about raising the issue of weight and weight gain with women. One of them was largest Australian survey (n=2338) conducted over in 2015 of pregnant women attending antenatal clinics at four maternity hospitals, examining knowledge of expected weight gain in pregnancy, understanding of risks associated with excess GWG. It revealed only half the cohort (51.0%) understood the potential impact of excess GWG [10].

In our study a pregnant women express their experience in counselling about these guidelines, small percentage (16.8%) has been received counselling and discussed about weight gain during pregnancy and readiness for healthy change. Only 7.5% (n=31) has been assisted for that and 89.2% (n=371) had not been received any good action from caregivers towards their weight in pre-pregnancy and in first 3 months of pregnancy. Likewise in the recent cross-section study finding in the UK-the MAGIC study (MAnaging weiGht In pregnanCy) that sought to examine women's self-reported experiences of usual-care antenatal weight management in early pregnancy. In considering the sample (n=193) is not wholly representative of the population, 50.3% of participants (n=97) could be classified as overweight or obese and 69.4% of highest weight women ($\geq$ 30 kg/m^2) did not report receiving advice about weight [11].

The increasing prevalence of preconception overweight and obesity and excessive gestational weight gain is recognized as significant risk factor for adverse maternal and infant outcomes. The risks may involve the pregnancy, birth, and later life for both the woman and her infant. As well as an increase in the risk of diabetes and cardiovascular disease in later life has also been reported among women with excessive pregnancy weight gain [1].

In order to overcome the main risk factors for maternal obesity (i.e., sedentary lifestyles and unhealthy diet intake), lifestyles Interventions targeting maternal obesity are a health priority. We might consider pregnancy a chance to reverse the threat to opportunity for the promotion of healthy lifestyle behaviours, as many women are concerned about the health of their babies and are in frequent contact with prenatal care providers as well as to minimize other comorbidities.

This study reveals that 76.9% (n-320) know that obesity has an adverse effect on pregnancy outcome, the majority (above 80%) think a pregnancy is an opportunity for the promotion of healthy lifestyle behaviours and encourage is an important factor for that with the importance of providing counselling in nutrition and physical activity. Although the avoidance of excess gestational weight gain is a high-value aim in the management of obesity in pregnancy, around 38.9% of pregnant in this study agree with that and 45.2% know the recommended gestational weight gain in obese pregnant women.

Management of maternal obesity prior to and during pregnancy is crucial care. This includes dietary measures and encouraging the modest increase in exercise. Ideally, the mother should achieve closer to an ideal body mass index prior to pregnancy using lifestyle intervention (e.g. routine physical activity (in those without contraindications); providing nutritional guidance and caloric literacy, maintain a food diary and physical activity log and tracking gestational weight gain) [12] but possibly with pharmacological therapy or bariatric surgery. The ideal weight gain for an obese mother is less than the ideal weight gain for non-obese mother [13]. Institute of Medicine recommendation for optimal weight gain during pregnancy recommended total weight gain range (13 to 18 kg) for underweight (BMI<18.5 kg per m^2), (11 to 16 kg) for normal weight (BMI 18.5 to 24.9 kg per m^2), (7 to 11 kg) for overweight (BMI 25.0 to 29.9 kg per m^2) and (5 kg to 9 kg) for obese (BMI $\geq$ 30.0 kg per m^2) [14].

Around 67.5% (n=281) in this study have poor awareness regarding nutrition guidance and 85.3%, 70.7% think the drugs and surgery for obesity are not safe in pregnancy respectively, but 86.5% think the herbal for obesity are safe in pregnancy. Although 65.9% think that obese pregnant at moderate risk of neural tube defect as it proved in recent guidelines [15], only 18.3% and 25.7% know the role of folic acid and the recommended dose in the management of obesity and weight gain during pregnancy, respectively. This is an example of many an interventions and procedures that may not well clarified for the client.

As there are numerous effective interventions for women who are overweight or obese, a systematic review found that medically supervised programs are more expensive and have higher rates of attrition, but are associated with greater weight loss (15% to 25%), compared with other types of commercial diets programs [16]. In Belgium, one randomized controlled trial design study evaluated the effect of lifestyle intervention in helping obese pregnant women limit their weight gain during pregnancy and improving their psychological comfort. Of the 235 eligible obese pregnant women randomized to a control group, a brochure group receiving written information on healthy lifestyle and an experimental group receiving lifestyle intervention sessions by a midwife trained in motivational lifestyle intervention. It concluded that a targeted lifestyle intervention programme based on the principles of motivational interviewing reduces gestational weight gain (GWG) and levels of anxiety in obese pregnant women [17].

However, for more effective antenatal interventions, the literature stated some strategies - including: engage prenatal care providers to develop consistent messages, train and prepare prenatal care providers to counsel women about healthy weight gain in pregnancy and address weight bias attitudes among prenatal care providers and motivational dialogue between pregnant women and prenatal care providers is needed before and throughout pregnancy [12]. In the USA, at the University of Illinois at Chicago investigate perceptions of minority pregnant women and providers about obesity and gestational weight gain (GWG). Sixteen obese pregnant women and 19 prenatal care providers participated in focus groups about prenatal care of body weight. Although, women were interested in learning about nutrition and reported self-encouragement, providers expressed discomfort-discussing GWG and they noted the challenges they faced during prenatal care including time constraints, cultural myths, and system issues. Providers considered a group setting with social support an ideal environment to address health behaviours in obese women [18]. Arguably, a shortage in medical staff, overcrowded clinical practice and complex health providing systems rather than doctor-patient dialogue should be taking account.

Four risk factors emerged from multiple logistic regression analysis are significant predictors. Employed women have good awareness and experience (Adjusted OR=2.7, p=0.001), Saudi woman have good awareness and experience more than two folds than non-Saudi (Adjusted OR=2.4, p=0.015), women enrolled in regular ANC have good awareness and experience in comparison with those have irregular follow up (Adjusted OR=1.7, p=0.049) as well as those get high level of education (Adjusted OR=1.3, p=0.009). The probable justification of the contribution of previous independent predictors for good awareness and experience among pregnant women attending Maternity and Children Hospital in Najran city towards the management of obesity and weight gain during pregnancy, women who have high education level and employed are willing to compensate their medical demands. Moreover, citizenship preferences for free access to health service either health education or counselling sessions as well as the benefits of regular and accumulative antenatal care.

Conclusion

- The antenatal period offers a unique opportunity to counter the current unsatisfied management for obesity and weight gain where bodyweight should be an issue to be addressed during pregnancy
- Moreover, exploring why women are not being served appropriately regarding obesity and overweight in the antenatal care and the solutions for that are strongly proposed
- Further works are needed to move away from the current low level of awareness to better-informed society
- Build the capacity of practitioners to deliver evidenced based individualized weight-related counseling

Acknowledgement

I would like to thank our colleagues from Maternity and Children's Hospital, Najran who provided support that greatly assisted in conduction of the research. I thank Health Research Consultancy Office (Research) for assistance with data analysis.

Disclosure of Interests

The researcher is faculty member of college of medicine in Najran University. He received administrative support from family and community medicine department at college of medicine and Maternity and Children's Hospital in Najran city, while the budget is researcher dependent.

Author Contribution

All of work including-substantial contributions to conception and design, or acquisition of data, or analysis and interpretation of data; and drafting the article or revising it critically for important intellectual content; and final approval of the version to be published; and accountability for all aspects of the work-was managed by the researcher and under his responsibility.

References

1. Dodd JM, Grivell RM, Louise J, Deussen AR, Giles L, et al. (2017) The effects of dietary and lifestyle interventions among pregnant women who are overweight or obese on longer-term maternal and early childhood outcomes⊠: Protocol for an individual participant data (IPD) meta-analysis 6: 1-12.
2. Spencer L, Rollo M, Hauck Y, Wicks L, Wood L, et al. (2015) The effect of weight management interventions that include a diet component on weight-related outcomes in pregnant and postpartum women: A systematic review protocol. JBI Database System Rev Implement Rep 13: 88-98.
3. Flynn A, Dalrymple K, Barr S, Poston L, Goff L, et al. (2016) Dietary interventions in overweight and obese pregnant women: A systematic review of the content, delivery, and outcomes of randomized controlled trials. Nutr Rev 74: 312-328.
4. Hafez AS, Sabra AA (2012) Prevalence of maternal obesity and pregnancy outcome among normal and high risk pregnant women in Al-Khobar city, Eastern region, Saudi Arabia 1: 11-9.
5. Demographic Survey 2016, General Authority for Statistics, KSA.
6. Asmari B, Alsaleem S, Shahrani A, Khaldi Y, Alqahtani M, et al. (2015) Weight status among pregnant women in Aseer region, Saudi Arabia. Saudi J Obes 3: 55.
7. Meher N, Aslam M, Ahmed SR, Rajab M, Kattea L (2009) Impact of obesity on fetomaternal outcome in pregnant Saudi females. Int J Heal Sci 3: 187-195.
8. Hafez S, Hafez SK, Dorgham L, Sayed SA (2014) Profile of high risk pregnancy among Saudi women in Taif, KSA. World Journal of Medical Sciences 11: 90-97.
9. Gilany AH, Wehady A (2009) Prevalence of obesity in a Saudi obstetric population. Obes Facts 2: 217-220.
10. Cheney K, Berkemeier S, Sim KA, Gordon A, Black K (2017) Prevalence and predictors of early gestational weight gain associated with obesity risk in a diverse Australian antenatal population: A cross-sectional study. BMC Pregnancy Childbirth 17: 296.
11. Swift JA, Pearce J, Jethwa PH, Taylor MA, Avery A, et al. (2016) Antenatal weight management: Women's experiences, behaviours, and expectations of weighing in early pregnancy. J Pregnancy P: 8454759.
12. Institute SP (2014) Interventions for weight management in pregnancy interventions for weight management in pregnancy: Overview of systematic review and meta-analysis studies executive summary.
13. Shaikh H, Robinson S, Teoh TG (2010) Management of maternal obesity prior to and during pregnancy. Semin Fetal Neonatal Med 15: 77-82.
14. Garrison AW (2013) Obesity in pregnancy. Am Fam Physician 87: 607-608.
15. https://www.rcog.org.uk/globalassets/documents/guidelines/cmacercogjointguidelinemanagementwomenobesitypregnancya.pdf
16. Farahi N, Zolotor A (2013) Recommendations for pre-conception counselling and care. Am Fam Physician 88: 499-506.
17. Bogaerts AFL, Devlieger R, Nuyts E, Witters I, Gyselaers W, et al. (2012) Effects of lifestyle intervention in obese pregnant women on gestational weight gain and mental health: A randomized controlled trial. Int J Obesity 37: 81421.
18. Kominiarek MA, Gay F, Peacock N, Medicine F (2016) Obesity in pregnancy: A qualitative approach to inform an intervention for patients and providers 19: 1698-1712.

12

Factors Affecting Women-Willingness to Pay for Maternal, Neonatal and Child Health Services (MNCH) in Gombe State, Nigeria

Muhammad Basheer Yahya* and Tepanata Pumpaibool

Department of Clinical Pharmacy and Pharmaceutical Care, Faculty of Pharmaceutical Sciences, Gombe State University, Gombe, Nigeria

***Corresponding author:** Muhammad Basheer Yahya, Lecturer, Department of Clinical Pharmacy and Pharmaceutical Care, Faculty of Pharmaceutical Sciences, Gombe State University, Gombe, Nigeria, E-mail: mybasheer@yahoo.com

Abstract

Background: Gombe State in North Eastern Nigeria is one of the states in the region that records the highest maternal and new-born death rates in the world. The region has a maternal mortality ratio of 1549/100,000, child mortality rate of 260/1,000 and neonatal mortality rate of 43/1,000. With a poverty incidence of 72.2% in the state and the displacement due to insurgency, a great deal of women in the villages is vulnerable to more poverty and maternal deaths. Establishing the factors that affect the willingness to pay (WTP) for maternal services will help to improve maternal health services thereby reducing maternal deaths in the state. This study looked at the factors that affect women's willingness to pay for maternal services in relation to antenatal care (ANC), delivery in health facilities and post-natal care (PNC) through a baseline survey.

Methods: This study was cross sectional where data were collected from women groups (including women not registered with the groups) in two purposively selected Local Government Areas (LGAs) of the state. Seven hundred and fifty (750) women were sampled for the survey in the two LGAs. The main outcome variables are utilization of maternal service (specifically improved antenatal care attendance, facility delivery and postnatal care) and WTP for these services by the women. Descriptive statistics of the respondents were analysed using IBM SPSS 22 software. Logistic regression analysis was done to determine the factors affecting WTP for the maternal services.

Results: The findings from this study have shown statistically significant association between WTP for maternal health care and several factors. Women are more likely to be willingness to pay for ANC and delivery in the health facility if they belong to the savings and loans group ($p<0.05$), had an average of 1-10 visits to a facility, married ($p<0.05$), can read and write in English ($p<0.05$) and live near health facilities ($p<0.05$). Income and employment ($p<0.05$) are additional factors affecting WTP for delivery. Post-natal care on the other hand was only associated with membership of savings and loans group.

Conclusions: Factors associated with the willingness to pay ANC and delivery in health facilities according to the findings of this study were membership of savings and loans group, closeness to a health facility, education, income and marital status. Number of previous visits to the health facility and occupation were also found to be significant predictors of willingness to pay for maternal services. Further studies on the association of WTP and PNC are suggested in order to improve PNC in the state.

Keywords: Maternal health; Poverty; Pregnancy; Delivery; Immunization

Introduction

Women have pivotal roles to play in the traditional and cultural lives of African societies. They have greater burden in carrying pregnancies, childbirth, rearing children and ensuring their adequate parenting as well as balancing their social contracts with their husbands. These burdens exert economic and social pressure on women who do not have any tangible means of livelihood apart from heavily relying on their husbands for their upkeep. This is a reality especially in our rural communities in North Eastern Nigeria where a mixture of religion, culture and low literacy all combine to shape the image of women in this region. The consequence therefore, is a pool of women who cannot afford to cater for their needs including the uptake of basic health-services for themselves and their children. This puts them at greater risk of maternal deaths from pregnancy related complications and deliveries attended to by unskilled personnel. Hence, it is not surprising that Gombe State in North Eastern Nigeria is one of the states in the region that records the highest maternal and new-born death rates in the world [1]. The National Health Insurance Scheme (NHIS) that is supposed to cover the general population has very low coverage and mostly enjoyed by urban and more educated women. Less than 2% of women age 15-49 have health insurance in Nigeria and that covers employees in the formal sector [2]. Women are therefore, left with no choice but to use out of pocket expenses to pay for their health needs further depleting their meagre resources and plunging them into more impoverishment. The logical thing to do is to empower these women economically to be able to have the independence to cater for their own basic needs, which include the utilization and payment for their maternal, neonatal and child health services [3]. A number of international donor organizations have supported some women groups in Northern Nigeria to improve access and utilization of maternal and child health services. This support came through different models of empowerment, which included provision of matching grants, training on small income generating activities and facilitation of access to loans.

Targeted States High Impact Project (USAID funded) supported the formation of 100 Women groups in Bauchi and Sokoto states with the aim of helping women to increase their voices and gain more control of local decisions within communities and in households [4]. The groups later introduced internal savings and lending components within them enabling them to engage in trading activities. Gombe State is one of the 36 states of the federal republic of Nigeria, located in the Centre of the North Eastern part of the country (Figure 1).

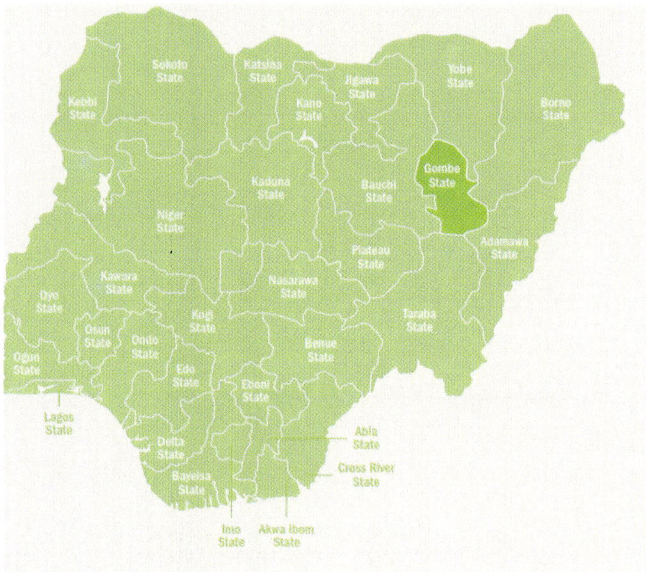

Figure 1: Map of Nigeria showing the study state.

The State has a population of 2,587,159 of which 50.1% (1,296,166) is male while 49.9% (1,290,993) is female and has a population growth of 3.2% annually [5] and the vegetation is guinea-savannah grassland. The budgetary allocation for health in the state stands at 2.1% of the total budget for the state, which is grossly inadequate for the effective delivery of health care in the state. Considering the poor maternal and child indicators, the Gombe State Strategic Health Development Plan (GSSHDP) for 2010-2015 had identified priority intervention areas to focus attention on. Maternal, perinatal and under five mortality will be addressed and reduced through implementing high impact public health interventions including the use of long lasting insecticidal treated nets (LLINs), intermittent preventive treatment (IPT), scaling up obstetric services, improved immunization and treatment of childhood illnesses [6]. Poverty incidence in the state is very high at 72.2%; this is coupled with the high out-of-pocket expenditures as citizens are not covered by NHIS in the state. ANC attendance for women is 58.2%, delivery in health facility is 27.6% and PNC check up by women in the first two days after birth is 32.8% [2]. A number of factors have been found to be significantly associated with WTP for health care from some studies. Age, education, income, quality of health care services and location (urban/rural) [7] were some of the factors documented to be influencing health care services. Information on cost to clients and their perception about the good quality of care was also essential factors found to be affecting changes in WTP [8]. This study conducted a baseline survey of the women groups to determine their "willingness to pay" for maternal and child health services (ANC, delivery and PNC), and to also determine the factors associated with the women's WTP from the baseline results.

Methods

Design

The design of the study was cross-sectional where data from baseline survey were collected. The methodology was quantitative involving data collection from members and non-members of women's savings and loan groups on their maximum willingness to pay for ANC, delivery at health facility and PNC and their utilization of maternal health services.

Study area

The study area was the north eastern state of Gombe, Nigeria. The choice of the state was based on the implementation of women groups in the state and its poor health indices, poverty exacerbated by the ongoing insurgency in the region further worsening the utilization of health services. Gombe (urban) and Kaltungo (rural/semi-urban) LGAs of the state were chosen for the study (Figure 2).

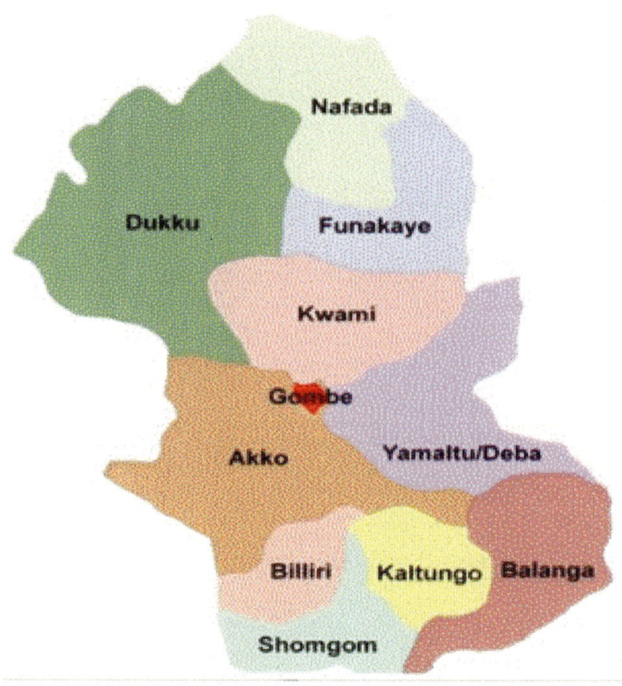

Figure 2: Map of Gombe State showing the local LGAs.

Two political wards in each the two LGAs were selected and women groups members from each of the two political wards were enrolled for the study. In each of the two LGAs, one ward was selected where women not participating in the women groups were enrolled.

Study period

The period of the study was for one month in August 2016 within which the baseline data on women groups were collected and analyzed.

Study population

The population for this study was the women in Gombe state registered as Mothers Groups that engaged in voluntary savings and loans schemes managed and supported by the state, civil society organizations and Non-Governmental Organization (NGO) partners. Women who did not belong to the women savings groups were also included for the purpose of comparison.

Sample and sample size

For the purpose of WTP estimation using Contingent Valuation Method (CVM), there is no literature on the standard formula for estimation of the sample size. However, previous studies on CVM have found out that at least 600 samples and 400 samples are required each for single bound and double bound CV methods respectively in order to ensure the statistical reliability of WTP estimations [9]. Considering the fact that the target population is the women groups and each group had between 25-30 members, and the two wards selected had five groups each, the sample size for one LGA was estimated at 250. The sample size for the 2 LGAs was therefore 500 taking the lower limit of 25 members per group. In the control wards, 125 women were sampled each based on the availability of five groups in each of the intervention wards.

Sampling technique

Purposive sampling was used in this study. Two LGAs Gombe (urban) and Kaltungo (rural/semi-urban) were purposively selected for the study. This was to allow for a mix of urban and rural characteristics of the women to be studied. Out of these two LGAs, the number of existing and registered women groups in the political wards of the LGA were identified and documented. Gombe LGA had 30 registered mothers Groups in six wards while Kaltungo LGA had 30 in 5 wards. Each ward had an average of five groups with minimum membership of 25 members. Two political wards were randomly selected from each of the two LGAs-Herwa Gana and Shamaki in Gombe LGA and Awak and Ture in Kaltungo LGA. All the women groups from each of the two wards were enrolled for this study. This gave 500 members in the two study LGAs within the 4 sampled wards. One ward in each of the sampled LGAs that did not have registered women groups for the intervention was randomly selected to serve as control (Bolari East ward in Gombe LGA and Kaltungo West in Kaltungo LGA). In each of the control wards, 125 women were sampled for the survey (Figure 3).

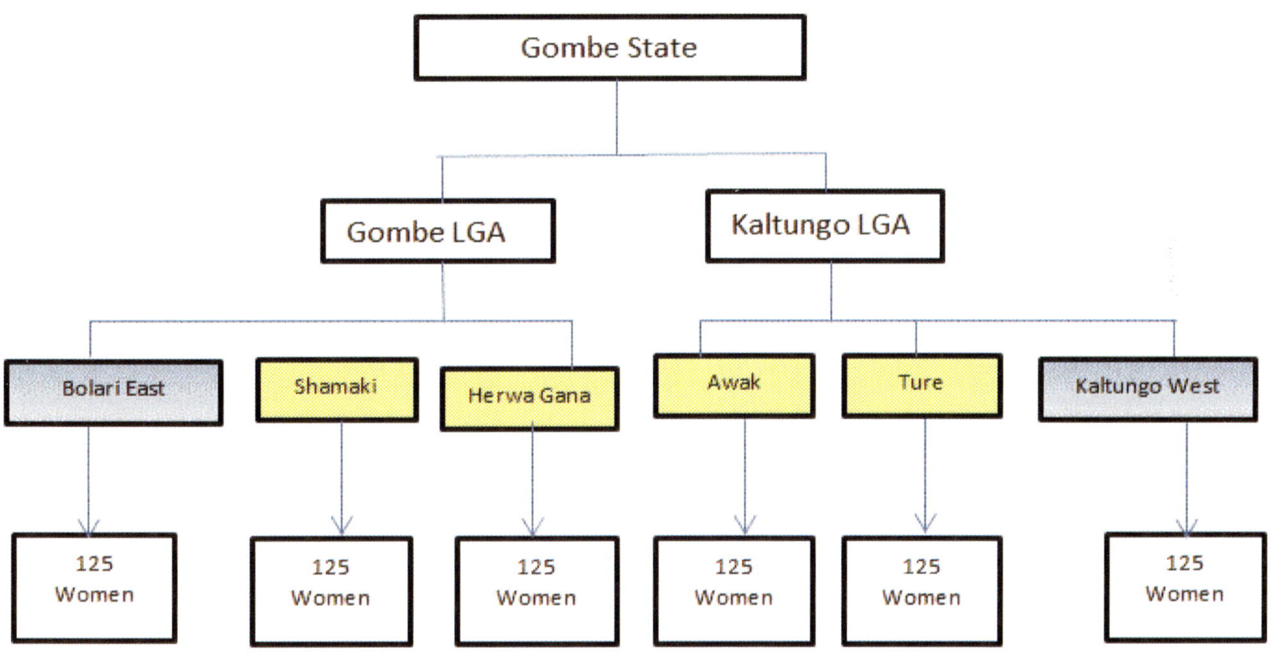

Figure 3: Flow chart for the sampling strategy.

These women were also of childbearing ages that did not belong to any women savings group but with similar demographic and socio-economic characteristics.

Data collection

Trained survey assistants through questionnaires collected data and the process was paper-based. The questionnaire had three sections containing questions on background and household characteristics of the women, their knowledge of vital maternal health issues, literacy and numeracy skills and WTP for maternal care. The household survey tools used by IDEAS project of the London School of Hygiene and Tropical Medical in their evaluation of MNCH interventions in Gombe were adapted [10]. Questions on WTP for maternal services for the women's saving groups were also adapted from willingness to pay surveys manual [11]. The questionnaires were in three parts and covered socio-economic and demographic data of the women, their knowledge and utilization of maternal health, educational level as well as their WTP for ANC, Delivery and PNC. The questionnaires were first translated into Hausa language, pretested and deployed in the field.

Data analysis

Quantitative data were collected and entered into Microsoft Excel and analysed using IBM SPSS Statistics 22 software. Descriptive statistics for the two groups were analysed at baseline. Binary logistic regression analysis was used for selected demographic and socio-economic factors to determine their relationship with the respondents' WTP for ANC, delivery in health facility and PNC.

Results

Seven hundred and fifty (750) women were sampled for the survey in two LGAs of the state one hundred kilometers apart and 689 responded (response rate of 91.9%). Women aged between 25-34 years constituted 41.2% of the sample. Islam is the religion of 65% of the women and 80% were pregnant before but 22.8% were currently pregnant. Only 25.1% of the women had ability to read and write in English but 52% could read and write in Hausa and Arabic. In terms of decision to spend the money they earn, 34.8% of the respondents take decision on their own, while on health care decisions only 12.5% take those decisions independently. The average monthly income of 48.9% of the women was below N500.00 (Nigeria Naira=$1.38) and 77.8% of them were unemployed and 84.8% married. Almost 90% of the respondents had Primary Health Care (PHC) centres available near them and 78% of them had course to visit the facilities at least once in the last six (6) months before the survey. Out of the 22% that gave reasons for their visit, 2.8% was for ANC, less than 1% for delivery and 1.5% for PNC. Walking was the major means of getting to the facilities for 81.7% of the women and 86% of them took between one and thirty minutes to reach the health facility from their houses (Table 1).

Variables		Frequency	Percentage (%)
Marital Status	Married	584	84.8
	Single	24	3.5
	Widowed/divorced	81	11.8
Age	15-24 years	229	33.2
	25-34 years	284	41.2
	35-44 years	154	22.4
	45-49 years	22	3.2
Religion	Islam	448	65
	Christianity	241	35
Pregnancy history	Previously pregnant	551	80
	Currently pregnant	157	22.8
Literacy	Ability to read or write in English	173	25.1
	Ability to read or write in other language	358	52
Decision on money spending	Respondent	240	34.8
	Husband/Partner	242	35.1
	Respondent and Husband/partner jointly	172	25
	Someone else	10	1.5
	Other	25	3.6
Decision on Health Care	Respondent	86	12.5
	Husband/Partner	287	41.7
	Respondent and Husband/partner jointly	276	40.1
	Someone else	16	2.3
	Other	24	3.5
Monthly Income	<N500	337	48.9

	N501-N1000	102	14.8
	N1001-N1500	40	5.8
	N1501-N2500	77	11.2
	>N2500	133	19.3
Occupation	Employed	21	3
	Self-employed	132	19.2
	Unemployed	536	77.8
PHC Facility	Availability	611	88.7
Number of visits to PHC Facility (last six months)	0 visit	153	22.2
	1-10 visits	527	76.5
	11-20 visits	6	0.9
	21-30 visits	3	0.4
Reasons for last visit to PHC	No response	538	78.1
	Family Planning	48	7
	Child Immunization	1	0.1
	Antenatal care	19	2.8
	Delivery care	4	0.6
	Post-Partum Care	10	1.5
	Neonatal Care	9	1.3
	Campaign	13	1.9
	Child Health Check	47	6.8
Reasons for non-visit	No reasons	153	22.2
	No illness in the family/No birth	314	45.6
	Facility too far away	140	20.3
	Costs too much money to go to health facility	82	11.9
Means of transportation to PHC Facility	Walking	563	81.7
	Bicycle	9	1.3
	Motor Vehicle	41	6
	Motor Bike	67	9.7
	Donkey/Horse/Cart	9	1.3
Time to PHC	1-30 minutes	592	86
	31-60 minutes	87	12.6
	61-120 minutes	10	1.5

Table 1: Demographic and socio-economic characteristics of the women.

The maximum willingness to pay for the women varied significantly based on the maternal health service sought (Table 2). PNC was found to be having the lowest value of N6000 ($16.48) with a mean of N552.60 followed by ANC with a value of N10000 ($27.47) and a mean of N786.79. Delivery services had the highest willingness to pay value at N50000 ($137.37) with a mean of N1013.34. Mean monthly income for the women was N1958.65 ($5.38).

Variables	WTPMAX for ANC	WTPMAX for Delivery	WTPMAX for PNC
Mean	786.79	1013.34	552.6
Median	500	500	500
Mode	1000	1000	500
std. deviation	1025.16	2628.67	576.44
Maximum	10000	50000	6000

Table 2: Descriptive statistics for the willingness to pay for ANC, Delivery and PNC (WTPMAX is the maximum willingness to pay).

To investigate the factors affecting WTP for ANC, Delivery and PNC, the following independent variables of interest from the socio-economic and demographic data were entered into the regression models: Marital Status, Age, Education, Religion, Average minimum income and decision on money spending and health care. Others were history of previous pregnancy, number of visits to the PHC facility as well as reasons for visit and non-visit. Willingness to pay for ANC, delivery and PNC were the three dependent variables for the three separate binary logistic regression models. The results of the regression analysis in Table 3 below show that Education (ability to read and write in English ($p<0.05$, OR=0.519), membership of savings and loans group ($p<0.001$, OR=0.149), occupation (Employed, p=0.02, OR=0.218) and marital status (p=0.005, OR=2.159) were found to have significant relationship with WTP for ANC.

Similarly, availability of PHC facility near the respondents ($p<0.001$, OR=0.163), higher monthly income (p=0.023, OR=0.463) and an average of one to ten previous visits to the facility (p=0.003, OR=0.511) were all significant predictors of WTP for ANC. WTP for Delivery was also found to be significantly associated with education of the women ($p<0.005$, OR=0.512) and membership of savings and loans group (p=0.005, OR=0.515). At least one to ten previous visits to the PHC facility ($p<0.001$, OR=0.299) and Marital status (p=0.018, OR=1.897) were also found to predict WTP for delivery significantly. Willingness to pay for PNC was found to be associated with membership of savings and loans groups only amongst all the other variables (p=0.048, OR=1.535) (Table 3).

Variables		ANC			Delivery			PNC		
		B	S.E.	OR	B	S.E.	OR	B	S.E.	OR
Membership of Savings and loans group		-1.904	0.266	0.149*	-0.663	0.235	0.515*	0.429	0.216	1.535*
Marital Status (Married)		0.77	0.274	2.159*	0.64	0.271	1.897*	-0.008	0.238	0.992
	English	-0.656	0.21	0.519*	-0.669	0.222	0.512*	0.211	0.187	1.235
Education	Other Languages	-0.333	0.18	0.717	-0.036	0.181	0.964	-0.069	0.161	0.934
	Availability of PHC facility nearby	-1.815	0.468	0.163**	-0.311	0.28	0.733	-0.275	0.272	0.759
	Transport means to PHC (Walking)	0.263	0.26	1.301	-0.083	0.24	0.92	0.008	0.22	1.008
PHC Facility	Number of Visits to PHC facility (1-10 visits)	-0.672	0.225	0.511*	-1.208	0.216	0.299*	-0.1	0.205	0.905
Pregnancy history	Previously Pregnant	0.237	0.297	1.267	-0.168	0.267	0.845	-0.47	0.257	0.625
	Currently Pregnant	0.182	0.224	1.2	-0.35	0.229	0.705	-0.07	0.195	0.932
	N0-N500	-0.383	0.243	0.682	-0.285	0.237	0.752	-0.027	0.215	0.973
	N501-N1000	-0.384	0.309	0.681	0.017	0.295	1.017	-0.015	0.274	0.985
Monthly income	N1001-1500	-0.656	0.427	0.519	-0.84	0.459	0.432	0.124	0.374	1.132
	N1501-2500	-0.77	0.338	0.463*	-0.542	0.337	0.582	0.395	0.305	1.484
	Employed	-1.522	0.606	0.218*	-0.77	0.661	0.463	0.073	0.469	1.075
	Self-employed/Unemployed	0.06	0.225	1.062	0.172	0.229	1.188	-0.221	0.201	0.802
Occupation	Constant	4.836	1.382	125.966	5.105	1.434	164.902	1.019	1.351	2.769
Calculation Index										

Model Chi-square	181.558 (p-value<0.001)	99.827 (p<0.001)	16.953 (p=0.568)
-2 log likelihood	764.521	780.85	913.144
Cox and Snell R^2	0.232	0.109	0.135
Nagelkerke R^2	0.31	0.152	0.189

Table 3: Logistic regression analysis results for factors affecting WTP for ANC, Delivery and PNC (*p<0.05, **p<0.001).

Discussion

In this study, we found several factors having relationship with women's willingness to pay for maternal services from their demographic and socio-economic characteristics. WTP for ANC was associated with more factors as compared to WTP for delivery and PNC. Membership of savings and loan groups, availability of primary health care facility close to the women, education (reading and writing in English) and employment were significant factors predicting WTP for ANC. Marital status, average monthly income and number of visits to the health facility was also found to have relationship with WTP for ANC. These results are consistent with findings from previous studies where living within 5 km radius of a facility was associated with ANC use [12].

Past experience of childbirth, distance and cost of transportation to health facility were equally associated with ANC use [13]. Previous studies found that Income and education for women affect WTP for maternal health [6,14]. Since maternal health information, education and communication materials are in English, women especially in the urban and rural areas who can read and write in English are likely to have more WTP for ANC in comparison to the women who do not have that ability. In the same vein, membership of savings and loans group, marital status, education and number of previous visits to the facility in the last 6 months were also found to be significant predictors of WTP for delivery in a health facility from the regression results. Women that had at least 1-10 visits to the health facility were more likely to be willing to pay more for delivery services as compared to those with more visits.

This could be due to the additional out of pocket expenses with each additional visit to the health facility. Interestingly, the respondents' independent decision on money spending and seeking health were not found to have any relationship with WTP for pregnancy in this study. This is in contrast to what Fawsitt and colleagues found out that if women were involved in decision-making actively during labour, it increased their willingness to pay more in order to have improvement of maternity services [15]. Mohale and colleagues documented the relationship between women's literacy and improved utilization of maternity care [16]. This agrees with the significant relationship of education in this study as a factor affecting WTP for delivery.

The regression model for willingness to pay for PNC and socio-demographic variables did not show any significant association between the variables and willingness to pay for PNC except membership of saving and loans group. The lack of association between the women's willingness to pay for PNC and their socio-economic and demographic characteristics on the other hand might be an indication of their ignorance on the importance of PNC in preventing maternal and child mortality.

This confirms the findings of Nigeria demographic and health survey where the percentage of women with a post-natal check up in the first two days after birth was only 32.8% [2]. This is also in agreement with the findings of Albers where they identified postpartum care as the most neglected component of maternity services [17]. In a recent qualitative study, low post-natal visits have been associated with limited value placed on post-natal care by women and providers [18]. All these might explain why willingness to pay for PNC has not been found to be associated with any of the variables tested apart from membership of savings group. However, we suggest further studies on the association of WTP and PNC and the prompt intervention of the State Government towards more funding and political support to improve PNC in the state.

Ethical Considerations

Ethical clearance was obtained from the Gombe state Ministry of Health Ethical Research Committee prior to the commencement of the study. All eligible women who participated in the survey signed consent forms describing this study and providing sufficient information for them to make an informed decision about their participation.

Conclusion

In conclusion, the most important factors associated with the willingness to pay maternal services according to the findings of this study are membership of savings and loan group, closeness to a health facility, education, income and marital status. Occupation and number of previous visits to the health facility were equally found to be significant predictors of willingness to pay for maternal services.

References

1. Schellenberg JA, Avan BI (2012) Data informed platform for health feasibility study report, Gombe State, Nigeria.
2. National Population Commission (2014) Nigeria and ICF International: Nigeria demographic and health survey 2013. Abuja, Nigeria, and Rockville, Maryland, USA: NPC and ICF International.
3. Chiang C, Elshair IH, Kawaguchi L, Fouad NA, Abdou NM, et al. (2012) Improvements in the status of women and increased use of maternal health services in rural Egypt. Nagoya J Med Sci 74: 233.
4. 100 women group movement: A platform for increased women's empowerment, stronger voice in governance, and accelerated access to health services.
5. National Population Commission. Population and housing census of the Federal Republic of Nigeria. Priority tables (2006).
6. Gombe State Government Strategic Health Development Plan (2010-2015).
7. El-Shiekh B, Kwaak A (2015) Factors influencing the utilization of maternal health care services by nomads in Sudan. Pastoralism 5: 23.
8. Gartoulla P, Liabsuetrakul T, Pradhan N (2010) Change in willingness to pay for normal delivery and caesarean section during pregnancy and after delivery in Kathmandu. Trop Med Int Health 15: 1227-1234.

9. Marchant T (2013) Maternal and newborn health care. Baseline findings from Gombe State, Nigeria. Interactions between families and frontline workers (their frequency, quality, and equity), and coverage of interventions for mothers and newborns. Project Report, LSHTM Research online.
10. Fujita Y, Fujii A, Furukawa S, Ogawa T (2005) Estimation of willingness-to-pay (WTP) for water and sanitation services through contingent valuation method (CVM): A case study in Iquitos City, The Republic of Peru. JBICI review pp: 59-87.
11. Foreit KG, Foreit JR (2004) Willingness to pay surveys for setting prices for reproductive health products and services: A user's manual.
12. Allegri M, Ridde V, Louis VR, Sarker M, Tiendrebéogo J, et al. (2011) Determinants of utilisation of maternal care services after the reduction of user fees: A case study from rural Burkina Faso. Health Policy 99: 210-218.
13. Kyokan M, Whitney-Long M, Kuteh M, Raven J (2016) Community-based birth waiting homes in Northern Sierra Leone: Factors influencing women's use. Midwifery 39: 49-56.
14. Ternent L, McNamee P, Newlands D, Belemsaga D, Gbangou A, et al. (2010) Willingness to pay for maternal health outcomes. Appl Health Econ Health Policy 8: 99-109.
15. Fawsitt CG, Bourke J, Lutomski JE, Meaney S, McElroy B, et al. (2017) What women want: Exploring pregnant women's preferences for alternative models of maternity care. Health Policy 121: 66-74.
16. Mohale H, Sweet L, Graham K (2016) Maternity health care: The experiences of Sub-Saharan African women in Sub-Saharan Africa and Australia. Women and Birth p: 9.
17. Albers LL (2000) Health problems after childbirth. J Midwifery Womens Health 45: 55-57.
18. Tao F, Huang K, Long X, Tolhurst R, Raven J (2011) Low postnatal care rates in two rural counties in Anhui Province, China: Perceptions of key stakeholders. Midwifery 27: 707-715.

13

Complementary and Alternative Medicine Use in a Heterogeneous Sample of Women

Lisa B Phipps[1], **Allison Sepulveda**[2], **Nicole Karjane**[3], **Donna Miles**[4], **Susan Kornstein**[5], **Kristopher J Pickens**[1] **and Dace S Svikis**[6*]

[1] *Office of Learning Innovation and Student Success and Institute for Women's Health, Virginia Commonwealth University, Virginia, USA*

[2] *Institute for Women's Health, Virginia Commonwealth University, Virginia, USA*

[3] *Department of Obstetrics and Gynecology, Virginia Commonwealth University, Virginia, USA*

[4] *Carolina Population Center, University of North Carolina at Chapel Hill, North Carolina, USA*

[5] *Department of Psychiatry, Institute for Women's Health, Virginia Commonwealth University, Virginia, USA*

[6] *Department of Psychology, Psychiatry, Obstetrics and Gynecology, Virginia Commonwealth University, Virginia, USA*

[*] **Corresponding author:** Dace S Svikis, Professor and Deputy Director, Department of Psychology, Psychiatry, Obstetrics and Gynecology, Institute for Women's Health, Virginia Commonwealth University, P.O. Box 980343, Richmond, Virginia 23298, USA, E-mail: dssvikis@vcu.edu

Abstract

This study examined prevalence of biologically-based Complementary and Alternative Medicine (CAM) use in adult women receiving care at three different sites in a health care system and to explore associated use of caffeine, alcohol, and tobacco. The Complementary and Alternative Medicine Prevalence Survey (CAMPS) assessed frequency, quantity and reason for use of 36 biologically-based CAMs and communication with a physician/pharmacist about use. CAMPS also assessed depressive symptoms and prior week use of alcohol, tobacco and caffeine. Of 289 participants, 83% reported CAM use in their lifetime, with 64% of respondents reporting regular use of at least one CAM. Only 51% of those using CAM reported informing their physician/pharmacist about it. African American women were less likely to report use than Caucasian women. Use was more prevalent among women reporting regular alcohol and/or caffeine use. Use of CAM is prevalent in this diverse sample of women. Under-reporting to medical providers suggests a need for screening in healthcare settings. Failure to do so could increase risk for interactions between CAM and prescribed medications. Further, the association between CAM use and regular or problematic use of alcohol or caffeine consumption warrants further study focusing on potential consequences.

Keywords: Alternative medicine; Health care; Screening; Pregnancy; Multivitamin; Vitamin C

Introduction

Health care approaches that are developed and used outside of modern western medicine are often considered complementary and/or alternative medicines. According to the National Center for Complementary and Integrative Health (NCCIH), complementary medicine is used together with conventional medicine and alternative medicine is used in place of conventional medicine [1]. Examining trends in National Health Interview Survey (NHIS) data, Clarke et al. found 32.3% of adults used complementary health approaches in 2002, and 35.5% in 2007. Rates have remained high; with the 2012 National Health Interview Survey reporting 33.2% of adults having used CAM therapy in the past year [2]. A secondary analysis examining sex differences in CAM use found that 59.1% of CAM users were women [3]. Further, rates of biologically based CAM, (i.e. herbal medicines such as vitamins, minerals, and other "natural products") are higher in Caucasians *vs.* African Americans [1,4].

Anecdotal reports of more patients using CAM recently triggered practitioner concern within the Virginia Commonwealth University (VCU) Health System for two main reasons. First, dietary supplements are regulated as foods and therefore subject to different regulations than prescription and over-the-counter drugs (e.g., manufacturers do not have to prove safety or efficacy of dietary supplements before marketing) [1]. Such supplements are readily accessible in health food stores and over the internet. Second, even if the substance is properly identified on the label, little may be known of the potential side effects and/or interactions with other medications [5]. Although some forms of CAM present little to no risk to patients, others have been found to produce serious side effects and/or interact with conventional medicines, in many cases increasing drug toxicity, inducing or inhibiting drug-metabolizing enzymes, and even leading to fatality [5,6]. In other instances, interactions may occur between the herbal medicines themselves, affecting blood sugar levels or increasing risk of bleeding [6]. Most CAM users do so in addition to conventional medical care, however 63-72% of these patients fail to inform their providers about their CAM use [7]. Disclosure of CAM use is particularly low among minority populations [8]. Even if physicians are aware their patients are taking herbal products, the need for more validated herbal medicine claims through randomized clinical trials [6] coupled with the lack of comprehensive federal regulations and standards further inhibits physicians from advising patients appropriately. As a result, this may put patients at risk.

The present study was conducted by a team of investigators from the VCU Institute for Women's Health (IWH), a National Center of Excellence. The topic area was identified by a group of physicians treating women seen in one of the VCU Health System clinics. Specifically, the physicians expressed concern that patients' use of CAM could interact with other prescribed medications. The three VCU Health System clinics were intentionally selected because they represented diversity with regard to age, race and socio-economic status. The purpose of the present cross-sectional study was to:

1) Establish the recent and lifetime prevalence of biologically based CAM use in women attending one of three clinics in the VCU Health System, and 2) Explore potential correlates of CAM use (such as demographics, use of other licit substances such as caffeine, alcohol and tobacco, and depressive symptomatology).

Materials and Methods

Study population and setting

Women were eligible to participate in this study if they were 18 years or older, English-speaking, and able to read and understand informed consent and survey documents. The survey was administered at three university-affiliated outpatient medical clinics with diverse populations: A suburban women's health practice serving predominantly middle to upper class women; a University student health clinic serving male and female students; and an urban, hospital-based gynecological clinic serving predominantly lower income women. The goal sample size was 300, with up to 100 completed surveys at each of the three clinics.

Procedure

Prior to their medical appointment, women at all three sites were approached in their clinic waiting area by a member of the research team. They were given a short introduction to the study by a research assistant, who indicated the survey assessed use of biologically based CAM therapies (defined as substances found in nature such as herbs, foods and dietary supplements). Informed consent was obtained from all participants who were eligible and expressed interest in the study. Participants were given a 10-15 minute self-administered, CAMPS survey, which was completed either prior to or following their medical appointment. Upon completing the survey, women were thanked for their participation. No monetary compensation was provided. This study was approved by the VCU Institutional Review Board.

Survey instrument

The Complementary and Alternative Medicine Prevalence Survey (CAMPS) was designed by the study team, with input from physicians providing care at the clinics. The CAM therapies listed in the survey were identified from a list of most commonly used biologically based CAM found on the website of the National Center for Complementary and Alternative Medicine (now the National Center for Complementary and Integrative Health). Section 1 focused on demographics (age, race, education, employment status, and insurance status), religious affiliation, pregnancy status, reason for that day's clinic visit, and use of prescription medications.

Section 2 comprised the crux of the survey and focused on biologically based CAM usage including age of first use, frequency and quantity of use, and the primary reason for using each CAM. Participants were asked to report any use, regular use, and current use (within the past 30 days) for 36 commonly used CAM therapies. Respondents were then asked to indicate the primary reason for use of each CAM therapy from a list of 20 potential health reasons (e.g., back pain, anxiety, insomnia, menopause, etc.). Perceived efficacy of CAM use was assessed using a 5-point scale from 'not at all effective' to 'extremely effective'. Additional space was provided for participants to report use of any additional CAM not listed in the survey. Participants who indicated ever using one or more CAM therapies were then asked why they chose CAM, if they informed their health care practitioner or pharmacist about their CAM use, how they learned about CAM, where they purchased it, why they discontinued CAM use (if applicable), and if any other family members also use CAM.

Section 3 focused on use of alcohol, tobacco and caffeine. Respondents were asked to report regular use of these substances, current use (within the past 30 days), age of first use, and frequency and quantity of use. The final section of the survey contained questions about the respondent's depressive symptomatology during the past week, utilizing the Center for Epidemiologic Studies Depression Scale (CES-D). This validated 20 item scale is widely used to measure depressive symptomatology in the general population [9]. Respondents recorded how they felt during the past week (e.g., I was bothered by things that don't usually bother me, I felt I was just as good as other people, I had trouble keeping my mind on what I was doing) on a 4-point Likert type scale (Rarely-less than 1 day, Some or a Little-1 to 2 days, Occasionally or Moderately 3 to 4 days, and Most or All of the time-5 to 7 days). Total scores range from 0 to 60; with scores of 16 and above indicative of depression.

Statistical analyses

Statistical analyses used SPSS software 14.0 (February 16, 2006). Continuous variables (e.g. age) were described with means or medians as appropriate based on normality, while categorical variables were described with frequencies. Demographic variables and higher frequency (>10% at a site) CAM use patterns were then compared across the three clinic sites using Chi-square and Kruskal-Wallis. CAM use frequencies as a function of regular use of other substances (alcohol, caffeine, and tobacco) and past week depressive symptoms were also compared.

Results

Demographic characteristics

The overall sample consisted of 289 women, with 98 at the urban clinic, 101 at the student clinic, and 90 at the suburban clinic. The median age was 29 years overall (range 18-74 years). A Kruskal-Wallis test indicated a statistically significant difference in age across the three clinic settings ($p<0.001$), with median ages of 34.5, 21, and 46 years at the urban, student, and suburban clinics, respectively. Of the total study sample, 175 were Caucasian, 91 were African American, and 23 were other races. A Chi-Square analysis of race indicated a difference in race distribution across the clinics, with fewer proportion of Caucasians in the urban clinic (n=41 *vs.* 67 in each of the other two clinics). There were more African Americans in the urban clinic (n=53) than in either the student (n=16) or suburban clinic (n=22). Races marked as "other" occurred at higher frequency in the student clinic (n=17) than in the urban (n=5) and suburban (n=2) clinics.

CAM use

Prevalence of ever and regular CAM use, CAM use excluding vitamins and minerals (CAM-EVM), and use of specific CAMs reported on the survey are presented in Table 1.

Dietary supplement (CAM)	Ever tried (%)	Regular use (%)
Any CAM	83	63.6
CAM-EVM	61.9	33.7
Multivitamin	67	44.6
Vitamin C	39.8	22.1
Echinacea	26.5	6.1
Vitamin B12	21.1	9.5
Vitamin E	20.7	10.5
Green Tea	20.4	7.5
Ginseng	19.4	6.1
Fish oil	18.4	10.2
Garlic	15.3	5.4
Chamomile	14.6	6.1
St. John's Wort	13.6	3.7
Gingko	12.9	4.1
Soy	12.6	6.1
Zinc	12.6	4.8
Vitamin B6	11.6	4.4
Ginger	10.2	3.1
Mint	9.2	2.7
Glucosamine	8.8	4.4
Magnesium	7.8	3.4
Vitamin B1	6.1	2
Vitamin A	5.8	2.4
Vitamin B3	5.4	1.7
Royal Jelly	5.1	1.7
Valerian	5.1	2.7
Metabolite	4.4	1
Ephedrine	3.4	1.7
Beta carotene	3.1	0.7
Manganese	3.1	1
Alfalfa	2.7	0
Kava Kava	2.4	0
Lycopene	2.4	0.7
Saw Palmetto	2	0.7
Ragweed	1	0

Cat's Claw	1	0
Choline	1	0
Barberry	1	0

Table 1: Participant's reported use of CAM.

Overall, 83% of respondents had ever tried CAM and 63.6% had used at least one CAM on a regular basis in their lifetime. Most regularly used CAMS were a Multivitamin (44.6%) or Vitamin C (22.1%). Sixty-two percent of participants reported CAM-EVM use, with 33.7% reporting using at least one on a regular basis. The top five reasons for trying CAM were: For improved health (43.6%), curiosity (33.3%), conventional medicine practitioner suggested it (22.5%), conventional medicine too costly (7.9%), and conventional medicine failed (6.7%). Among participants using CAM (n=227), 51.1% had not informed their physicians of their CAM use.

Table 2 using bivariate analyses, depicts statistically significant differences in proportions for CAM use that was at least 10% prevalent by at least one of the sites. While the student clinic site showed the highest percentage of having tried any CAM or CAM-EVM, *Echinacea*, glucosamine, fish oil, and soy had been tried with higher frequency at the suburban clinic site. Ginkgo, ginger, chamomile, and vitamins A, B6, and C were tried with higher frequency at the student site. There were no instances where a CAM was tried most frequently by patients at the urban site, and in fact, the urban site had the lowest reported frequency for ever trying CAM for all but Vitamin C (30.8% at the urban site, 26.5% at suburban site and 42.7% at student clinic).

	Urban Clinic	**Student clinic**	**Suburban clinic**	
Variable	**(n=98)**	**(n=101)**	**(n=90)**	**p-value**
Any CAM	76 (77.6%)	91 (90.1%)*	77 (85.6%)	0.011
Any CAM-EVM	46 (46.9%)	71 (70.3%)*	65 (72.2%)	<0.001
Glucosamine	4 (4.08%)	4 (3.96%)	18 (20.0%)*	<0.001
Fish oil	9 (9.18%)	19 (18.8%)	26 (28.9%)*	0.002
Ginger	4 (4.08%)	14 (13.9%)*	12 (13.3%)	0.034
Soy	5 (5.1%)	14 (13.9%)	18 (20.0%)*	0.007
Chamomile	8 (8.2%)	20 (19.8%)*	15 (16.7%)	0.046
Vitamin A	5 (5.1%)	11 (10.9%)*	1 (1.1%)	0.013
Vitamin B6	5 (5.1%)	16 (15.8%)*	13 (14.4%)	0.032
Vitamin C	36 (36.7%)	50 (49.5%)*	31 (34.4%)	0.048
Regular CAM use	50 (51.0%)	76 (75.2%)*	61 (67.8%)	<0.001
Regular CAM-EVM use	21 (21.4%)	43 (42.6%)*	35 (38.9%)	0.002
Regular Soy use	3 (3.1%)	4 (4.0%)	11 (12.2%)*	0.016
Regular Multivitamin use	33 (33.7%)	54 (53.5%)*	44 (48.9%)	0.007
Regular Vitamin C use	14 (14.3%)	28 (27.7%)*	23 (25.6%)	0.038

Table 2: Frequency (and percent) for lifetime CAM use by health clinic site [Note: Only CAM with a reported prevalence of at least 10% at one or more sites are included in the table (*Indicates significantly higher CAM use)].

Similar trends were found for regular use, with the highest frequency of regular use of any CAM and CAM-EVM reported at the student clinic, and lowest frequencies reported at the urban clinic. Regular use of Multivitamins and Vitamin C were reported with highest frequency at the student clinic, while regular use of glucosamine, fish oil, and soy were reported with highest frequency at the suburban setting. The urban site had the lowest reported frequency for regular use of CAM in all categories where CAM use had a prevalence of at least 10%. CAMs that had reported prevalence of at least 10% at one or more sites but were not statistically significantly different between sites were ginseng, garlic, St. John's Wort, Mint, Green tea, Multivitamin, Vitamins B12 and E, and zinc, as well as regular use of Vitamins B12 and E.

For CAMs with at least 10% use at one or more sites, statistically significant age differences were found for fish oil, green tea, and Vitamin C, as well as for regular use of fish oil. Those who had tried fish oil were older than those who had not (median age 37.5 years *vs.* 29.0 years, p=0.014). This was also the case for those who had regularly used fish oil (median age 42.5 years *vs.* 29.0 years, p=0.004). Conversely, those who had tried green tea or Vitamin C were younger than those who had not (median age 24.0 years *vs.* 32.0 years, p=0.009 and 26.0 years *vs.* 32.0 years, p=0.036, respectively).

African Americans had the lowest prevalence of CAM use for all categories, with 67.0% reporting use of any CAM and 46.2% reporting use of CAM-EVM (Table 3). Likewise, 42.9% of African Americans reported regular use of any CAM, and 20.9% reported using CAM-EVM. Frequency was highest for the "other" race category for trying CAM-EVM and zinc, and for regular use of CAM-EVM.

Variable	Caucasian (n=175)	African American (n=91)	Other (n=23)	p-value
Any CAM	160 (91.4%)	61 (67.0%)	20 (83.3%)	<0.001
Any CAM-EVM	119 (68.0%)	42 (46.2%)	18 (75.0%)	0.001
Tried *Echinacea*	59 (33.7%)	13 (14.3%)	5 (20.8%)	0.002
Tried St. John's Wort	33 (18.9%)	5 (5.5%)	2 (8.3%)	0.008
Tried Multivitamin	137 (78.3%)	44 (48.4%)	14 (58.3%)	<0.001
Tried Zinc	28 (16.0%)	4 (4.4%)	4 (16.7%)	0.02
Regular use of Multivitamin	98 (56.0%)	23 (25.3%)	10 (41.7%)	<0.001
Regular use of Vitamin C	49 (28.0%)	12 (13.2%)	4 (16.7%)	0.018
Regular use of any CAM	131 (74.9%)	39 (42.9%)	15 (62.5%)	<0.001
Regular use of CAM-EVM	68 (38.9%)	19 (20.9%)	10 (41.7%)	0.009

Table 3: Differences in CAM use by race [Note: Only CAM with a reported prevalence of at least 10% at one or more sites are included in the table].

CAM and other licit substance use

Regular caffeine use was reported by 62.2% of women surveyed, regular tobacco use by 29.9%, and regular alcohol use by 26.2%. Regular users of alcohol and caffeine were more likely to report any CAM-EVM use, as well as regular CAM and CAM-EVM use (Table 4). No differences were found between regular tobacco users and the rest of the sample for either CAM or CAM-EVM use.

Substance	Regular user of substance (%)	Non-regular user of substance (%)	p-value
CAM			
Alcohol			
Tried CAM-EVM	72.7	58.3	0.025
Tried *Echinacea*	39	22.2	0.004
Tried Ginseng	31.2	15.3	0.002
Tried St. Johns Wort	20.8	11.1	0.034
Tried Chamomile	23.4	11.6	0.012
Tried Multi vitamin	77.9	63.4	0.02
Tried Vitamin B6	18.2	9.3	0.036
Tried Vitamin C	50.6	36.1	0.025
Tried Vitamin E	35.1	15.7	<0.001
Tried Zinc	19.5	10.2	0.035
Regular CAM use	79.2	58.3	0.001

Regular CAM-EVM	42.9	30.6	0.05
Regular Multi vitamin	61	38.9	0.001
Regular Vitamin C	35.1	17.6	0.002
Regular Vitamin E	18.2	7.9	0.012
Caffeine			
Triedany CAM	89.1	73.6	0.001
Triedany CAM-EVM	67.8	52.7	0.01
Tried *Echinacea*	30.6	20	0.047
Tried St. Johns Wort	18.6	5.5	0.002
Tried Multi vitamin	72.1	59.1	0.021
Tried Vitamin C	47	28.2	0.001
Tried Vitamin E	24.6	14.5	0.04
Regular CAM	76	43.6	<0.001
Regular CAM-EVM	41	21.8	0.001
Regular Multi vitamin	53.6	30	<0.001
Regular Vitamin C	28.4	11.8	0.001

Table 4: Significant differences of CAM use by regular users of alcohol and caffeine.

CAM and depressive symptoms

A valid CES-D score was calculated for n=254 respondents. Of these, a depression score ≥ 16 was reported by 35.8% of women (n=91). Within this group there were no significant differences found between women who reported having ever used CAM as compared to those who reported no CAM use (36.9% *vs.* 29.7%, p=0.404). Although not statistically significant, a higher percentage of women in this group did report CAM-EVM use as compared to no CAM-EVM use (40.1% *vs.* 28.3%, p=0.058).

Discussion

In this study, we report a high prevalence of lifetime CAM use (83%) in a diverse population of women. Further, 3 out of every 4 women who ever tried CAM (77%) report using at least one CAM regularly. Rates of CAM use varied across the 3 sites, with the highest percentage of participants having ever tried or used CAM regularly occurring at the student and suburban clinics. The higher use of CAM excluding vitamins and minerals in the suburban clinic (average age 46) is consistent with national survey data, which shows the highest rates (44%) of CAM use occurring among people aged 50-59 [10]. We observed African Americans reporting lower regular CAM use (21.1%) than Caucasians (70.8%), which has also been previously demonstrated in the literature [4].

Women who used alcohol and caffeine regularly were more likely to use CAM, while no differences were found among regular tobacco users. Holden et al. [10] also found an association between CAM use and patterns of moderate to heavy alcohol consumption. Future research on the interaction of CAM with these substances, in addition to prescribed medications, is warranted. While not statistically significant, a trend was observed toward higher CAM-EVM use among women with depressed mood.

Among the top five reasons indicated for using CAM, three of these were in response to, or dissatisfaction with, conventional medicine, yet the majority (51%) of CAM users had not informed their physician or pharmacist that they were using CAM. This is consistent with previous findings which estimate as many as 63-72% of patients using CAM in addition to conventional medical care do not inform their healthcare providers of their CAM use [7]. National survey data further demonstrate that among the largest adult age group reporting CAM use (ages 50-59), two-thirds (67%) had not discussed their use with a healthcare provider [11].

These findings indicate a need for physician screening tools, particularly within clinics providing services to older suburban patients, and student populations. While many physicians are concerned about their patients' use of CAM and potential interactions with prescription medications, the reality of adding additional screening tools to lengthy assessment batteries in busy clinical settings poses a challenge. These findings may be useful in identifying risk groups where additional CAM screening is warranted. Associations found between CAM use and regular use of alcohol or caffeine also warrant further attention; in particular, quantity of use data should be examined to determine if heavier alcohol or caffeine use is related to CAM use.

If so, such women may represent a unique subgroup; one that might benefit from follow-up assessment and/or education about heavy/regular alcohol or caffeine consumption and potential interactions with CAM use [12]. To minimize practitioner time needed to screen for tobacco, alcohol, and other drug use, computer-delivered measures have been developed, with the goal of promoting integration with routine medical care [13]. Such methods may promote more routine screening for CAM use, which in turn, can better alert practitioners to any risks associated with CAM and other medication interactions.

Limitations

This study is descriptive and taken from a convenience sample in three clinics within the same health system; thus, generalizability may be reduced due to selection bias. In addition, the cross-sectional study design does not allow for causal inference. Third, measures of alcohol, tobacco, and caffeine use were limited to frequency, with no estimates of quantities consumed. Finally, study participants were adult women; findings may not generalize to other groups such as men or adolescents. Such populations may warrant future research, with subsequent comparisons to present study findings.

Conclusion

Use of CAM is common among women seeking healthcare and is often not reported to clinicians. Given the potential for untoward interactions between CAM and prescribed medications, coupled with the lack of reported CAM use to medical professionals, a need for physician screening is apparent. Public health strategies that promote patient disclosure of CAM use to health care providers may be of benefit. The association between CAM use and the use of alcohol and caffeine found in this study provides additional support for future exploration of concurrent use of CAM with alcohol and caffeine.

Acknowledgements

This research was supported by the Virginia Commonwealth University Institute for Women's Health, a designated National Center of Excellence by the U.S. Department of Health and Human Services.

References

1. Complementary, alternative, or integrative health: What's in a name? U.S. National Center for Complementary and Integrative Health. National Institutes of Health (NIH), U.S. Department of Health and Human Services.
2. Clarke TC, Black LI, Stussman BJ, Barnes PM, Nahin RL (2015) Trends in the use of complementary health approaches among adults: United States, 2002-2012. Natl Health Stat Report 10: 1-16.
3. Zhang Y, Leach MJ, Hall H, Sundberg T, Ward L, et al. (2015) Differences between male and female consumers of complementary and alternative medicine in a national US population: A secondary analysis of 2012 NHIS data. eCAM pp: 413173.
4. Barnes PM, Griner E, McFann K, Nahin RL (2004) Complementary and alternative medicine use among adults: United States, 2002. Advance data from vital and health statistics no. 343. National Center for Health Statistics. Hyattsville, Maryland.
5. Hu Z, Yang X, Ho PC (2005) Herb-drug interactions: A literature review. Drugs 65: 1239-1282.
6. Skalli S, Zaid A, Soulaymani R (2007) Drug interactions with herbal medicines. Ther Drug Monit 29: 679-686.
7. Eisenberg DM, Kessler RC, Rompay MI (2001) Perceptions about complementary therapies relative to conventional therapies among adults who use both: results from a national survey. Ann Intern Med 135: 344.
8. Chao MT, Wade C, Kronenberg F (2008) Disclosure of complementary and alternative medicine to conventional medical providers: Variation by race/ethnicity and type of CAM. Natl Med Assoc 100: 1341-1349.
9. Radloff LS (1977) The CES-D Scale: A self-report depression scale for research in the general population. App Psych Meas 1: 385-401.
10. Holden SC, Gardiner P, Birdee G (2015) Complementary and alternative medicine use among women during pregnancy and childbearing years. Birth: Issues in Perinatal Care 42: 261-269.
11. https://nccih.nih.gov/news/camstats/2010/introduction.htm
12. Svikis D, Henningfield J, Gazaway P (1997) Tobacco use for identifying pregnant women at risk for substance abuse. J Reprod Med 42: 299-302.
13. McNeely J, Wu L, Sharma G, Cathers L (2016) Performance of the tobacco, alcohol, prescription medication, and other substance use (TAPS) tool for screening in primary care patients. Ann Int Med 165: 690-699.

A Quantitative Analysis Explaining the Aetiology of Body Weight Concerns and Physical Appearance Dissatisfaction among Undergraduates at The University of Mauritius

Khan NM*, Rampat S and Sannassee L

Faculty of Social Sciences and Humanities, University of Mauritius, Moka, Mauritius

**Corresponding author: Naushad Ali Mamode Khan, Lecturer, Faculty of Social Sciences and Humanities, University of Mauritius, Moka, Mauritius,*

E-mail: n.mamodekhan@uom.ac.mu

Abstract

The idea of thinness in today's society is omnipresent and is leading to body dissatisfaction thereby encouraging unhealthy eating and exercise practices in not only women, but also in men who are increasingly focusing on their appearance. This study aimed at identifying the risk factors for weight concerns and physical appearance displeasure among 300 students, aged 18 to 25 years, at the University of Mauritius. Factor analysis was used to identify the following common weight loss behaviors which the participants adopt: "Concern about dieting and weight", "Physical Activities" and "Controlling the amount of food intake". Binary logistic regression analyses revealed that age, gender and region had an impact on one's willingness to maintain the ideal body weight and shape. There was also an interaction between age and region on body dissatisfaction.

Keywords: Depression; Prevalence; Anorexia nervosa; Dieting; Fitness

Introduction

In today's world, our society and media defines our physical appearance and determines what constitutes 'beauty', although these 'perfect' images to which we aspire are more often than not digitally enhanced (airbrushed) and manipulated before final production. Thus, it is not surprising that, instead of accepting and embracing our unique physique and morphology, we tend to focus on an illusory and unattainable perfection which can only be detrimental to us [1,2]. Various factors such as poor body image, negative body weight perception, media influence, and health problems have been linked to our obsession with thinness [3-6]. In particular, body image, defined as the way people see or think about their bodies and how they are viewed by others [7], has attracted lots of attention recently as people are very determined to improve their appearance when they perceive a gap between their own body and their "ideal" body. This gap results in body dissatisfaction, defined as a person's negative thoughts about his or her own body [8], low self-esteem [3,9,10] and also results in a significant increase in state depression [11,12]. Furthermore, distortions in body image and the resulting body dissatisfaction can be used to explain the prevalence of eating disorders such as Anorexia Nervosa and Bulimia Nervosa [13].

Individuals' weight management practices such as diet or exercise control is determined by one's body weight perception [14], which is one's self-evaluation of one's weight as underweight or normal weight or overweight irrespective of actual weight [15]. This perception of one's own body [8] is influenced by factors such as age, gender, family, peers, media, and ethnicity [16]. Indeed, children as young as 8 year olds reported body image concerns [17], with the notion of an ideal body becoming more salient in adolescence [18].

Additionally, body weight perception varies across different ethnicities [19] with white Americans and Japanese idealizing the ultra-thin body while African-Americans preferring larger bodies [20,21]. Past research on body weight perception was focused mainly on females because of the sociocultural accentuation given to skinny appearance for females [22]. However, recently body dissatisfaction has affected adolescent boys as well [23]. Yet, negative body image is expressed differently between the sexes-with women displaying an obsession with thinness [24,25], and men displaying an aspiration to lower body fat [26] or gain weight to look muscular [2]. Despite the contradictions, research suggests that the average weight boy is satisfied with his body mass and has a positive body weight perception [27]. Dieting has always been considered as the perfect strategy towards weight loss [28] among not only people who are normal and over-weight, but also those who are underweight. Yet, research demonstrates that, in the long run, restricting caloric intake will anticipate weight gain, instead of weight loss [25,29]. Whilst it is commonly known that females, as young as 13 years, consistently diet, males also diet to decrease body fat and gain lean muscles [30]. The quest for the ideal body has not left Mauritians unaffected. Fitness facilities are mushrooming around Mauritius, highlighting a drastic increase in the practice of physical activities in adults aged 35 to 54 years [31].

Additionally, weight loss programs, such as "Weigh-Less", proposing specific diet and/or exercise plans catered to individuals' needs have experienced sustained success in the country. Weight loss supplements such as 'Slim & Trim', 'Dr. Ernst' and 'BioSlim' have also proved to be quite popular among the population since they are perceived to provide quick results. Since individuals worldwide experience societal pressure to be thin and consequently experience body dissatisfaction, this study aimed at investigating the perception of body image, strategies of weight reduction and management, and the social factors influencing body dissatisfaction among male and female students at the University of Mauritius.

Data was collected using standardized questionnaires. Factor analysis technique was used to obtain the set of factors that influence perception of body image, strategies for weight control and social pressure to be thin. Stepwise logistic regression analysis was done to assess whether the factors Gender, Age, Region, Ethnicity, Faculty, Waist Circumference, and Body Mass Index predict body dissatisfaction amongst the youth of University of Mauritius. The organization of the paper is as follows: in the next section, the methodology part is described in detail consisting of the sampling strategy, the factor analyses and the step-wise regression analysis. The conclusion is presented in the following section.

Methodology

In this section, three important components are discussed. Firstly, the data collection and sampling layout are presented followed by the results of the factor analysis and lastly, the Generalized Linear Regression Model (GLM) is established to measure the contributory effects of the different factors influencing whether an undergraduate student is satisfied with his/her body image.

Data collection and sampling strategy

The target population was the undergraduate students who were enrolled at the University of Mauritius (UOM) for the academic year 2015/2016. Using the sampling strategy, an unbiased sample of students aged 18 and above was selected from the sampling frame that comprises of students from the different cohorts via a list submitted to us by the UOM registrar.

The table below provides the details on the sampling selection exercise from the different faculties at the University of Mauritius with FOA: Faculty of Agriculture; FOE: Faculty of Engineering; FOS: Faculty of Science; FLM: Faculty of Law and Management; FSSH: Faculty of Social Studies and Humanities (Table 1).

FOA	318	318/8013 × 300 ≈ 12
FOE	2265	2265/8013 × 300 ≈ 85
FOS	868	868/8013 × 300 ≈ 33
FLM	2867	2867/8013 × 300 ≈ 107
FSSH	1695	1695/8013 × 300 ≈ 63
Total	8013	300

Table 1: Sample determination.

Factor analyses for the different likert scales questions

The results from the factor analysis yield the followings (Table 2-4):

Strategies of weight control	
Factor 1: Physical Activities is Important	**Factor 5:** Not wasting Food
V8 Physical Activity	V28 Do not read calorie content
V12 Weight Control	V29 Eat due to frustration
V11 Duration Of Physical Activity	**Factor 6:** Emotional Eating
V13 Feeling Refreshed	V15 Eat less
V9 Exercise is Important	V17 Leave food on plate
Factor 2: Control the amount of food you consume	**Factor 7:** Controlling your food consumption
V20 Feeling Hungry	V22 Avoid fried foods
V21 Tasty Food	V30 Eat less
V19 Large Portion	V31 Eat due to depression
V18 Love for Food	**Factor 8:** We can eat dessert and still look healthy
V16 Overeat	V33 Eat more due to relationship problems
Factor 3 : Concern about weight control and Dieting	V32 Eat more when depressed
V2 Eating less when breaking diet	**Factor 9:** We consume more junk foods when we are anxious

V3 Preoccupied with Weight and Shape	V24 Eat dessert
V1 Rewarding oneself when losing weight	V35 Stress Eating
V4 Not worrying about weight gain	**Factor 10:** We eat more sweets when we are frustrated
Factor 4: Pastries	V27 No junk foods
V7 Not worried about gaining weight	V34 Anxiousness
V23 Avoid butter	**Factor 11:** How emotions affect your eating
V25 Eat sweets	V14 Avoid sporting activities
V10 Healthy without exercise	V26 Avoid ready -made foods

Table 2: Strategies of weight control.

Factor 1: How you feel about your body
V1 Should diet
V5 Feel fat due to pastries
V8 Worrying about body shape
V6 Feel large
V4 Feel fat
V14 Need for exercise
V9 Lack of self-conscious
V10 Seeing rolls of flesh
Factor 2: How you see your body
V7 Ashamed
V12 Reflection
V13 Among friends
V3 Bad shape
V11 Unfair
V2 Self-conscious about your shape

Table 3: Perception of the body image.

Factor 1: Pressure from family and friends
V11 Look thinner
V12 Improve appearance
V16 Develop appearance
V15 Get thinner
V13 Decrease body fat level
V17 Look in better shape
V14 Get in better shape
V18 Decrease level of body fat
Factor 2: Athletic Profile
V7 Look athletic
V6 Look More athletic
V2 Looking muscular
V1 Important to look athletic
V10 Look more muscular
Factor 3: Media pressure
V21 Good appearance
V19 To be in better shape
V22 Less body fat
V20 be thinner
Factor 4 : Thinness
V3 Look thin
V5 Thinking to look thin
V4 Little fat
V9 Little body fat
V8 Look very lean

Table 4: The Social factors.

Binary logistic regression analysis

In this subsection, the outcome variable (binary) which is "satisfied' or 'not satisfied" is regressed on a set of predictor variables. The explanatory variables that may influence the response variable are as follows: Gender, Age, Region, Ethnicity, Faculty, Waist Circumference, and Body Mass Index.

The below table illustrates the variables with their p-value and their reduction in deviance represented by the G-statistics (Table 5).

Explanatory	G-statistics	P-value	Significance
Gender	8.913	0.003	Significant
Age	35.586	0	Significant
Region	28.261	0	Significant
Ethnicity	3.015	0.083	Insignificant
Faculty	0.675	0.411	Insignificant
Waist circumference	3.789	0.052	Insignificant
Body Mass Index	3.558	0.059	Insignificant

Table 5: Reduction in deviance.

The first three variables listed were significant, namely: Gender, Age and Region with their p-value<0.005 and higher decrease in deviance (Table 6). The best model is defined as follows:

Satisfaction with body image=Constant+Gender+Age+Region +Age*Region

$logit\pi_{ijk} = \eta + \alpha_i + \beta_j + \gamma_k + (\beta\gamma)_{jk}$ where 1=Male, 2= Female j: 1=18-21, 2= 22-25

k: 1= Rural, 2= Urban

Variable and Category	Symbol	Estimate	Odds Ratio
Constant	η	1.8685	$e1.8685=6.4786$
Gender: Male	α_1	-0.4364	$e-0.4364=0.6464$
Age: 22-25	β_2	-2.2172	$e-2.2172=0.1089$
Region: Urban	γ_2	-1.8436	$e-1.8436=0.1583$
Age-Region: 22 to 25-Urban	$\beta\gamma_{22}$	1.1826	$e1.1826=3.263$

Table 6: Best model estimates.

The odds ratio and the probability that a student is in the age group of 22-25, male and living in an urban region and including an interaction effect between age and region is shown below:

Odds Ratio, 1.8685(1)–0.4364(1)–2.2172(1)–1.8436(1)+1.1826 = 0.236

Probability:

$$\pi i = \frac{e1.8685(1) - 0.4364(1) - 2.2172(1) - 1.8436(1) + 1.1826}{1 - e1.8685(1) - 0.4364(1) - 2.2172(1) - 1.8436(1) + 1.1826}$$
$$= 0.308$$

About 30.80% of the student is satisfied with their body image if they fit in the age category 22-25, being a male and living in an Urban region and with an interaction effect of age and region.

Conclusion

This study was designed to explore the reasons for weight concerns and physical appearance dissatisfaction among undergraduate students at the University of Mauritius. 300 questionnaires were distributed to the students through PPS sampling technique where 183 of the respondents were female and 117 were male. In this study, we observed that both males and females are preoccupied with thoughts of their weight and shape. The response rate was 6% for "Strongly Disagree", 13% "Disagree", 10% were "Neutral" and the highest rate was 46% for "Agree" and 25% for "Strongly Agree". It is noteworthy that 40% of the respondents who agreed being worried about their weight and shape also agree that they engage in physical activities for their health. This is consistent with the reasonable BMI of 62.3% of the students falling in the normal weight range which is between 18.5 and 24.9.

The effect of gender on body shape concerns was justified with female respondents being more dissatisfied with their body shape with a response rate of 67% "Usually True" for "Have you been so worried about your shape that you have been feeling that you ought to diet". As expected though, male respondents rated this question equally with 20% "Almost Never True" and 20% "Usually True". Next, the body image perception, when asked to compare their profile with the body image contouring drawing, 26% opted for profile 4 and 24% profile 5 which represent the average body profile. Hence we conclude that most students perceived themselves as having an average profile. Only 1% of the sample perceived themselves as having the extreme body type that is profile 1 and profile 9 representing extremely underweight and extremely obese.

Results from the sociocultural attitude test revealed that male counterparts favour a muscular body with 51 out of the 117 respond "Mostly Agree". Whereas for majority of females which was 61 out of 187 responded "Neutral". However, the response rate for a thin body was highest as expected with 75 "Mostly Agree" among females and only 41 from males. The power of the media was justified with the highest records for "I feel pressure from the media to improve my appearance" being 54 "Mostly Agree" for female and 35 "Mostly Agree" for male. The results of the first factor analysis performed showed that "Physical Activities", Control of amount of food consumed" and "concern about weight and shape" are the 3 most popular weight loss behaviors to maintain the ideal weight. The second factor confirmed the fact that the way we feel and see our body influences our willingness to lose weight.

The Last factor analysis was about sociocultural attitude which demonstrate that the "Pressure from family and friends", "Athletic Profile", "Thinness" and "Media Pressure" have a direct impact on body dissatisfaction. Binary Logistic regression was performed to assess whether University of Mauritius students experience body satisfaction or not. The variables Age, Gender and Region were found to be significant and were the risk factors for body image.

It is also worth noting that as age increases body dissatisfaction decreases. The best model consists of Gender, Age, Region with an interaction between Age and Region. The data collected and the findings only show the causes of body image dissatisfaction in the sample and their willingness to maintain an ideal profile in society. Further research should aim at clarifying body image disturbance in early stages of childhood and more efforts could be made to sensitize individuals against these false ideologies about beauty.

References

1. Sztainer DN, Paxton SJ, Hannan PJ, Haines J, Story M (2006) Does body dissatisfaction prospectively predicts depressive mood and low self-esteem in adolescent girls and boys. J Clin Child Psychol 35: 539-549.
2. Smolak L, Levine M, Thompson JK (2001) The use of the sociocultural attitudes towards appearance questionnaire with middle school boys and girls. Int J Eat Disord 29: 216-223.
3. Paxton SJ, Sztainer D, Hannan PJ, Eisenberg ME (2006) Body dissatisfaction prospectively predicts depressive mood and low self-esteem in adolescent girls and boys. J Clin Child Adolesc Psychol 35: 539-549.
4. Berg P, Paxton SJ, Keery H, Wall M, Guo J, et al. (2007) Body dissatisfaction and body comparison with media images in males and females. Body image 4: 257-268.
5. Zaccagni L, Masotti S, Donati R, Mazzoni G, Russo EG (2014) Body image and weight perceptions in relation to actual measurements by means of a new index and level of physical activity in Italian University students. J Transl Med 12: 42-45.
6. Goldfield GS, Moore C, Henderson K, Buchholz A, Obeid N, et al. (2010) Body dissatisfaction, dietary restraint, depression and weight status in adolescents. J Sch Health 80: 186-192.
7. Khor GL, Safiza MN, Jamalludin AB, Jamaiyah H, Geeta A, et al. (2009) Nutritional status of children below five years in Malaysia: Anthropometric analyses from the third National Health and Morbidity Survey III (NHMS, 2006). Malays J Nutr 15: 121-136.
8. Grogan S (2008) Body image: Understanding body dissatisfaction in men, women and children (2nd edition), Hove, UK, Routledge.
9. Silberstein LR, Striegel RH, Timko, C, Rodin J (1988) Behavioural and psychological implications of body dissatisfaction: Do men and women differ? Sex Roles 19: 219-232.
10. Tiggemann M (2005) Body dissatisfaction and adolescent self-esteem: Prospective findings. Body Image 2: 129-135.
11. Durkin SJ, Paxton SJ (2002) Predictors of vulnerability to reduced body image satisfaction and psychological wellbeing in response to exposure to idealized female body images in adolescent girls. J Psychosom Res 53: 995-1005.
12. Orbach S (1986) Hunger Strike. London, Faber and Faber.
13. Media, Body image and eating disorders. In National Eating Disorders Association [NEDA].
14. Cash TF (2004) Body image: Past, present, and future. Body Image 1: 1-5.
15. Cheung PC, Ip PL, Lam ST, Bibby H (2007) A study on body weight perception and weight control behaviours among adolescents in Hong Kong. Hong Kong Med J 13: 16-21.
16. Gregory CO, Blanck HM, Gillespie C, Maynard LM, Serdula MK (2008) Health perceptions and demographic characteristics associated with underassessment of body weight. Obesity (Silver Spring) 16: 979-986.
17. Welch C, Gross S, Bronner Y, Dewberry D, Paige D (2004) Discrepancies in body image perception among fourth-grade public school children from urban, suburban and rural Maryland. J Am Diet Assoc 1040: 1080-1085.
18. Chen LJ, Fox KR, Haase AM, Ku PW (2010) Correlates of body dissatisfaction among Taiwanese adolescents. Asia Pac J Clin Nutr 19: 172-179.
19. Dorsey RR, Eberhardt MS, Ogden CL (2009) Racial/ethnic differences in weight perception. Obesity (Silver Spring) 17: 790-795.
20. Fitzgibbon ML, Stolley M, Schiffer L, Sharp L, Singh V, et al. (2008) Obesity Reduction Black Intervention Trial (ORBIT): Design and baseline characteristics. J Womens Health 17: 1099-1110.
21. Kagawa M, Kuroiwa C, Uenishi K, Mori M, Dhaliwal S, et al. (2007) A comparison of body perceptions in relation to measured body composition in young Japanese males and females. Body Image 4: 372-380.
22. Rosenblum GD, Lewis M (1999) The relations among body image, physical attractiveness, and body mass in adolescence. Child Dev 70: 50-64.
23. Jones DC (2004) Body image among adolescent girls and boys: A longitudinal study. Dev Psychol 40: 823-835.
24. Kostanski M, Fisher A, Gullone E (2004) Current conceptualization of body image dissatisfaction: Have we got it wrong? J Child Psychol Psychiatry 45: 1317-1325.
25. Barker ET, Galambos NL (2003) Body dissatisfaction of adolescent girls and boys: Risk and resource factors. J Early Adolesc 23: 141-165.
26. Frederick DA, Buchanan GM, Sadeghi-Azar L, Peplau LA, Haselton MG, et al. (2007) Desiring the muscular ideal: Men's body satisfaction in the United States, Ukraine and Ghana. Psychol Men Masc 8: 103-117.
27. Richards MH, Boxer AM, Petersen AC, Albrecht R (1990) Relation of weight to body image in pubertal girls and boys from two communities. Dev Psychol 26: 313-321.
28. Enriquez E, Duncan GE, Schur EA (2013) Age at dieting onset, body mass index, and dieting practices: A twin study. Appetite 71: 301-306.
29. Stice E, Presnell K, Shaw H, Rohde P (2005) Psychological and behavioural risk factors for obesity onset in adolescent girls: A prospective study. J Consult Clin Psychol 73: 195-202.
30. McCabe MP, Ricciardelli LA, Banfield S (2001) Body image, strategies to change muscles and weight, and puberty: Do they impact on positive and negative affect among adolescent boys and girls? Eat Behav 2: 129-149.
31. Ministry of Health and Quality of Life (2004). Mauritius Non-Communicable Diseases Survey 2004.

15

Early Postnatal Care Service Utilization and Associated Factors among Mothers Who Gave Birth in the Last 12 Months in Aseko District, Arsi Zone, South East Ethiopia in 2016

Teklehaymanot AN*, Niguse D and Tesfay A

Department of Population and Family Health, College of Health Sciences, Jimma University, Ethiopia

***Corresponding author:** Teklehaymanot AN, Department of Population and Family Health, College of Health Sciences, Jimma University, Ethiopia, E-mail: aderajewnu@gmail.com

Abstract

Background: Even though early postnatal care visit is one of the strategies to reduce maternal and new-born morbidity and mortality, it is the weakest of all reproductive and child health interventions in Africa and receives much less attention from healthcare providers than pregnancy and childbirth.

Objective: To assess early postnatal care service utilization and associated factors among mothers who gave birth in the last 12 months in Aseko district, Arsi zone, South East Ethiopia, 2016.

Method: Community based cross-sectional study was conducted from May 10th-May 20th 2016 in Aseko district, Ethiopia. A total of 382 mothers who gave birth in the last 12 months were identified using random number generated by computer from six kebeles selected by simple random sampling techniques were included in the study. Data were collected using structured questionnaire through face to face interview and entered to Epi data version 3.1 and exported to SPPS version 20. Descriptive statistics, principal factor analysis (PCA), bivariate and multivariable logistic regression analysis were used for the analysis and a P-value<0.05 was declared a statistically significant in this study. Finally, the result was presented using texts, tables and figures.

Results: The level of early postnatal care service utilization was 23.7%. The reasons for not to use early PNC services were: Having no information on the importance of early PNC services 140 (48.5%) followed by lack/no transportation access 76 (26.3%). In multivariable logistic regression analysis; experience of early postnatal care utilization for previous child (AOR=4.211; 95% CI: 1.548, 11.458), Institutional delivery (AOR=2.778; 95% CI: 1.386, 5.568), Women decision making power (AOR=4.103; 95% CI: 2.087, 8.067), Information/advise about early postnatal care services from health profession (AOR=5.049; 95% CI: 2.074, 12.289), Distance/time took to arrive health facility on foot (AOR=0.458; 95% CI: 0.231, 0.908) and Access to transportation (AOR=2.655; 95% CI: 1.322, 5.330) were found to be predictors of early PNC service utilization.

Conclusion and Recommendations: Less than quarters (23.7%) of the respondents were utilizing early postnatal care services in the district. Experience of early PNC utilization, place of delivery, decision making power, information/advice from health profession, distance of health facility and access to transport were statistically significant for early postnatal care utilization. Strengthening health facilities to enhance service provision and information education and communication, decision making power of the women, improving transportation service and encouraging institutional delivery are necessary measures to enhance early PNC service utilization in the district.

Keywords: District; Early PNC; Early PNC utilization; Comprehensive care

Introduction

Women's health and involvement in health care are essential keys to health for all. Postnatal care is regarded as one of the most important Maternal and child healthcare services for the prevention of impairments and disabilities resulting from childbirth. The Postpartum period starts from one hour after the birth of placenta and ends 42 days of delivery [1].

Lack of appropriate care during this period could result in significant ill health and even death. Rates of provision of skilled care are lower after childbirth when compared to rates before and during childbirth [2]. Most maternal and infant deaths occur during this time [3].

Globally, more than 500,000 women die each year due to complications of pregnancy and childbirth and most deaths occur during or immediately after childbirth [4]. Every year three million infants die in the first week of life, and another 900,000 die in the next three weeks [5].

Bleeding and infection following childbirth account for many maternal deaths, while preterm birth, asphyxia and severe infections contribute to two thirds of all neonatal deaths [6]. A large number of women in the sub-Saharan region do not have access to health care during the early postnatal period which puts them at risk of diseases and mortality [7].

The harsh reality is that about 4 million infants do not live through the immediate postnatal period, and a large number of them are disabled due to pregnancies and births that are poorly monitored or handled [8].

And the deaths within the first week of life account for almost 40% of all deaths among children under the age of five. Also, about 700 babies die (around 30 every hour) on a daily basis which has the highest number of new-born deaths in Africa, and the second highest in the world [9].

Maternal and new-born deaths occur mostly during pregnancy, delivery, or within the first week after delivery [10-12]. WHO estimates that 50% of maternal and 40% of new born deaths occur within the first 24 hours after delivery [13]. In developing countries also shows 50% to 71% of maternal deaths happen during postpartum period, particularly in the first few hours [4].

Early postnatal care (EPNC) visits can reduce maternal and new born morbidity and mortality, and enhance survival, particularly through early detection and management of postpartum complications [14]. However, it is the weakest of all reproductive and child health interventions in Africa and receives much less attention from healthcare providers than pregnancy and childbirth [13].

As WHO global database on maternal health indicators, globally, only 48% of the mothers are following the postnatal care within two days of child birth [15]. Based on an analysis of Demographic and Health Surveys in 23 African countries, no more than 13% receive a postnatal care visit within two days of delivery [11]. The level of postnatal care coverage is extremely low in Ethiopia. Only 7% of women received postnatal care within two days, as recommended [16].

Studies in developing countries indicates that factors affect utilization of early postnatal care services such as distance from health services, access to transportation, socio-economic status, geographical location, maternal education, multiple demands on women's time, women's lack of power in decision making within the family and poor quality of services including poor handling by health providers [17]. Even though early PNC service utilization plays a critical role in reducing maternal and new born child mortality, little is known about its determinants. Thus, understanding the factors related with early PNC utilization is critical for countries like Ethiopia with alarmingly high maternal mortality.

Therefore, such adequate postnatal care utilization is mandatory to reduce mortality and morbidity among mothers' and their babies. Postnatal care is important for mothers for treatment of complications arising from delivery, especially for births that occurred at home.

For non-institutional births particularly, postnatal care enables detection of complications that may threaten the survival of the mother. Yet, despite the benefits of PNC, most new born and mothers do not receive postnatal care services from a skilled health care provider during the critical first few days after delivery [3]. In Ethiopia, where the largest proportions of births take place at home, postnatal care by health professionals is extremely low and uncommon [10]. Therefore, this study aims to identify factors affecting early PNC utilization and recommend increasing the service in the study area (Figure 1).

Materials and Methods

The assessment was conducted in Aseko district, Arsi zone, Oromia region, South East Ethiopia, which is 244 km far from Addis Ababa and 186 km from Arsi zone, Asella. Aseko district is bounded by Western Haraghe from East, Fentale/East shewa from south, Merti woreda from West and Gololcha woreda from North. The weather condition of the district is characterized by 44% Weyna dega, 33% Kolla and 22% Dega.

The district has 18 Kebeles with one urban and seventeen rural kebeles. According to the 2007census population projection, the total populations of the district are estimated 107,376 out of which 53,258 are females. The total numbers of women of reproductive age group are 23,730, pregnant women are 3,726 and surviving infants are 3,458.

95% of the district has rural population. There are three public health center, 18 health posts, six private clinics and three private drug venders and it has 53 health professional workers and 39 health extension workers. The district had planned 3,726 women for postnatal care services by 2015/2016 [18].

The required sample size determined by using single population proportion formula based on the following assumption. The prevalence of early postnatal care (P) was considered to be 34.5% (P=0.345) with 95% level of confidence, 5% margin of error and 10% none response rate was considered. The district has a total of 18 kebeles. First 6 kebeles named Iftu Bulala, Haro Alle, Aseko 01, Dirre Oda, Nano Aseko and Komicha kebeles were chosen by simple random sampling technique. Then after consultation with local administrators and district health office, a census of the sampled six Kebeles with the help of health extension workers was conducted and frames of all households with women who gave childbirth from May 2015 to May 2016 was made [19-23].

From the result of census, the number of woman who gave birth in the past 12 months in each kebele were; Iftu Bulala (367), Haro Alle (288), Aseko 01 (207), Dirre Oda (300), Nano Aseko (129) and Komicha (133). The total sample size of 382 was distributed proportionate allocation to size to each kebele. Finally, the participants were selected by simple random sampling using random number generated by computer from the existing sampling frame of households. Structured interview questionnaire had been developed by reviewing pertinent literatures using English language then translated into the local language, Afan Oromo and used to collect the data after back translating to English by different experts to check its consistency [16,24-31].

The questionnaires were designed to capture demographic and socio-economic characteristics or household assets and equipment's, water supply, power supply, sanitary facility, residential homes, farmlands and livestock ownership to compute wealth index, maternal status including ten question of maternal knowledge on early PNC and danger sign of postpartum, three questions for women's decision making power which was adopted from EDHS, 2011, experience on ANC, PNC, health care factors and utilization of early postnatal care.

Six diploma nurses who are fluent in the local language and familiar with the local customs had been trained for the purpose of data collection. The data was collected from the respondents by using face to face interview. One BSc. nurse was assigned as a supervisor to check for the daily activity, consistency and completeness of the questionnaire and to give appropriate support during the data collection process.

The questionnaire was pre-tested on 19 (5%) of the total sample size and a necessary adjustment was made before used for actual data collection. During data collection when the selected households were closed, the interviewers revisit the house holds three times at different time intervals.

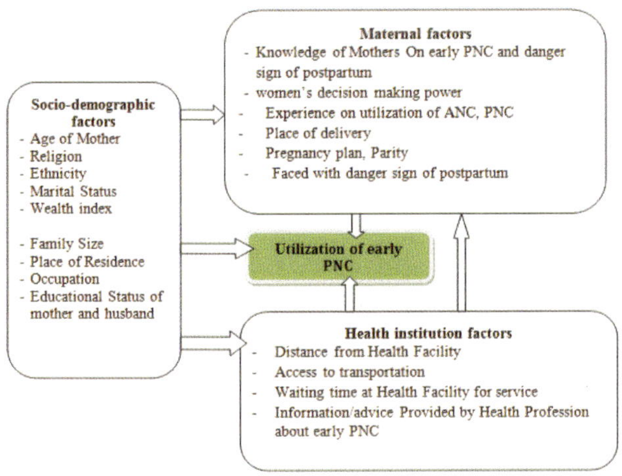

Figure 1: Conceptual framework developed from review of different literatures.

The questionnaires were designed to capture demographic and socio-economic characteristics or household assets and equipments, water supply, power supply, sanitary facility, residential homes, farmlands and livestock ownership to compute wealth index, maternal status including ten question of maternal knowledge on early PNC and danger sign of postpartum, three questions for women's decision making power which was adopted from EDHS in 2011, experience on ANC, PNC, health care factors and utilization of early postnatal care.

Six diploma nurses who are fluent in the local language and familiar with the local customs had been trained for the purpose of data collection. The data was collected from the respondents by using face to face interview. One BSc. nurse was assigned as a supervisor to check for the daily activity, consistency and completeness of the questionnaire and to give appropriate support during the data collection process. The questionnaire was pre-tested on 19 (5%) of the total sample size and a necessary adjustment was made before used for actual data collection. During data collection when the selected households were closed, the interviewers revisit the house holds three times at different time intervals.

The data were coded, edited and entered into Epi data version 3.1 software package. Then exported to SPSS version 20.0 statistical software package and recoded, cleaned for inconsistency and missing value and finally analysed. Descriptive statistics such as frequencies, percentages, means, standard deviations, crosstabs and chi-square were computed to describe the study population in relation to relevant variables (age, residence, ethnicity, religion, marital status, educational status, occupational status, parity, family size, ANC, distance from health facility and place of delivery) and to show the prevalence of early postnatal care utilization.

Wealth index was determined by quintiles using Principal Component Analysis (PCA). Bivariate and multivariable logistic regression analysis was used to determine the association between dependent and independent variables and controlling the confounding effect.

Those factors that were significant at p-value<0.25 level in the Bivariate logistic regression analysis were considered for the multivariable logistic regression analysis. The crude and adjusted odds ratio together with their corresponding 95% confidence interval was computed. A P-value<0.05 was considered declaring a result as statistically significant in this study. Finally the result was presented using texts, tables and figures.

Operational Definitions

Early postnatal care

In this study healthcare services that are given immediately after delivery to the end of first week of delivery both for the mothers and new born babies by health workers and health extension workers.

Early postnatal care utilization

In this study mothers or their new born babies those who had at least one early postnatal care check-up for the current delivery by health workers and health extension workers within first week of delivery.

Good knowledge

Mothers those who are capable of answering >5 out of 10 knowledge question on utilization of early postnatal care and danger sign of postpartum.

Fair knowledge

Mothers those who are capable of answering 4-5 out of 10 knowledge question on utilization of early postnatal care and danger sign of postpartum.

Poor knowledge

Mothers those who are capable of answering <4 out of 10 knowledge question on utilization of early postnatal care and danger sign of postpartum.

Women decision making power

Women are considered to participate in a decision if they usually make that decision alone or jointly with their husbands on households [16].

Autonomous

In this study if women are usually make decision alone or jointly with their husbands on household's three out of three decision making question.

Non-autonomous

In this study if women are usually make decision alone or jointly with their husbands on households' less than three out of three decision making question.

Poorest women

Woman lives in a household with the 1st quintile or the 1st 20% from the score of wealth index.

Poor women

Woman lives in a household with the 2nd quintile or the 2nd 20% from the score of wealth index.

Middle women

Woman lives in a household with the 3rd quintile or the 3rd 20% from the score of wealth index.

Rich women

Woman lives in a household with the 4th quintile or the 4th 20% from the score of wealth index.

Richest women

Women lives in a household with the 5th quintile or the 5th 20% from the score of wealth index [10,16].

Ethical Considerations

Ethical clearance and approval was obtained from the Ethical Review Committee of the College of Health Sciences, Jimma University. Permission was obtained from district administrative office, district health office and local administrative. Written and verbal consent was obtained from each participant after explaining the purpose and nature of the research. Participation in the study was on a voluntary basis and participants were informed their right to quit/ refuse their participation at any stage of the study if they did not want to participate. Moreover, confidentiality and privacy of study participants were assured during the interview.

Results

Socio-economic and demographic characteristics of respondents

Of the total 379 sample respondents, 134 (35.4%) of them were at the age group 25-29 years and 254 (67%) of them were Muslim. Oromo was the predominant ethnic group, 280 (73.9%) and majority of respondents 358 (94.5%) are currently married.

Regarding educational status, 176 (46.4%) of them attended primary school. The great majority, 278 (73.4%) of them were housewives (Table 1).

Variable Name and Category		Frequency	Percentage (%)
Age of the mothers	15-19	19	5
	20-24	89	23.5
	25-29	134	35.3
	30-34	84	22.2
	≥5	53	14
Religion	Muslim	254	67
	Orthodox	119	31.4
	Protestant	6	1.6
Ethnicity	Oromo	280	73.9
	Amhara	99	26.1
Marital status	Married	358	94.5
	Single	4	1.1
	Divorced	9	2.3
	Widowed	8	2.1
Place of residence	Rural	314	82.8
	Urban	65	17.2
Maternal educational status	Unable to read and write	148	39.1
	Primary school (1-8)	176	46.4

	Secondary school (9-12)	47	12.4
	Above secondary	8	2.1
Husband educational status	Unable to read and write	102	28.3
	Primary school (1-8)	167	46.4
	Secondary school (9-12)	66	18.3
	Above secondary	25	7
Maternal occupational status	Housewife	278	73.4
	Farmer	54	14.2
	Merchant	24	6.3
	Employed	17	4.5
	Daily labour	6	1.6
Husband occupational status	Farmer	273	75.8
	Merchant	30	8.3
	Employed	38	10.6
	Daily labour	19	5.3
Family size	<5	165	43.5
	05-Jul	176	46.5
	>7	38	10
Wealth index	Poorest	75	19.8
	Poor	76	20.05
	Middle	76	20.05
	Rich	76	20.05
	Richest	76	20.05

Table 1: Socio-demographic characteristics of respondents, Aseko district, Arsi zone, South east Ethiopia, 2016.

Early PNC service utilization

The level of early postnatal care service utilization was 23.7% of which 58 (15.3%) were within 24 hours of postpartum, 23 (6.1%) within 24-48 hours of postpartum and about 9 (2.3%) within 49 hours-6 days of delivery and 65 (72.2%) of them had got services at health centre.

The reasons that the participants responded for not to use early PNC services were; having no information on the importance of early PNC services 140 (48.5%) followed by lack /no transportation access 76 (26.3%) (Table 2).

Variables		Frequency	Percentage (%)
Frequency of early PNC utilization	One	79	87.8
	Two	11	12.2
Time of Early PNC utilization	Within 24 hours	58	64.4
	24-48 hours	23	25.6
	49-72 hours	1	1.1
	4-6 days	8	8.9

Place of early PNC service utilization	Health post	7	7.8
	Health centre	65	72.2
	Hospital	11	12.2
	Home	7	7.8
The reason for not to use early PNC	Lack/no transportation	76	26.3
	Far from health facility	28	9.7
	I don`t know the benefit	140	48.5
	It is not customary	35	12.1
	Others	10	3.4

Table 2: Early PNC utilization and the reasons participants responded for not to use the service in Aseko district, 2016.

Maternal factors

Out of the total respondents, 164 (43.3%) of them had fair knowledge on early postnatal care services and danger sign of postpartum.

From the total respondents only 36 (9.5%) of them had experience on early PNC service utilization for previous child (Figure 2).

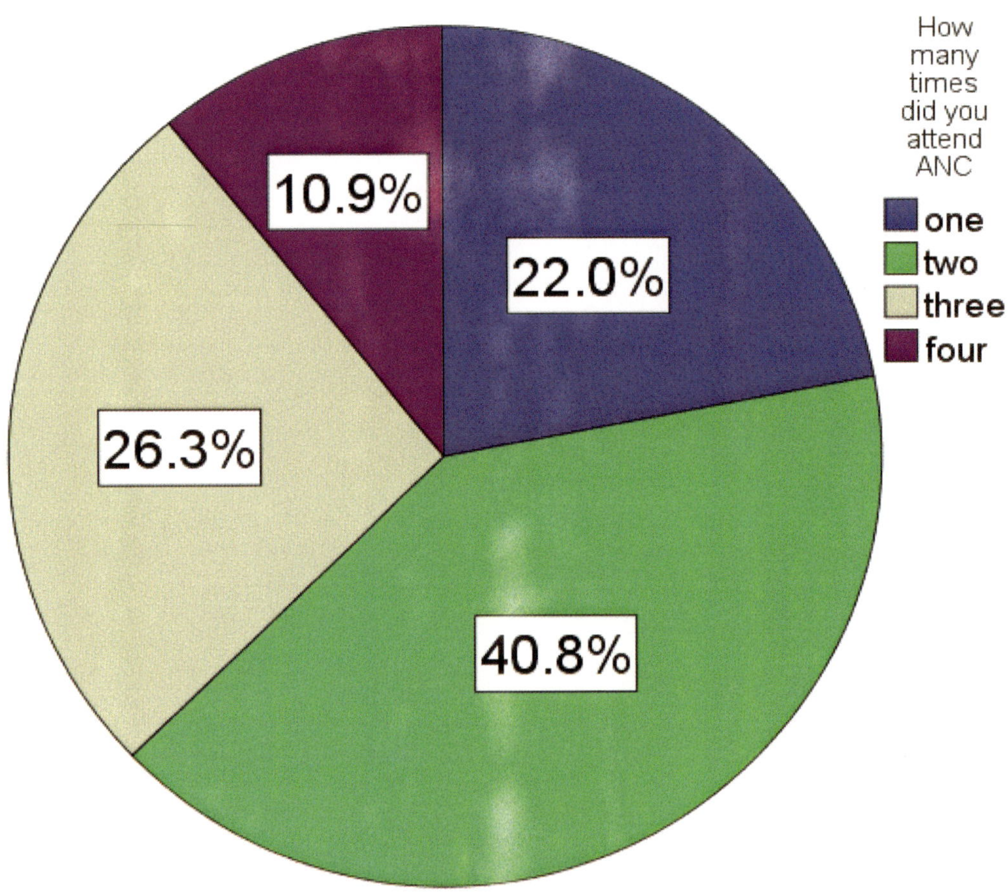

Figure 2: Number of ANC visit follow up for the respondents in Aseko district, 2016.

Place of delivery

Regarding Place of delivery, 96 (25.3%) of respondents gave births their last child in health institution and 86 (89.6%) of them were attended by Midwife/Nurse/Health officer. From those gave birth at health facility, 50 (52.1%), 29 (30.2%) and 17 (17.7%) of them had stayed at health institution for 24 hours, for less than 24 hours and for more than 24 hours, respectively.

From sampled women, only 57 (15%) of them experienced/faced any health problem related to last delivery during postpartum with 20 (35.1%) of the health problem was vaginal bleeding (Table 3).

Institutional factors for early PNC services utilization

From the total respondents, 237 (62.5%) of them had got information/ advice from health profession for early PNC check-up. For 256 (67.5%) of participants, took two hours and more to arrive to the nearest health facility and majority 270 (71.2%) of respondents had no access to transportation (Table 4).

Variables		Frequency	Percentage (%)
Number of live birth	01-Mar	261	68.9
	4-5	85	22.4
	≥6	33	8.7
Level of maternal knowledge on early PNC and danger sign during postpartum	Poor knowledge	71	18.7
	Fair knowledge	164	43.3
	Good knowledge	144	38
Early PNC service utilization for previous child	Yes	36	9.5
	No	343	90.5
ANC follow up	Yes	304	80.2
	No	75	19.8
Place of current delivery	Health facility	96	25.3
	Home	283	74.7
Experienced/faced with any health problem related to last delivery	Yes	57	15
	No	322	85
Health problem faced	Vaginal bleeding	20	35.1
	Fever	11	19.3
	Lower abdominal pain/cramp	19	33.3
	Foul smelling of vaginal Discharge	7	12.3
Pregnancy planed/wanted	Yes	259	68.9
	No	120	31.1
Women decision making power	Autonomous	164	43.3
	Non-autonomous	215	56.7

Table 3: Maternal factors of sample respondents, Aseko district, Arsi zone, south east Ethiopia, 2016.

Variables		Frequency	Percentage (%)
Information/ advice from health profession for early PNC check up	Yes	237	62.5
	No	142	37.5
Place for information/ advice for early PNC service	At Health Post	107	45.2
	At Health Centre	93	39.2

	At Hospital	9	3.8
	At the community level	28	11.8
Think/perceived services given at health facility having a long Waiting time problem	Yes	39	10.3
	No	340	89.7
Distance/time took to arrive to the nearest health facility from house on foot	<2hours	123	32.5
	≥2hours	256	67.5
Access to transportation to reach health facilities	Yes	109	28.8
	No	270	71.2

Table 4: Health institutional factors for early PNC utilization among respondents in Aseko district, Arsi zone, South East Ethiopia, 2016.

Factors associated with early postnatal care utilization

Using principal component analysis (PCA), the wealth index score was made by 8 variables with 3 components that explained a total variance of 67.9% and measure of sampling adequacy 0.734.

Out of a total 28 variables, 14 variables namely: place of residence, mother's educational status, husband educational status, husband occupation, wealth index, knowledge of mothers on early postnatal care and danger sign of postpartum, experience of early PNC utilization for previous child, place of delivery, experienced/faced with any health problem related to last delivery, pregnancy plan, decision making power of the women, getting information/advice about early postnatal care follow up from health profession, distance/time took to arrive on foot to the nearest health facility and access to transportation were considered for multivariable logistic regression analysis.

Finally, after adjusting for confounders using multivariable logistic regression model, 6 variables namely, experience of early PNC utilization for previous child, place of delivery, decision making power of the women, getting information/advice about early postnatal care follow up from health profession, distance/time took to arrive on foot to the nearest health facility and access to transportation were found to be statistically significant predictors for early postnatal care utilization.

Mothers with experience of early postnatal care utilization for previous child were 4.2 times more likely to utilize early postnatal care than mothers with had no experience (AOR=4.211; 95% CI: 1.548, 11.458). Similarly mothers who gave births their last child at health institution were significantly better in early postnatal care utilization than those gave births at home (AOR= 2.778; 95% CI: 1.386, 5.568).

Early Postnatal care service utilization also increased with increasing decision making power of mothers. Mothers who have been able to decide on health care service by themselves were 4.1times more likely to attend early postnatal care as compared with mothers whose health care service was decided by other people (AOR=4.103; 95% CI: 2.087, 8.067). In addition, mothers who got information/advise about early postnatal care services from health profession were 5 times more likely to utilize early postnatal care than mothers who didn't get information/advice (AOR=5.049; 95% CI: 2.074, 12.289). The result also revealed that, mothers who travelled for two and more hours on foot to the nearest health facility were 54% less likely to utilize early postnatal care than mothers who travelled less than two hours (AOR=0.458; 95% CI: 0.231, 0.908).

Moreover, mothers who had access to transportation were 2.6 times better in attending early postnatal care as compared with those had no access of transportation to reach health facility (AOR=2.655; 95% CI: 1.322, 5.330) (Table 5).

Variables		Early PNC utilization		COR 95% CI	AOR 95% CI
		Yes	No		
Place of residence	Rural	62	252	1	1
	Urban	28	37	3.076 (1.750, 5.407)	0.955 (0.221, 4.126)
Mother's education	Unable to read and write	1 7	131	1	1
	Primary school	39	137	2.194 (1.183, 4.069)	0.937 (0.337, 2.602)
	Secondary school	29	18	12.415 (5.718, 26.957)	1.54 (0.348, 6.814)
	Above secondary school	5	3	12.843 (2.815, 58.599)	0.944 (0.37, 23.852)
Husband education	Unable to read and write	12	90	1	1
	Primary school	32	135	1.778 (0.870, 3.634)	0.637 (0.236, 2.063)

	Secondary school	32	34	7.059 (3.262, 15.274)	0.949 (0.231, 3.892)
	Above secondary school	12	13	6.923 (2.575, 18.616)	0.096 (0.008, 1.100)
Husband occupation	Farmer	45	228	1	1
	Employed	25	13	9.744 (4.637, 20.474)	6.085 (0.742, 49.885)
	Merchant	15	15	5.067 (2.314, 11.095)	1.542 (0.225, 10.56)
	Daily labourer	3	16	0.950 (0.266, 3.396)	0.97 (0.100, 9.443)
Wealth index	poorest	10	65	1	1
	poor	12	64	1.219 (0.492, 3.020)	0.261 (0.060, 1.135)
	Middle	16	60	1.733 (0.730, 4.115)	0.237 (0.056, 1.002)
	Rich	25	54	3.009 (1.329, 6.814)	0.692 (0.192, 2.496)
	Richest	27	46	3.815 (1.684, 8.645)	1.576 (0.469, 5.292)
Knowledge of mothers on early PNC and danger sign of postpartum	Poor knowledge	10	61	1	1
	Fair knowledge	24	140	1.046 (0.471, 2.319)	3.076 (0.683, 13.862)
	Good knowledge	56	88	3.882 (1.837, 8.201)	4.287 (0.972, 18.915)
Experience of early PNC utilization	No	63	280	1	1
	Yes	27	9	13.333 (5.977, 29.744)	4.211 (1.548, 11.458)*
Place of delivery	Home	35	248	1	1
	Health institution	55	41	9.505 (5.554, 16.268)	2.778 (1.386, 5.568)*
Experience/faced with any health problem related to delivery during postpartum	No	70	252	1	1
	Yes	20	37	1.946 (1.063, 3.563)	2.749 (1.057, 7.145)
Pregnancy plan	No	9	111	1	1
	Yes	81	178	5.612 (2.709, 11.626)	1.356 (0.484, 3.802)
Decision making power	Non-autonomous	17	198	1	1
	Autonomous	73	91	9.343 (5.214, 16.742)	4.103 (2.087, 8.067)**
Getting information/advice about early PNC from health profession	No	8	134	1	1
	Yes	82	155	8.861 (4.136, 18.984)	5.049 (2.074, 12.289)**
Distance/time took to arrive on foot to the nearest health facility	<2hours	45	78	1	1
	≥2hours	45	211	0.370 (0.227, 0.602)	0.458 (0.231, 0.908)*
Access of transportation	No	30	240	1	1
	Yes	60	49	9.796 (5.736, 16.730)	2.655 (1.322, 5.330)*

Table 5: Multivariable logistic regression analysis result of factors affecting early PNC service utilization of respondents in Aseko district, Arsi zone, Southeast Ethiopia, 2016.

Discussion

This study primarily aimed to assess early postnatal care service utilization and associated factors among mothers who gave birth in the last 12 months in Aseko district, Arsi zone, South East Ethiopia. The study revealed that the level of early PNC service utilization was 23.7%. This figure is low compared with the study findings in Nepal, 2011, where 43.2% of the mothers had attended immediate postnatal care within 24 hours of delivery [19] and Kingdom of Cambodia, 2013, where 77% of urban and 58% of rural attended postnatal care within the first 24 hours [20].

This difference of service provision may be attributed due to the difference in socio-economic status, geographical barriers and accessibility of services, information and health education between countries.

Moreover, a community based cross sectional study in Ethiopia, Dembecha district in 2013 revealed still a higher figure that show 34.5% of women utilized the service [27]. However, this study showed the early PNC service utilization in the district to be slightly higher than the case of Soroti district, eastern Uganda in 2015, where only 15.4% of women used early PNC [30]. In addition, the result of the current study indicates the service utilization to be higher than EDHS in 2011, study results that show only 7% of women received postnatal care within two days [16].

This difference may be explained by the time period difference for early PNC service reported by EDHS and this study as well the study time difference that there could be improvement in accessing and utilizing health care service through time. This low coverage of service provision indicates that a lot needs to be done in the study area as well as in the country to increase service utilization to the desired target.

In this study, the maternal status and institutional factors were found to be important determinants of early postnatal care utilization. Among maternal status, experience of early PNC for previous child, place of delivery and decision making power of the women were significant predictors of dependent variable. Mothers with experience of early postnatal care for previous child were 4.2 times more likely to utilize early postnatal care than mothers with had no experience.

This finding was consistent with cross-sectional study done in Gondar Zuria in the year 2014 [32]. This may be explained by experienced mothers may had a better opportunity to get information/advice provision on the importance of early postnatal care service follow up during previous child from health care providers.

Moreover, mothers who gave births their last child at health institution had 2.78 times more chance of getting early postnatal care service compared with mothers who gave births at home. This finding is in line with study results done in Kenya, DHS in 2014 [22] and with cross sectional study results in Ethiopia namely, in Jabitena district in 2013, Dembecha district in 2013 and Enderta district in 2013 [26,27,31].

For instance in Jabitena district, mothers who gave birth their last child in health institutions were about 4 times more likely to utilize postnatal care service utilization. This can be attributed to the fact that women who gave their last birth in health institution have greater opportunity and access of health education and advice or counselling received on early postnatal care follow up provided by health care providers during stayed in health facility.

The other variable that has significant and positive effect on mothers' early postnatal care service utilization was decision making power of the mothers themselves. Mothers who had autonomy to make decision in the household were 4.1 times more likely to attend early postnatal care than counterparts. This finding agrees with the results of study done in Jabitena district in 2013, Abi-Adi town in 2013 and Gondar Zuria district in 2014 [26,28,32].

For instance, in Jebitena district mothers who were autonomous to make health care decision by themselves were about 13 times more likely to utilize postnatal care service than those whose health care decision was made by others. This may be explained by the fact that gender inequality or women often have unequal access to health services, education and economic resources and thus influences of socio-economic inequality for women result in unable to make informed decision for their health care services.

Among institutional factors, information/advice on early postnatal care follow up from health profession, distance/time taken to arrive on foot to the nearest health facility and access to transportation were found to be significantly associated variables with early postnatal care utilization. Mothers who have information/advice on early postnatal care services were 5 times more likely to utilize the service than mothers who didn't have information/advice. This finding is also in line with findings of study done in Enderta district, 2013 and Abi-Adi town, 2013 [28,31]. Women who had got information about postnatal care services from health extension workers and Midwife/Nurse were more likely to attend postnatal care service than counter parts. This implies unequal access or dissemination of information, education and communication/advice provision on the importance of early postnatal care services for all women at all part of the study area.

With regard to distance from health institution, the study showed that mothers who travelled for two and more than two hours on foot to arrive at nearest health facility were less likely to utilize early postnatal care than mothers who travelled for less than two hours. This finding is consistent with study outcomes done in Dembecha and Gondar zuria districts, Ethiopia in 2013 and 2014, respectively [27,32,33]. This may be explained due to the reason that having nearby health facility increases access to health information and reduces distance barriers leading to better utilization.

The analysis result also identified that mothers who had access to transportation service were 2.6 times more likely to utilize early postnatal care as compared with those had no access to transport to reach health facility. Again this finding is line with findings of study conducted in Dembecha district in 2013 [27]. This could be the main reason why mothers did not use early postnatal care especially for those live in rural areas and no road for transportation.

Conclusion

The findings of this study show that early postnatal care service utilization in the study area was 23.7%. This implies that less than a quarter of the participants were using early PNC services. This figure is low compared with most of study findings conducted in other parts of the country and in other countries. The main reasons stated by mothers for not using early postnatal care service were: having no information on the importance of early postnatal care, it is not customary to go out of home before a week after delivery, lack/no transportation access to reach health facility and distance of health facility from their residence implying the need to travel longer distances on foot to get the service.

The multivariable logistic regression analysis estimation result revealed that, mother's experience of early PNC utilization for previous child, place of delivery, decision making power of the women, getting information/advice about early postnatal care follow up from health profession and access to transportation were positively associated factors while distance/time took to arrive on foot to the nearest health facility was negatively associated factor with early postnatal care service utilization.

Recommendations

Based on the findings of the study, the following recommendations are forwarded to respective responsible bodies to enhance early postnatal care service utilization in the study area:

For district level administrative office

Should give strong attention to improve transportation service in the study area by connecting kebeles of the district through road construction.

For district level women and children affairs office

Encourages women to practice more and strengthening to optimize their ability to make informed decisions about their own health care service utilization.

For district level health office

Increasing the access and strengthening health facilities to enhance service provision and information, education and communication both at the facility and at the community level to improve early PNC service.

For health workers and health extension workers

- Strengthening community based Information, Education and communication on the importance and availability of the services as well as on postpartum danger signs for all women at all part of the study area.
- Should take the opportunities to encourage mothers who attend delivery and ANC on the importance and availability of early PNC services.
- Strengthening institutional delivery service and encouraging mothers to attend skilled delivery in health institutions to improve the early postnatal care service utilization in the study area.
- Strengthening the service through home visit for those travelling more hours on foot to the nearest health facility.

For researchers

Researchers should conduct further studies which are supported by qualitative studies.

References

1. Ebun A, Wally C, Guillermo C, Conde A, Indra M, et al. (2013) WHO recommendations on Postnatal care of the mother and newborn. Geneva: WHO p: 58.
2. http://www.who.int/whosis/mme_2005.pdf
3. WHO/RHT/MSM/983 (2004) Postpartum care of the mother and newborn: a practical guide. Geneva: WHO Document Production Services p: 49-58.
4. Van WL, Annick M, Zoe M (2005) Make every mother and child count. WHO p: 219.
5. Ahman E, Zupan J (2007) Neonatal and perinatal mortality. Country, regional and global estimates (2004) p: 14.
6. Ronsmans C, Graham WJ (2006) Maternal mortality. Who, when, where, and why? 368: 1189-1200.
7. Lawn JE, Cousens S, Bhutta ZA, Darmstadt GL, Martines J, et al. (2004) Why are 4 million new born dying each year? Lancet 362: 399-401.
8. Moreen L (2003) Desire for pregnancy and prenatal and postnatal care in California women who recently delivered a live infant. Women's Health Issues. The 131st Annual Meeting of APHA.
9. UNFPA, UNICEF, WHO, World Bank (2012) Trends in maternal mortality: 1990-2010. WHO p: 44.
10. Ethiopian Society of Population Studies (2005) Maternal health care seeking behaviour in Ethiopia: Findings from EDHS 2005. In-depth: Analysis of the Ethiopian demographic and health survey p: 29.
11. Charlotte W, Pat D, Lalla T, Pyande M, Joy L, et al. (2006) Postnatal care, in opportunities for Africa's newborn. Partnership for maternal newborn and child health. Save the Children, UNFPA, UNICEF, USAID, WHO and partners III: 79.
12. Sines E, Syed U, Wall S, Worley H (2007) Postnatal Care. A critical opportunity to save mothers and newborns.
13. Mathai M, Xylander SV, Zupan J (2008) WHO technical consultation on postpartum and postnatal care. Geneva, Switzerland: WHO Document production services p: 52.
14. Habiba SN (2012) National health policy in postnatal care in Bangladesh: gap between policy and practice.
15. World Health Statistics. WHO: 2014
16. Central Statistical Agency (Ethiopia) and ICF International (2012) Ethiopia demographic and health survey 2011. Addis Ababa, Ethiopia and Calverton, Maryland, USA p: 275.
17. Cunningham F, Garry ED (2002) Williams Obstetrics. New York, McGraw Hill p: 89-96.
18. Aseko District Health Office (2015) District health department report.
19. Vishnu K, Mandira A, Rajendra K, Tania G (2014) Factors associated with the utilization of postnatal care services among the mothers of Nepal: analysis of Nepal Demographic and Health Survey 2011. BMC Women's Health p: 13.
20. Net K, Mengseang T, Dararith Y, Verakpheap S (2013) Early postnatal care and its determinants in Cambodia: Further analysis of the Cambodia demographic and health survey. Phnom Penh, Cambodia: National Institute of Statistics, Ministry of Planning and Directorate General for Health, Ministry of Health p: 21.
21. Nankwanga A (2004) Factors influencing utilization of postnatal services in Mulago and Mengo Hospitals Kampala, Uganda 11394: 237.
22. Daniel A, Diana M, Mark K (2014) Determinants of postnatal care use in Kenya. UAPS 28: 1457.
23. Muturik P (2014) Factors affecting utilization of postnatal care services In Kenya. South Am J Public Health 2: 522.
24. Shegaw M, Sue L, Vincentas G (2014) Determinants of maternal health service utilization in Ethiopia: Analysis of the 2011 Ethiopian Demographic and Health Survey. BMC Pregnancy Childbirth 14: 161.
25. Berhe H, Tilahun W, Aregay A, Bruh G, Gebremedhin H (2013) Utilization and associated factors of postnatal care in Adwa Town, Tigray, Ethiopia. A cross sectional study. ARPB 3: 359.
26. Yinager G, Desta A (2014) Factors affecting utilization of postnatal care service in Jabitena district, Amhara region, Ethiopia. SJPH 2: 169-176.
27. Mulatu A, Samrawit S, Molla G, Habte B (2015) Postnatal care service utilization and associated factors among women in Dembecha District, Northwest Ethiopia. Sci J Public Health 3: 686-692.
28. Hailemariam A, Huruy A, Yohannes A (2014) Prevalence and factors associated with post natal care utilization in Abi-Adi Town, Tigray, Ethiopia: A Cross Sectional Study. IJPBSF 8: 1.
29. Katusiime A (2015) Factors affecting the utilisation of postnatal services among mothers attending Kitagata Hospital in Sheema District. Healthcare p: 1-46.
30. Izudi J, Amongin D (2015) Early postnatal care among postpartum women in Eastern Uganda. Int J Gynecol Obstet 129: 161-164.
31. Asfawosen A, Mussie A, Huruy A, Wondeweson T (2014) Factors associated with maternal health care services in Enderta District, Tigray, Northern Ethiopia: A cross sectional study. Am J Nurs Sci 3: 117-125.

Assessment of Knowledge and Attitudes of Men and Women Aged between 15-49 Years towards Legalization of Induced Abortion in Mizan Aman Town, Bench Maji Zone, South West Ethiopia, 2016

Asrat Meleko Mara*, **Mengistu Ayenew, Haile Haftu and Binyam Aregay**

Department of Public Health, Mizan-Tepi University, Mizan Aman, Ethiopia

***Corresponding author:** Asrat Meleko Mara, Department Of Public Health, Mizan-Tepi University, College Of Health Sciences, Ethiopia, E-mail: melekoasrat@gmail.com

Abstract

Background: Countries with narrow bases for legal abortion are vulnerable for burden of unsafe abortion and related mortality. Globally, 26% of populations live where abortion is prohibited or permitted on certain circumstances where majorities are in developing countries.

Objectives: To assess knowledge and attitudes of men and women aged 15-49 years towards legalization of abortion in Mizan Aman town, South West Ethiopia.

Methods: Community based cross-sectional study was conducted from October 2015 to June 2016. Data collection tool used was structured questionnaire. Data entry and analysis was done using EpiData V3.1 and SPSS V20. The result was displayed using tables and figures. Verbal consent was obtained from study participant.

Result and Discussion: Total of 422 individuals were included in this study. Majority, 238 (56.4%), of them preferred legalization of induced abortion. Only, 24 (5.7%), respondents know current legal status of abortion. Knowledge about abortion complication and preference to terminate unwanted pregnancy has association with attitude towards legalization of abortion ($P<0.005$).

Conclusions and Recommendation: Low number of respondents knows current legal status of abortion. Professionals and other influential individuals should be involved in improving community perception towards legal aspects of abortion.

Keywords: Abortion; Legalization; Maternal mortality; Pregnancy

Introduction

Unsafe abortion as described by World Health Organization (WHO) is considered as a procedure for terminating unwanted pregnancy either by persons lacking the necessary skills or in an environment lacking the medical standards, or both [1]. Countries with narrow bases for legal abortion are highly vulnerable for large burden of unsafe abortion and related mortality. Globally, 26% of the world's population lives where abortion is prohibited altogether or permitted only on certain circumstances like to save the woman's life. Of those peoples, majority of them are found in the developing world [2].

Each year, about 585,000 women die every year worldwide due to pregnancy and childbirth related complications, out of which 99% of them occur in developing countries. The leading causes of maternal death include hemorrhage (25%), infection (15%) and unsafe abortion (13%) [3].

The World Health Organization (WHO) estimates that every year, nearly 5.5 million African women have an unsafe abortion. As many as 36,000 of these women die from the procedure, while millions more experience short or long term illness and disability. The unsafe abortion mortality ratio (the number of unsafe abortion-related deaths per 100 000 live births) varies across regions. About half of all deaths from unsafe abortion are in Asia, with most of the remainder (44%) in Africa. Generally, in Africa maternal mortality is estimated as high as 900/100,000 live births [4]. Many studies identified that the foremost determinants of unsafe abortion in different settings include level of utilizing family planning, emergency contraceptive, and legalization of abortion and the skill of the health professionals [5].

Legal abortion service markedly reduces deaths from abortion complications and the overall maternal mortality [6]. For instance a case from Romania confirmed that, due to legalization of abortion in 1989, maternal mortality ratio was dropped from 170/100,000 live births in 1989 to 60/100,000 live births in 1992, which was mainly attributed to the improved safety of abortion after the legalization [7].

In Ethiopia, one in seven women die from pregnancy-related causes, and of this unsafe abortion contribute for maternal deaths of more than half of the 20,000 that occur annually. Also other studies revealed that Ethiopia has the fifth highest number of maternal deaths in the world: One in 27 women die from complications of pregnancy or childbirth annually [8]. To make unsafe abortions safe, national policies including making induced abortion legal reforms are the prerequisites [1].

However, for much of Ethiopia's modern history, safe abortion services were unavailable. Currently, motivated by the growing death toll from unsafe abortion and other related causes, the Ethiopian government made abortion to be allowed by law in certain conditions. By considering its significance, in 2005, Ethiopia expanded its abortion law, which had previously allowed the procedure only to save the life of a woman or protect her physical health [5].

It is fact that only setting Legal reforms alone in a given country cannot reduce abortion related deaths especially in Ethiopia. Creating awareness within the community through different campaigns are crucial to modify society's attitude towards abortion, prevent unsafe and illegal practices, and inform about legal and safe abortion care services. If government did not work on improving knowledge and attitude of peoples they are not likely to benefit from the legal reform and services.

Therefore' this study was aimed to fill the existing information gap by assessing knowledge and attitudes of men and women towards legalization of induced abortion.

Objectives

General objective

To assess knowledge and attitudes of men and women aged between 15-49 years towards legalization of induced abortion in Mizan Aman Town, Bench Maji zone, South West Ethiopia.

Specific objectives

- To assess knowledge of men and women aged between 15-49 years towards induced abortion and its legalization in Mizan Aman Town, Bench Maji zone, 2016.
- To assess attitudes of men and women aged between 15-49 years towards legalization of induced abortion in Mizan Aman Town, Bench Maji zone, 2016.
- To assess factors affecting knowledge and attitudes of men and women aged between 15-49 years towards legalization of induced abortion in Mizan Aman Town, Bench Maji zone, 2016.

Methods and Materials

Study area

Mizan-Teferi is found in bench Maji zone located at the south western part of Ethiopia, about 561 kilometers south west from Addis Ababa and 849 km from Hawassa which is capital city of SNNP region. The zone is bordered in north and north east with Kaffa zone and North West with Sheka zone, in south east with Debub Omo zone, south west with Gambella region and south Sudan.

According to the Ethiopian censes 2007 Bench Maji zone a total population of 760313 (male 450106 and female 310210). Currently the name Mizan Teferi is changed into Mizan Aman which consists of two sub cities Mizan and Aman 6 km apart from each other.

Study design and study period

Community based cross-sectional design was conducted from October 2015 to June 2016 to assess the attitudes of 15-49 year old women and men towards legalization of abortion, in Mizan-Aman town, Bench Maji zone, SNNP region.

Source population

All men and women with age of 15-49 years old that are found in Mizan Aman town was the source population.

Study population

Men and women aged 15-49 years old that are found in Mizan Aman town and who are available during data collection were the study population.

Inclusion and Exclusion Criteria

Inclusion criteria

Those who are men and women aged between 15-49 years old, those who are volunteers and who are relatively healthy to provide information were included in this study.

Exclusion criteria

Those who are severely ill could not talk and hear, and who were involuntary and not available at time of study were excluded from this study.

Sample size determinations

The sample size was determined by using single population proportion formula using 95% confidence interval at 5% margin of error and since there was no research done on attitude and knowledge towards legalization of abortion in this locality.

The sample size was calculated by taking value of population proportion (50%) for maximum sample size, using the following formula:

$N= (Z\alpha/2)^2\ p\ (1-p)\ /d^2$

$n= (1.96)^2 \times 0.5\ (1-0.5)/(0.05)^2=0.96604/0.0025=384$

Then we add non response rate of 10%, so n=422

Where, z=value of 95% from z table (1.96) p=proportion of the population (50%) and d=margin of error (5%)

Sampling technique

Systematic random sampling method was used for this study to select households.

Study Variables

Dependent variables

- Knowledge and attitudes towards legalization of induced abortion

Independent variables

- Socio demographic characteristics of respondents (Age, sex, educational level, marital status, religion, occupation and income status)
- Previous experience related to unsafe abortion

- Knowledge about complication of unsafe abortion

Operational Definitions

Knowledge: Awareness about current legal status of abortion in Ethiopia context and post abortion complication. Also it includes those who are aware of the possible measures to prevent morbidity and mortality which is caused by abortion.

Attitude: It is the way to which clients are thinking or behaving about legalization of abortion.

Abortion: is termination of pregnancy before viability of fetus (<28) weeks of gestation in Ethiopia OR <20 weeks of gestation in USA and according to WHO).

Unsafe abortion: World Health Organization (WHO) definition, "as a procedure for terminating unwanted pregnancy either by persons lacking the necessary skills or in an environment lacking the medical standards, or both".

Data collection tools

Questionnaire that was prepared after reviewing similar literature and modified to our context was used to collect data. Two weeks earlier to the actual data collection period, pretest/pilot study was carried out in other nearby town to check its reliability.

Data was collected by three 4th year public health students.

Data quality control

Data collectors were trained by instructors in public health department. Daily checking of the completeness of questions was made by supervisors.

Data processing and analysis

Data entry and analysis was done using Epi Data V3.1 and SPSS V20. The data was summarized using descriptive statistics and chi square test for significant association between dependent and explanatory variables.

Finally, the result was displayed using tables, graphs, and figures as well.

Plan for result dissemination

The copy of the research was disseminated to Mizan Aman health bureau, Mizan Tepi university teaching hospital and Mizan Tepi University.

Result

Socio-demographic profile of respondents

A total of 422 individuals were included in this study, of those, male participants constitutes 224 (53.1%) of the total and the remaining 198 (46.9%) were female respondents.

Majority of respondents, 89 (21%), were found in the age range of between 26-30 years of old.

The ethnic groups which have large number in Mizan Aman town were Bench and Amhara with a value of 179 (42.5%) and 128 (30.5%) respectively (Table 1).

Variables	Category	Frequency	Percentage (%)
	Male	224	53.1
Sex	Female	198	46.9
	15-20	46	11.3
	21-25	63	14.7
	26-30	89	21
	31-35	76	18
	36-40	72	17.2
Age (year)	41-45	76	18
	Illiterate	101	24
	Only read and write	93	22
	Grade 1-8	51	12
	Grade 9-10	67	16
Educational level	College and university	110	26
	Orthodox	194	44.9
	Protestant	142	33.8
	Muslim	74	17.7
Religion	Other	13	3.05
	Married	173	41
	Unmarried	194	46
	Divorced	38	9.7
Marital status	Widowed	17	3.3
	Civil servant	55	23
	Student	93	22
	Daily labourer	76	18
	Merchant	107	26
	House wife	63	15
Occupation	Farmer	25	6

Table 1: Socio demographic status of respondents in Mizan Aman town, Bench Maji zone, SWE, 2016.

History of abortion among interviewed reproductive age women in past pregnancies

The result of this study discovered that women's who had history of terminating pregnancy constitutes 28 (14.1%) of total women's interviewed.

Most, 21 (75%) and 20 (71.4%), of women who have terminated their pregnancy were identified premarital pregnancy and unintended sex as a major reason for undertaking abortion respectively.

Majority of abortions, 23 (82.1%), were induced by health professional and 18 (64.3%) of abortions were done using oral drug (modern) method.

Eighteen, 18 (64.3%), of abortions made were induced in hospital.

Majority, 20 (71.5%), of women who did induced abortion faced mainly abdominal pain (Table 2).

Variable	Category	Frequency	Percentage (%)
Ever had history of abortion (terminating pregnancy)	Yes	28	14.1
	No	170	85.9
Reason of terminating pregnancy*	Become pregnant while using FP	1	3.5
	Didn't want more child	18	64
	Last child too young	6	21
	Couldn't afford to rear child	16	57
	Too young to have child	12	43
	Stay in school	13	46.4
	Pre-marital pregnancy	21	75
	Extra marital pregnancy	3	10.7
	Become pregnant after being raped	2	7.1
	Become pregnant after unintended sex	20	71.4
	Partner didn't want	14	50
	Fear of family	13	46.4
	Fear of society	7	25
	Health problem	5	17.8
Who else induced that particular abortion	Health professional	23	82.1
	Traditional abortionist	3	10.7
	Myself	2	7.1
	Relative	0	0
	peer	0	0
Where were that particular abortion induced	Patients home	2	7.1
	Abortionist home	3	10.7
	Hospital	18	64.3
	Health center	5	17.9
Any problem you have following that particular abortion*	Heavy bleeding	2	7.1
	Abdominal pain	20	71.5
	Genital/uterine trauma	2	7.1
	Fever	11	39.2
	Incomplete abortion	1	3.5

Table 2: History of abortion and reason for termination among reproductive age women in Mizan Aman town, Bench Maji zone, SWE, 2016 [*Multiple responses were allowed and hence totals could be greater than actual size].

Knowledge and attitudes respondents on induced abortion, and legalization of induced abortion

Attitude of respondents towards legalization of induced abortion

Out of the total respondents, 238 (56.4%) preferred legalization of induced abortion in Ethiopia. Of those who preferred legalization of induced abortion majority, 41.9%, of respondents considered unsafe abortion as a major health problem on the contrary of those who opposed legalization of induced abortion, 54.9%, of them had perceptions that termination of pregnancy was homicide. Out of the total, 234 (55.6%) believed that people would use legal abortion services, if induced abortion were legalized in Ethiopia.

Also 234 (55.6%) of respondents replied that they would encourage a friend other individuals who are in need to go for an abortion if abortion is legalized (Table 3).

Variable	Category	Frequency	Percentage (%)
Do you believe that abortion should be legalized	Yes	238	56.4
	No	179	42.4
	I don't mind	5	1.2
Reason why abortion should be legalized*	Abortion is major health problem	177	41.9
	Reduce morbidity and mortality	147	34.9
	Can facilitate to get service in safe area	101	24
	Solve problems of unwanted pregnancy	67	16
	Reduce cost for inducing abortion	34	8.1
	Other	7	1.7
Why do you prefer abortion not to be legalized*	Abortion is homicide to the fetus	232	54.9
	Abortion is homicide to the fetus	232	54.9
	My religion doesn't allow	107	25.4
	Encourage un wanted pregnancy	96	22.8
	Culturally not accepted	31	7.3
	Encourage pre or extra marital sex	33	7.9
	Other	7	1.7
Would advise or encourage a friend to go for an abortion if abortion is legalized	Yes	234	55.6
	No	149	35.4
	I don't know	39	9.2

Table 3: Attitude of respondents towards legalization of abortion in Ethiopia, in Mizan Aman town, Bench Maji zone, SWE, 2016 [*Multiple responses were allowed and hence totals could be greater than actual size].

Out of those who preferred legalization of abortion, 360 (85.2%) preferred hospitals. Of all, 200 (47.5%) and 127 (30.1%), said both partners, and the pregnant woman should have equal right to make decision to terminate pregnancy, respectively. Majority, 148 (35%), of respondents replied that unmarried women should have allowed to make abortion in legal way other than other groups. Of all respondents, 156 (36.9%) believed that a woman has the right to terminate her pregnancy, if she wants, while 266 (63.1%) of them were against it (Table 4).

Variable	Category	Frequency	Percent (%)
Preferred place to provide safe abortion service	Hospital	360	85.2
	Health center	49	11.6
	Clinic	6	1.4
	Private clinic	3	0.8

	Other	3	0.8
Who should decide on termination of pregnancy	Both partners	200	47.5
	Pregnant women	127	30.1
	Health worker	78	18.4
	Relatives	27	6.4
	Husband	22	5.3
	Pregnant women and health worker	20	4.7
	Other	1	0.2
	Do not know	11	2.6
What type of women should be allowed for abortion	Unmarried	148	35
	Have medical indication	96	22.7
	Students	76	18
	All women	68	16.1
	Married	26	6.2
	All should not be allowed	14	3.31
	Do not know	33	7.9
	other	4	1.5
Respondents opinion towards the right to decide termination of pregnancy	Yes	156	36.9
	No	266	63.1

Table 4: Respondents preferred places to abortion, who should decide and what type of women should be allowed to terminate pregnancy in Mizan Aman town, Bench Maji zone, SWE, 2016 [*Multiple responses were allowed and hence totals could be greater than actual size].

Out of all respondents, 359 (85%) of them had awareness about the complication of abortion. Health problems related to unsafe abortion, which were mainly mentioned by respondents include, death 321 (76.1%) and HIV/AIDS transmission. Majority, 99%, of respondents suggested at least one solution to solve the problem related with unsafe abortion, while 1% of them responded that they did not know. Out of the total, 288 (68.3%) respondents believed that legalization of induced abortion would reduce problems related to unsafe abortion (Table 5).

Variables	Category	Frequency	Percentage (%)
Respondents knowledge about complication of abortion	Yes	359	85
	No	50	11.9
	Do not know	12	3.1
Anticipated health problems due to abortion	Bleeding	131	31.4
	Infection	120	28.4
	Transmission of HIV/AIDS	178	42.2
	Incomplete abortion	13	3.1
	Infertility	72	17.1
	Death	321	76.1
	Extra cost	11	2.6
	Do not know	13	2.9

Suggested measures to prevent health problems due to unsafe abortion	Use of modern/traditional FP method	219	52
	Legalization of induced abortion	72	17.1
	Safe abortion service	31	7.3
	Avoiding sex if unmarried	63	15
	Give birth if once pregnant	20	4.7
	Health education	160	38
	I do not know	2	1
Did you think legalization of induced abortion reduce the problem associated with it	Yes	288	68.3
	No	112	26.4
	I don't know	23	5.4

Table 5: Knowledge of respondents towards the health effect of unsafe abortion in Mizan Aman town, Bench Maji zone, SWE, 2016 [*Multiple responses were allowed and hence totals could be greater than actual size].

Knowledge of respondents towards the current legal status of induced abortion in Ethiopia

Only 24 (5.7%) of respondents replied that the country law allow induced abortion for specific peoples who are in need.

On the contrary 346 (82%) of them replied as induced abortion was currently illegal in Ethiopia (Figure 1).

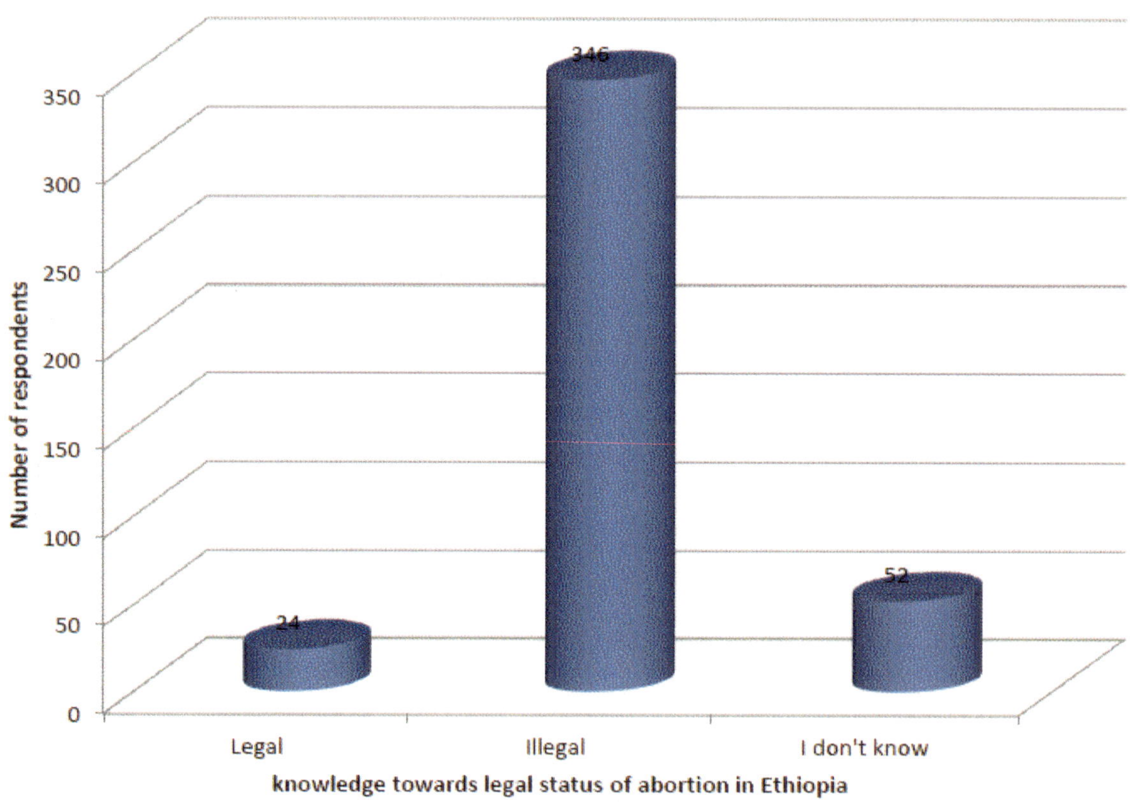

Figure 1: Knowledge of respondents towards current legal status of abortion in Ethiopia, Mizan Aman town, Bench Maji zone, SWE, 2016.

Factors affecting attitudes of respondents towards legalization of abortion

According to the finding of this study knowledge of respondents about complication of abortion has an association with an attitude towards legalization of abortion, where X^2=6.89, p=0.008 which was P<0.05. Respondents preference to terminate unwanted pregnancy and their belief whether legalization of abortion would reduce associated complication have a significant association with attitudes towards legalization of induced abortion with X^2=77.36, and X^2=86.37 respectively where both have P<0.005.

The remaining variables such as sex, marital status, religion and educational status of respondents did not showed any significant association with attitudes of respondents towards legalization of induced abortion (Table 6).

Variable	Category	Attitude towards legalization		X^2, OR (95% CI)	P-value
		Supported	Unsupported		
Sex	Male	122 (54.4%)	102 (45.6%)	0.726, 0.846 (0.575, 1.244)	0.394
	Female	116 (58.5%)	82 (41.5%)		
Marital status	Married	102 (59.3%)	71 (40.7%)	0.933, 1.213 (0.819, 1.796)	0.334
	Currently not married	135 (54.9%)	114 (45.1%)		
Educational level	Literate	58 (57.5%)	43 (42.5%)	3.315, 1.519 (0.967, 2.385)	0.068
	Illiterate	151 (47.9%)	170 (52.1%)		
Religion	Christians	197 (56.5%)	151 (43.5%)	0.036, 1.050 (0.634, 1.74)	0.849
	Muslim	41 (55.8%)	33 (44.2%)		
Prefer abortion if pregnancy is unwanted*	Yes	216 (92.9%)	17 (7.1%)	77.39,9.949 (5.619,17.614)	0
	Other	106 (56%)	83 (44%)		
knowledge about complication of abortion*	Yes	212 (59.1%)	147 (40.9%)	6.89, 2.052 (1.191,3.536)	0.008
	Other	26 (41.3%)	37 (58.7%)		
Legalization of abortion would reduce associated complication*	Yes	213 (74.1%)	75 (25.9%)	86.37, 8.033 (5.037-12.811)	0
	Other	35 (18.4%)	99 (81.6%)		

Table 6: Factors affecting attitude of respondents towards legalization of abortion, in Mizan Aman town, Bench Maji zone, SWE, 2016 [OR-Odds ratio, *-variables which were found to have significant association with attitude towards legalization of abortion].

Discussion

Lack of awareness about the current abortion law can influence individual decision making regarding contraceptive use, lead to accessing unsafe abortion and unsafe post abortion care. Recently, the Ministry of Health (MoH) has emphasized that increasing of knowledge and vital safe abortion care information at grass-root level are crucial to provide the required service especially for women in areas of the country where the level of awareness and service is low [5].

The result of this study revealed that only 24 (5.7%) of respondents had knowledge of current legal status of abortion by law while, majority, 346 (82%), of them were replied as induced abortion was illegal in Ethiopia. This study was comparably similar with a result obtained in Jimma town where only 10.8% of respondents replied as the country had legalized abortion with some circumstances [9] and Sri Lanka where only 11% of the respondents knew the situations in which abortion was legal in [10].

Also, despite the liberalized abortion law Ethiopian women are facing major obstacles such as lack of awareness of the liberalized abortion law and access to safe abortion services. Moreover, health professionals also lack awareness about the new law. This may be attributed to poverty, lack of services, religion, culture, and fear of health risks are the possible reasons [11].

Unsafe abortion complications are most common in poor women and younger age women, who are also the ones with limited access to abortion care and family planning services and with higher proportion of unwanted pregnancies [12]. The result of this study estimated that from women's who had history of terminating pregnancy which constitutes 28 (14.1%) of total women's interviewed, most, 21 (75%) and 20 (71.4%), of women who have terminated their pregnancy were mentioned premarital pregnancy and unintended sex as a major reason for undertaking abortion respectively.

Majority of abortions, 23 (82.1%), were induced by health professional which was similar with a result obtained in Gambella Hospital where among patients admitted to Gynecological ward during the period from June 1997 to May 1998, 70% of all were reported to be cases of abortion, of which 35.7% were induced [5].

Informants' attitudes toward the abortion law varied widely depending on a lot of factors. Having negative attitudes towards abortion and lack of skills and information for termination of pregnancy were found to be the two commonest reasons for not providing services as required as possible [13]. Out of the total respondents, 238 (56.4%) preferred legalization of induced abortion in.

Of those who preferred legalization of induced abortion majority, 41.9%, of respondents considered unsafe abortion as a major health problem, on the contrary of those who opposed legalization of induced abortion, 54.9%, of them had perceptions that termination of pregnancy was homicide.

This result was comparatively better than a result obtained in Nigeria, where more than one-third of informants opined that abortion should not be legal under any circumstance, and a significant proportion suggested that the solution to unsafe abortion is not to legalize the procedure but to provide sexuality education. Religious and moral concerns were the most common reasons for opposing liberalization of abortion laws [14].

Public perceptions on induced abortion can influence not only the outcome of the unwanted pregnancy but also health sector policy response. In this study area more than 234 (55.6%) of total respondents, believed that people would use legal abortion services, and they would encourage a friend or other individuals who are in need to go for an abortion which was indicator of positive perception towards induced abortion.

Women right to undertake decision on their fetus can be significant factor that play a critical role to enhance utilization of abortion services [13]. In this study of all, 200 (47.5%) and 127 (30.1%), said both partners, and the pregnant woman should have equal right to make decision to terminate pregnancy, respectively. As well, 156 (36.9%) believed that a woman has the right to terminate her pregnancy, if she wants, while 266 (63.1%) of them were against it.

From this study a significant proportion of participants, 359 (85%), of them had awareness about the complication of abortion. Health problems related to unsafe abortion, which were mainly mentioned by respondents include, death 321 (76.1%) and HIV/AIDS transmission. Majority, 99%, of respondents suggested at least one solution to solve the problem related with unsafe abortion.

Out of the total, 288 (68.3%) respondents believed that legalization of induced abortion would reduce problems related to unsafe abortion. This result was similar with a result obtained in Uganda [15] and Ethiopia [16] where more than 90% knew at least one complication of an induced abortion and 75% of respondents knowing the complications of induced abortions respectively.

This study showed that knowledge of respondents about complication of abortion, (X^2= 6.89, p=0.008), respondents preference to terminate unwanted pregnancy (X^2=77.36, p<0.005) and their belief whether legalization of abortion would reduce associated complication (X^2=86.37, P<0.005) has an association with an attitude towards legalization of abortion. This finding was coherent with other similar study in Argentina [17], Uganda [15], Ethiopia [17] and Jimma [9].

Also this study discovered that there were not have statistically significant association between sex, marital status, religion and educational status of respondents and their attitudes towards legalization of induced abortion. This result was similar with a finding in Jimma where educational status has no association with an attitude towards legalization X^2=7.217 which P=0.301 [9].

But it is different from a result obtained from a study conducted in Ethiopia where the educational status has a statistical significant association with an attitude that is X^2= 69.84 which P value is P<0.05 [18].

Strengths

Since this study was the first conducted on knowledge and attitudes of men and women towards legalization of induced abortion in the country which was a community based, gives strength to this study.

Limitations

- The study conducted only in urban settings and thus it is difficult to generalize both for urban and rural community.
- The study was cross sectional, thus, under reporting of induced abortion might exist.

Conclusions

- In contrast to other studies attitudes of respondents towards legalization of abortion were good, where more than half of the people in the study area had positive attitudes towards legalization of induced abortion.
- Also more respondents believed that people would use legal abortion services, and they would encourage a friend or other individuals who are in need to go for an abortion which was the main reflection of positive attitude towards legalization of induced abortion.
- Large number of respondents in the studied area prefers induced abortion to be legalized in their locality. Majority of them were aware of any complications related with unsafe abortion and thus most of them consider unsafe abortion as a major health problem.
- The result of this study revealed low number of respondents had knowledge of current legal status of abortion in their country.
- Knowledge of respondents about complication of unsafe abortion, respondent's preference to terminate unwanted pregnancy and their belief whether legalization of abortion would reduce associated complication has an association with an attitude towards legalization of abortion.
- Most of women who have terminated their pregnancy were mentioned premarital pregnancy and unintended sex as a major reason for undertaking abortion.

Recommendations

- It is very critical to increase awareness of community towards the current legal status of abortion and existing services. Thus concerned bodies such as professionals, CBOs and other influential individuals should be involved to enhance community knowledge and perception towards legal aspects of abortion otherwise since it can affect decision making on abortion legal reforms.
- It is better prepare discussion on the risk of unsafe abortion and current legal status of abortion in Ethiopia with the community particularly with reproductive age groups that are found in Mizan Aman town.
- Unintended pregnancy were identified as a common cause of unsafe abortion in the studied area and thus promotion of information and education on unsafe abortion related problems, the benefits of safe legal abortion services, family planning is very essential.

- The attitude of communities in Mizan town were in good status in contrast to other studies but since communities negative attitude can be a cause for failure of a countries policy it is expected to disseminate information on risks of unsafe abortion and prevention of unwanted pregnancies, and promotion legal abortion.
- The researchers suggested that further studies need to be conducted to assess the magnitude of problems related with unintended pregnancy.

Ethical Consideration

Ethical permission was obtained from Mizan Tepi University, college of health science. Verbal consent was obtained from each study subject included in the study. The participant who was included in the study was given enough information in order to make an informed decision. Each piece of information that was given by every responding subject was strictly kept confidential.

Acknowledgement

We would like to pass our heartily felt acknowledgement to Mizan Tepi University, College of health science for their cooperation in doing this research. Our sincere appreciation also goes to staff members of public health department for their support and encouragement. Finally we want to appreciate the cooperation of all concerned officials and respondents in Mizan Aman town.

References

1. Berrer M (2000) Making abortions safe: A matter of good public health policy and practice. The Int J Public Health 78: 569-714.
2. FORE/CSA (1999) The 1994 population and housing census of Ethiopia: Results at the country level. Analytical report II: 375.
3. http://www.who.int/whosis/mme_2005.pdf
4. World Health Organization (WHO) (2004) Unsafe abortion: Global and regional estimates of the incidence of unsafe abortion and associated mortality. Geneva, Switzerland.
5. Federal Ministry of Health (Ethiopia) (2006) Technical and procedural guidelines for safe abortion services in Ethiopia. Addis Ababa, Ethiopia.
6. Rahman A (1998) A global review of laws on induced abortion. Int Fam Plan Perspect 24: 56-64.
7. Sserbanescu F (1995) The impact of recent policy changes on fertility, abortion and contraception use in Romania. Stud Fam Plann 26: 76-87.
8. Population Reference Bureau (PRB) (2008) World population data sheet. Popul Today.
9. Tenkir L (1999) Induced abortion among Jimma comprehensive high school students. Knowledge, attitude and practice. Ethiop J Health science 9: 25-31.
10. Suranga MS (2016) Perception on the abortion laws in Sri Lanka: A community based study in the city of Colombo. Ceylon Med J 61: 171-175.
11. Goodman N (2008) Bridging the gaps: Implementation of comprehensive abortion care in Ethiopia.
12. Care for post abortion (1997) USA: Johns Hopkins School of public Health. Popul Rep D.
13. Ethiopian Society of Obstetricians and Gynecologists (ESOG) (2001) Knowledge, attitude and practice of health workers regarding the Ethiopian abortion law. In: East, Central and Southern African Association of Obstetrical and Gynecological Societies Conference, Addis Ababa, Ethiopia p: 3-4.
14. Friday E (2009) Perceptions of policymakers in Nigeria toward unsafe abortion and maternal mortality. Int Perspect Sex Reprod Health 35: 194-202.
15. Paluku JL (2013) Knowledge and attitudes about induced abortions among female youths attending Naguru teenage information and health centre, Kampala, Uganda. J Epidemiol Public Health 5: 178-185.
16. Senbeto E (2005) Prevalence and associated risk factors of induced abortion in northwest Ethiopia. Ethiop J Health Dev 19: 37-44.
17. Hestvik H (2014) Knowledge and attitudes towards abortion among medical students at the University of Buenos Aires, Argentina. Medical student research project p: 1-36.
18. Bitew S (2013) Knowledge and attitude of women of childbearing age towards the legalization of abortion, Ethiopia. J Sci Innov Res 2: 192-203.

Gender Differences in Verbal Behavior Style in Interviews in Family Medicine: Mars and Venus, or North Dakota and South Dakota?

Jose Luis Turabian*, Minier-Rodriguez LE, Moreno-Ruiz S, Rodriguez-Almonte FE, Cucho-Jove R and Villarin-Castro A

Specialists in Family and Community Medicine, Health Center Santa Maria de Benquerencia, Toledo, Spain

***Corresponding author:** Jose L Turabian, Specialist in Family and Community Medicine, Health Center Santa Maria de Benquerencia, Toledo, Spain, E-mail: jturabianf@hotmail.com

Abstract

Objective: To describe and compare the doctor-patient communication referred to the verbal behavior of the female patients *vs.* males in the family medicine consultation.

Participants and Methods: Secondary analysis of existing dataset coded to explore patient-clinician verbal communication during ambulatory visits in a family medicine office in a health Centre in Toledo (Spain) was carried out. The audio recording of the consultations and verbal content analysis of the interviews, based on the identification of 6 categories of classification of behaviors of the interaction process (Proposing, Supporting/ Agreeing, Disagreeing, Giving Information, Seeking Information, and Building) was performed. A convenience sample was carried out. Other variables included were age, sex and duration of the consultation in minutes. Triangulation between different evaluators, and methodological (qualitative and quantitative) was used as a technique to control the reliability and biases. Once the qualitative study is completed, the results of the number of behaviors in the total of triadic and dyadic consultations were presented in a quantitative way (Frequencies: No, %). The bivariate comparisons were performed using the test of Chi squared and exact probability Fischer.

Results: 20 consultations were included in the analysis. In interviews with women *vs.* males, differed only in showing more "Supporting" (39% and 29%, respectively; $p=0.05$), and less "Disagreement" (3% and 11% respectively; $p<0.05$). There were no differences in the verbal behaviors of the physician in the consultations with female *vs.* male patients. There were also no differences in the duration of the consultation among female patients *vs.* males (7': rank: 3'-15' *vs.* 7'; rank: 4'-12').

Conclusion: The verbal behavior in interview in the family medicine consultation with female patients *vs.* males shows only small differences. Neither men are of Mars nor the women of Venus; may be men are from North Dakota and women from South Dakota.

Keywords: Family practice; Physician-patient relations; Methodology; Gender differences; Verbal behavior style; Communication; Language

Introduction

Communication refers to the process of human beings responding to the symbolic behavior of other persons. Verbal communication is the conscious effort of expression that tries to facilitate the understanding of the message on the part of the other through the use of the words. On the most obvious level, language allows us to satisfy basic functions such as describing ideas, making requests, and solving problems. But beyond these functions, the way we use language also influences others and reflects our attitudes in more subtle ways.

Any language is a collection of symbols governed by a variety of rules and used to convey messages between people. Because of its symbolic nature, language is not a precise tool: meanings rest in people, not in words themselves. In order for effective communication to occur, it is necessary to negotiate meanings for ambiguous statements. Language not only describes people, ideas, processes, and events; it also shapes our perceptions of them in areas including status, credibility, and attitudes about gender and ethnicity. Along with influencing our attitudes, language reflects them. The words we use and our manner of speech reflect power, responsibility, affiliation, attraction, and interest [1].

The clinical interview is a technique or channel and place of communication, where the doctor-patient relationship is produced and developed. And communication in the doctor-patient relationship points out signalizes (like signaling a path in the forest, so that we can focus our field study on the natural values of the place) the clinical setting [2]. Communication is increasingly essential in clinical practice. Since the end of the eighteenth century a process of recovery of the word in medicine has been consolidated, culminating in Freud, who introduces the term "talking cure", a cure through the word [3]. The cornerstone of general practice is the consultation. Communication is an important component of patient care [4], maybe the most important aspect of practice that health care professionals have to master [5]. The physician-patient interview is the key component of all health care, particularly of primary medical care [6].

Studies have linked physicians' communication skills to a variety of positive outcomes, including patient and physician satisfaction, higher levels of adherence to therapeutic recommendations, improved physiological indicators of disease control, and enhanced physical and mental health status. Previous research has displayed, a physician's communication style is an essential factor predicting patient satisfaction and compliance. Furthermore, a good physician-patient relationship and high communication quality seem to be crucial elements fostering the activation of patients' self-healing powers [7,8]. The patients' amount of talking using their own words in the medical history segment of the health center visit was significantly correlated with reductions in blood pressure from clinic to home visit, but not with blood pressure levels at the clinic or the home interview [9].

About communication much has been written, from psychology to sociology, psychiatry and anthropology. As doctors and patients communicate during medical interactions they both offer accounts and respond to them. The medical interview is characterized by a moment-to-moment battle that mirrors and largely sustains the institutional authority and status of doctors and the reality of genders [10-14].

Men and women differ, and numerous academic and lay books have exploited those differences [4]. The relationship between gender and language is a confusing one. There are many differences in the ways men and women speak: The content of their conversations varies, as do their reasons for communicating and their conversational styles [1]. About gender and language, so far it has been discussed language use as if it were identical for both sexes. Some theorists and researchers, though, have argued that there are significant differences between the way men and women speak, whereas others have argued that any differences are not significant. What are the similarities and differences between male and female language use? These differences begin early in childhood. A variety of sociolinguistic studies show that boys use talk to assert control over one another, whereas girls use talk to maintain harmony. Women behave differently in conversations than do men. For example, women ask more questions in mixed-sex conversations than do men [15,16].

Gender is often thought of in terms of bipolar categories. On the basis of this gender assignment, naturalized norms and expectations about verbal behavior are imposed upon people. There is a strong tendency for gender stereotyping. Stereotyping involves a reductive tendency: to "stereotype someone is to interpret their behaviour, personality and so on in terms of a set of common-sense attributions which are applied to whole groups. Like caricatures, they focus obsessively on certain characteristics, real or imagined, and exaggerate them [17].

So, stereotypes about men and women's conversational styles abound. It has been suggested that men and women come from different planets-men are from Mars, women are from Venus, and that they have different ways of talking, thinking, different brain organizations, etc. [18]. Research has supported these theories-at least in some cases. In one study women's talk was judged more aesthetic, whereas men's talk was seen as more dynamic, aggressive, and strong. In another, male job applicants were rated more fluent, active, confident, and effective than female. Despite the differences in the ways men and women speak, the link between gender and language use isn't as clear-cut as it might seem. Despite the differences identified earlier, several research reviews have found that the ways women and men communicate are much more similar than different. In light of the considerable similarities between the sexes and the relatively minor differences, some communication scholars suggest that the "*men are from Mars, women are from Venus*" claim should be replaced by the metaphor that "*men are from North Dakota, women are from South Dakota*." [1,19], and the overall difference made by gender is either small or close to zero [20].

However, it is accepted that communication is more or less cross-cultural [21], and numerous studies have been done using this approach, and while the results have been mixed, the commonest finding is that men talk more than women [22]. On the other hand, patients vary in their willingness and ability to actively participate in medical consultations. Patient participation in medical interactions is influenced by:

- The patient's personal characteristics (e.g., age, gender, education, ethnicity)
- The physician's communication style (e.g., use of partnership-building and supportive talk)
- The clinical setting (e.g., the health condition, medical specialty) [23].

The influence of the physician's gender or the gender agreement of the physician and the patient has also been studied to some extent [24-33], but much less the gender influence of the patient in the doctor-patient interview. It has been found that there is a lack of research using patient gender as a meaningful variable in health communication research. Furthermore, because of poor research designs in many studies, many of the conclusions about the role of gender in health communication interaction were found to be suspect. Suggestions for improving future research are:

- Including patient gender as a significant variable in research designs
- Using research procedures appropriate to the research being conducted
- Using a more descriptive, rules-based epistemological approach to forming research questions [34].

Communication during medical encounters can be analyzed by using different interaction analysis systems. These systems differ with regard to their clinical relevance, observational strategy, reliability/validity and channels of communicative behavior. There are several communicative behaviors that occur in consultations: instrumental (cure oriented) *vs.* affective (care oriented) behavior, verbal *vs.* non-verbal behavior, high *vs.* low controlling behavior, and medical *vs.* everyday language vocabularies [35].

Existing research is limited because of lack of consensus of what to measure, conflicting findings, and relative lack of empirical studies [6]. The dynamics of communication, which has been tried to measure on the basis of verbal participation questionnaires [36], as well in relation with some aspects of patient-centered communication [37], as well using the Rotter interaction analysis [38], or by studying different aspects of the biopsychosocial model in the clinical interview [39], or by measuring whether family history and family problems were being taken into account during the visit [40], by the percent of total visit speech [36], by physician statements that were analyzed and coded as social talk, physician-centered statements, patient-centered statements, and discussion of patient affect, family, health promotion, and patient education [39], by cluster analysis [41], by means of coding what physicians say when they are trying to influence patients' behaviors [42], by audio recorded, and categorized using the Medical Communications Behavior System and using Synote, a freely available application enabling synchronization of audio recordings with transcripts and coded notes [8], or by Revised Maastricht History-Taking and Advice checklist (MAAS-R) [25], by the VR-MICS/D (Verona-Medical Interview Classification System/Doctor) [43,44], using Stiles' Verbal Response Mode coding system (VRM) [9,45], by Bales Interaction Process Analysis [46], by means of focusing upon the relational aspects of communication to interpret the diversity of patients' verbal communications to the female interviewer [26], and the classification of Byrne and Long [47], among other.

In this context, we carried out a qualitative and quantitative study with the objective of describe and compare the doctor-patient communication referred to the verbal behavior of the female patients *vs.* males at the family practice clinic, and to assess the implications that these possible differences may have in clinical management and interpersonal relationship.

Patients and Methods

Design and variables

Secondary analysis of existing dataset coded to explore patient-clinician verbal communication during ambulatory visits in a family medicine office was carried out [48]. A qualitative, observational, narrative study was conducted during the months of November and December 2016, through the audio recording of the consultation, and verbal content analysis of the interviews, based on the identification of 6 categories of classification of the behaviors in meetings that describe the class or behavioral style of the interaction process, not its content, proposed by its simplicity by open university, and based on the principles of Bales and Flanders, reviewed from a study by Huthwaite Research Group [49]:

- **Proposing:** A behavior that advances a new concept or suggests a course of action
- **Supporting or agreeing:** A behavior that includes a conscious and direct statement of support or agreement with another person or their concepts
- **Disagreement:** A behavior that involves a conscious and direct statement of difference of opinion, or criticism of the concepts of another person
- **Giving information:** A behavior that offers facts, opinions or clarifications to other individuals
- **Seeking information:** A behavior that seeks facts, opinions or clarifications of another individual or individuals
- **Building:** A behavior that extends or develops a proposal that has been made by another person.

Other variables were also collected like age, sex, and time in minutes of the consultation. The study is descriptive in its approach since it aims at describing an existing phenomenon and it is qualitative in nature although the study uses a quantitative method for data collection.

In all cases the doctor was the same professional, a family doctor who remains in the same consultation for over 25 years. The location was a family medicine office, in the Health Center Santa Maria de Benquerencia, Toledo, Spain, which has a list of 2,000 patients. Patients of both sexes over 14 years old were included (In Spain family doctors attend patients over 14 years old). The phrases of courtesy of initial and final greetings were not included in the content analysis of the interview.

Sample

A non-random sampling, intentional of convenience was carried out by the investigators. A suitable sample number was considered when saturation occurred, i.e. no new data were obtained [50]. The criterion of maximizing the diversity in obtaining the sample was taken into account, and all types of interviews were included, with the widest possible situations.

Ethical aspects

The informed consent of all patients and companions for using of data in research was obtained. There was an ethical approval of the institution (Teaching unit of Family Medicine).

Analysis

The interview was recorded in audio, and later transcribed to Microsoft® Word. With the written text of the interview, their content was subsequently analyzed, classifying the interaction in the doctor-patient interview, according to the 6 proposed categories [51,52]. Once the qualitative study is completed, the results of the number of behaviors in the total of consultations are presented in a quantitative way.

Only as an orientation, because the size of the sample was not calculated as a quantitative, but qualitative, the bivariate comparisons were performed using the test of chi-square and exact probability Fischer.

But the sample is reasonably no different from the one randomly selected. Besides, it would be very strange if there were individuals over represented or absent in the sample studied. So, with all cautions, quantitative results could be extrapolated to the population of family medicine consultations [49,53].

Control of validity and reliability of the study

- **Internal validity (credibility):** A qualitative study has internal validity when it is credible. We present a description and interpretation of a human experience or phenomenon such that people who live that experience immediately recognize the descriptions and interpretations as their own.
- **External validity (applicability):** Although it is not an objective of the qualitative studies, that do not pretend to generalize findings, to the extent that the researchers have respected the criterion of maximizing the diversity in obtaining the sample and make a detailed description of the context and participants, the findings may be applicable in similar contexts.

Technique to control bias

Triangulation (it is to get different perspectives of the phenomenon studied).

Among different evaluators: The written transcripts of voice recordings of the interviews were read by the research team to reach agreements on the categories that were used. The process was as follows:

- Each researcher made several individualized readings of each interview, obtaining the frequency of each of the 6 categories, until obtaining a file of categories of each journal.
- A group agreement of categories was made for each interview-assigning phrase of original data to new categories-and thus forming a file of definitive categories for each interview. To facilitate this process, it was worked from the categories of a researcher, which were compared with those of the rest in group work. And finally, the results were interpreted.

Methodological triangulation: The integration of qualitative and quantitative findings, help researchers to clarify their theoretical propositions and the basis of their results [54].

Results

About 20 consultations were included in the analysis. In interviews with women *vs.* males, differed mainly in showing more "Supporting" (39% and 29%, respectively; p=0.05), and less "disagreement" (3% and 11%, respectively; p<0.05) (Table 1).

There were no differences in the verbal behaviors of the physician in the consultations with female *vs.* male patients (Table 2).

There were also no differences in the duration of the consultation among female patients *vs.* males.

Table 3 presents some "verbatims" (literal phrases) in relation to the behaviors of each actor in consultations.

Patients behavior styles	Female patients (N=12) No (%)	Male patients (N=8) No (%)	Statistical Significance
Proposing	8(3%)	9(6%)	X^2=2.5211, p=0.112332, NS
Supporting/ Agreeing	104(39%)	42(29%)	X^2=3.8335, p=0.05
Disagreeing	8(3%)	16(11%)	X^2=11.2697, p=0.000788
Giving information	125(47%)	65(46%)	X^2=0.0884, p=0.766177, NS
Seeking information	18(7%)	5(4%)	X^2=1.8743, p=0.170987, NS
Building	3(1%)	6(4%)	Fisher Exact test= 0.071202, NS
Total	266(100%)	143(100%)	
Age	X=43 (Range: 14-54)	X=51 (Range: 20-70)	

Table 1: Comparison of verbal behavior between patients female/male.

Doctor behavior styles	Female patients (N=12) No (%)	Male patients (N=8) No (%)	Statistical Significance
Proposing	44(16%)	28(16%)	X^2=0.907, p=0.340914, NS
Supporting/Agreeing	32(12%)	25(14%)	X^2=2.8276, p=0.092657, NS
Disagreeing	7 (2%)	3(2%)	X^2=0.0747, p=0.784558, NS
Giving information	108(39%)	67(39%)	X^2=2.3996, p=0.121363, NS
Seeking information	65(23%)	36(21%)	X^2=0.1508, p=0.69774, NS
Building	21(8%)	13(8%)	X^2=0.2889, p=0.590917, NS
Total	277(100%)	143(100%)	

Table 2: Comparison of verbal doctor behavior between patients female/male.

Behaviour styles	Female Patients	Male Patients	Doctor
Proposing	That, make me a study, I do not know why...	You have to measure me the blood pressure...	You can try...
	Yes, let me have a complete analysis	I ... I want to take...better... pills	This drug that I am going to change you does not make that potassium is lost...
Supporting/ Agreeing	Okay, I'll try to quit smoking	Yes, yes, it's three weeks that's left...	Let's see... you're right.
	All right, we'll have to try them	Exactly...	All right, nothing happens
Disagreeing	No, nothing	No, I have not seen her; that was yesterday...	No, no, I think you cannot...
	No, no ... No, it was to be warned before February, but now it is not...	No ... I do not trust in this	It should not because it is the same...

Giving information	Well the truth... I did not know whether to come or not, because I have always been a little delicate...,but I have been many years that I noticed that my gut swells a lot and …	He gave me some drops here and then yesterday... Well, I'll explain what about these patches ...	Well, I'll explain what about these patches ...
	He gave me some other little pills and I almost died	He says that I have the eyes, dry, dry, dry, dry...	What you can take at meals while there is pain or fever
Seeking information	He has prescribed these patches for me and I have not bought them because ... I'm afraid to wear them, and I'm waiting for your opinion...	A question: can you prescribe...?	For pain do you have something at home, ibuprofen?
	And if it goes more?"...	And then they told me that I have to make me an x-ray to...	You need to tell me if you want....
Building	A complete blood test that the doctor of the skin sent me because of the problem that I have, so I guess ...	.. Better ... in mid-January because he wants to have it fairly recent	It's related....
	... actually it is so...I tell you, because sometimes ... I say these are nerves, I'm very nervous	... or the same is a fastitis of those...	You are already a veteran.... well, although it usually tends to cure alone, an antibiotic is usually taken...

Table 3: Some "verbatims" (literal phrases) in relation to the behaviors of each actor in consultations.

Discussion

Ways to measure verbal communication in the doctor-patient interview

The clinical interview is an essential competence of the family doctor and communication a key piece in the doctor-patient relationship. Health care and its outcomes depend on how the professional and the consultant communicate, since profitable communication is a major component in health recovery [4,7-9].

In our study, a proposed Open University classification, though based on similar principles to Bales and Flanders, was used. It was chosen from other existing ones because it is a much simpler system and consist an abbreviated system devised originally to study management skills and behaviour by the Huthwaite Research Group [49].

Gender and language: gender differences in patients' verbal behaviors

What are the similarities and differences between male and female language use? In our study, interviews with women *vs.* males differ very little, these differences being found only in showing more "Supporting", and less "disagreement" in women (Table 1), which coincides with what was previously reported.

Research shows that the notion that men and women communicate in dramatically different ways is exaggerated. Men are more likely than women to emphasize making conversation fun. By contrast, women's conversations focus more frequently on feelings, relationships, and personal problems. Because women use conversation to pursue social needs, female speech typically contains statements showing support for the other person, demonstrations of equality, and efforts to keep the conversation going. With these goals, it's not surprising that traditionally female speech often contains statements of sympathy and empathy: "I've felt just like that myself", "The same thing happened to me!" Women are also inclined to ask lots of questions that invite the other person to share information: "How did you feel about that?" "What did you do next?" The importance of nurturing a relationship also explains why female speech is often somewhat powerless and tentative. Saying "This is just my opinion..." is less likely to put off a conversational partner than a more definite "Here's what I think..." Men's speech is often driven by quite different goals than women's. When someone else is sharing a problem, instead of empathizing, men are prone to offer advice: "That's nothing to worry about ..."or "Here's what you need to do..." Besides taking care of business, men are more likely than women to use conversations to exert control, preserve their independence, and enhance their status. This explains why men are more prone to dominate conversations and one-up their partners. Men interrupt their conversational partners to assert their own experiences or point of view. (Women interrupt too, but they usually do so to offer support: quite a different goal) [1]. Table 3 presents some "verbatims" (literal phrases) in relation to the behaviors of each actor in consultations of our study.

It has been reported that women consult with more problems, usually give more information, and ask more [55], but no in our study. The sociolinguistic research of communication indicates that before a problem, men prefer to solve it by their account, while the women look for suggestions and solve it consensually, and women are the more supportive [56]. We found similar findings. In addition, the fact that in our study women show more behaviors of agreement and support makes us think about the possibility of achieving better health outcomes in those consultations. Verbal behaviors positively associated with health outcomes included empathy, reassurance and support and the therapeutic alliance is based in rapport, trust, communicative success and agreement [57]. Although other authors report that women were more likely than men to refuse medication [58].

Duration of the consultations

Who speaks more, women or men? The results of the investigations seem contradictory. It may depend on where the conversation is: public or private. For women the language of communication tends to establish connections and negotiate relationships. For men, communication tends to preserve independence and maintain status and hierarchy [59]. Female callers are more verbose than male callers for open style prompts [60]. Older men and women were significantly more verbose than young men and women [61]. And it may be interpreted that longer consultations are associated with more adequate diagnoses, at least in psychological problems [62]. But, we found no differences in the duration of the consultation among female patients *vs.* males (Figure 1).

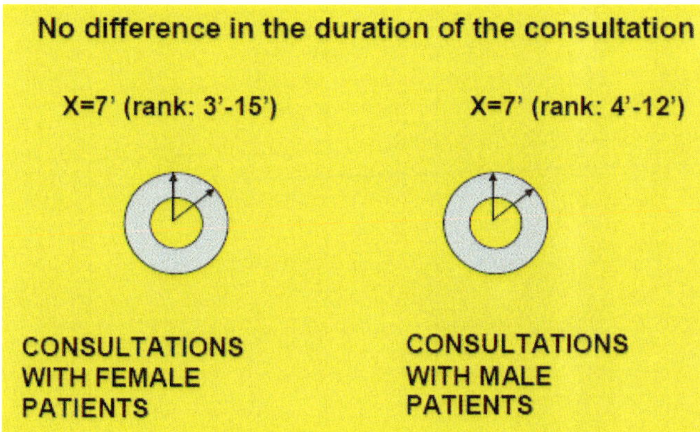

Figure 1: Duration of consultation in female and male patients.

A growing body of research explains some of the apparent contradictions between the similarities and differences between male speech and female speech. They have revealed other factors that influence language use as much or more than does gender. Orientation toward problem-solving also plays a role in conversational style. The cooperative or competitive orientations of speakers have more influence on how they interact than does their gender. The speaker's occupation and social role also influence speaking style [1].

The gender of the care providers

In our study it was the same male doctor in all the interviews, and in this way they have not influenced differences by gender nor social gradient, etc. Although with contradictions, as there are authors who communicate that male and female doctors use a speech style which is not gender specific [24], or the gender of the care providers was not an issue for patients regarding communication about some issues [26], most of the data show patient-doctor gender concordance/discordance is associated with their agreement/disagreement on advice given during the consultation. Physicians need to be conscious that their own demographic characteristics and perceptions might influence the quality of prevention counseling delivered to their patients [27]. The authors hypothesize that physician gender could have an effect on patient satisfaction, compliance, and health status through the mechanisms of the physician patient relationship and gender-specific communication strategies to explore the patient's agenda [7,28-30,32,33,63]. On the other hand, it has been reported that physicians make more efforts to communicate with female patients than with men, and give more time to consultations with women [55], but this is not reproduced in our study.

Verbal behavior of the physician

The doctor-patient discourse is characterized by the asymmetry that emerges in the encounter, the distribution of turns in the conversation and the type of language strategies that are used. While the doctor has at his disposal more linguistic alternatives to participate in the speech, the patient has more restricted possibilities of using the same linguistic resources in that event. The physician, in his role, searches for information about the patient, makes a diagnosis, proposes and evaluates a treatment. The patient tends to give personal information about his psycho-social identity and to initiate, according to the need and possibility, subjects that he considers relevant.

Michael Balint suggested that the patient begins the consultation by offering one or more problems and issues to the doctor. The doctor respond to these offers, indicating his acceptance or rejection of them, until some kind of compromise is worked out. In consequence, while the matters that are discussed in the consultation reflect the problems presented by the patient, they include only those aspects that the doctor indicates that are allowable [47].

In our study, the verbal behaviors of the physician (male) in females and males patient's consultations were similar [Table 2], and coincides with that reported by other authors. Although there may be much variability among physicians in their verbal behavior in the consultation, this does not change individually according to gender of the patients attended [47].

Limitations of the Study

Coding difficulties: There may be difficulties in sorting, since in one sentence more than one category can be observed. A disagreement phrase can also be a proposal, and a proposition can also give information. Many phrases can be considered either as giving or requesting information, but once the technique has been learned, and biases have been avoided through the triangulation of researchers, it can provide useful data on the behavior of individuals and groups [49,53].

The question of representativeness of the sample: How "typical" was the behavior of the participant? Will the "typical" activity be found if the sample were larger? Is the activity collected subject to fluctuations? Interviews were recorded on normal consultation days, communication was not subject to fluctuations, and we thought that by maximizing the diversity of the participants, they represented the patients usual of the consultation. It may be thought that the size of the sample is small, but in qualitative studies this usually is small, and sample size was given by the saturation of the data [50]. Once the qualitative study was completed, the results of the number of behaviors in were presented in a quantitative way, and only as an orientation.

The content of the interviews was not collected: Only the class or behavioral style of the interaction process. The conceptualization of the disease is another point of interest that can vary between males and females. A different understanding of the origin of a disease, for example, can cause communication problems and lead to misunderstandings. Although there is a great deal of variation within each gender, on the average, men and women discuss a surprisingly different range of topics. These differences can lead to frustration when men and women try to converse with one another. Male patients tended to describe their ailments with performance-oriented statements, whereas the female patients usually used emotional-oriented statements [64,65], and more women indicate symptoms of fatigue than men did [34] and consult with more problems [55]. All these possible differences in verbal content were not studied in our study.

Silences have not been collected: we could interpret the silence that the patients assume, in some segments of the conversation, is a reflection of the emotional load they feel with the situation they are living. But when picking up the audio recording it was not possible to know when the patient's voice was silenced.

Non-verbal communications have not been collected: verbal and nonverbal messages should be studied as inseparable phenomena they happen together [65].

Conclusion

In the 90's of the twentieth century, a book was published in the United States that was successful sales; *"Men are from Mars, women are from Venus"* [18]. This book argues that men and women were destined not to understand us because we assume that the other will react as we do. The book revolves around the argument that men find it easier to deal with specific issues, aggressiveness and competition (Mars was the god of war in Greek mythology) and women are more accustomed to dealing with The affective issues, which have to do with human bonds and communication (Venus was the goddess of love).

The book has been criticized for placing human psychology into stereotypes. Men and women are not fundamentally different, contrary to what Gray suggests in his book. The idea that men and women "speak different languages" has itself become a dogma, treated not as a hypothesis to be investigated. The idea that men and women differ fundamentally in the way they use language to communicate is a myth in the everyday sense [20].

The verbal behavior in interview in the family medicine consultation with female patients *vs.* males shows very small differences. There is a weak indication of a profile of verbal behavior that may facilitate the work of the physician. Neither men are of Mars nor the women of Venus; maybe men are from North Dakota and women from South Dakota [1,19]. Anyway, he results of communication are more complex than what these results may indicate. Communication is an extremely important but underexplored dimension of the patient-therapist relationship [8], and the methods described here could provide a useful model for further research and reflective practice, although they need further refinement. However, our data, showing that consultations with female patients show more agreement/support, which coincides with other authors [66], suggest that this type of interview can achieve better results [4].

Why is the research on gender differences so confusing? In some studies, male speech and female speech seem identical, whereas other studies reveal important differences. As we have already said, one reason for the confusion is that factors besides gender influence the way people speak: the setting in which conversation takes place, the expertise of the speakers, their social roles (husband/wife, boss/employee, and so on). Also, female roles are changing so rapidly that many women simply don't use the conversational styles that characterized their older sisters and mothers. But in addition to these factors, another powerful force that influences the way individual men and women speak is their sex role-the social orientation. Research suggests that neither a stereotypically male style nor female style is the best Choice. As opportunities for men and women become more equal, we can expect that the differences between male and female use of language will become smaller [1].

References

1. Adler RB, Rodman G (2006) Understanding human communication (9th Edn) Oxford University Press, New York.
2. Turabian JL, Perez Franco B (2008) The effect of seeing the sea for the first time. An attempt at defining the family medicine law: The interview is clinical medicine. Aten Primaria 40: 565-566.
3. Ibor JJ (2008) Learning to communicate with the patient and the people around them. Educ Med 11: 1.
4. Teutsch C (2003) Patient-doctor communication. Med Clin North Am 87: 1115-1145.
5. Roberts L, Bucksey SJ (2007) Communicating with patients: What happens in practice? Phys Ther 87: 586-594.
6. Beck RS, Daughtridge R, Sloane PD (2002) Physician-patient communication in the primary care office: A systematic review. J Am Board Fam Pract 15: 25-38.
7. Roter DL, Hall JA, Aoki Y (2002) Physician gender effects in medical communication: A meta-analytic review. J Am Medical Assoc 288: 756-764.
8. Roberts LC, Whittle CT, Cleland J, Wald M (2013) Measuring verbal communication in initial physical therapy encounters. Phys Ther 93: 479-91.
9. Orth JE, Stiles WB, Scherwitz L, Hennrikus D, Vallbona C (1987) Patient exposition and provider explanation in routine interviews and hypertensive patients' blood pressure control. Health Psychol 6: 29-42.
10. Troike SM (2003) The ethnography of communication: An introduction (3rd edn.) Blackwell Publishing, Malden, USA.
11. Fisher S, Groce S (1990) Accounting practices in medical interviews. Language in society 19: 225-250.
12. Fisher S (1984) Doctor-patient communication: a social and micro-political performance. Sociol Health Illn 6: 1-29.
13. Fisher S, Groce SB (1985) Doctor-patient negotiation of cultural assumptions. Sociology of Health and Illness 7: 342-374.
14. Zola K (1972) Medicine as an institution of social control. Sociological Review. 20: 487-504.
15. Giles H, Street RL (1985) Communication characteristics and behaviour: In Knapp ML and Miller GR. Handbook of interpersonal communication. Beverly Hills, CA. Sage pp: 205-261.
16. Kohn A (1988) Girl talk, guy talk. Psychology Today 22: 65-66.
17. Talbot M (2003) Gender stereotypes: Reproduction and challenge. In: The handbook of language and gender. Edited by Janet Holmes and Meyerhoff. Blackwell Handbooks in Linguistics MA, USA.
18. Gray J (1992) Men are from mars, women are from venus. New York: HarperCollins.
19. Canary DJ, Dindia K (1998) Sex differences and similarities in communication: Critical essays and empirical investigations of sex and gender in interaction. LEA's communication series. Mahwah, NJ.
20. Cameron D (2007) The Myth of Mars and Venus: Do men and women really speak different languages? Oxford University Press, Oxford.
21. Suciu G. Why don't you understand? Male-Female communication. University of Oradea.
22. James D, Drakich J (1993) understanding gender differences in amount of talk. In: Tannen D. Gender and conversational. New York: Oxford studies in sociolinguistics. Oxford University Press.
23. Street RL, Gordon HS, Ward MM, Krupat E, Kravitz RL (2005) Patient participation in medical consultations: why some patients are more involved than others. Med Care 43: 960-969.
24. Skelton JR, Hobbs FD (1999) Descriptive study of cooperative language in primary care consultations by male and female doctors. BMJ 318: 576-579.
25. Christen RN, Alder J, Bitzer J (2008) Gender differences in physicians' communicative skills and their influence on patient satisfaction in gynaecological outpatient consultations. Soc Sci Med 66: 1474-1483.
26. Kummer K, Doren M, Kuhlmey A (2008) Communication about incontinence between affected individuals and health care providers-the patients' perspective. Z Gerontol Geriatr 41: 267-273.
27. Schieber AC, Delpierre C, Lepage B, Afrite A, Pascal J, et al. (2014) Do gender differences affect the doctor-patient interaction during

consultations in general practice? Results from the intermede study. Fam Pract 31: 706-713.

28. Weisman CS, Teitelbaum MA (1985) Physician gender and the physician-patient relationship: recent evidence and relevant questions. Soc Sci Med 20: 1119-1127.
29. Sandhu H, Adams A, Singleton L, Carter D, Kidd J (2009) The impact of gender dyads on doctor-patient communication: A systematic review. Patient Educ Couns 76: 348-355.
30. Meeuwesen L, Bensing J, Muinen A (2002) Communicating fatigue in general practice and the role of gender. Patient Educ Couns 48: 233-242.
31. Hall JA, Roter DL (2002) Do patients talk differently to male and female physicians? A meta-analytic review. Patient Educ Couns 48: 217-224.
32. Roter DL, Hall JA (2004) Physician gender and patient-centered communication: a critical review of empirical research. Ann Rev Publ Health 25:497-519.
33. Roter DL, Lipkin M, Korsgaard A (1991) Sex differences in patients and physicians communication during primary care medical visits. Medical Care 29: 1083-1093.
34. Alley AS (2009) Health communication and gender: A Review and Critique. Journal Health Communication: 35-54.
35. Ong LML, Haes JCJM, Hoos AM, Lammes FB (1995) Doctor-patient communication: A review of the literature. Soc Sci Med 40: 903-918.
36. Schmidt KL, Lingler JH, Schulz R (2009) Verbal communication among Alzheimer's disease patients, their caregivers, and primary care physicians during primary care office visits. Patient Educ Couns 77: 197-201.
37. Shields CG, Epstein RM, Fiscella K (2005) Influence of accompanied encounters on patient-centeredness with older patients. Am Board Fam Med 18: 344-354.
38. Rotter J (1954) Social learning and clinical Psychology. Englewood Cliffs, New York: Prentice-Hall.
39. Marvel K, Major G, Jones K, Pfaffly C (2000) Dialogues in the exam room: Medical interviewing by resident family physicians. Fam Med 32: 628-632.
40. Main DS, Holcomb S, Dickinson P, Crabtree BF (2001) The effect of families on the process of outpatient visits in family practice. J Fam Pract 50: 888.
41. Roter DL, Stewart M, Putnam SM, Lipkin M, Stiles W (1997) Communication patterns of primary care physicians. JAMA 277: 4.
42. Smith VA, DeVellis BM, Kalet A, Roberts JC, DeVellis RF (2005) Encouraging patient adherence: primary care physicians' use of verbal compliance-gaining strategies in medical interviews. Patient Educ Couns 57: 62-76.
43. Saltini A, Cappellari D, Cellerino P, Piccolo L, Zimmermann C (1998) An instrument for evaluating the medical interview in general practice: VR-MICS/D Verona-Medical Interview Classification System/Doctor. Epidemiol Psichiatr Soc 7: 210-223.
44. Piccolo L, Saltini A, Zimmermann C, Dunn G (2000) Differences in verbal behaviours of patients with and without emotional distress during primary care consultations. Psychol Med 30: 629-643.
45. Meeuwesen L, Schaap C, Staak C (1991) Verbal analysis of doctor-patient-communication. Soc Sci Med 32: 1143-1150.
46. Stewart M (1984) Patient characteristics which are related to the doctor-patient interaction. Fam Pract 1: 30-36.
47. Usherwood T (2009) Understanding the consultation. Evidence, theory and pactice. Open University Press. Berkshire, UK.
48. Turabian JL, Rodriguez LE, Ruiz SM, Almonte FE, Jove R, Castro A (2017) Qualitative and quantitative study of verbal behavior style in interviews with patient's companion in family medicine: understanding and measuring. Scientific Pages of Family Medicine.
49. Bell J (1997) Doing your research project. A guide for first-time researches in education and social sciences. Open University Press, Buckingham.
50. Malterud K, Siersma VD, Guassora AD (2016) Sample size in qualitative interview studies. Guided by information power. Qual Health Res 26: 13.
51. Bowling A (2000) Research methods in health. Investigating health and health services. Open University Press, Philadelphia.
52. Burnard P, Gill P, Stewart K, Treasure E, Chadwick B (2008) Analysing and presenting qualitative data. Br Dent J 204: 429-432.
53. Flanders NA (1970) Analysing teaching behavior. Cambridge, MA: Addison-Wsley.
54. Ostlund U, Kidd L, Wengströn Y, Dewar N (2010) Combining qualitative and quantitative research within mixed method research designs: A methodological review. Int J Nurs Stud 48: 369-383.
55. Thompson V, Waitzkin H (1999) Differences in clinical communication by gender. JGIM 14: 112-121.
56. Flaherty J, Richman J (1989) Gender differences in the perception and utilization of social support: Theoretical perspectives and an empirical test. Soc Sci Med 28: 1221-1228.
57. Pinto RZ, Ferreira ML, Oliveira VC, Franco MR, Adams R, et al. (2012) Patient-centred communication is associated with positive therapeutic alliance: a systematic review. J Physiother 58: 77-87.
58. Haskell SG, Bathulapalli H, Pham T, Goulet J, Skanderson M, et al. (2014) Sex differences in patient and provider response to elevated low-density lipoprotein cholesterol. Women's Health Issues 24: 575-580.
59. Tannen D (1990) You just don't understand: women and men in conversation. New York, NY: Ballantine Books.
60. Jonsson H, Eklund R (2011) Gender differences in verbal behaviour in a call routing speech application. Fonetik p: 51.
61. Ruffman T, Murray J, Halberstadt J, Taumoepeau M (2010) Verbosity and emotion recognition in older adults. Psychol Aging 25: 492-497.
62. Hutton CM, Gunn J (2007) Do longer consultations improve the management of psychological problems in general practice? A systematic literature review. BMC Health Serv Res 7: 71.
63. Verlinde E, Laener N, Maesschalck S, Deveugele M, Willems S (2012) The social gradient in doctor-patient communication. Int J Equity Health 11: 12.
64. Piccolo L, Mazzi M, Saltini A, Zimmermann C (2002) Inter and intra individual variations in physicians' verbal behaviour during primary care consultations. Soc Sci Med 55: 1871-1885.
65. Hedegaard J, Ahl H, Johansson A, Siouta E (2014) Gendered communicative construction of patients in consultation settings. Women Health 54: 513-529.
66. Jones SE, LeBaron CD (2002) Research on the relationship between verbal and nonverbal communication: Emerging integrations. J Commun 52: 499-521.

O-Shot: Platelets Rich Plasma in Intimate Female Treatment

Neto JB*

Department of Aesthetic Vaginal Surgery, Centro Clínico Mãe de Deus, Brazil

***Corresponding author:** João Brito Jaenisch Neto, Surgeon, Department of Aesthetic Vaginal Surgery, Centro Clínico Mãe de Deus, Brazil, E-mail: jaenisch2402@yahoo.com.br

Abstract

Background and objectives: This pilot study measures the response of women with stress incontinence, overactive bladder, lubrication and sexual dysfunction (libido, arousal, dyspareunia) to evaluate the safety, tolerability and clinical efficacy of "O-Shot" Platelets Rich Plasma (PRP) of the vulvo vaginal field. PRP has recently been shown to accelerate rejuvenate aging skin by various growth factors and cell molecular adhesions. Each patient received two sessions at the intervals of two months apart.

Material and methods: This is a first prospective study in Brazil, in a private clinic, non-randomized controlled, in non-selected 68 women performed by the same doctor (author) between August 1st 2016 to February 1st 2017. All Patients were fully informed of the therapeutic innovation of the PRP injection (O-Shot) and consented to the procedure. Sixty-eight women, non-select ages of 32-97 (average: 62.8 years old) were included in this pilot study and self-reported having stress incontinence (13 patients), overactive bladder (15 patients), mixed (22 patients), lack of lubrication and sexual dysfunction (libido, arousal, dyspareunia). Detailed history, physical examination, questionnaire, neurological tests, urine sample, Q-tip test and stress test were performed. All patients were followed by the author each two weeks until the end of protocol. The protocol was based on two sessions of Platelet Rich Plasma (O-Shot) two months apart, no matter if the patient was satisfied or not with the first session.

Results: About sixty-eight women in the age ranging from 32 to 97 (average: 62.8 years old) were enrolled in this study. Of the sixty-eight patients, 94% of them were satisfied, only 6% of them with overactive bladder did not have any improvement with this treatment.

Conclusion: Platelet Rich Plasma, "O-Shot" is an in-office treatment that is safe, effective, non-surgical, and non-hormonal option for women having stress incontinence, overactive bladder, lack of lubrication, and sexual dysfunction, such as lack of libido, arousal or dyspareunia.

Keywords: Dyspareunia; Neurological tests; Rejuvenation; Anorgasmy; Stem cells

Introduction

Platelet Rich Plasma (PRP) has been used over last 20 years as an effective treatment in various medical and surgical fields [1]. There are publications about the use of PRP in wound treatment, maxillofacial surgery, soft tissue injuries, orthopedic, gastrointestinal surgeries, burns, and in cosmetic procedures [1,2]. PRP has been demonstrated to be effective with no serious side effects and activates pluripotent cells in the area of injection resulting in rejuvenation [3,4].

Since PRP is autologous, there are no known contraindications and also offers the advantage of flowing into tissue. There are several growth factors and cytokines [5,6] in the platelets that are released to cellular damage starting to work together stimulating process of fibroblast collagen synthesis. This pilot study measures the responses of women with stress incontinence, overactive bladder, varying degrees of sexual dysfunction (libido, orgasm, and dyspareunia) and lack lubrication.

Material and Methods

About 68 non-selected women, ages 32-97 (average: 62.8 years old) G 60/Para 48/Abortation 27 were enrolled in this pilot study from August 1st 2016 to February 1st 2017 with complaints of urinary problems such as urinary stress incontinence, overactive bladder (OAB), lack of lubrication and sexual dysfunction (lack of libido, decreased arousal, dyspareunia and anorgasmy) (Table 1).

All sixty-eight women were treated by the author and underwent to have a Platelet Rich Plasma "O-Shot" (Dr. Charles Runels Patent) as proposal protocol treatment getting two session two months apart.

All patients work up:

- Detailed history
- Physical examination (by the author)
- Answer a questionnaire (Figure 1)
- Neurological exam (abdominal reflexes, sensorial problems)
- Urine sample (urinalysis and culture)
- Q-tip test and stress test

Cure to urinary complaints was defined as complete subjective relief of urinary incontinence (stress/overactive bladder) and absence of loss urine on physical examination. Those complaints of lack of lubrication and sexual dysfunction a subjective improvement of their symptoms and a questionnaire answered were used as a treatment response.

Symptoms	Patients	Age	Average
USI+OAB+LUB	15	56-88	75.6
OAB	4	46-75	67
USI+OAB+2° ANORG+LUB+AROU+LIB+DYSP	7	36-67	53.4
OAB+2° ANORG+LUB+LIB+AROU	5	45-87	64
OAB+LUB+AROU+LIB	6	69-97	83.1
USI+LUB+AROU+LIB	13	38-74	55.3
ATR+LUB+DYSP	10	33-73	59.7
1° ANORG+LUB+AROU+LIB+DYSP	2	32-64	48
2° ANORG+LUB+AROU+LIB+DYSP	6	55-77	63
Total	68	32-97	62.8

Table 1: List of patients with different complaints (USI: Urinary Stress Incontinence; LUB: Lack of Lubrication; AROU: Arousal; DYSP: Dyspareunia; OAB: Overactive Bladder; ANORG: Anorgasmy; LIB: Lack of Libido; ATR: Atrophy).

Symptoms	Yes	No
Stress Incontinence		
Over active Bladder		
Lack of Lubrication		
Lack of Libido		
Atrophy		
Anorgasmy 1° or 2°		
Dyspareunia		
Arousal		

Figure 1: Questionnaire indicating symptoms.

Your goals were achieved with this protocol-Very pleased: Yes/No; Not pleased: Yes/No

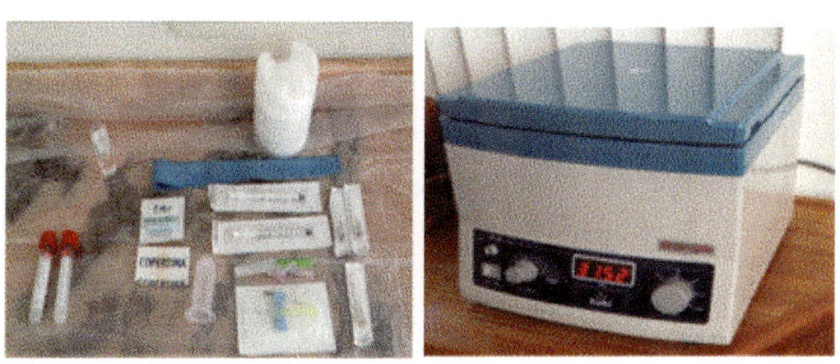

Figure 2: Syringes to be used and Centrifuge used for separation of blood cells.

Equipment's used for the procedure include 5 cc syringes (Figure 2), 30 G ½ needles,10% calcium chloride, Vacutainer kit-vacuum collection tube with separator gel, Butterfly 23 G, Centrifuge (Figure 2), Numbing cream (topic anesthesia): 20% Benzocaine, 6% Lidocaine and 4% Tetracaine.

Technique

Peripheral blood was drawn from the arm (Figure 3) and a numbing cream Benzocaine 20%; Lidocaine 6%; Tetracaine 4% was used in the vulvo vaginal area.

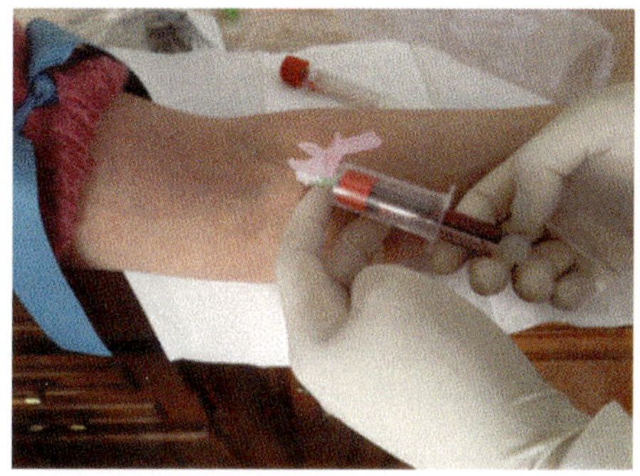

Figure 3: Collection of peripheral blood from the arm.

The kit was equipped with a butterfly 23 G needle, Vacutainer Kit, 10% calcium chloride, 5 cc syringe and 30 ½ needle. 8 cc blood sample was aspirated from the patient's peripheral vein in vacuum collection tube with separator gel, which is centrifuged separating red and white cells at 3.100 RPM for 9 minutes. Platelet cells were on top of the tube and the 4 cc of cells suspension are called Platelet Rich Plasma (PRP) (Figure 4).

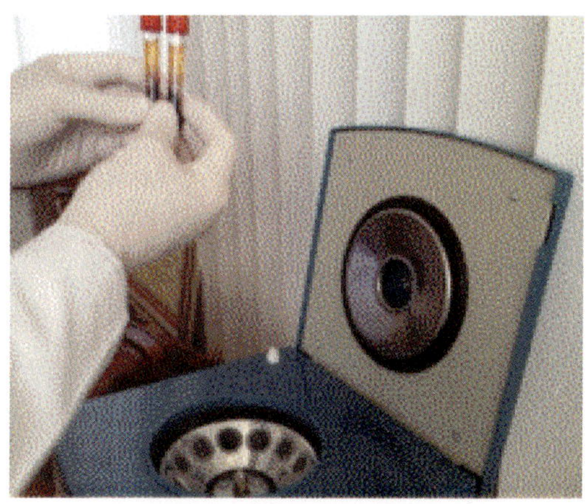

Figure 4: Centrifuged blood sample.

After isolation of the PRP, 10% of calcium chloride 0.2 cc is added to the 4 cc of PRP (Figure 5) and injected by a 5 cc syringe with 30 G ½ needle into the following anatomic areas: 2 cc in Pubocervical fascia (G-Spot); 0.5 cc in Skene's gland each and 1 cc in to the clitoral area (button part of the clitoris) (Figure 6).

The average procedure time was 15 minutes and no prophylaxis antibiotics were used.

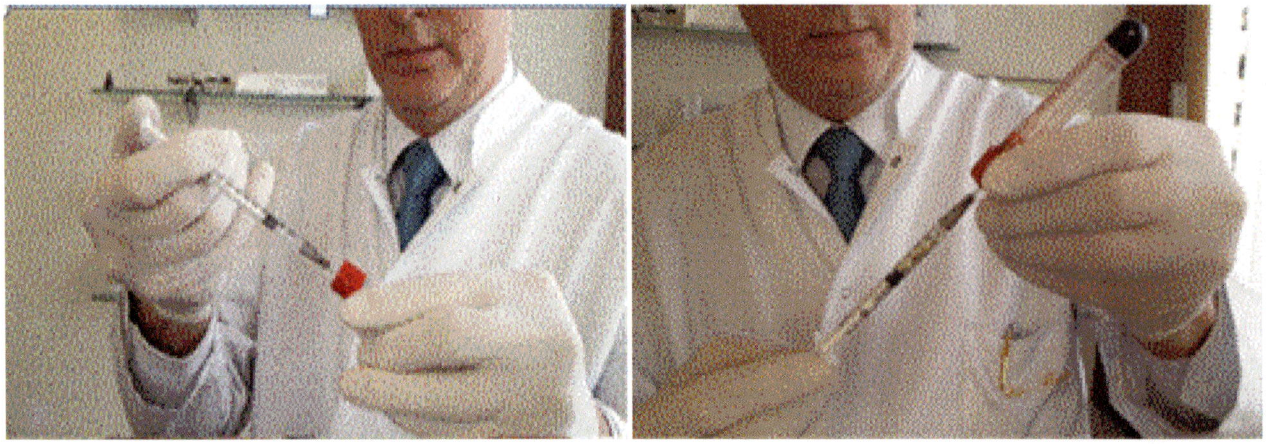

Figure 5: Addition of 10% Calcium chloride to the PRP.

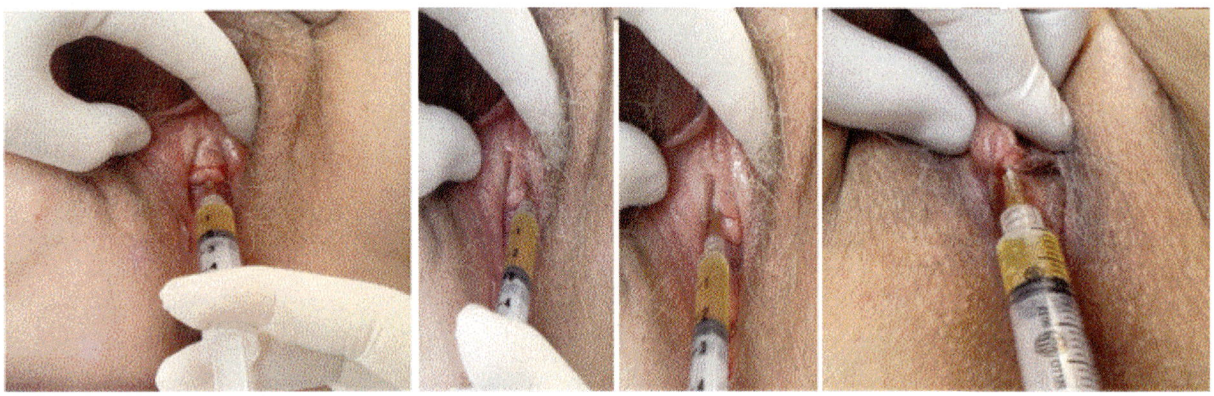

Figure 6: Procedure for PRP injection.

Results

About sixty-eight women were treated by PRP ("O-Shot" 2 sessions, 2 months apart) in the first non-randomized pilot study in the Southern Brazil, from August 1st 2016 to February 1st 2017 in a private clinic, in Porto Alegre, RS-Brazil. Around 94% (64 patients) were satisfied with the outcome reporting subjectively and by a questionnaire improvement of lubrication and sexual dysfunction (arousal, libido, dyspareunia and anorgasmy) on the first session and getting better after the second PRP Shot. Those complaints stress urinary stress urinary incontinence (13 patients) reported more than 90% of relief of the symptoms. It was amazing and surprising that these patients related great deal of benefits after 2 weeks of the first "O-Shot". Patients with overactive bladder (15 patients) had 74% of relief of symptoms and 6% (4 patients) have no treatment response. All females with mixed urinary incontinence (22 patients) were satisfied with the results. Cure was defined (urinary problems: stress incontinence, overactive bladder and mixed incontinence) as complete subjective relief of urinary incontinence, questionnaire and absence of loss urine on physical examination.

Side-effects

We have no extreme sexual arousal or ejaculating problem. None of our patients were lost within the 6 month follow up period, and the procedure was well tolerated without serious side effects. Burning sensation were exposed by 100% of our patients when injection in para urethral areas and clitoris.

Discussion

The use of Platelet Rich Plasma (PRP) has been known in aesthetic medicine. PRP is an autologous preparation of platelets in concentrated plasma that contains a mixture of bioactive agents derived from both platelet and plasma. When PRP is activated (calcium chloride), and injected in to the anatomic areas such as clitoris; pubo-cervical fascia; G spot; Skene's glands, then growth factors may cause differentiation of pluripotent stem cells resulting in neo-angiogenesis, fibroblast growth, and neuronal growth, improving physiologic responsiveness. PRP is non-antigenic and contains no synthesis agents that could cause an untoward local or systemic reaction. We could find no reports of granuloma formation, infections, or local tissue necrosis. The body will not react to it immunologically [7]. No allergic reactions. PRP induces regrowth of new tissues by of the activation of pluripotent stem cells. [7,8] Improved vascularity and neuronal regrowth in the vagina and in the clitoral area could restore or possibly enhance sexual responsiveness and sensitivity by increasing blood flow. Collagen and sensory nerve regrowth might relieve coital discomfort as well as enhance vaginal sensitivity. It is a great benefit to those suffering with stress incontinence and overactive bladder, rejuvenating the entire surrounding area to the urethra, pubo-cervical fascia and Skene's glands. It seems to last around 1-2 years.

Conclusion

Platelet Rich Plasma is a safe non-surgical, cost-effective procedure to be utilized as a new tool to help patients with stress incontinence, overactive bladder and sexual dysfunctions.

References

1. Redaelli A (2010) Face and neck revitalization with Platelet Rich Plasma (PRP): Clinical outcome in a series of 23 consecutively treated patients. J Drugs Dermatol 9: 466-472.
2. Banihashemi M, Nakhaeizadeh S (2014) An introduction to application of PRP in skin rejuvenation. Rev Clin Med 1: 38-43.
3. Shin MK, Lee JH, Lee SJ, Kim NI (2012) Platelet Rich Plasma combined with fractional laser therapy for skin rejuvenation. Dermatol Surg 38: 623-630.
4. Sclafani AP, Steven A, Cormic SA (2011) Induction of dermal collagenesis, angiogenesis and adipogenesisis human skin by injection of platelet rich fibrin matrix. Arch Facial Plast Surg 14: 132-136.
5. Sclafani AP (2011) Safety, efficacy and utility of platelet rich fibrin matrix in facial plastic surgery. Arch Facial Plastic Surg 13: 247-251.
6. Runels C, Melnick H, Debourbon E, Roy L (2014) A pilot study of the effect of localized injections of autologous Platelet Rich Plasma (PRP) for the treatment of female sexual dysfunction. J Womens Health 3: 169.
7. Nakudo N, Minakata T, Mitsui T, Kushida S, Notodihardjo FZ, et al. (2008) Proliferation promoting effect of PRP on human adipose- derive stem cells and human dermal fibroblast. Plast Reconstr Surg 122: 1352-1360.
8. Anitua E, Sanchez M, Zalduendo MM, Prado R, Orive G, et al. (2009) Fibroblastic response to treatment with different preparations rich in growth factors. Cell Prolif 42: 162-170.

Is Gestational Weight Gain and Early Postpartum Weight Retention Associated with Clinician Advice in First Time Mothers?

van der Pligt P [1*], Ball K [1], Hesketh KD [1], Teychenne M [1], Crawford D [1], Dodd J [2,3] and Campbell K [1]

[1] *Institute for Physical Activity and Nutrition (IPAN), School of Exercise and Nutrition Sciences, Deakin University, Geelong, Australia*

[2] *The University of Adelaide, School of Paediatrics and Reproductive Health, Robinson Research Institute, Adelaide, South Australia, Australia*

[3] *Department of Perinatal Medicine, The Women's and Children's Hospital, Women's and Babies Division, North Adelaide, South Australia, Australia*

***Corresponding author:** van der Pligt P, Institute for Physical Activity and Nutrition (IPAN), School of Exercise and Nutrition Sciences, Deakin University, Geelong, Australia, E-mail: p.vanderpligt@deakin.edu.au

Abstract

Objective: Excess gestational weight gain (GWG) and postpartum weight retention increase risk for multiple maternal and child health complications. It is necessary to determine factors which influence maternal weight across the perinatal period. The aim of this study was to describe change in maternal body mass index (BMI) from pre-pregnancy to early postpartum, document weight advice provided by clinicians and assess associations of advice received with maternal weight gain during and following pregnancy.

Methods: First-time mothers (n=448) and their newborns who attended first-time parent groups at their local Maternal and Child Health Centres were recruited to the InFANT Extend cluster randomised controlled trial. Baseline data collection occurred when women were approximately three months postpartum. Women completed a written questionnaire assessing their own health and the provision of weight-related advice received by clinicians. Pre-pregnancy weight and GWG were self-reported. Postpartum height and weight were objectively measured.

Results: Mean GWG was 14.0 ± 6.08 kg and 41.0% of women experienced excess GWG. Mean PPWR was 4.3 ± 5.75 kg and mean BMI increased from 24.8 ± 4.9 kg/m² pre-pregnancy to 26.2 ± 4.9 kg/m² at three months postpartum. The proportion of women classified obese (BMI≥ 30kg/m²) almost doubled from pre-pregnancy (11.8%) to three months postpartum (21.7%) (p<0.001). 54.4% of all women reported receiving advice regarding how much weight to gain during pregnancy and 42.6% reported receiving advice to avoid excess GWG. During the postpartum period, just 5.8% of women reported receiving advice about how much they should weigh and 8.3% reported receiving advice about programs to support weight loss. No associations were found between provision of clinician advice with GWG or postpartum weight retention.

Conclusion: More intensive approaches are required, opposed to provision of advice alone, to influence healthy maternal weight across the perinatal period in the interest of best maternal and child health outcomes.

Keywords: Clinician; Gestational weight gain; Postpartum; Weight; Maternal; Obesity; Body mass index; Perinatal; Pregnancy

Introduction

The US Institute of Medicine (IOM) 2009 guidelines [1,2] provide clinical guidance as to the amount of weight women should gain during pregnancy and have been adopted in the absence of country specific gestational weight gain (GWG) guidelines (Figure 1) [3,4]. Women who gain within these recommendations have been shown to have better perinatal outcomes than women who exceed them [5].

Excess GWG places the mother and child at increased risk of multiple pregnancy complications [1,6-12] and has been shown to adversely impact offspring birth weight (both large for gestational age and small for gestational age [13,14] and higher long term BMI [13]. Postpartum weight retention (PPWR) has been associated with an increased risk for complications during subsequent pregnancies [15], the development of maternal overweight and obesity [16,17] and future cardiovascular disease [16,18].

Moreover, a 20-40% increased risk for babies being born large for gestational age, has been shown to exist, with an increase of 1-2 maternal BMI units between pregnancies [19].

Advice provided by antenatal clinicians may be an effective means to assist women to achieve best maternal weight outcomes. Women are in frequent contact with a wide range of health professionals during the antenatal period [20-22].

This study aimed to assess change in maternal BMI from pre-pregnancy to the postpartum period, document weight advice provided by clinicians during and following pregnancy, and assess associations of the advice received with maternal GWG, PPWR and postpartum BMI.

Pre pregnancy weight category	Pre pregnancy BMI	Recommended total weight gain Range (kg)	Recommended rate of weight gain*2nd and 3rd Trimester Range (kg/week)
Underweight	<18.5kg/m²	12.5 – 18kg	0.51 (0.44 – 0.58)
Normal weight	18.5 – 24.9kg/m²	11.5 – 16kg	0.42 (0.35 – 0.50)
Overweight	25 – 29.9kg/m²	7 – 11.5kg	0.28 (0.23 – 0.33)
Obese	≥30kg/m²	5 – 9kg	0.22 (0.17 – 0.27)

Figure 1: Institute of Medicine (IOM) 2009 guidelines for total gestational weight gain^ (* Calculations assume a 0.5-2 kg weight gain during the first trimester, ^Adapted from the IOM's 2009 report Weight Gain During Pregnancy: Re-examining the Guidelines).

Materials and Methods

Participants were from the three year, extended Melbourne Infant Feeding Activity and Nutrition Trial Program (InFANT Extend) (Trial registration: (InFANT Extend) Australian New Zealand Clinical Trials Registry (ACTRN12611000386932 13/04/2011)), a cluster-randomised controlled intervention trial which recruited first-time mothers who attended first-time parent groups at their local Maternal and Child Health Centres in Victoria, Australia [23]. The InFANT Extend trial was a community based, early obesity prevention program whereby first-time parent groups received 6x2 hour sessions, delivered quarterly from when infants were three months of age up until 18 months [24]. Sessions were based on anticipatory guidance and were focussed on child feeding, active play, screen time alternatives, parent modelling, physical activity and sedentary behaviours [24].

Women allocated to the control group received usual care as part of the Maternal and Child Health system and mailed newsletters regarding general information (e.g. dental health and sun protection) [24]. A two-stage random sampling design was used to select first-time parent groups across all socio-economic areas [23].

As described elsewhere, [23] to ensure inclusion of a broad representation of socio-economic areas, each Local Government Area (LGA) was classified by socio-economic position (SEP) classified by the Australian Bureau of Statistics Socio-Economic Indices for Areas (SIEFA). Local Government areas with SEIFAs in the lowest quintile throughout the state of Victoria were eligible for selection. Firstly, nine LGAs met criteria to be approached for recruitment and seven LGAs agreed to take part. Secondly, 62 first-time parent groups were selected from the seven LGAs.

To be eligible, parents needed to be English literate. A minimum of eight participants per group needed to consent within mid and higher SEP LGAs and six participants per group were required to consent within the lower SEP LGAs. This lower number required for lower SEP areas was because participation rates tend to be low in health behaviour interventions for vulnerable population groups or low socio-economic areas [25]. Groups that provided written consent, administered by trained researchers at the recruitment visit were then randomly allocated to intervention or control arms.

The InFANT Extend trial was approved by the Deakin University Human Research Ethics Committee (2011-029) (2007-175) (11/02/2011) and the Victorian Government Department of Human Services, Office for Children Research Co-ordinating Committee.

Questionnaires including demographic information and questions regarding practitioner advice were distributed to all mothers when they were approximately three months postpartum at the recruitment visit. Surveys were completed prior to women being allocated to either the control or interventions groups. Postpartum weight was measured by trained research staff when women were approximately three months postpartum. As detailed in a previously published study [23], weight in light clothing and without shoes was measured once using Tanita digital scales (Model 1582) and recorded to the nearest 0.01 kg.

Height was measured using a Victar stadiometer. Two measurements were taken separately and were recorded to the nearest 0.1cm. If the two measurements disagreed by 0.5cm or more, a third measurement was taken. The average of the height measurements was used to calculate maternal pre-pregnancy BMI and postpartum BMI (weight (kg)/height (m^2)). Body Mass Index classification was according to World Health Organization criteria [26].

Excess GWG was defined as weight gain exceeding the 2009 IOM recommendations [2], a universally used reference for multiple studies which have assessed pregnancy weight gain [12,27-30]. Postpartum weight retention was calculated as the difference between objectively measured weight at three months postpartum and self-reported pre-pregnancy weight. While this method does not take into account the possibility of maternal weight gain during the first few months following childbirth [31], this method has been used for calculating PPWR in multiple studies of varying design assessing maternal PPWR [17,32-35], as well as a recent, large, Norwegian, prospective cohort pregnancy study which assessed PPWR of approximately 95, 200 women [36]. This method is considered a standard method for calculating PPWR [2].

Provision of advice given by clinicians during pregnancy was measured by two items requiring a yes/no response which asked women if during their pregnancy, a doctor, nurse or other healthcare practitioner talked with them about weight advice: 'how much weight you should gain during pregnancy' and 'avoiding gaining too much weight during pregnancy'.

Provision of advice given by clinicians during the postpartum period was measured by two items requiring a yes/no response which asked women if, since delivering their baby, they had they received advice from their doctor, nurse or other healthcare worker about 'how much you should now weigh' and 'programs or resources to help you lose weight after pregnancy'.

Data were analysed using SPSS statistical package version 21, and for regression analyses assessing associations of clinician advice with maternal weight, Stata Version 12 was used to allow controlling for clustering. Adjustment for clustering within the analysis is necessary when assessing a cluster-randomised trial such as the Melbourne InFANT RCT [37] and accounts for the design effect and expected intra-cluster correlations of maternal characteristics within a first-time parent group.

Analyses included descriptive statistics to characterize the sample and distributions of key variables. The change in the proportion women classified as overweight/obese and underweight/healthy weight was assessed via paired t-tests. Chi square tests were conducted to detect differences in the proportion of women who reported receiving advice during pregnancy compared to during the postpartum period.

For associations of clinician advice with maternal weight both during and following pregnancy, linear regression was conducted for these continuous outcomes. Such outcome measures were checked for normality and when found to be non-normally distributed, were transformed using root or log transformations. Binomial or multinomial logistic regression analyses were conducted for categorical outcomes.

Statistical significance was set as $p<0.05$ for all analyses and maternal age, education, income and BMI or GWG were adjusted for in the analyses. The rationale for adjusting for various confounding factors in the analyses was based on previously established predictors of the outcome variables. Pre-pregnancy BMI has been frequently associated with GWG [38-40] and GWG has consistently been shown to be the strongest predictor of PPWR [2,41-45]. In addition and consistent with other studies which have previously assessed maternal weight both during and following pregnancy, age, education, and income were also adjusted for [46-51].

Results

A total of 477 women from 62 first-time parent groups were recruited to the InFANT Extend RCT from 531 women approached (90%). Of the 62 groups, 28 were classified as low SEP, 20 were medium and 14 were high SEP. The present analysis excluded mothers with non-singleton pregnancies (n=6) and those who did not provide detail regarding parity (n=6).

Those women who were not first-time mothers (n=15) were also excluded and survey data were missing for two women. Data for 448 women were included in the analysis. Sample characteristics are presented in Table 1.

Variables	Mean ± SD	Range
Maternal age (years)	31.9 ± 4.25	19.3-43.5
Pre-pregnancy weight (kg) (n=445)	67.1 ± 14.34	35.0-155.0
Pre-pregnancy BMI (kg/m²) (n=430)	24.8 ± 4.88	16.3-55.0
Postpartum BMI (kg/m²) (n=416)	26.2 ± 5.00	17.1-46.8
	Percentage (%)	
Marital status		
Married	74.1	
De facto	22.3	
Separated/Divorced	1.3	
Never married	2.2	
Birth country		
Australia	75.9	
UK	3.3	
New Zealand	2.2	
Other	18.5	
Weekly household income (n=433)		
$1-1499	36.7	
$1500-1999	22	
$2000 or more	29.7	
Unsure/Don't want to answer	11.6	
Education (n=447)		
No qualification/up to year 12	11.6	
Trade/apprenticeship/certificate/diploma	30	
University degree/Higher degree	58.4	
Employment status (n=446)		
Full time work	3.4	
Part time work	6.3	
Keeping house/raising children full time	88.6	
Studying full time/Unemployed	1.8	
Smoking during pregnancy		
Yes	3.8	
No	96.2	
Smoking currently		
Yes	5.4	
No	94.7	
Breastfeeding		
Exclusive breastfeeding	49.6	
Combined breastfeeding	28.1	
Formula feeding only	22.3	

Table 1: Maternal weight status across the perinatal period and characteristics at 3 months Postpartum (n=448 unless otherwise stated).

Two thirds (60.0%) of women had a healthy pre-pregnancy BMI. Just over one third of women were classified as either overweight or obese pre-pregnancy (37.7%) (Table 2). The proportion of women classified as overweight and obese (combined) women increased significantly from pre-pregnancy to three months postpartum by 30%. Mean GWG was 14.0 ± 6.08 kg.

Overall, 41.0% of women exceeded IOM recommendations. Compared with healthy women (n=258), those who were overweight (n=110) or obese (n=52) pre-pregnancy, were more likely to exceed IOM recommendations for weight gain during pregnancy (OR=4.3, 95% CI=2.7, 7.0 and OR=3.2, 95% CI=1.7, 6.0 respectively). Mean PPWR was 4.3 ± 5.75 kg.

Women who were obese pre-pregnancy retained significantly less weight, on average (1.9 ± 6.41 kg) compared to women with a healthy BMI (4.4 ± 5.51) and women who were overweight (5.0 ± 5.84) (p=0.023 and p=0.009 respectively) (Table 2).

	Pre-Pregnancy (n=430)		3 months postpartum (n=416)		Combined BMI category	Change pre-pregnancy to 3 months postpartum (+/-n)	p-value
BMI category	n	%	n	%			
Underweight	10	2.3	5	1.2			
Healthy	258	60	200	48.1	Underweight/Healthy*	-63 (-24%)	<0.001
Overweight	110	25.6	121	29.1			
Obese	52	12.1	90	21.6	Overweight/ Obese*	+49 (+30%)	<0.001
GWG (kg)~	n				%		
Below recommendations	88				21.1		
Within recommendations	158				37.9		
Exceeded recommendations	171				41		
	Mean ± SD				**Range**	**p-value^**	
GWG (kg) (n=434)	14.0 ± 6.08				-11.0-47.0		
Underweight	14.8 ± 7.40				4.5-30.0	0.217^	
Healthy	14.4 ± 5.07				2.0-40.0	0.001^	
Overweight	14.4 ± 6.50				0.0-47.0	0.003^	
Obese	10.9 ± 7.54				-7.0-30.0		
PPWR (kg) (n=415)	4.3 ± 5.75				-12.0-32.9		
Underweight	4.9 ± 4.91				-2.3-12.5	0.994^	
Healthy	4.4 ± 5.51				-6.7-32.9	0.023^	
Overweight	5.0 ± 5.84				-8.2 ± 26.9	0.009^	
Obese	1.9 ± 6.41				-12.0-16.8		

Table 2: Change in maternal BMI, gestational weight gain and postpartum weight retention across the perinatal period (*change in number of women in the combined underweight/healthy weight BMI category and overweight/obese category from pre-pregnancy to three months postpartum, ^the difference in GWG (kg) and PPWR (kg) when 'obese' was used as the reference category, ~ GWG compared to IOM recommendations based on pre-pregnancy BMI).

Approximately half (54.4%) of all women reported receiving advice regarding how much weight to gain during pregnancy, while 42.6% reported receiving advice to avoid excess GWG (Table 3). During the postpartum period, just 5.8% of women reported that they had received advice about how much they should now weigh and 8.3% reported receiving advice about programs to support weight loss, during the postpartum period.

There were no significant associations found between clinician advice regarding how much weight to gain or how to avoid excess weight gain received during pregnancy, and either GWG (kg) or gaining weight within IOM recommendations (Table 3).

During pregnancy (#) did a doctor, nurse, or other health care worker talk with you about?		n	%	Gestational Weight Gain (n=448)	β-coef (95%CI)	p-value	OR/RRR (95%CI)	p-value
How much weight you should gain during pregnancy?	Yes	244	54.5	GWG (kg)	-0.17 (-1.30, 0.97)	0.765		
	No	204	45.5	GWG within IOM recommendations			0.87 (0.57, 1.33)	0.506

Avoiding gaining too much weight during pregnancy?	Yes	191	42.6	GWG (kg)	-0.48 (-1.63, 0.67)	0.405		
	No	257	57.4	GWG within IOM recommendations			0.91 (0.57, 1.44)	0.679
Since delivering this baby (##) Has a doctor, nurse, or other health care worker talked with you about:		**n**	**%**	**Postpartum Weight (n=448)**	**β-coef (95%CI)**	**p-value**	**OR/RRR (95%CI)**	**p-value**
How much you should now weigh?	Yes	26	5.8	PPWR (kg)	0.81 (-0.47, 2.08)	0.21		
	No	422	94.2	Postpartum BMI				
				Overweight			1.67^ (0.66, 4.23)	0.278
				Obese			2.46^ (1.00, 6.06)	0.049
Programs or resources to help you lose weight after pregnancy?	Yes	37	8.3	PPWR (kg)	1.12 (-1.05, 3.29)	0.306		
	No	411	91.7	Postpartum BMI				
				Overweight			0.93^ (0.34, 2.56)	0.887
				Obese			1.01^ (0.43-2.36)	0.983

Table 3: Associations of weight advice received by mothers with gestational weight gain and postpartum weight retention (#Analyses controlled for maternal age, education, income, pre-pregnancy BMI and/or GWG and clustering by first-time mother's group, ##Analyses controlled for maternal age, education, income, postpartum BMI and/or GWG and clustering by first-time mother's group, ^where healthy weight was used as the reference category; OR (odds ratio); RRR (relative risk ratio) for measures of association from regression analyses).

Discussion

This study showed a shift in maternal weight across the perinatal period, whereby mean BMI increased by over one whole unit from pre-pregnancy to three months postpartum. Moreover, the proportion of women who were classified as either overweight or obese increased by roughly 30%, both likely explained by a combination of excess GWG and/or PPWR experienced by many women. Furthermore, while a much higher proportion of women reported having received weight related advice from antenatal clinicians during pregnancy, compared to the postpartum period, provision of advice did not appear to influence weight outcomes.

Nearly half of all women exceeded IOM recommendations for GWG. These results are consistent with findings from other studies [5,52]. Interestingly, overweight and obese women in this study were more likely to experience excess GWG. Considering almost half of all women enter pregnancy already overweight or obese [53,54] and that excess GWG is the strongest predictor of PPWR [55,56], the need to focus on the promotion of healthy weight gain for women with high BMIs is further highlighted.

Despite the high rate of women experiencing excess GWG in this study, less than half of all women reported receiving advice to avoid excess GWG. While detail of the advice provided to women regarding recommendations for GWG was not assessed, it might be reasonable to assume that advice was varied among healthcare providers as there are no formal guidelines in Australia to advise targets for GWG. This could promote inconsistent advice being given; a hypothesis supported by the results of other studies assessing management of GWG [38,57]. This is an important consideration, as when healthcare practitioners do use target GWG as part of their practice, women have been shown to adhere to guidelines [58].

Of the few studies that have assessed postpartum weight management provided by healthcare practitioners, provision of maternal weight advice does not appear to be a priority [59]. For example, in North Carolina, as part of a prospective cohort study, Ferrari et al. (2010) assessed clinician advice regarding postpartum weight-loss in women (n=688) at three months postpartum [59]. The majority of women in that study (89%) reported receiving no weight-loss advice during the postpartum period. Likewise, results of this study showed that weight was not a focus of care received in the postpartum period, whereby less than one in ten women reported receiving advice regarding suitable weight loss programs and even fewer women reported receiving advice about how much they should weigh.

The lack of advice received during the postpartum period may not necessarily reflect a new mother's level of interest or motivation in wanting to lose weight. For example, in a study of 179 women at four months postpartum, approximately half (53%) of normal weight women, 79% of overweight women and 81% of obese women reported plans to seek weight-loss information, despite the fact that 85% of the women received no such information from healthcare providers [60]. Moreover, many women have been found to report that they perceived their weight as less important during pregnancy compared with following childbirth [45,61].

However, provision of advice alone may not be sufficiently rigorous to influence maternal weight as suggested by our results. Implementation of alternate support strategies such as healthy lifestyle intervention programs may be promising approaches to assist women. To date, successful lifestyle programs which have been shown to reduce excess GWG [43,57,62,63] and limit PPWR [64-67] have included more than provision of education or information alone. It is encouraging that healthcare practitioners themselves have previously acknowledged the need for lifestyle interventions to assist in promoting healthy maternal weight gain during pregnancy and following childbirth [68,69] and future work should aim to further identify healthy weight strategies while being conducive to the unique life stage encountered by women both during and following pregnancy.

A strength of this study was the assessment and comparison of frequency of advice both during pregnancy and following childbirth. This comparison enabled identification of gaps in current management strategies to be identified, and showed that the postpartum period can be considered a missed opportunity at present, for provision of healthy weight advice, thereby supporting the need for greater provision of support in the months following childbirth. This study was limited by the inability to determine what specific advice regarding weight was provided to women. This is an important consideration as if women were following advice received from clinicians, differences in the type of advice given may account for variations in weight gain or weight loss and the lack of associations observed in this study. Further, the type of advice provided may have influenced maternal weight, yet this is unable to be determined.

Further, this sample of women were predominately highly educated and over half of the sample of women had moderate to high household income therefore limiting the generalizability of the results. Future research would ideally consider advice provided to low income women to enable specific delivery of support amongst different population groups across the perinatal period. A final limitation was the method of self-reported pre-pregnancy weight used in this study.

Yet with studies having previously shown that under-reporting of weight and BMI tends to be common amongst overweight adults [70,71], rather than weight overestimations, expected inaccuracies in self-reported data in this study would have been towards more favourable outcomes (under-reporting of body weight). It could be possible that rate of excess GWG and maternal obesity have been underestimated or that if overweight or obese women were misclassified at pre-pregnancy, the increased rates of obesity from pre-pregnancy to three months postpartum could have been less.

With the many adverse health implications resulting from excess GWG, PPWR and maternal overweight and obesity, there is a need to better influence women to attain and maintain a healthy weight status across the perinatal period. Future work should seek to identify strategies which are most likely to be successful in promoting healthy maternal weight.

This study has provided valuable insight into maternal weight change across the perinatal period and the potential for BMI to increase significantly in first time mothers as a result of weight gained during pregnancy. As is stands, provision of advice alone may be inadequate for promoting healthy maternal weight during a period whereby many women are vulnerable to weight gain. The findings from this study have raised the importance of exploring alternate strategies (e.g. behavioral interventions) to assist in facilitating healthy maternal weight across the perinatal period. Successful approaches should be embedded in the current antenatal system, which at present, seemingly does not sufficiently support many women to attain a healthy weight both during and following childbirth. With the many adverse health implications resulting from excess GWG, PPWR and maternal overweight and obesity, there is a need to better influence women to attain and maintain a healthy weight status across the perinatal period.

Acknowledgements

The InFANT-Extend study, within which this study was nested, was funded by a World Cancer 452 Research Fund grant (2010/244). PV was funded by a National Health and Medical Research Council (NHMRC) Postgraduate Scholarship at the time of drafting this paper; KB is supported by a NHMRC Principal Research Fellowship, ID 1042442 (the contents of this work are the responsibility of the authors and do not reflect the views of NHMRC); KDH is supported by an Australian Research Council Future Fellowship (FT130100637) and Honorary National Heart Foundation of Australia Future Leader Fellowship (100370). We would like to thank Dr Gavin Abbott for his expertise and assistance with the statistical analysis conducted in formulating this paper. Thank you to all staff who worked on the InFANT Extend RCT.

Authors' Contributions

PV and KC conceived this study and KC, KB, KH, MT and DC advised on the study design. PV assisted with study recruitment, data collection and conducted the statistical analysis. PV drafted the manuscript together with JD. All authors contributed to the critical revision of the paper and approved the final manuscript. All authors have approved the final manuscript.

References

1. Rasmussen K, Yaktine A (2009) Weight Gain during Pregnancy: Reexamining the Guidelines USA.
2. Institutue of Medicine (2009) Weight Gain During Pregnancy: Reexamining the Guideliens.
3. Willcox J, Campbell K, McCarthy E, Lappas M, Ball K, et al. (2015) Gestational weight gain information: seeking and sources among pregnant women. BMC Pregnancy & Childbirth 15: 164.
4. Oteng-Ntim E, Varma R, Croker H, Poston L, Doyle P (2012) Lifestyle interventions for overweight and obese pregnant women to improve pregnancy outcome: systematic review and meta-analysis. BMC Medicine 10: 47.
5. Stotland NE, Gilbert P, Bogetz A, Harper CC, Abrams B, et al. (2010) Preventing excessive weight gain in pregnancy: How do prenatal care providers approach counseling? Journal of Women's Health 19: 807-814.
6. Abrams B, Altman SL, Pickett KE (2000) Pregnancy weight gain: still controversial. Am J Clin Nutr 71: 1233S-1241S.
7. Brennand EA, Dannenbaum D, Willows ND (2005) Pregnancy outcomes of first nations women in relation to pregravid weight and pregnancy weight gain. J Obstet Gynaecol 27: 936-944.
8. Oken E, Kleinman KP, Belfort MB, Hammitt JK, Gillman MW (2009) Associations of gestational weight gain with short- and longer-term maternal and child health outcomes. Am J Epidemiol 170: 173-180.
9. Ramachenderan J, Bradford J, McLean M (2008) Maternal obesity and pregnancy complications: A review. Aust NZ J Obstet Gynaecol 48: 228-235.
10. McGuire W, Dyson L, Renfrew M (2010) Maternal obesity: consequences for children, challenges for clinicians and carers. Semin Fetal Neonatal Med 15: 108-112.
11. Guelinckx I, Devlieger R, Beckers K, Vansant G (2008) Maternal obesity: pregnancy complications, gestational weight gain and nutrition. Obes Rev 9: 140-150.
12. Guelinckx I, Devlieger R, Mullie P, Vansant G (2010) Effect of lifestyle intervention on dietary habits, physical activity, and gestational weight gain in obese pregnant women: a randomized controlled trial. Am J Clin Nutr 91: 373-380.

13. Einerson BD, Huffman JK, Istwan NB, Rhea DJ, Joy SD (2011) New gestational weight gain guidelines: An observational study of pregnancy outcomes in obese women. Obesity 19: 2361-2364.
14. Siega-Riz AM, Viswanathan M, Moos MK, Deierlein A, Mumford S, et al. (2009) A systematic review of outcomes of maternal weight gain according to the Institute of Medicine recommendations: Birth weight, fetal growth, and postpartum weight retention. Am J Obstet Gynecol 201: 339e1-339e14.
15. Bogaerts A, Van den Bergh BRH, Ameye L, Witters I, Martens E, et al. (2013) Interpregnancy weight change and risk for adverse perinatal outcome. Obstet Gynecol 122: 999-1009.
16. Rooney BL, Schauberger CW, Mathiason MA (2005) Impact of perinatal weight change on long-term obesity and obesity-related illnesses. Obstet Gynecol 106: 1349-1356.
17. Shrewsbury V, Robb K, Power C, Wardle J (2009) Socioeconomic differences in weight retention, weight-related attitudes and practices in postpartum women. Matern Child Health J 13: 231-240.
18. Willett WC, Manson JE, Stampfer MJ, Colditz GA, Rosner B, et al. (1995) Weight, weight change, and coronary heart disease in women. JAMA: The J Am Med Ass 273: 461-465.
19. Riley H (2011) Weight management before, during and after pregnancy-what are the 'rules'? Nutr Bull 36: 212-215.
20. Draper A, Swift JA (2011) Qualitative research in nutrition and dietetics: data collection issues. J Human Nutr Diet 24: 3-12.
21. Wiltheiss GA, Lovelady CA, West DG, Brouwer RJN, Krause KM, et al. (2013) Diet quality and weight change among overweight and obese postpartum women enrolled in a behavioral intervention program. J Acad Nutr Diet 113: 54-62.
22. Streuling I, Beyerlein A, Rosenfeld E, Hofmann H, Schulz T, et al. (2011) Physical activity and gestational weight gain: a meta-analysis of intervention trials. 2011 BJOG: An Int J Obstet Gynaecol 118: 278-284.
23. Van der Pligt P, Olander EK, Ball K, Crawford D, Hesketh KD, et al. (2016) Maternal dietary intake and physical activity habits during the postpartum period: associations with clinician advice in a sample of Australian first time mothers. BMC Pregnancy Childbirth 16: 27.
24. Campbell KJ, Hesketh KD, McNaughton SA, Ball K, McCallum Z, et al. (2016) The extended Infant Feeding, Activity and Nutrition Trial (InFANT Extend) Program: a cluster-randomized controlled trial of an early intervention to prevent childhood obesity. BMC Public Health 16: 166.
25. World Health Organization (2008) Waist Circumference and Waist-Hip ratio: Report of WHO Expert Consultation. Geneva.
26. WHO (2011) Global Strategy on Diet, Physical Activity and Health. What is overweight and obesity?
27. Duthie EA, Drew EM, Flynn KE (2013) Patient-provider communication about gestational weight gain among nulliparous women: a qualitative study of the views of obstetricians and first-time pregnant women. BMC pregnancy childbirth 13: 231.
28. Skouteris H, Hartley-Clark L, McCabe M, Milgrom L, Kent B, et al. (2010) Preventing excessive gestational weight gain: A systematic review of interventions. Obes Rev 11: 757-768.
29. Jeffries K, Shub A, Walker SP, Hiscock R, Permezel M (2009) Reducing excessive weight gain in pregnancy: a randomised controlled trial (Clinical report). Med J Aust 191: 429-433.
30. Fowles ER, Walker LO (2006) Correlates of dietary quality and weight retention in postpartum women. J Comm Health Nurs 23: 183-197.
31. Lipsky LM, Strawderman MS, Olson CM (2012) Maternal weight change between 1 and 2 years postpartum: The importance of 1 year weight retention. Obesity 20: 1496-1502.
32. Heslehurst N, Russell S, Brandon H, Johnston C, Summerbell C, et al. (2013) Women's perspectives are required to inform the development of maternal obesity services: a qualitative study of obese pregnant women's experiences. Health Expect 18: 969-981.
33. Evenson KR, Moos MK, Carrier K, Siega-Riz AM (2009) Perceived barriers to physical activity among pregnant women. Matern Child Health J 13: 364-375.
34. Althuizen E, Van Poppel MNM, De Vries JH, Seidell JC, Van Mechelen W (2011) Postpartum behaviour as predictor of weight change from before pregnancy to one year postpartum. BMC Public Health 11: 165-171.
35. Backe B (2001) Overutilization of antenatal care in Norway. Scand J Public Health 29: 129-132.
36. Goodrich K, Cregger M, Wilcox S, Liu J (2013) A Qualitative Study of Factors Affecting Pregnancy Weight Gain in African American Women. Matern Child Health J 17: 432-440.
37. Lioret S, Campbell KJ, Crawford D, Spence AC, Hesketh K, et al. (2012) A parent focused child obesity prevention intervention improves some mother obesity risk behaviors: the Melbourne inFANT program. IJBNPA 9: 100.
38. Phelan S, Phipps MG, Abrams B, Darroch F, Schaffner A, et al. (2011) Practitioner advice and gestational weight gain. J Women's Health 20: 585-591.
39. Streuling I, Beyerlein A, von Kries R (2010) Can gestational weight gain be modified by increasing physical activity and diet counseling? A meta-analysis of interventional trials. Am J Clin Nutr 92: 678-687.
40. McIntyre HD, Peacock A, Miller YD, Koh D, Marshall AL (2012) Pilot study of an individualised early postpartum intervention to increase physical activity in women with previous gestational diabetes. Int J Endocrinol p: 892019.
41. Brown WJ, Trost SG (2003) Life transitions and changing physical activity patterns in young women. Am J Prev Med 25: 140-143.
42. Gore S, Brown D, West D (2003) The role of postpartum weight retention in obesity among women: a review of the evidence. Ann Behav Med 26: 149-159.
43. Polley BA, Wing RR, Sims CJ (2002) Randomized controlled trial to prevent excessive weight gain in pregnant women. Int J Obes Relat Metab Disord 26: 1494.
44. Walker LO (2007) Managing excessive weight gain during pregnancy and the postpartum period. J Obstet, Gynecol, Neonatal Nurs 36: 490-500.
45. Olander EK, Atkinson L, Edmunds JK, French DP (2011) The views of pre-and post-natal women and health professionals regarding gestational weight gain: An exploratory study. Sex Reprod Healthc 2: 43-48.
46. Mamun A, Callaway L, O'Callaghan M, Williams G, Najman J, et al. (2011) Associations of maternal pre-pregnancy obesity and excess pregnancy weight gains with adverse pregnancy outcomes and length of hospital stay. BMC Preg Childbirth 11: 62.
47. Crane J, White J, Murphy P, Burrage L, Hutchens D (2009) The effect of gestational weight gain by body mass index on maternal and neonatal outcomes. J Obstet Gynaecol Can 31: 28-35.
48. Cedergren M (2006) Effects of gestational weight gain and body mass index on obstetric outcome in Sweden. Int J Gynecol Obstet 93: 269-274.
49. Oken E, Taveras EM, Popoola FA, Rich-Edwards JW, Gillman MW (2007) Television, walking, and diet: Associations with postpartum weight retention. Am J Prev Med 32: 305-311.
50. Oken E, Taveras EM, Kleinman KP, Rich-Edwards JW, Gillman MW. Gestational weight gain and child adiposity at age 3 years. Am J Obstet Gynecol 196: 322e1-322e8.
51. Nicklas JM, Zera CA, Seely EW, Abdul-Rahim ZS, Rudloff ND, et al. (2011) Identifying postpartum intervention approaches to prevent type 2 diabetes in women with a history of gestational diabetes. BMC Preg Childbirth 11: 23.
52. Cogswell ME, Scanlon KS, Fein SB, Schieve LA (1999) Medically advised, mother's personal target, and actual weight gain during pregnancy. Obstet & Gynecol 94: 616-622.
53. Dodd J, Turnbull D, McPhee A, Wittert G, Crowther C, et al. (2011) Limiting weight gain in overweight and obese women during pregnancy to improve health outcomes: the LIMIT randomised controlled trial. BMC Preg Childbirth 11: 79.

54. Dodd JM, Grivell RM, Nguyen AM, Chan A, Robinson JS (2011) Maternal and perinatal health outcomes by body mass index category. Aust NZ J Obstet Gynaecol 51: 136-140.
55. Walker LO (1996) Predictors of weight gain at 6 and 18 months after childbirth: A Pilot Study. J Obstet, Gynecol, Neonatal Nurs 25: 39-48.
56. Linné Y, Neovius M (2006) Identification of women at risk of adverse weight development following pregnancy. Int J Obesity 30: 1234-1239.
57. Hui A, Back L, Ludwig S, Gardiner P, Sevenhuysen G, et al. (2012) Lifestyle intervention on diet and exercise reduced excessive gestational weight gain in pregnant women under a randomised controlled trial. BJOG: An Int J Obstet Gynaecol 119: 70-77.
58. Stotland NE, Haas JS, Brawarsky P, Jackson RA, Afflick EF, et al. (2005) Body mass index, provider advice, and target gestational weight gain. Obstet Gynecol 105: 3.
59. Ferrari RM, Siega-Riz AM, Evenson KR, Moos M, Melvin CL, et al. (2010) Provider advice about weight loss and physical activity in the postpartum period. J Women's Health 19: 397-406.
60. Ohlendorf J, Weiss M, Ryan P (2012) Weight-management information needs of postpartum women. Am J Matern Child Nursing 37: 57-63.
61. Tovar A, Chasan-Taber L, Bermudez O, Hyatt R, Must A (2010) Knowledge, Attitudes, and beliefs regarding weight gain during pregnancy among hispanic women. Matern Child Health J 14: 938-949.
62. Phelan S, Phipps MG, Abrams B, Darroch F, Schaffner A, et al. (2011) Randomized trial of a behavioral intervention to prevent excessive gestational weight gain: the Fit for Delivery Study. Am J Clin Nutr 93: 772-779.
63. Claesson IM, Sydsjö G, Brynhildsen J, Cedergren M, Jeppsson A, et al. (2008) Weight gain restriction for obese pregnant women: a case-control intervention study. BJOG: Int J Obstet Gynaecol 115: 44-50.
64. O'Toole ML, Sawicki MA, Artal R (2003) Structured diet and physical activity prevent postpartum weight retention. J Women's Health 12: 991-998.
65. Leermakers E, Anglin K, Wing R (1998) Reducing postpartum weight retention through a correspondence intervention. Int J Obes 22: 1103-1109.
66. Tripette J, Murakami H, Gando Y, Kawakami R, Sasaki A, et al. (2014) Home-based active video games to promote weight loss during the postpartum period. Med Sci Sports Exerc 46: 472-478.
67. Colleran HL, Lovelady CA (2012) Use of my pyramid menu planner for moms in a weight-loss intervention during lactation. J Acad Nutr Diet 112: 553-558.
68. Oteng-Ntim E, Pheasant H, Khazaezadeh N, Mohidden A, Bewley S, et al. (2010) Developing a community-based maternal obesity intervention: a qualitative study of service providers' views. BJOG: Int J Obstet Gynaecol 117: 1651-1655.
69. Heslehurst N, Moore H, Rankin J, Ells LJ, Wilkinson JR, et al. (2011) How can maternity services be developed to effectively address maternal obesity? A qualitative study Midwifery 27: e170-e177.
70. Dekkers JC, Van Wier MF, Hendriksen IJM, Twisk JWR, Van Mechelen W (2008) Accuracy of self-reported body weight, height and waist circumference in a Dutch overweight working population. BMC Med Res Methodol 8: 69.
71. Niedhammer I, Bugel I, Bonenfant S, Goldberg M, Leclerc A (2000) Validity of self-reported weight and height in the French GAZEL cohort. Int J obes Relat Metab Disord 24: 1111-1118.

Magnitude of Unintended Pregnancy and its Determinants among Pregnant Women Visiting Dilla University Referral Hospital, South Ethiopia

Mohammed Feyisso[1*], **Alebachew Girma**[1], **Hamid Yimam**[2] **and Sileshi Hailu**[3]

[1]*Department of Public Health, College of Health Sciences and Medicine, Dilla University, Dilla, Ethiopia*

[2]*Department of Public Health, College of Health Sciences and Medicine, Mizan Tepi University, Mizan, Ethiopia*

[3]*Department of Anesthesia, College of Health Sciences and Medicine, Dilla University, Dilla, Ethiopia*

[*]**Corresponding author:** Mohammed Feyisso, Department of Public Health, College of Health Sciences and Medicine, Dilla University, Dilla, Ethiopia, E-mail: mamfys8@gmail.com

Abstract

Background: Unintended pregnancy is important maternal public health concern both in the developing and developed world. The proportion of unintended pregnancies is alarmingly high in Ethiopia and there is enormous information gap on the determinants of unwanted and mistimed pregnancy.

Objectives: To determine magnitude of unintended pregnancy and its determinants among pregnant women visiting antenatal and postnatal care clinic at Dilla University Referral Hospital.

Methods: Institution based cross-sectional study was conducted on 290 women attending antenatal clinic and Postnatal women at Dilla University Referral Hospital from February to June, 2016. Using consecutive arrival of client systematic sampling technique was conducted based on the patient flow per month. A structured questionnaire survey was used to collect data the data was entered and processed by IBM SPSS statistics version 20 for analysis. Descriptively frequencies and percentage was used and association between unintended pregnancy and independent variables were assessed using logistic regression.

Results: The prevalence of unintended pregnancy is 36.9%. The study revealed that women less than 20 years old were about 2 times higher risk of having unintended pregnancy compared to 30 years and above women (AOR=1.84, CI: 1.02-4.29). Likewise, compared to married women singles were 2 times more likely to have unintended pregnancy (AOR=1.78; CI: 1.048- 5.078) and illiterate women were found to be less likely to have unintended pregnancy (AOR=0.074; CI: 0.021-0.263) according to multi-variable analysis.

Conclusion: From the finding significant proportion of women (36.9%) had unintended pregnancy. Age of women, marital status and educational status were the variables significantly affecting the level of unintended pregnancy.

Keywords: Pregnant women; Unintended pregnancy; Prevalence; Antenatal care

Abbreviations: ANC: Ante-natal Care; DHS: Demographic and Health Survey; DURH: Dilla University Referral Hospital; FP: Family Planning; GC: Gregorian Calendar; ICPD: International Conference Population and Development; IUD: Intra Uterine Device; KAP: knowledge Attitude and Practice; SNNPR: South Nation Nationality of People Region; TFR: Total Fertility; WHO: World Health Organization; AOR: Adjusted Odd Ratio; COR: Crude Odd Ratio

Background

Unintended pregnancy is a pregnancy that is either mistimed or unwanted at the time of Conception. It is one of the leading factor contributing to high level of maternal and child morbidity and mortality [1]. Globally, nearly 80 million unintended pregnancies occur each year [2] and one in every 10 of the outcome of pregnancies is unsafe abortions [3]. In the year 2008, about 13% of deaths were occurred as a result of unsafe abortion of which 62% were happened in Africa [2]. Many of the unintended pregnancies were unsafely aborted [4]. About 6.2 million African [nearly 90% from Sub-Saharan] women face unsafe abortion per year and 29,000 of them die due to risks related with procedure [2]. Unintended pregnancy and births are global social and health burdens and they have serious health consequences to the mother and family [2,5,6]. Unintended pregnancies mainly due to non-use or erroneous use of contraceptive methods and it could also be due to noticeable contraceptive failure [7,8]. In Africa more than one in every five women of reproductive age had unmet need for family planning during the year of 2007. Five percent of the family planning users encounter unexpected pregnancy as a result of method failure [2].

In developing countries 20-40% of births are mistimed or unwanted at all endangering the health and life of millions of women and children. Yearly about 50 million induced abortions are done and nearly 20 million of those conducted in unsafe condition or by unskilled providers. Each year pregnancy related causes halt the life of nearly 600,000 women and 99% of these women are from developing countries. Pregnancy related complication(s) occur among 40% of pregnant women and life threatening complication(s) that require obstetric care occur in 15% of all Pregnant women [9,10]. To avoid the burden of unwanted or unplanned births considerably large proportion of women goes for induced abortion. This occurs both in countries where abortion is legal and where it is illegal [11]. Unintended pregnancy in Africa was estimated to reach up to 57 per 1000 women. The rates of intended and unintended pregnancy are highest in Africa (136 and 86 respectively) compared to other regions [12]. Ethiopia has an old population policy developed in 1993 just before the International Conference on Population and Development in 1994, which adopted the principle that every pregnancy should be planned and wanted [13,14].

In Ethiopia the uses of contraceptive methods upsurge from 4.0% to 27%; and the TFR declined from 7.7 to 4.8 between 1990 and 2011. In rural area modern contraceptive method use was far below the national average. Currently modern contraceptive use prevalence rate in Ethiopia is encouraging news for improving the health of women and their families. Nevertheless, it is difficult to meet women's reproductive goals with current large number of unintended pregnancies, high unmet need for family planning and high maternal mortality (673 deaths per 100,000 live births) [15]. In Ethiopia the fertility of is among the highest in sub-Saharan Africa. Ethiopian woman have an average of 4.6 children each. The high total fertility rate for women has led to high population growth rate of 2.6 percent per year [16]. The proportion of unintended birth was 37%, 35% and 28% during 2000, 2005, and 2011 respectively [15]. In study from Eastern Ethiopia the most recent pregnancies of 33.3% of sexually active women was unintended and the proportion of unintended childbirth was 14.4% [10].

Another study from the same region shows a 27.9% unintended pregnancy level [17]. In Ethiopia previous studies focus on unintended pregnancy and forgo unintended childbirths and relied on data from history of pregnancy and the status of that pregnancy. Additionally the selected study area is characterized by high fertility rate and it is the most densely populated area in Ethiopia. Hence this study was planned to delineate the prevalence of unintended pregnancy and its determinants among women visiting ANC and post natal clinic in Dilla University Referral Hospital.

Methods and Materials

Study design and study area

Institution based descriptive cross-sectional study was conducted among pregnant women and postnatal women attending Dilla University Referral Hospital antenatal and post natal clinic from February 05 to May 29, 2016. The hospital was located in Gedeo zone, South Ethiopia 360 km from Addis Ababa, the capital city of Ethiopia, and 90 km from Hawassa, the capital city of SNNPR. Currently the hospital serves around 3 million peoples in the catchment area.

Sample size determination

The sample size is determined using single population proportion formula. The following assumptions were used: p=proportion of unintended pregnancy in Amhara region (22.1%) [15], 95% confidence level of certainty and 5% margin of error.

$$n=(Z\alpha/2)^2 \times P\,(1-P)/(d)^2$$

$$(1.96)^2 \times 0.221(1-0.221)/(0.05)^2=264$$

The calculated sample size becomes 264 and adding 10% non-response rate final sample size is 290.

Data collection

For selecting of the study participant systematic sampling technique was used based on the consecutive arrival of clients and considering the patient flow per month in the institution. In addition the usual date in week on which the client flow is higher was also taken into consideration. The questionnaire was adopted from previously published literatures on the subject area and the tool was pretested on 5% of the sample size before field data collection to harmonize the content and concepts of the tool with the local context and corrections were made accordingly. The tool contains structured questionnaire prepared in English and later translated into local language was used through face to face interview to collect data from the respondents. The data collectors were female final year midwifery students in Dilla University.

Data analysis plan

For data processing and analysis IBM SPSS Statistics version 20 was used. Descriptive statistics computed for prevalence of unintended pregnancy. For bivariate analysis chi-square test was employed and binary logistic regression was used to select variables for multivariable analysis. A multivariable logistic regression was used to assess determinants of unintended pregnancy and unintended birth. The crude and adjusted odds ratios together with their corresponding 95% confidence intervals were computed. A P-value ≤ 0.05 was considered statistically significant in this study.

Result

Socio-demographic characteristics

About 290 pregnant and postnatal women were participated study of which 178(61.4%) were in the age group of 21-29. The majority of respondents 175(60.3%) were Gedeo in ethnicity and 174(60.0%) were protestant by religion. Regarding the educational status of the study participants 125(43.1%) have attended elementary school and occupationally 104 (35.9%) of the study participants were house wives, 77(26.6%) were government employee and 44(14.1%) of the respondents were self-employed (Table 1).

Socio-demographic characteristics	Frequency	Percentage (%)
Age	287	100
<20	54	18.6
21-29	178	61.4
30-39	55	18.9
Ethnicity	282	100
Amhara	42	14.5
Oromo	65	22.4
Gedeo	175	60.3

Religion	284	100
Orthodox	83	28.6
Muslim	27	9.3
Protestant	174	60
Marital status	290	100
Married	265	91.4
Single	16	5.5
Income	290	100
<500	88	30.3
501-1000	162	55.9
1001-1500	19	6.6
1501-2000	21	7.2

Table 1: Socio-demographic characteristics of survey respondents DURH, June, 2016.

Reproductive history of pregnant women

Women were asked about the total number of live children they have. Accordingly about 111 of study participants have 1-2 and for 52 of the women their most recent pregnancies at the time of data collection was their first pregnancy (Figure 1).

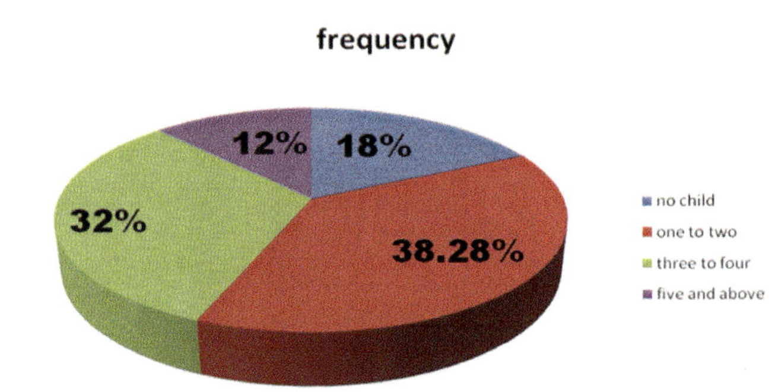

Figure 1: Number of alive children among ANC attendants at Dilla University Referral Hospital, Dilla, Ethiopia, June, 2016.

Regarding the status of current pregnancy or child about 107(36.9%) of women reported that their recent pregnancy was unintended and about 58(20%) of the women also have previous history of unintended pregnancies. According to the report from the mothers the reasons for failure to avoid such pregnancies were contraceptive method failure 63(21.7%), lack of knowledge of contraceptive method 14(4.8%), partner disapproval 10(3.4%) and lack of access to contraceptive methods 3(1%).

Knowledge and practice on contraceptive use

There are 3 multiple-choice questions which are prepared to assess knowledge of respondents about modern contraceptive method and these questions assess about awareness about at least one contraceptive method, its advantage and the place where they get it. All of the respondents (100%) are aware about at least one contraceptive method. Majority of the respondents, 278(95.9%) are knowledgeable about contraceptive method (Figure 2).

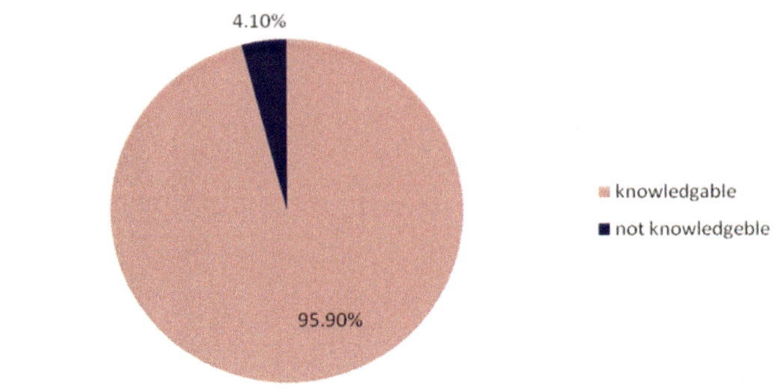

Figure 2: Distribution of overall knowledge about contraceptive among respondents.

Variables	Frequency	Percentage (%)
Place to get FP	290	100
Hospital	110	37.9
Health centre	164	56.5
Community health post	8	2.8
None	8	2.8
Advantages of modern contraceptive	290	100
To avoid unwanted pregnancy	273	94.1
To delay mistimed pregnancy	10	3.4
To prevent STDS	3	1
None	4	1.4
Heard of EC	290	100
Yes	250	86.2
No	40	13.8
Effective use of EC	250	100
Immediately after sex	71	28.4
Within 24 hours	32	12.8
Within 48 hours	34	13.6
Within 72 hours	77	30.8
Any time	36	14.4
Ever use of modern contraceptive method	290	100
Yes	245	84.5
No	45	15.5

FP used by the respondents	245	100
Pills	12	4.5
Condom	2	0.7
Injectable	170	58.6
Implant	61	21

Table 2: knowledge and practice of respondents on contraceptive use.

Of the total respondents, 245(84.5%) reported to have ever used contraceptives and among these 170 (69.3%) were used as injectable followed by implants 61(24.8%). Majority 250 (86.2%) of the study respondents have heard of emergency contraceptives and about 110(37.9%) of the respondents mentioned that Emergency contraceptives should be used within 48 hours after unprotected sexual intercourse (Table 2).

Associations between unintended pregnancy and its determinant factors

From the result of bivariate analysis, age of the women (x^2=11.5, p<0.05), marital status (x^2=6.45, p<0.05), educational status (x^2=2.16, p>0.05 and income(x^2=11.6, p<0.05 were significantly associated with unintended pregnancy (Table 3).

Variables	Yes	No	x^2	p=value
Age category (287)				
<20	41(14.3)	13(4.5)	X^2=11.5	P=0.09
21-29	104(36.2)	74(25.8)		
30-39	38(13.2)	17(5.9)		
Ethnicity (282)				
Amhara	22(7.8)	20(7.1)	X^2=31.3	P=.000
Oromo	25(8.9)	40(14.2)		
Gedio	128(45.4)	47(16.7)		
Religion (284)				
Orthodox	48(16.9)	35(12.3)	X^2=11.96	P=0.08
Muslim	11(3.8)	16(5.6)		
Protestant	118(41.5)	56(19.7)		
Marital status (281)				
Married	166(59.1)	99(35.2)	X^2=6.45	P=0.039
Single	8(2.8)	8(2.8)		
Educational status (290)				
Illiterate	24(8.3)	22(7.6)	X^2=10.7	P=0.03
Read or write	22(7.6)	7(2.4)		
Elementary school	87(30.0)	38(13.1)		
Junior or high school	23(7.9)	24(8.3)		
Higher education	27(9.3)	16(5.5)		
Occupation (290)				
Farmer	28(9.6)	5(1.7)	X^2=10.7	P=0.03
Government employee	33(11.4)	44(15.1)		
Student	18(6.2)	8(2.8)		
House wife	70(24.1)	34(11.7)		
Self-employed	27(9.3)	14(4.8)		

Jobless	4(1.4)	5 (1.7)		
Income (290)				
<500	63(21.7)	25(8.6)	X^2=11.6	P=0.009
501-1000	89(30.7)	73(25.1)		
1001-1500	16(5.5)	3(1.0)		
1501-2000	15(5.1)	6(2.1)		
Number of alive children (290)				
0	36(12.4)	16(5.5)	X^2=11.6	P=0.376
1-2	69(23.8)	42(14.5)		
3-4	60(20.7)	32(11.0)		
≥ 5	18(6.2)	17(5.9)		

Table 3: Unintended pregnancy, in relation to its determinant factors of respondents, DURH, Ethiopian, June, 2016.

Logistic Regression Analysis Result

According to the finding from multivariate analysis, age category, marital status and educational level of the respondents were found to be the determinants of unintended pregnancy. From the finding women in the age group below 20 years are about 2 times more likely to have higher risk of unintended pregnancy AOR=1.84, (CI:1.02,4.29). Similarly married women were found to be about 2 times higher risk of having unintended pregnancy when compared to married women AOR: 1.78, (CI: 1.05,5.08). Another variable that affect the level of unintended pregnancy in the study area was level of educational of the respondents.

The finding of the study shows that less educated women namely illiterate women and women with high school level education were found to be less likely to have unintended pregnancy when compared to women with higher education with AOR: 0.07, (CI: 0.02,0.26) and AOR: 0.22,(CI: 0.08,0.63) respectively. On the other hand number of currently alive children was found to have no significant effect on unintended pregnancy among mothers in this study both on bivariate and multivariable analysis. Variables like income, occupational status and knowledge of contraceptive method were found to be not associated with unintended pregnancy on multivariable analysis result (Table 4).

Determinant factor	Prevalence of unintended pregnancy		
	Frequency (%)	**COR(95% CI)**	**AOR(95% CI)**
Age			
<20	41(14.3)	1.13(0.78,1.7)	1.84(1.02,4.29)
21-29	104(36.2)	1.70(1.00,3.56)	1.20(0.72,1.88)
30-39	38(13.2)	1	1
Marital status			
Married	166(59.1)	1	1
Single	8(2.8)	1.83(1.304,4.12)	1.78(1.05,5.08
Educational status			
Illiterate	24(8.3)	1.55(0.66,3.61)	0.07(0.02,0.26)
Read or write	22(7.6)	0.54(0.19,1.54)	0.59(0.17,2.08)
Elementary school	87(30.0)	0.74(0.36,1.52)	0.43(0.16,1.12)
Junior or high school	23(7.9)	1.76(0.76,4.09)	0.22(0.08,0.63
Higher education	27(9.3)	1	1

Occupational status			
Farmer	28(9.6)	1	1
Government employee	33(11.4)	0.36(0.05,2.5)	2.41(0.30,19.41)
Student	18(6.2)	0.89(0.13,59)	0.62(0.019,1.36)
House wife	70(24.1)	0.97(0.17,5.57)	0.44(0.07,2.84)
Self-employed	27(9.3)	1.04(0.17,6.37)	0.30(0.04,2.21)
Jobless	4(1.4)	1.45(0.32,8.35)	0.41(0.05,3.12)
Income			
<500	63(21.7)	0.99(0.35,2.85)	0.277(0.07,1.09)
501-1000	89(30.7)	2.05(0.76,5.55)	0.24(0.065,1.882)
1001 1500	16(5.5)	0.47(0.99,2.22)	0.48(0.08.98)
1501-2000	15(5.1)	1	1
Knowledge of contraceptive			
Knowledgeable	180(64.7)	1	1
Not knowledgeable	3(25.0)	0.18(0.48,0.69)	0.195(0.51,1.751)

Table 4: Determinants of unintended pregnancy among pregnant women visiting Dilla University Referral hospital ANC clinic, South Ethiopia, June, 2016.

Discussion

In Ethiopia many women and couples lack knowledge, tools or support they need to enhance their reproductive health and to have the number of children they desire. As a result, large number of mothers have more children than they really want or can care for [18]. In this study the magnitude and determinants of unintended pregnancies was examined for a sample of 290 women attending ANC and post natal clinic at Dilla University Referral Hospital. From the findings of this study the most recent pregnancy of more than third, 36.9%, of women was unintended. This figure is lower than the finding from Damote Gale district, South Ethiopia, 42.4% [19] and the finding from Nepal, 41.2% [20].

The lower prevalence in this study could be due to the change in the awareness through the course of time and the difference in the level of facility in these areas. In this study all women participated on the study were knowledgeable about contraceptive method. However knowledge doesn't seem to assure the use of family planning in this study as about 37% of the women had unwanted pregnancy. About 84.5% of the women had ever used family planning method and the most reported method was injectable (58.6%) followed by implants (21.1%). When compared to older women, those women whose their age is less than 20 years were more likely to have unintended pregnancy. This might be due to the possible poor reproductive health knowledge and lesser opportunity to freely access family planning services by young women.

Likewise, older women are also mostly in a marital union and their pregnancies are more likely to be planned. The finding from other study done on correlates of unintended pregnancy other part of Ethiopia [19] also supports this finding where women between 25 to 29 years and 35 to 49 years have lower number of unintended pregnancy when compared women who are younger. This study also revealed that educational status of the women was also one of the factors determining the proportion of unwanted pregnancy. This finding is also supported by the findings other studies that revealed educational status playing considerable role in determining the prevalence of unwanted pregnancy [21].

However, the strange finding from this study is that less educated women were found to have lesser risk of having unintended pregnancy when compared to women in higher educational level. This may be the fact that less educated women always have need more number of children and are less likely to have pregnancies unintended when compared to educated women. Marital status of the respondents was another determinant factor significantly associated with unintended pregnancy. From the finding single women were about 2 times more likelihood of having unintended pregnancy when compared to married women. This may be attributed to the cultural influence on illegitimate birth to unmarried women in Ethiopia as this is culturally unacceptable in most of the communities.

Conclusion and Recommendations

According to the finding of this study large proportion of women had unintended pregnancy. From the findings of this study age of the women, marital status and educational status of women were independent predictors of unintended pregnancy among women attending Dilla University Referral Hospital, South, Ethiopia. Hence emphasis should be given to young women specially women empowerment needs due attention to reduce the women child bearing at young age. Furthermore, further in depth and large-scale study in order to explore underlying causes and design specific interventions is highly recommended.

Strength and Limitations of the Study

Strengths

- Strong sampling technique
- Successful participation of all expected respondents
- Use of same gender interviewers for increasing response rate

Limitations

- Lack of triangulation with qualitative enquiry to assess some hidden factors
- Recall bias
- Absence of participants from private facilities

Ethical Clearance

Ethical clearance was obtained from Dilla University College of Health Science and School of Medicine ethical review Committee. Letter of permission was obtained from Authorities in the study area and consent was also obtained from the study respondents for the collected data and for future consideration of the publication of the results of the study prior to data collection.

Acknowledgements

We acknowledge Dilla University that covered all the financial and material support for the research. We also acknowledge Gedeo Zone health department and respective health offices for providing us important materials. Lastly, we thank all participants for devoting their time to take part in this study.

Ethical Consideration

Written support letter was obtained from Dilla University, College of Medicine and Health Sciences. After explanation of the purpose of the study for the participants the right of the respondent not to be involved in the study or not to answer the question for which she is do not want was carefully. All interviews took confidentially at place and time chosen by the respondent.

Authors' Contributions

This work was a collaborative effort between all authors. MF, AG, HY and conceptualized the study, managed the literature searches, ran the statistical analysis, interpretation of the data, and wrote part of the first draft of the manuscript. SH assisted in literature searches, ran statistical analysis and managed write up of the result and manuscript. All authors read and approved the final manuscript.

Competing Interests

The authors declare that they have no competing interests.

References

1. Santelli J (2003) The measurement and meaning of unintended pregnancy. Perspectives on Sexual and Reproductive Health 35: 94-101.
2. World Health Organization (2011) Unsafe abortion, global and regional estimates of the incidence of unsafe abortion and associated mortality in 2008, Geneva.
3. World Health Organization (2012) Unsafe abortion incidence and mortality Global and regional levels in 2008 and trends during 1990-2008, Geneva.
4. http://www.who.int/reproductivehealth/publications/unsafe_abortion/9789241596121/en/
5. Frost JJ, Darroch JE, Remez L (2008) Improving contraceptive use in the United States, Guttmacher Institute, New York.
6. Singh S, Sedgh G, Hussain R (2010) Unintended Pregnancy: Worldwide Levels, Trends, and Outcomes. Stud Fam Plan 41: 241-250.
7. WHO (1992) The prevention and management of unsafe abortion. Report of a Technical Working Group.
8. Hussain R (2013) Unintended pregnancy and abortion in Uganda. Guttmacher Institute, New York.
9. WHO (1997) Population reference bureau improving reproductive health in developing countries. A Summary of finding from the National Research Council of US National Academy of science, Washington D.C pp: 1-32.
10. Solomon W, Mesganaw F (2006) Unintended pregnancy and induced abortion in a town with accessible family planning services: The case of Harar in Eastern Ethiopia. Ethiopian Journal of Health Redevelopment 20: 79-83.
11. Ross S (1998) Promoting quality maternal and newborn cares. A reference manual for a Program manager.
12. Sedgh G (2007) Legal abortion worldwide: Incidence and recent trends. International family planning perspectives 33: 106-116.
13. Nations U: Report of the International Conference on Population and Development: Cairo 5-13 September 1994. 1995, New York: United Nations.
14. https://cyber.harvard.edu/population/policies/ETHIOPIA.htm
15. https://dhsprogram.com/pubs/pdf/FR255/FR255.pdf
16. https://dhsprogram.com/pubs/pdf/PR81/PR81.pdf
17. Kassa N, Berhane Y, Worku A (2012) Predictors of unintended pregnancy in Kersa, Eastern Ethiopia, 2010. Reprod Health 9: 1-10.
18. Adu SA (1996) Bio-social profile of women of incomplete abortion in Ga-Rankuwa hospital Medunnsa. Cent Afr J Med 42: 198-202.
19. FMoH (2007) Health extension program in Ethiopia: Federal Ministry of Health. In: HeaE Addis Ababa.
20. Coeytaux FM (1988) Induced abortion in Sub-Saharan Africa: what we do and don't Know. Studies in Family Planning 19: 187-190.
21. Hulton LA, Cullen R, Khaloko SW (2000) Perception of sexual activity and their consequences among Ugandan adolescents. Studies in Family Planning 31: 35-10.

Male Partner Involvement on Prevention of Mother to Child Transmission of HIV and Associated Factors among Pregnant Mothers Attending Antenatal at Fantale District, Ethiopia

Lemma E[1#] and Husein G[2*#]

[1]Public Health Expert at Fantale District, Oromia Regional State, Fantale, Ethiopia

[2]Department of Public Health, College of Health Science, Arsi University, Assela, Ethiopia

[*]**Corresponding author:** Gebi Husein, Lecturer of Epidemiology, Department of Public Health, College of Health Science, Arsi University, Assela, Ethiopia, E-mail: gebihussein@gmail.com

Abstract

Background: Only screening pregnant mother is not adequate to prevent mother to child transmission of HIV. Thus, male partners' involvement has been considered as a first priority to focus intervention to be intensified in prevention of mother to child transmission of HIV. But it remained one of the biggest challenges in Ethiopia.

Objective: Assess the extent of male partner's involvement in prevention of mother to child transmission of HIV and identify associated factors in Fentale district, Eastern Ethiopia.

Methods: Institution based cross-sectional study design was employed. Data was collected from random sample of 272 pregnant mothers at antenatal care clinic of Health facilities in Fentale district from 1st to 31st March, 2016. Data was analyzed using SPSS version 21.0. Multivariate logistic regressions were carried out, association between independent and dependent variables was measured using adjusted odds ratios and 95% confidence interval and P-value below 0.05 was considered statistically significant.

Result: Male partner involvement on Antenatal care/Prevention of Mother to Child transmission (PMTCT) of HIV was 14.0%. Pregnant mothers living in urban were 3.8 times more likely to be accompanied by their partner on Antenatal care/Prevention of Mother to Child transmission of HIV compared to those from rural (AOR=3.8, 95% CI: 1.24, 7.86). On the other-hand mothers not having negative cultural belief about accompanying their partner at Antenatal care were 2.3 times more likely to involve their partner compared to those having negative beliefs (AOR=2.3, 95% CI: 1.94, 9.66).

Conclusion: Male partner involvement on Antenatal care/Prevention of Mother to Child transmission of HIV was 14.0% which is very low. Residence and cultural beliefs about accompanying pregnant mother at Antenatal care were found to be the independent predictors of male partner involvement. Hence, comprehensive strategy should be put in place to improve male partner involvement giving special focuses for pastoralists.

Keywords: Male partner involvement; Pregnant mothers; Public health; Treatment

Abbreviations: ANC: Antenatal Care; ART: Anti-retroviral Treatment; ARV: Anti-retroviral; AIDS: Acquired Immune Deficiency Syndrome; CSA: Central Statistical Agency; HC: Health Center; HCT: HIV Counseling and Testing; HIV: Human Immune Virus; MCH: Maternal and Child Health; MTCT: Mother-to-Child Transmission of HIV; MPH: Master in Public Health; PMTCT: Prevention of Mother-to-Child Transmission of HIV; VCT: Voluntary Counseling and Testing; WHO: World Health Organization

Introduction

Globally about 370,000 children became infected with HIV yearly and more than 1000 every day. Nearly all of these children acquired HIV through mother-to-child transmission (MTCT). Worldwide an estimated 2 million HIV-positive women become pregnant every year. Among those women, 20% to 30% of them are in absence of prevention of mother to child transmission (PMTCT) program and infect their children with HIV [1]. PMTCT can be more successful in reducing HIV infections among infants when it is required early in pregnancy and continues through delivery and infant care [2]. It is estimated that about 25 million HIV-infected people are living in sub-Saharan Africa. Among those, 2 million of them are children below the age of 15 years and account for about 90% of all HIV-infected children worldwide. In excess of 95% of them acquire HIV through mother-to child transmission [2,3]. Countries with high HIV prevalence contribute for a high incidence of HIV infection in women during pregnancy or in the postpartum period. Certainly, in this period, women particularly are vulnerable to become HIV infected. At the time of HIV positive mother being pregnant and eligible for Antiretroviral Treatment (ART), she should begin treatment and antiretroviral (ARV) prophylaxis needs to be initiated as early as 14 weeks of gestational age [4].

HIV is the leading cause of death for women of reproductive age, and in countries with a high burden of the disease, such as South Africa and Zimbabwe, HIV is now the leading cause of maternal mortality. It is estimated that in 2009 between 42,000 and 60,000 pregnant women died because of HIV. In 2009, an estimated 26% of pregnant women in low and middle-income countries were tested for HIV, and 53% of the estimated HIV-positive pregnant women received at least some type of ART prophylaxis [5].

Male partner involvement is expected to lead to better adoption of HIV prevention practices by a well-informed couple [6]. Berhumbiize, revealed that, lack of male partner support, socio-economic characteristic, cultural fear of domestic violence, desertion and stigmatization remain the main problem that made male partner not to involve on ANC/PMTCT uptake [7-9]. For this reason, ANC/PMTCT is the only opportunity to capture pregnant mothers and their male partners on the process of prevent transmission of HIV during pregnancy, labor and breast feeding (Figure 1) [10,11].

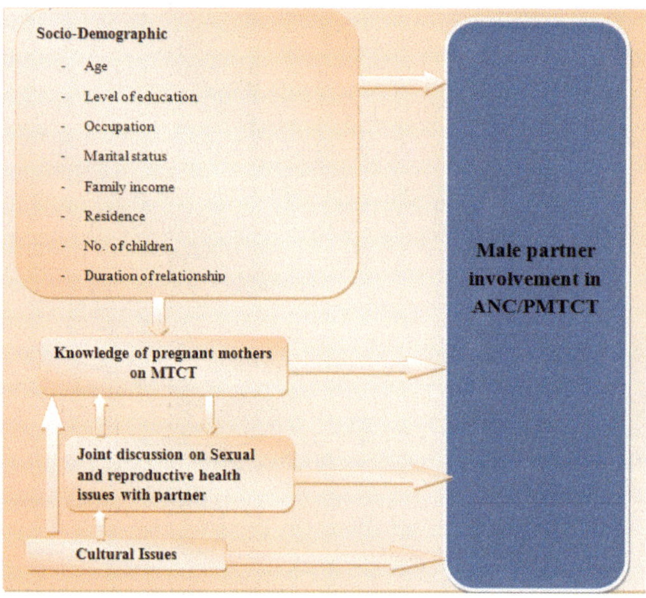

Figure 1: Conceptual framework of male partner involvement on the prevention of ANC/PMTCT, Fantale district, Eastern Ethiopia March 1-31, 2016.

It needs engagement of male partner in their wives ANC/PMTCT service. To do so, awareness creation at community level, enhancing potential service provider's commitment, enhancing intervention to increase male partner involvement and looking for systematic approach to mitigate obstacles for the engagement of male is very important to protect children being affected by HIV.

Yet, it is achieved insufficiently [11-13]. Studies in Ethiopia and other parts of the world indicate that HIV testing acceptance is encouraging to improve the PMTCT uptake. Stigma and discrimination, husbands' negative reactions and fear of positive test result were reasons that impede higher acceptance of the test. Majority of the pregnant women do not decide independently for acceptance of HIV testing. Decision-making authority is commonly referred to their male partners [13,14].

In Sub Saharan Africa, AIDS has now become the leading cause of deaths for fewer than five thousand children per year. In the absence of any intervention, incidence of HIV via MTCT is estimated to be from 25-40% in developing countries. Male partner involvement plays a fundamental part in decision-making within the home.

In Ethiopia, 13,008 children are infected with HIV annually and evidence shows that most common transmission is via MTCT. So, male partner contribution is a critical element to enhance PMTCT service [15]. The significant problem encountered in this issue is that, screening pregnant mother only isn't enough to prevent mother to child transmission of HIV. Male partner involvement is neglected in many health facilities and continued to be one of the potential program gaps adversely affecting PMTCT services uptake [16,17].

To our knowledge, there is a limited scientific data with regards to male partner involvement on prevention of mother to child transmission of HIV and associated factors in such a purely pastoralist areas of Ethiopia. Therefore, the aim of this study was to assess male partner involvement on prevention of mother to child transmission of HIV and associated factors among mothers attending Antenatal/prevention of mother to child transmission [18-20].

Materials and Methods

Study area and period

This study was conducted in Fentale district, Eastern Ethiopia from March 1st-31st, 2016. The district is the resident for purely pastoralists of kereyu, the well-known tribe of Oromo Ethnic group. Metehara town, the capital of the district, is located at 196 km East of Addis Ababa. Fentale District is divided into two administrations: Fentale rural district administration having 18 rural kebeles and Metehara town administration which have 2 town kebeles.

According to CSA 2007, Fentale District has a total population of 114,562 of whom 71,662 are men and 42,900 are women. Fentale District has 6 health centers and 1 hospital which are providing HCT for the population in the District.

Study design

Facility based cross-sectional study design was employed.

Source population

Source population of the study were all pregnant mothers who were registered for ANC/PMTCT follow up in health facilities providing HCT and PMTCT services in the district during data collection period.

Study population

Study Population of the study were all randomly selected pregnant mothers attending ANC/PMTCT in Fentale district health facilities which are providing HCT and PMTCT services during data collection period.

Sample size determination

The sample size was determined using a single population proportion formula.

By taking 20.1% of pregnant mothers who have been accompanied by their male partner to the ANC/PMTCT service [10], 5% precision, 95% confidence interval and non-response of 10%, the calculated sample size was 272 pregnant mothers.

$n = z\,\alpha/2^2 \times p\,(1-p) / d^2$

$= (1.96)^2 \times 0.201\,(1-0.201) / (0.05)^2$

$= 0.7721616 \times 0.799 = 0.6169 / 0.0025$

$= 246.8 \sim 247 \times 0.1$

$= 24.7 + 247$

$= 271.7 \sim 272$

Where, $z\,\alpha/2$=Standard normal value at 0.05 level of significance (1.96); d=Margin of error; p=Estimated population proportion

The sample size was 272 pregnant mothers who attend ANC/PMTCT in a given period of time.

Sampling procedure

All the 6 public health centers and 1 district hospital providing ANC/ PMTCT in Fentale district are included. The number of study units to be sampled from each health facility was determined using proportional allocation to size based on the number of client flow in the current year of total average case load of the selected health facilities. Systematic random sampling was employed to select and approach each study subjects. The sampling fraction of the Kth interval was calculated (N/n=2695/272=9.9~10).

Based on the patients' card number a starting woman was determined by using lottery method from the first 10 from the record and every tenth pregnant woman was included as a study unit until the allocated number of study subjects for each facility reached (Figure 2).

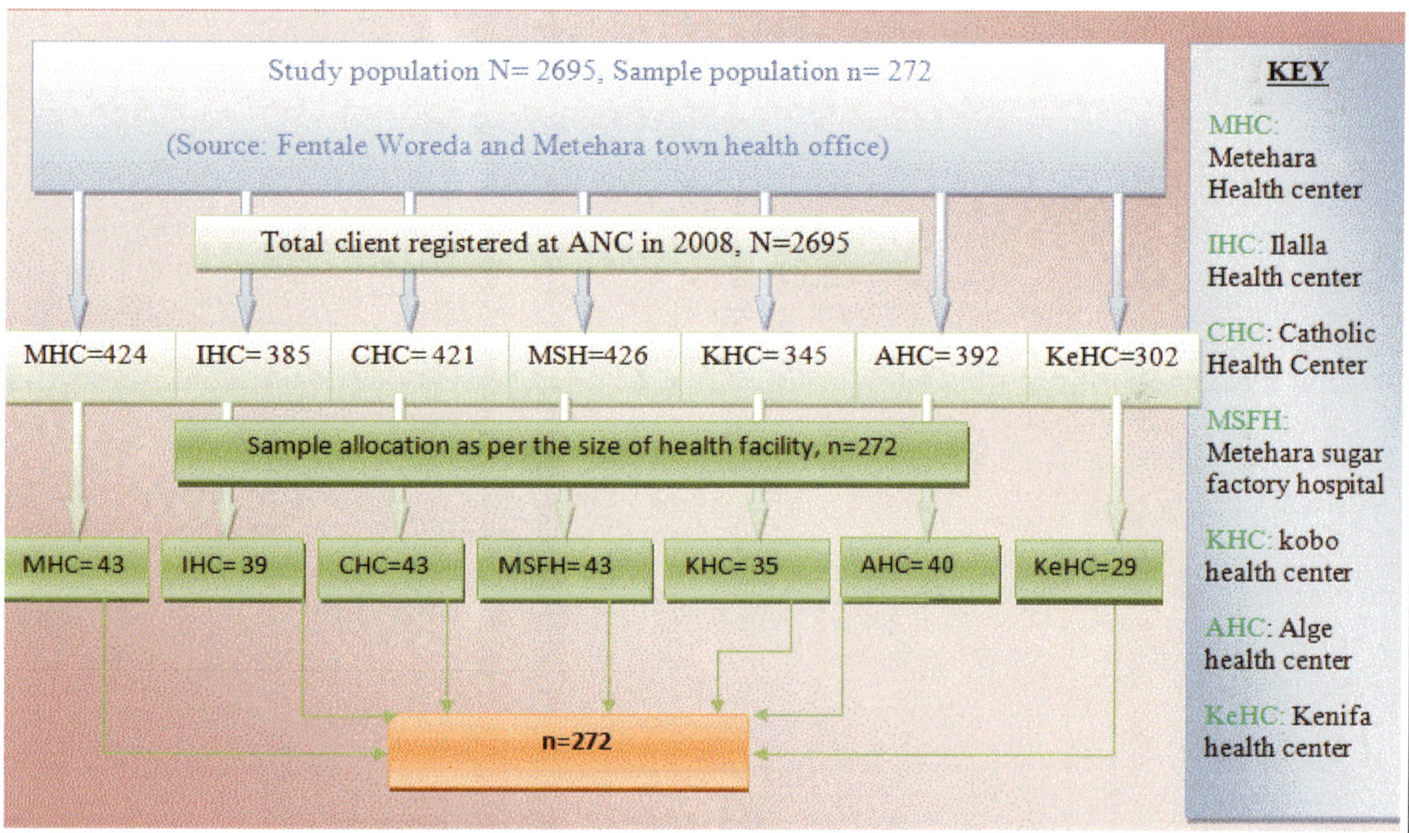

Figure 2: Thematic presentation of sampling procedure for the selection of study units in selected health facilities, Fantale district, Eastern Ethiopia March 1-31, 2016.

Data collection instrument

Interviewer administered structured questionnaires in English language was adapted from different similar studies and modification was made according to local context by the investigators. All data collection instruments were translated into local languages (Amharic and Afaan Oromo) by legal translators who are native speakers and then back translated to English by two other competent translators to check for consistency.

The questionnaires were pretested on 5% of the total sample size in similar settings (health centers in Boset District) which is outside the study area. Amendments were made after pre-testing. The questionnaires were designed to obtain information like characteristics of pregnant women and their male partners and determinants of male involvement in ANC/PMTCT.

Data collection

Face to face interview was conducted to collect data from ANC attending pregnant women after the interviewers explained the purpose of the study and obtained the participant's verbal consent to participate in the study.

Data quality control

Seven interviewers and 3 supervisors were recruited for the survey and were trained on the data collection and interview techniques. All the data collectors are diploma nurses and the supervisor is degree holder nurse who are providing ANC services and are competent in Amharic and Afaan Oromo languages. The completeness and consistency of data was assured through direct and daily supervision by the supervisors and principal investigators. They returned to interviewers if the data were incomplete and inconsistent. Interviewers re-administered the questionnaire to the respondent under supervision by the supervisor. To avoid double counting each card of interviewed mothers was marked using green marker on the top of the card.

Study Variables

Dependent variable

Male partner involvement.

Independent variable

Independent variables for this study were age of mothers and their male partner, Educational status of mothers and their male partner, family income, residence of mother and their male partner, religion, occupation, marital status, previous experience of information sharing about sexual and reproductive issues, previous knowledge of Male partner about their wife HIV sero status, partner informed about the availability of VCT in the ANC, Couples HIV sero status, cultural issues with regards to accompanying pregnant mother at ANC and Fear of being identified to undergo HCT at ANC clinic with partner.

Data processing and analysis

Data was entered into Epi-Info software version 3.5.2 then checked for completeness, inconsistency and outliers by looking at their distribution. Incomplete and inconsistent data were excluded from the analysis. Data were properly filed and stored in electronic copies with back up. Data were then, edited, cleaned and analyzed using SPSS for Windows version 16.0. Male involvement is determined by the proportion of male partners accompanying their pregnant wives during ANC/PMTCT service. Descriptive statistics such as frequencies and proportion was used to describe the study population in relation to relevant variables.

Bivariate logistic regression was carried out to see the association of each independent variable on the dependent variables and those which have p-values below 0.25 remained in to the final models i.e., multivariate logistic regressions. Odds Ratios (OR) was generated for each variable and the independence of any association was controlled by entering all variables into the model using backward stepwise method for adjustment of confounding effect between independent variables. The magnitude of the association between the independent variables in relation to male partner involvement was measured using, Adjusted Odds Ratios (AOR) and 95% Confidence Interval (CI) and P-values below 0.05 was considered statistically significant.

Operational definition

Knowledge

The result for this section was categorized as inadequate knowledge if the respondents answer below and equal to 5 correct answer for the questions asked under this section (number of ANC visit, type of ANC visit and mode of MTCT of HIV) and adequate knowledge if the respondents answer correctly for the similar question asked.

Male partner involvement

The result was put as high level of male involvement if there are more than 4 correct answers for the questions asked for this section and categorized as low level of male involvement, if there are less than 4 correct answer for the questions asked for this section. All questions have an equal weight of score. For all items, a score of 1 is given for "Yes" responses for positive answer and 0 (zero) for "No" or "Uncertain" responses for negative.

Male partner support on ANC/PMTCT

The result for this section was put as adequate support if the mother got two or more support from her male partner listed in the questionnaire and inadequate support if she got less than two or no support from her male partner through-out her pregnancy period.

Result

Socio-demographic characteristics of study participants

A total of 272 pregnant mothers attending ANC/PMTCT in selected health facilities of Fantale district were interviewed and responded to the questionnaire, making the response rate 100%. The majority 182 (66.9%) of the respondents were mothers from rural area. One hundred nine (40.1%) of mothers were in the age range of 25-29 years old with mean age of 26 years. A higher proportion of mothers 166 (61.0%) were Muslim and 97% of them were married and living with their current male partner. A higher proportion 137 (50.4%) of mothers were unable to read and write and 116 (42.6%) of their male partner were also unable to read and write (Table 1).

	Mother accompanied by her partner in Num (%)		
Variables	Yes	No	Frequency (%)
Residence			
Rural	18 (9.9)	164 (90.1)	182 (66.9)
Age			
15-19 years	7 (15.2)	39 (84.8)	46 (16.9)
20-24 years	9 (14.1)	55 (85.9)	64 (23.5)
25-29 years	19 (17.4)	90 (82.6)	109 (40.1)
30-34 years	5 (11.9)	37 (88.1)	42 (15.4)
35-44 years	2 (18.1)	9 (81.9)	11 (4.0)
Marital Status			
Married	36 (13.5)	230 (86.5)	266 (97.8)
Level of Education			

Can't read and write	11 (8.0)	126 (92.0)	137 (50.4)
Read and write only	8 (18.6)	35 (81.4)	43 (15.8)
Primary	4 (13.8)	25 (86.2)	29 (10.7)
Secondary	11 (28.2)	28 (71.8)	39 (14.3)
Post-secondary	4 (16.7)	20 (83.3)	24 (8.8)
Male Partner Educational Status			
Can't read and write	9 (7.8)	107 (92.2)	116 (42.6)
Read and write only	8 (20.0)	32 (80.0)	40 (14.7)
Primary	3 (9.7)	28 (90.3)	31 (11.4)
Secondary	11 (26.8)	30 (73.2)	41 (15.1)
Post-secondary	7 (15.9)	37 (84.1)	44 (16.20)
Religion			
Muslim	118 (71.1)	48 (28.9)	166 (61.0)
Orthodox	13 (7.8)	53 (92.2)	66 (24.3)
Protestant	5 (3.0)	26 (97.0)	31 (11.4)
Catholic	2 (1.2)	2 (98.8)	4 (1.5)
Other*	0 (0.0)	5 (100.0)	5 (1.8)
Occupation			
House wife	9 (9.5)	86 (90.5)	95 (34.9)
Farmer	7 (9.5)	67 (90.5)	74 (27.2)
Self employed	11 (22.4)	38 (77.6)	49 (18.0)
Daily laborer	5 (18.5)	22 (81.5)	27 (9.9)
Government employed	1 (5.0)	19 (95.0)	20 (7.4)
Other**	5 (71.4)	2 (28.6)	7 (2.6)
Family Income			
100-500 birr	21 (15.4)	116 (84.6)	137 (50.4)
501-1000 birr	12 (12.6)	83 (87.4)	95 (34.9)
≥ 1000 birr	7 (17.5)	33 (82.5)	40 (14.7)
Live Together with Partner			
Yes	34 (12.9)	230 (87.1)	264 (97.1)
Number of Children			
01-03	29 (15.6)	157 (84.4)	186 (68.4)
04-07	7 (10.6)	59 (89.4)	66 (24.3)
>8	2 (10.0)	18 (90.0)	20 (7.3)

Table 1: Socio-demographic characteristics of pregnant mothers attending ANC/PMTCT, Fantale district, Eastern Ethiopia March 1-31, 2016 (Others* include Wakefeta and local beliefs; Others** include different kinds pity trades).

Knowledge of pregnant mothers about ANC/PMTCT

Only 72 (26.5%) of the study participants responded that pregnant mothers should visit ANC at least four times up to delivery time and only 148 (54.4%) of them could list four different types of services provided for pregnant mothers in ANC clinic. On the other hand 209 (76.8%) of the study participants responded that their male partner should accompany them and go through HCT at ANC/PMTCT.

Majority 247 (90.8%) of the interviewed mothers responded that HIV can transmit from mother to child but only 91 (36.8%) of these mothers could list that HIV can transmit from mother to child during pregnancy, labor and delivery and breastfeeding and only 94 (38.1%) of them responded that transmission during the mentioned period can be prevented (Table 2).

Variables	Frequency (%)
Recommended Frequency (number) of ANC visit	
Twice	44 (16.2)
Three times	151 (55.5)
Four times	72 (26.5)
I don't know	5 (1.8)
Types of ANC services	
Listed at least four different types of services provided for pregnant mothers in ANC clinic	148 (54.4)
About who should go for HCT ANC/PMTCT	
Pregnant mother only	63 (23.2)
Pregnant mother and her male partner	209 (76.8)
I don't know	27 (9.9)
HIV transmit from mother to child	
Yes	247 (90.8)
No	14 (5.1)
I don't know	11 (4.0)
Duration of mother to child transmission of HIV	
Could list the three duration of mother to child transmission (during pregnancy, labour and delivery and breastfeeding)	91 (36.8)
Couldn't list the three duration of mother to child HIV transmission	156 (65.4)
Transmission of HIV from mother to child can be prevented	
Yes	94 (38.1)
Means of PMTCT (list at list three)	
Could list at list three means of PMTCT	120 (44.1)

Table 2: knowledge of pregnant mothers about ANC/PMTCT, Fantale district, Eastern Ethiopia, March 1-31, 2016.

Perception of pregnant mothers about their male partner involvement in ANC/PMTCT

About Fifty eight (21.3%) of the study participants thought that their male partner was wasting time that they could have use for their normal job when they accompanied them during ANC/PMTCT follow-up.

On the other hand 171 (62.9%) of the respondents thought they must obtain permission from their male partner to undergo HIV-test during ANC/PMTCT follow-up (Table 3).

Variables	Frequency (%)
Accompanying their wives during ANC/PMTCT is considered as wasting time that he could have use for his normal work	
Strongly agree	8 (2.9)
Agree	58 (21.3)
Undecided	8 (2.9)
Disagree	121 (44.5)
Strongly disagree	77 (28.3)
Pregnant women can undergo HCT in ANC/PMTCT without permission of her male partner	
Strongly agree	70 (25.7)
Agree	171 (62.9)
Undecided	8 (2.9)
Disagree	20 (7.4)
Strongly disagree	3 (1.1)
Both pregnant mother and her male partner should undergo HCT in ANC/PMTCT together	
Strongly agree	133 (48.9)
Agree	127 (46.7)
Undecided	3 (1.1)
Disagree	6 (2.2)
Strongly disagree	3 (1,1)
Male partners should accompany their wives during ANC/PMTC	
Strongly Agree	122 (44.9)
Agree	134 (49.3)
Undecided	4 (1.5)
Disagree	11 (4.0)
Strongly disagree	1 (0.4)

Table 3: Perception of pregnant mothers about their male partner involvement in ANC/PMTCT, Fantale district, Eastern Ethiopia, March 1-31, 2016.

Male partner involvement in ANC/PMTCT

Only 83 (30.5%) of the study participants were accompanied by their male partner at the ANC/PMTCT.

Among male partners who accompanied their pregnant wives, 51 (18.8%) had counseled and tested for HIV at ANC/PMTCT in the current pregnancy or showed their test results done elsewhere (Table 4).

Variables	Frequency (%)
Had an experience of sharing information about sexual and reproductive health like mother to child HIV transmission	
Yes	112 (41.2)
Couple have Joint plan to visit ANC/PMTCT	
Yes	99 (36.4)
Male partner accompanied their wife at ANC/PMTCT	
Yes	83 (30.5)
Male partners counseled and tested for HIV in ANC/MPTCT	
Yes	51 (18.8)
Male partner knew his wife sero status	
Yes	88 (32.4)
Got support from her male partner (at least two different kind of supports)	
Yes	86 (31.6)
Reasons of male partner for not accompanying their wife at ANC/MPTCT	
Lack of interest	73 (33.0)
Being busy with his regular duty	119 (53.8)
Not important	29 (13.2)

Table 4: Male partner involvement in ANC/PMTCT, Fantale district, Eastern Ethiopia, March 1st -31st, 2016.

Independent predictors of male partner involvement at ANC/PMTCT

In this study residence of respondents showed statistically significant association with male partner involvement.

Which explains that pregnant mothers living in urban were 3.8 times more likely to be accompanied by their partner on ANC/PMTCT compared to those from rural (AOR=3.8, 95% CI: 1.24, 7.86) (Table 5).

Similarly, cultural issues with regards to accompanying pregnant mother at ANC was found to be significantly associated with male partner involvement.

Which means mothers not having negative cultural belief about accompanying their partner at ANC were 2.3 times more likely to involve their partner on ANC/PMTCT compared to those having negative beliefs (AOR=2.3, 95% CI: 1.94, 9.66) (Table 5).

Variables	Male partner involvement on ANC/PMTCT		COR (95% C.I)	AOR (95% C.I)
	Yes Num (%)	No Num (%)		
Residence of the respondent				
Urban	20 (22.2)	70 (77.8)	2.68 (1.04,5.64)	3.80 (1.24,7.86)*
Rural	18 (9.9)	164 (90.1)	1	
Education of respondent				
No formal education	11 (8.0)	126 (92.0)	1	
Read and write	8 (18.6)	35 (81.4)	2.61 (0.97, 7.00)	3.34 (0.39,8.16)
Primary	4 (13.8)	25 (86.2)	3.82 (0.54,6.22)	1.42 (0.07,12.62)
Secondary	11 (28.2)	28 (71.8)	4.55 (1.77, 11.41)	4.98 (0.18,7.54)
Post-secondary	4 (16.7)	20 (83.3)	2.26 (1.66, 7.89)	8.10 (0.16,10.89)
Husband Education				
No formal education	9 (7.8)	107 (92.2)	1	
Read and write	8 (20.0)	32 (80.0)	2.90 (0.06, 8.33)	3.14 (0.19,9.79)
Primary	3 (9.7)	28 (90.3)	3.26 (0.32, 5.01)	2.50 (0.04.5.04)
Secondary	11 (26.8)	30 (73.2)	4.31 (0.65, 11.49)	2.19 (0.17,6.56)
Post-secondary	7 (15.9)	37 (84.1)	3.25 (2.78, 6.46)	5.415 (0.02,8.57)
Religion				
Orthodox	18 (27.3)	48 (72.7)	1	
Muslim	13 (7.8)	153 (92.2)	1.21 (1.10,7.49)	1.25 (0.84,1.64)
protestant	5 (16.1)	26 (83.9)	2.54 (1.17, 10.59)	2.43 (0.95,4.14)
Catholic	2 (50.0)	2 (50.0)	3.62 (1.34, 20.34)	4.37 (0.80,9.83)
Other	0 (0.0)	5 (100.0)	3.03 (2.01, 11.32)	3.06 (0.88. 14.99)
Occupation of respondent				
Daily labourer	5 (18.5)	22 (81.5)	1	
Government employee	1 (5.0)	19 (95.0)	2.20 (1.02, 7.16)	4.32 (0.04,25.27)
Self-employee	11 (26.4)	38 (77.6)	1.23 (0.39, 4.14)	2.73 (0.68,6.97)
Farmer	7 (9.5)	67 (90.5)	0.46 (0.13, 1.59)	3.28 (0.81,5.63)
House wife	9 (9.5)	86 (90.5)	0.49 (0.14, 1.51)	1.56 (0.08,3.88)
Other	5 (71.4)	2 (28.6)	11.0 (0.64. 73.97)	1.12 (0.26,8.15)
Live together with partner				
Yes	34 (12.9)	230 (87.1)	6.70 (1.61, 28.32)	6.98 (0.87,12.97)
No	4 (50.0)	4 (50.0)	1	
Family income				
100-500 birr	21 (15.4)	116 (84.6)	1	
501-1000 birr	12 (12.6)	83 (87.4)	1.82 (.038, 4.67)	0.97 (0.28,3.3.37)

≥ 1000 birr	7 (17.5)	33 (82.5)	2.51 (1.98, 6.87)	4.11 (0.98, 12.03)
Cultural issues with regards to accompanying pregnant mother at ANC				
Shameful	36 (15.6)	195 (84.4)	1	1
No	2 (4.9)	39 (95.1)	3.6 (2.83, 15.57)	2.3 (1.94, 9.66)*

Table 5: Association between male partner involvement in ANC/PMTCT and each independent variable (Crude, adjusted OR and its 95% CI), Fentale district, Eastern Ethiopia, March 1st-31st, 2016 (*statistically significant at P-value).

Discussion

In this study, the level of male partner involvement in ANC/PMTCT is 14.0%. The finding is consistent with a cross-sectional study done in Kibaale District, Uganda [7], a cross-sectional study done in eastern Uganda [9] and Kenya [21,22] which showed level of male involvement in the ANC/PMTCT was 16%, 15% and 15% respectively. But it is not supported by the study conducted in Northern Ethiopia, Mekele which revealed the level of male partner involvement in ANC/PMTCT services was 20% [6]. The later mentioned study was conducted in big town (Mekele) but our study participants were from pastoralist rural area which could be explanation of the inconsistency.

In our study, pregnant mothers living in urban were 3.8 times more likely to be accompanied by their partner on ANC/PMTCT compared to those from rural (AOR=3.8, 95% CI: 1.24, 7.86). This finding is in agreement with studies conducted in Rural Baluchistan Province, Pakistan [3]. Accompanying female partner in Antenatal care services is more likely to be higher among urban dwellers and those with higher socioeconomic status than by rural residents and groups with a lower socioeconomic status in developing countries [23]. But our finding is inconsistent with the study conducted in a cross-sectional study, Mekelle, Northern Ethiopia [6]. Possible reasons for the inconsistency may be the mentioned study was done in ANC clinics in urban areas which may not be applicable in rural pastoralist settings.

On the other hand finding of this study also showed that cultural issues with regards to accompanying pregnant mother at ANC was found to be significantly associated with male partner involvement i.e. mothers not having negative cultural belief about accompanying their partner at ANC were 2.3 times more likely to involve their partner on ANC/PMTCT compared to those having negative beliefs (AOR=2.3, 95% CI: 1.94, 9.66). This finding is consistent with the study conducted in Kibaale District, Uganda [7]. The referred study revealed that African men have been found to hold onto certain traditional cultural beliefs which inhibit their active involvement in reproductive health programmes [24-27].

Traditionally, men have the pride of always being consulted in matters of family health, yet are very hesitant in seeking medical care. A majority of women declined routine HIV testing mainly because they required partner's consent. A similarly, social and cultural barriers such as fear of their partners and parents deter pregnant women from accessing PMTCT services. Furthermore, a study the mentioned study reported that source of information and who relays it seemed to affect utilization since men still regard themselves as 'bringers' of health information to the family and usually trusted information more from health workers than their female partners [7,28-30].

The result of our study is also in line with the result of reviews from different studies conducted in Sub-Saharan African countries [4]. It revealed that cultural standards were identified as barriers for male involvement. It reported negative perceptions towards men attending ANC services. Men who accompanied their wives to ANC services were perceived as being dominated by their wives. Frequently men perceive that ANCs services are designed and reserved for women, thus are embarrassed to find themselves in such "female" places. Certain women too, do not like to be seen with their male partner attending the ANC service [4].

Strength and Limitation of the Study

Strength of the study

The study was conducted and tried to assess factors affecting male partner involvement in rural pastoralist area which could be mentioned as strength of the study.

Study limitations

This study assessed level of male partner involvement at ANC/PMTCT in the view of pregnant mothers which may affect the trustworthiness of the information about male character like, age, reasons why not to involve on ANC, educational status and VCT test and result. In addition, presence of male partner in the ANC was used to measure male involvement in ANC/PMTCT which may underestimate male involvement. Other point which could be mentioned as a limitation of this paper is the psychometric property aspects of our questionnaire was not validated as to the standard, even though its internal validity was carefully considered.

Conclusion

In this study the level of male partner involvement in ANC/PMTCT was low at 14%. Residence of respondents and cultural issues with regards to accompanying pregnant mother at ANC were found to be independent predictors of male partner involvement at NC/PMTCT. Pregnant mothers living in urban were 3.8 times more likely to be accompanied by their partner on ANC/PMTCT compared to those from rural and mothers not having negative cultural belief about accompanying their partner at ANC were 2.3 times more likely to involve their partner on ANC/PMTCT compared to those having negative beliefs.

Other variables like age of mothers and their male partner, educational status of mothers and their male partner, Family income, religion, occupation, marital status, Previous experience of information sharing about sexual and reproductive issues, previous knowledge of Male partner about their wife HIV sero status and partner informed about the availability of VCT in the ANC didn't show statistically significant association with male partner involvement.

Recommendation

Based on the findings of the study the following recommendations are forwarded to responsible organizations like federal MOH, Oromia regional health bureau, East shoa zone health department, Fentale District, Metahara town health office and health institutions in the district.

Efforts should be given for intensive and continued information dissemination to both pregnant mother and their partners about MTCT of HIV, the role of HIV counseling and testing (HCT) on the prevention of mother-to-child transmission of the virus, and about the existence of intervention that reduce the possibility of prenatal transmission of the HIV virus giving special emphasis for pastoralists. Moreover, efforts must be made to achieve full attendance of ANC by all pregnant mothers. For this to be realized effective health promotion programs need to be emphasized.

Health centers should use couple counseling as a strategy to improve male involvement. Couple counseling facilitated through couple-friendly ANC services could be taken as a strategy to boost male involvement. We also recommend encouraging counseled pregnant women to invite their partners in the next visit if they were not accompanied with their partners. We again recommend strengthening male friendly counseling at PMTCT institutions.

We also recommend future studies preferably community-based that examine male partner involvement at ANC/PMTCT using of both partners as a study subject during pregnancy period.

Ethical Consideration

Ethical clearance was obtained from Arsi University College of Health Sciences research ethical and review committee. Then permission paper was obtained from deferent concerned authorities after discussion of the purpose of the study. Permission to conduct the study was obtained from all the sampled seven health facilities as well. Verbal consent was obtained from each study participant. All interviewers are oriented on how to obey the rules of strict confidentiality practices for all clients both during and after data collection.

Competing Interest

The authors declare that they have no competing interests

Acknowledgments

We authors extend our very genuine appreciation to Arsi University College of Health Science for sponsoring the study. We are also very grateful to all health workers in the selected health facilities for their unreserved support they made during data collection. We also appreciate all study participants for sharing the information cooperatively. Last but not least, we are grateful to all data collectors and supervisors for handling their duties responsibly.

Funding

The entire research fund was covered by Arsi University. However, the university had no role in the design of the study, collection, analysis, interpretation of data and in writing the manuscript.

Authors' Contribution

EL involved in proposal writing, designing, recruitment and training of supervisors and data collectors, analysis and write-up of the paper. GH contributed in the designing of the project proposal and methodology, led the study, design of questionnaires, supervised and involved in the analysis stage of the project, final approval of the paper and preparation of the manuscript. Both authors read and approved the final manuscript.

References

1. UNAIDS (2012) Report on the global AIDS epidemic: Joint United Nations program on HIV/AIDS. Geneva.
2. World Health Organization (2007) Prevention of mother-to-child transmission of HIV. HIV technical briefs for use, Geneva.
3. Abdul G (2012) Provision and utilization of routine antenatal care in rural Baluchistan province, Pakistan: A survey of knowledge, Attitudes, and practices of pregnant women. J Applied Med Sci 1: 93-116.
4. Ditekemena J (2012) Determinants of male involvement in maternal and child health services in Sub-Saharan Africa a review. BMC Report health 9: 32.
5. World health organization (2012) Male involvement in the prevention of mother-to-child transmission of HIV. Geneva.
6. Fisaha H (2014) Male partner involvements in PMTCT. BMC Pregnancy and Childbirth 14: 65.
7. Behumbiize P (2009) Factors influencing male's involvement in prevention of mother to child transmission (PMTCT) services in Kibaale District, Uganda. Magister Public Health p: 2683.
8. Stefanie T (2009) Male involvement in PMTCT service. J AIDS Behav 13: 92-102.
9. Fatch W (2012) Male partner involvement in prevention of mother to child transmission of HIV in sub-Saharan Africa, Malawi. Open J Prev Med 1: 35-42.
10. Falnes Eli F (2011) It is her responsibility: Partner involvement in prevention of mother to child transmission of HIV program. J Int AIDS Soc 14: 21.
11. Robert B (2010) Determinants of male involvement in the prevention of mother-to-child transmission of HIV program. BMC Report Health 7: 11.
12. Nkuoh G, Meyer D (2010) Barriers to Men's participation in antenatal prevention of mother-to-child HIV transmission care in Cameroon. J Midwifery Womens Health X 55: 363-369.
13. Tweheyo R (2010) Male partner attendance of skilled antenatal care in peri-urban Gulu district. BMC Pregnancy Childbirth 10: 53.
14. Yohannes A (2014) Male involvement in prevention of mother to child transmission of HIV and associated factors among males in Addis Ababa, Ethiopia. Am J Health Research 2: 338-343.
15. Anteneh A (2014) Prevention of mother-to-child transmission (PMTCT) of HIV services in Adama town, Ethiopia. BMC Pregnancy Childbirth 14: 1471-2393.
16. Endawoke A (2013) Level of male partner involvement and associated factors in prevention of mother to child transmission of HIV/AIDS services in Debremarkos town, Northwest Ethiopia. Afr J AIDS HIV Res 1: 16-25.
17. Federal Ministry of Health (2010) The Ethiopian Health Sector Development Program IV.
18. https: //www.unicef.org/ethiopia/ET_2011_EDHS.pdf

19. Manzi M (2005) High acceptability of voluntary counseling and HIV-testing but unacceptable loss to follow up in a prevention of mother to-child HIV transmission program in rural Malawi. J Trop Med Int Health 10: 1242-1250.
20. Marina M (2002) Counselors' perspective on antenatal HIV testing and infant feeding: dilemmas facing women with HIV in northern Tanzania. J Reprod Health Matters 10: 144-156.
21. Neil A (2011) Male responsibility and maternal morbidity: a cross-sectional study in two Nigerian states. BMC Health Services Research 11: S7.
22. Reece M (2010) Assessing male spousal engagement with prevention of mother-to-child transmission of HIV programs in western Kenya. AIDS Care 22: 743-750.
23. Tilaye T (2010) Factors affecting acceptance of HIV testing among antenatal care attendees with emphasis on role of male partners. Extracts on HIV/AIDS, Wolaita Zone, SNNPR, Ethiopia.
24. Takele A (2007) Assessment of male partner influence on pregnant women towards voluntary HIV testing and support on PMTCT in Hospitals of Addis Ababa, Ethiopia.
25. Ayehu M (2010) Knowledge and attitude towards MTCT and its prevention methods among mothers attending the antenatal care clinics. EPHA Maternal and Newborn health abstract book, October 26-28, Mekelle, Ethiopia.
26. Adera A (2015) Assessment of male partner's involvement in prevention of mother-to-child transmission of HIV and associated factors among males in PMTCT services. Am J Health Research 3: 221-231.
27. Central Statistical Agency, ORC Macro (2006) Ethiopia Demographic and Health Survey 2005. Addis Ababa and Calverton.
28. Katz DA (2009) HIV testing men in the antenatal setting: understanding male non-disclosure. Int J STD and AIDS 20: 765-767.
29. Msuyaabc SE, Mbizvoad M (2008) Low male partner participation in antenatal HIV counseling and testing. AIDS Care 20: 700-709.
30. https: //www.duo.uio.no/handle/10852/30108

22

Health Care Providers' Perception and Associated Factors towards Safe Abortion in Selected Health Facilities in Adama, Ethiopia

Yitagesu Sintayehu[1*], **Birhanu Hordofa**[2] **and Kasiye Shiferaw**[1]

[1]*Department of Midwifery, College of Health and Medical Sciences, Haramaya University, Ethiopia*

[2]*Department of Nursing and midwifery, College of Health and Medical Sciences, Addis Ababa University, Ethiopia*

[*]**Corresponding author:** Yitagesu Sintayehu, Department of Midwifery, College of Health and Medical Sciences, Haramaya University, Ethiopia, E-mail: yitagesu.sintayehu@gmail.com

Abstract

Background: Every year it is estimated that worldwide, from 210 million pregnancies, maternal deaths are 3,58,000 and unsafe abortions are estimated to be between 21 million and 22 million. Half of abortions globally are unsafe. Almost all of them occur in developing countries, with the higher number of deaths concentrated in Africa, especially Sub-Saharan Africa, and South Asia. Unsafe abortion is still common and demands a heavy toll on women in Ethiopia.

Objective: To assess health providers' perception and associated factors towards safe abortion in health facilities.

Method: Institution based cross-sectional study was conducted in March 2016, by using pre-tested and structured self-administered questionnaire. A total of 394 health providers were selected by systematic random sampling. Logistic regression was used to analyze the association between the dependent and independent variables.

Result: A total of 383 health care providers participated in the study making the response rate 97%. About 48% of the respondents were found to have favorable perceptions towards safe abortion care. Preference of current legislation and institutional regulation (AOR=6.902 [95% CI=3.553, 13.406]), access to quality abortion service (AOR=6.628 [95% CI=2.122, 20.698]), preference of full legalization to safe abortion (AOR=8.862[5.008, 15.682]) and availability of adequate and functional equipment in the facilities (AOR=2.270[95% CI 1.245, 4.141]) were significantly associated with perceptions of health care providers towards safe abortion.

Conclusion: Health care providers' perception toward safe abortion care services was low. Therefore, sensitizing health providers about the essential nature of safe abortion services and the law governing abortion and equipping health facilities with essential supplies and accessibility of safe and legal termination of pregnancy are mandatory.

Keywords: Abortion; Health care; Pregnancy; Public health; Reproductive age

Introduction

Unsafe abortions are of major public health significance. Half of abortions globally are unsafe or estimated to be between 21 million and 22 million, therefore around one in ten pregnancies ends in an unsafe abortion. Almost all of them occur in developing countries, with the higher number of deaths concentrated in Africa, especially Sub-Saharan Africa, and South Asia. At the same time, there is a global shortage of health care providers with many countries prioritizing scarce human resources for a variety of pressing health problems. Therefore, there is a general consensus among various bodies that legalization of abortion is central in preventing the suffering and death of women [1,2]. Unsafe abortion is still common and demands a heavy toll on women in Ethiopia and 382,000 induced abortions occurred in 2008 and abortion rate is 23 per 1,000 women in reproductive age; 11-15 abortions occurred per 100 live births [3]. To address the large number of maternal deaths caused by unsafely performed abortions, as part of law reform in Ethiopia in 2005, the penal code was revised to broaden the indications under which abortion is permitted. Termination of pregnancy by recognized medical institution within the period permitted by the profession is not punishable or legal when the pregnancy results from rape or incest, when continuation of the pregnancy endangers the health or life of the woman or the fetus, in cases of fetal impairment, for women with physical or mental disabilities, for minors who are physically or psychologically unprepared to raise a child and in cases of grave and imminent danger that can be averted only through immediate pregnancy termination. A second, related change was made on 2006 publication, to "translate the law into actionable measures" and to inform "women, health professionals, law enforcement agencies and all sectors of society" about implementation of the law [4].

In addition to serious negative health consequences, unsafe abortion also has a severe economic impact, especially in poor countries with already overburdened health systems. Direct costs include skilled personnel, medications, blood, supplies, equipment's and hospitalization expenses associated with treating women who suffer complications of unsafe abortion [5,6]. The outcome of complications of unsafe abortion depends not only on the availability and quality of emergency abortion care, but also on a women's willingness to turn to medical services, and the readiness of medical staff to deal promptly with the complications. Even where abortion is legally permitted, technical and policy barriers related to healthcare personnel, facilities, medical equipment and supplies, and other factors commonly inhibit access to safe abortion care [1]. Many women needing abortion care are in vulnerable situations that make it difficult for them to exercise autonomous decision making. In some settings, health providers may agree to provide an abortion only in exchange for high fees or insist the woman to use a particular contraceptive method, including sterilization and some healthcare workers' negative attitudes and even punitive treatment towards women seeking safe abortion and others' refusal often on grounds of conscientious objection to provide in abortion care. A woman's access to services is determined in part by positive attitudes of health care providers for the better abortion related services in order to reduce maternal mortality and morbidity [5,7-9].

From the five top causes of maternal deaths in Ethiopia, one is abortion. The prevalence rates of abortion in general and induced abortion in particular are very high, 14.3% and 4.8%, respectively. To achieve a three-fourth decline in Maternal Mortality Rate (MMR) and to decrease the proportion of abortion-related deaths from 32% of all maternal deaths to 10% as set by Millennium Development Goal (MDG) plan, again about half a million pregnancies are estimated to end in abortion each year in Ethiopia indicating the need of comprehensive abortion care [10-13]. Increasing access to Comprehensive Abortion Care (CAC) requires careful consideration and understanding of the multilayered physical, legal, political, economic and cultural context of women's daily lives. Social status, level of education, community norms, standards, expectations and limited health services are all factors that determine the choices women have and their ability to exercise their right to make decisions relating to reproductive health. Two critical aspects of improving implementation of CAC are raising awareness and increasing access to resources for both women and health care providers [14]. Therefore this study designed to assess perception of health care providers towards safe abortion service and associated factors.

Methodology

Study setting and design

The study was conducted in Adama town, Oromiya Regional State which is found 100 km away from Addis Ababa to the east. According to the 2007 census by Central Statistic Authority (CSA) the town has a projected population of 337,556. There are 4 hospitals (1 government hospital and 3 private hospitals), 4 public health centers and 2 Non-Governmental Organization health facilities which are giving safe abortion services. The study involved both private and public health institutions in Adama which were providing safe abortion services. A facility based cross-sectional quantitative study design was used in March 2016.

Population and sampling

All health care providers who were working in Adama town health facility were source population and health care providers who were available during data collection time in selected institution were study population.

Sample size estimation

Single population proportion formula was used to determine the minimum sample size considering 95% confidence interval, margin of error 5% and 37% prevalence of positive attitude of health care providers towards safe abortion [15].

$n=(Z\alpha/2)^2p(1-p)/d^2$

$n=(1.96^2)0.37(1-0.37)/(0.05)^2$

$n=(3.8416)\ (0.2331)/0.0025=358$

Where: n=Initial minimum sample size; $Z\alpha/2$=Z value at 95% CI [1.96]; p=Estimated prevalence rate is 37%; d=Margin of error tolerable is 5% [0.05]; By considering 10% (36) non response rate, the total sample size was 394 health providers.

Sampling technique

The study was conducted in ten selected health institution of Adama town. After proportional allocation of health care providers for each health institutions, samples of health care provider were selected by systematic random sampling (SRS) method.

Study variables

- **Dependent variables:** Perception of health care providers.
- **Independent variables:** Individual factor: Education, experience, religion; Environmental factor: Law/policy (safe abortion liberalization), socio cultural issue; Institutional factor: Health facility policy and regulation, availability and accessibility of equipment's and supplies, type of health sector level of activity, availability of reference, availability of trained provider.

Data collection procedures

The study had employed self-administered questionnaires. The questionnaire was taken from other two similar study conducted in different part of Ethiopia [15,16]. The data collectors and supervisors were given training on how to collect the data, objective and method of the study and on issues of confidentiality and rights of respondents. A copy of the questionnaire was submitted to the expert to examine whether the number and type of items in the questionnaire measured the concept or construct of interest (objective of the study).

Data quality control

Before the actual data collection the questionnaires were pre-tested on 5% of the total sample size on similar health care providers groups in different facilities which is not sampled institution. Based on the findings of the pre-test, there were some modifications was made on the tool before administration to actual study participants. Data collectors were instructed to check the completeness of each questionnaire whether each and every question was completely answered and also the supervisors and principal investigator were recheck the completeness of the questionnaire immediately after submission.

Data processing and analysis

The questionnaire were cleaned, coded and entered into EPI data version 3.1. Then the data was exported to SPSS version 21 for cleaning and analysis. The descriptive analysis was used to determine frequency distribution, proportions and percentage. Logistic regressions were carried out between dependent and independent variables to determine their associations at 95% confidence interval.

Operational definitions

Perception: Refers to the participants' response as favorable or unfavorable attitudinal statement towards safe abortion care.

Favorable responses: Agreeing with the positive statements (respondents those answer greater than mean attitude score considered as favorable attitude).

Unfavorable responses: Disagreeing for positive statement (respondents those answer with a score below mean attitude score considered as unfavorable attitude).

Health care provider: Also known as health personnel, those professionals were Obstetrics and Gynecology specialists, Surgeons, General practitioner, Residences, Nurses, Midwives and Health officer.

Mean attitude score: the average of response on the attitudinal questions.

Results and Discussion

Socio-demographic characteristics

From total of 394 study participants about 383 of health care providers were participated in the study which makes response rate 97%. Among participants in the study, more than half, 225(58.7) were female and the median age of respondent was 29 years. About 229(59.8%) of the respondents were currently married. Of all respondents, 223 (58.2) were orthodox followers and 219(57.2%) of the respondents primary work place were government. From participants 191(49.9%) were nurses. About 65% of the respondents had less than or equal to 5 years of work experience (Table 1).

Variable	Frequency	Percentage
Sex		
Female	225	58.7
Male	158	41.3
Age		
15-24	23	6
25-34	291	76
35-44	69	18
Marital status		
Never married	146	38.1
Married	229	59.8
Divorced	7	1.8
Widowed	1	0.3
Religion		
Orthodox	223	58.2
Muslim	80	20.9
Protestant	73	19.1
Others	7	1.8
Profession		
Obstetrics and Gynecology specialist	8	2.1
General practitioner	39	10.2
Midwife	93	24.3
Health officer	46	12
Nurse	191	49.9
Emergency surgery	6	1.6

Year of professional experience		
Less than one year	35	9.1
1-3 years	89	23.2
3-5 years	125	32.6
6-10 years	84	21.9
More than 10 years	50	13.1
Primary work place		
Government hospital	175	45.7
Private hospital	135	35.2
Government health center	44	11.5
NGO health institution	29	7.6

Table 1: Socio-demographic characteristics of study participants, 2016, Adama, Ethiopia.

Attitude of health providers toward safe abortion care services

The study revealed that 184 (48%) of them had a favorable attitude towards safe abortion care services (Figure 1).

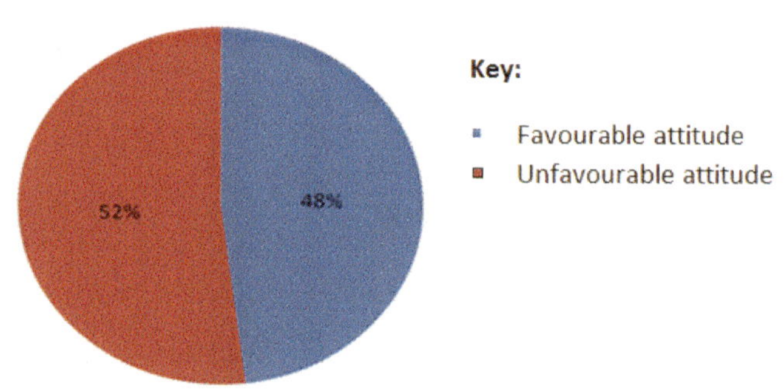

Figure 1: Pie-chart showing attitude of health providers towards safe abortion services at Adama, 2016, Ethiopia.

Views of respondents according to their attitude towards different characteristics of safe abortion

The respondents were asked to state their reasons why they are not comfortable working in site where safe abortion was done and their response were religion (42.3%), followed by personal value (15.1%). On the other hand, the respondents were asked about why they chose for legalization of safe abortion, and the majority of the respondents (44.6 %) said because it reduces morbidity and mortality which would occur due to unsafe abortion. The primary anticipated problem if abortion was fully legalized were, fear of opposition from religious group which account (82.8 %). Health care providers also asked their reason why they oppose fully legalization of safe abortion, and majority of them (88.8%) said it's due to their religion factors. Moreover, the respondents were asked to suggest conditions under which women should not be allowed to terminate their pregnancies. More than 4 of the respondents believed that the service should not be rendered for married women (Table 2).

Variables	Frequency	Percent (%)
Reason of respondents' not comfortable working in a site where abortion is done*		
Outside of their scope of practice	31	8.1
Against religious practice	162	42.3
Against personal value	58	15.1
Didn't have opportunity to trained	19	5
Reason for preference of legalization of safe abortion*		
Abortion is a health problem in our area	102	26.6
Facilitate to get service in safe area and trained provider	139	36.3

Reduce mortality and morbidity occur due to unsafe abortion	171	44.6
Solve problems of unwanted pregnancy	108	28.2
Reduce cost for inducing abortion	71	18.5
Reason for not opting to a full legalization safe abortion*		
My religion does not allow	165	43.1
Culturally not accepted	51	13.3
Homicide	80	20.9
Encourage to have unwanted pregnancies	52	13.6
Encourage pre/extra marital sex	46	12
Anticipated problem if abortion is fully legalized*		
Opposition from religious group	317	82.8
Opposition from the whole community	84	21.9
Opposition from the part community	159	41.5
Lack of trained man power	186	46.8
Lack of adequate service provision facilities	132	34.5
Shortage of fund	56	12
Reason of providers for not legalized safe abortion*		
Religion	340	88.8
Culture	176	46
Lack of facility/provider	165	43.1
Poverty	51	13.3
Women who were not allowed to have safe abortion*		
All women	46	12
With no medical indication	153	39.9
Married women	155	40.5
Unmarried woman	30	7.8
Student	42	11
Victims of incent	48	12.5
Victims of rape	72	18.8
Very young women	61	15.9
All should be allowed	61	15.9
Who else should involve in decision making, for women*		
Health provider	97	25.3
Partner/family	145	37.9

Table 2: Views of respondent according to their attitude towards different characteristics, 2016, Adama, Ethiopia (*total do not added to 100% because of multiple responses).

Factors associated with health care providers' attitude

Independently being male and being Physician/Ho were more likely had favorable attitude than their counterparts (COR=1.689[1.121-2.546]) and (COR=1.678[1.057-2.663]) respectively and participants who were works where there were trained staff in the facility, availability of essential supplies and drugs in the facility\and ready facility to give safe abortion were more likely had favorable attitude when compared to their counterparts (COR=1.849[1.215-2.816]), (COR=2.920[1.898-4.492]) and (COR=3.531[2.190-5.695]) respectively.

Variable	Favorable attitude score	Crude OR (CI)	Adjusted OR (CI)
Sex			
Female	96(42.7)	1	1.286(0.720-2.298)
Male	88(55.7)	1.689(1.121-2.546)	
Profession			
Nurse/midwife	127(44.7)	1	1.721(0.867-3.415)
Physician/Ho	57(57.6)	1.678(1.057-2.663)	
Preference of current legislation and institutional regulation			
No	17(11.9)	1	6.902(3.553-13.406)*
Yes	167(69.6)	16.956(9.529-30.171)	
Access to quality abortion service is a key step to reduce unsafe abortion			
No	5(8.1)	1	6.628(2.122-20.698)*
Yes	179(55.8)	14.370(5.612-36.80)	
Preference to safe abortion legalization			
No	34(17.5)	1	8.862(5.008-15.682)*
Yes	150(79.4)	18.0(10.858-30.171)	
Availability of adequate and functional equipment in the facility			
No	43(30.9)	1	2.270(1.245-4.141)*
Yes	141(47.8)	3.056(1.968-4.747)	
Availability of well trained staff in the facility			
No	56(38.6)	1	0.791(0.363-1.726)
Yes	128(53.8)	1.849(1.215-2.816)	
Availability of essential supplies and drugs in the facility			
No	48(32.2)	1	1.734(0.803-3.746)
Yes	136(58.1)	2.920(1.898-4.492)	
Facility readiness to give safe abortion			
No	31(27.2)	1	0.189(0.500-2.831)
Yes	153(56.9)	3.531(2.190-5.695)	

Table 3: Multivariate analysis for attitude of health care providers' (*statistically significant at 95% confidence interval).

Preference to fully legalization of safe abortion and preference of current legislation and institutional regulation of safe abortion associated with attitude of heath care providers towards safe abortion (AOR=8.862 [95% CI=5.008-15.682]) and (AOR=6.902 [95% CI=3.553, 13.406]) respectively. Accordingly, those who said access to quality abortion service is a key step to reduce unsafe abortion and where there were adequate and functional equipment in their facility associated with attitude of health care provider providers towards safe abortion (AOR=6.628 [95% CI=2.122-20.698]) and (AOR=2.270 [95% CI=1.245-4.141]) respectively. Our study results reveals 48% of providers had favorable attitude towards safe abortion. This was inconsistent with a study done in Mekele town which was 94.8% [16].

This difference might be due to setting difference and the study done in Mekele included only four public hospitals while our study had ten all levels of governmental and private facilities. But, this result was nearly in line with the study done in East Gojam Zone which was 56.7% [17]. This similarity might be due to both studies were done within one year deference and they incorporated both hospitals and health centers.

The vast majority of health care providers (91.9%) believed complications of unsafe abortion, including mortality was a "very serious" health problem in their setting, 87.7% of providers also agreed that access to safe abortion services could reduce maternal mortality and 83.8% agreed with expansion of access to quality of safe abortion services was a key step to reducing unsafe abortion. This result is slightly greater than study done on how provider attitudes towards abortion can impact the quality and access to abortion services in 6 Latin American and Caribbean Countries [18]. This might be due to setting and study time difference. Reasons of health care providers' not comfortable working in site where safe abortion was done were due to religious grounds, personal value, out of their scope of practices and lack of training (42.3%, 15.1%, 8.1 and 5%) respectively. This study result is also in line with the study done in Nepal, Ghana and Addis Ababa [15,19,20]. Those health care providers who were against the low, said that religious reason, cultural reason, lack of trained provider and lack of facility were the main factors to be against the law. The result was nearly similar with a study done at Mekele town and Addis Ababa [15,16]. This similarity might be due to these studies were done in urban facilities.

The respondents were asked to forward their agreement or disagreement on whether or not the woman herself should decide to have a legal abortion and 46.5% agreed, whereas 53.5% of respondents disagreed. This was similar with the same study done in Addis Ababa which shown 55.1% of respondents disagreed with the idea of women themselves should decide to have safe abortion [15]. This similarity might be due to both studies were done on nearly similar population characteristics. After adjustment of logistic regression the study have shown that those who preferred full legalization of safe abortion were found to had more favorable attitude compared to those who don't prefers full legalization of safe abortion (AOR=8.862 [95%=5.008, 15.682]). This result was in line with the study done in East Gojam, Ethiopia [17]. This might be due to both studies included both hospitals and health centers and the study period was not far apart.

Health care providers who prefers current legislation and institutional regulation to safe abortion found to had more likely favorable attitude than who don't prefer current legislation and institutional regulation to safe abortion (AOR=6.902 [95% CI=3.553, 13.406]) and the study participants who agreed with concept of access to quality abortion service as a key step to reduce unsafe abortion, found to had seven times more favorable attitudes than those who didn't agree (AOR=6.628 [95% CI=2.122, 20.698]). Moreover; health care providers working in a facility where there were adequate and functional equipment in the facility had more favorable attitude than those health care providers working in the health facilities where there were no adequate and functional equipment (AOR=(2.270 [95% CI=1.245, 4.141]). For the last three associated factors (variables) other studies were tested them and there were no studies found their association, but in this study these variables were associated as indicated above.

Ethical Considerations

Ethical clearance was obtained from institution review board (IRB) of Addis Ababa University, College of health science, School of allied health sciences, department of Nursing and Midwifery. Then formal letter of cooperation was written concerned bodies. Each study participant was adequately informed about the purpose, method, anticipated benefit and risk of the study. Informed voluntary written and signed consent was obtained from each study participants. Confidentiality and cultural norms of study participants were maintained. Considering the sensitivity of this research, all the basic principles of human research ethics (respect of persons, beneficence, voluntary participation, confidentiality and justice) was respected.

Conclusion

From the study findings the following conclusions are drown: Health care providers had low favorable attitudes towards safe abortion care. The finding also revealed that quality of safe abortion care, availability of basic supplies and functional equipment, preference to current legislation and institutional regulation of safe abortion and preference to fully legalization of safe abortion found to be significantly associated with providers' attitude toward safe abortion services.

Limitations

Ministry of health should increase health care provider awareness toward safe abortion and its importance in reducing maternal morbidity and mortality. The ministry should also equip the institutions with necessary supplies and have to increase number of trained health care providers. Moreover, the government should strengthen the existing abortion legislation of the country and support health care providers on its implementation. Further qualitative study should be done on perception of health care provider and associated factors.

Competing Interests

The authors declare that they have no competing interests.

Funding

The funding was obtained from Addis Ababa University, College of health science. There was no code for the budget and it was released by simple signature of the correspondent author.

Authors' Contributions

YS designed the study, performed the statistical analysis and drafted the manuscript. BH and KS participated in the study design, implementation of the study, and contributed to the draft manuscript. All authors contributed to the data analysis, read and approved the final manuscript.

Acknowledgement

We are very grateful to the Addis Ababa University for their technical and financial support of this study. Then, we would like to thank all respondents who participated in this study for their commitment in responding to our questionnaire.

References

1. World Health Organization (2011) Unsafe abortion: Global and regional estimates of incidence of unsafe abortion and associated mortality in 2008 (6th edtn.).
2. World Health Organization (2015) New WHO guidelines on health worker roles in safe abortion. Guttmacher Policy Review.
3. Singh S, Fetters T, Gebreselassie H, Abdella A, Gebrehiwot Y, et al. (2010) The estimated incidence of induced abortion in Ethiopia, 2008. Intl Perspect Sexual Reprod Health p: 16-25.
4. FMOH (2006) Technical and procedural guidelines for safe abortion services in Ethiopia.
5. Marie Stopes International (MSI), Ipas (2009) For women's lives and health: Report of the global safe abortion conference. Whose right? Whose choice? Who cares? London, England.
6. Vlassoff M, Fetters T, Kumbi S, Singh S (2012) The health system cost of post-abortion care in Ethiopia. Int J Gynecol Obstet 118(S2): S127-S133.
7. Hyman AG, Castleman L (2005) Woman-centered abortion care. Ipas. North Carolina, USA.
8. Rehan N (2003) Attitudes of health care providers to induced abortion in Pakistan. J Pak Med Assoc 53: 3.
9. Ahman E, Shah IH (2010) Generating national unsafe abortion estimates: Challenges and choices. Guttmacher Institute/IUSSP pp: 13-22.
10. Senbeto E, Alene GD, Abesno N, Yeneneh H (2005) Prevalence and associated risk factors of induced abortion in Northwest Ethiopia. EJHD 19: 37-44.
11. Abdella A (2010) Maternal mortality trend in Ethiopia. EJHD 24: 115-122.
12. Tadesse E, Yosephi S, Gasso A, Muletta E, Pogharian D, et al. (2001) Illegal abortion in Addis Ababa Ethiopia. East Afr Med J 78: 25-29.
13. FDRE (2006) National reproductive health strategy: 2006-2015. Department of Family Health. Addis Ababa: Ministry of health.
14. Neesha G, Anna S, Rachel V (2008) Bridging the gaps: Implementation of comprehensive abortion care in Ethiopia. Addis Ababa, Ethiopia.
15. Abdi J, Gebremariam MB (2011) Health providers' perception towards safe abortion service at selected health facilities in Addis Ababa. African J Reprod Health 15: 31-36.
16. Tadesse Z, Kahsay AB, Tilahun W, Berhe KK (2014) Assessment of health care providers attitude and associated factors to wards safe abortion at public hospitals, in Mekelle City, Tigray, Ethiopia: A cross-sectional study. Global J Med Res 14: 3.
17. Abebe M (2015) Assessement of health care providers 'attitude and associated factors towards safe abortion care at public health institiutions in East Gojjam Zone, Amhara, Ethiopia: Cross-sectional study.
18. Dabash R, Pena M, Koladycz R, Carino G, Mejia M, et al. (2004) How provider attitudes towards abortion can impact the quality of and access to abortion services: An assessment of IPPF/WHR provider knowledge, attitudes and practices in 6 Latin American and Caribbean Countries.
19. Puri M, Lamichhane P, Harken T, Blum M, Harper CC, et al. (2012) Sometimes they used to whisper in our ears: Health care workers' perceptions of the effects of abortion legalization in Nepal. BMC Public Health 12: 297.
20. Aboagye PK, Gebreselassie H, Asare GQ, Mitchell EM, Addy J (2007) An assessment of the readiness to offer contraceptives and comprehensive abortion care in the Greater Accra Eastern and Ashanti regions of Ghana. Ipas.

Pilates for Pregnant Women: A Healthy Alternative

Andrade Martin C, Fernandes Alvares R*, Reis Nascimento T, Waldemar Paranaiba SS, Karen da Silva Morais T and Carvalho Santos D

Physical Therapist, Studio-100 Pilates, Brasilia, Brazil

***Corresponding author:** Alvares RF, Physical Therapist (FARPLAC), Pharmacist (UNIPLAN), Owner Partner, Manager and Coach, Studio-100 Pilates, Brasilia, Brazil, E-mail: rachelalvares@hotmail.com

Abstract

Pregnancy is a specific stage in women's life, a time when they face physiological and biomechanical changes that, without proper monitoring, lead to the emergence of musculoskeletal discomforts. Most of these issues are associated with postural changes, balance, ligament laxity, body weight increase and cardiorespiratory disorders. The Pilates method provides several benefits such as increased respiratory capacity, improved muscle strength and the strengthening of torso-stabilizing muscles, flexibility, spine mobility, postural alignment, coordination, proprioception, balance and motor control. Given the specific condition of pregnant women and the variations derived from such condition, Pilates may positively contribute to these women's health within their physical and psychological limitations. The aim of the current study is to address the importance of Pilates, clinical guidelines and physical activities practiced in the main pregnancy periods (trimesters) through a bibliographical analysis. Pregnant women are known for the several physiological changes they go through; thus, Pilates can make important contributions to their health, such as the promotion of quality of life and wellbeing to improve their adaptation to each gestational week.

Keywords: Pregnancy; Pregnant women; Parturient; Pelvic floor; Perineum; Muscles; Movement; Physical exertion; Locomotor activity; Pilates

Introduction

As pregnancy evolves, women's physical capacity reduces. Therefore, exercising during pregnancy should be prioritized and encouraged [1,2].

According to the World Health Organization (WHO), 31% of the world population at the age of 15 years or older show insufficient physical activity level. This prevalence is even higher among pregnant women [1].

Choosing an adaptable and interesting physical activity increases the satisfaction and attendance degree and, consequently, decreases sedentariness. According to Tavares et al. the sedentary lifestyle affected 100% of the pregnant women participating in a study carried out with 118 pregnant, sedentary women in the 32nd gestational week [3].

Healthy pregnant women, who prioritize their well-being, during and after pregnancy, acknowledge the importance of this moment of great transformation in their bodies and seek to improve and keep their conditioning, strength and physical fitness. The main goal of Pilates lies on body strengthening and stabilization, pain relief, as well as on improved flexibility, concentration and breathing [4].

Nowadays, Pilates has been used as a physical or therapeutic activity technique, which applies well-oriented and optimized movements to generate physical and mental wellbeing [5,6].

The Pilates' philosophy and strategy may be applied to pregnant women because they strengthen the muscles responsible for lumbopelvic stabilization, improving postural alignment and respiratory pattern, and optimizing daily-living activity movements. Pregnancy is associated with several musculoskeletal and hormonal changes; thus, it is crucial orienting all pregnant women to avoid compensations, as well as to make them more aware of their bodies [3].

The Pilates method uses the resistance of the springs assembled in the equipment to quantify the exercises. Therefore, it is worth performing a force/time assessment, since force and time are important elements to be taken into consideration at the time to prescribe the exercises. The principles of Pilates, such as breathing, must be emphasized; after all, individuals who breath well can benefit from aspects such as maximum exercise attainment, concentration (which allows coordinating the thoughts and the energy to a certain body area) and centralization (which is essential to develop the muscles responsible for supporting the body, as well as to strengthen the torso-transverse abdomen, multifidus muscle, pelvic floor and latissimus dorsi). Stability-challenging exercises are introduced to the exercise program when these muscles are well developed. Therefore, the aim of Pilates exercises applied to pregnant women is to improve the physical, physiological and mental conditions of these women in order to assure both the mother and the baby's health [3,6].

During pregnancy, the female body goes through moments when all systems are provisionally involved. Thus, the Pilates method, which was first developed under the name "Contrology" by Joseph Pilates, has the overall philosophy of achieving and coordinating all systems-mind, spirit and body by taking into consideration the entire physiological process. Therefore, Pilates allows women to rapidly recover their silhouette after giving birth through abdominal and muscle strengthening exercises. One of the great causes of low self-esteem is the diastasis recti i.e., the rectus abdominis muscle separation, since it affects two-thirds of pregnant women [6,7].

The aim of the current study is to address the Pilates method efficacy and benefits during pregnancy [3].

Pilates' Special Conditions during Pregnancy

It is possible avoiding painful manifestations during pregnancy through the practice of physical exercises. Lumbar pain is common during this period and several factors must be taken into account; among them, the sedentary lifestyle, as well as the existence of previous pain and emotional factors, stand out. The pain may worsen due to increased muscle weakness, poor flexibility, poor joint mobility, poor posture and due to the compensations pregnant women experience during the gestational weeks [8,9].

Nowadays, pregnant women are concerned about keeping a good body weight so as not to develop pathologies such as Hypertension and Gestational Diabetes Mellitus. The Pilates method is one of the techniques extensively used by physical therapists, since it provides physical conditioning, as well as body control and awareness. In addition, it does not impose undue stress on the human body [8,10,11]. Good guidance enables pregnant women to maintain an adequate posture and reduce compensations in the lower back. Thus, it is possible reducing the pain episodes and, consequently, improving the quality of life of pregnant women, mainly in their daily-life activities [12,13].

Several hormonal, hemodynamic and biomechanical changes take place throughout the gestational trimesters, mainly in the second and third ones. The growth of the gravid uterus, and of body structures, results in increased pressure over the pelvic floor muscles, as well as in edema, weight gain, ligament laxity and postural changes [14].

The increased blood volume, heart rate and cardiac output, both at rest and during exercise, stand out among the changes taking place in the pregnant women's body during the first two trimesters.

There is increased compression in the inferior vena cava from the third gestational trimester on, and it may lead to arterial hypotension. Hormonal changes such as increased estrogen, progesterone and relaxin reduce the muscle tone, which is responsible for stabilizing the joints. The ligaments also undergo relaxation, mainly in the pelvic region. All these changes make it necessary adapting pregnant women's physical exercises in order to facilitate their movements. According to Balogh, the Pilates method has beneficial effects on pregnant women, since it allows increasing the thoracic cavity through respiratory exercises, as well as strengthening the abdominal muscles and improving urinary incontinence [15-21].

Women's quality of life should be one of the main goals of physical activity, which should address weight management, pains (mainly the postural-related ones), postpartum-depression risk reduction, and greater autonomy in labor. "It is essential assessing health-related quality of life in order to identify different wellbeing and health economics levels by investigating the efficacy, effectiveness, efficiency and usefulness of different therapies available for several types of diseases or conditions" [22].

The Pilates method is an exercise modality that can be therapeutically used to provide physical conditioning, since it exercises the body as a whole and is based on Contrology, i.e., the conscious control of body and joint movements. Studies have found that activities such as Pilates help rebalancing body muscles, as well as improving body awareness, breathing and wellbeing [14]. The principles in this method should focus on improving the efficacy of the exercises to be practiced during class through breathing, body alignment, torso control, as well as movement efficiency and fluency [7].

Another point of fundamental importance concerns the fact that pregnant women practicing Pilates should work in partnership with their physiotherapists in order to improve their training, as well as to be well informed about and more involved with the treatment, thus generating better conditions and resources for an integrated and collaborative treatment. Consequently, the individualized treatment becomes more effective. In addition, the role played by pregnant women is very important from the moment they describe their goals to the feedback they provide during and in the end of the treatment, since it allows them to be informed about the most favorable results, as well as to avoid risks, thus showing greater adherence to the practice of Pilates [23,24].

First Trimester

The physical activity should be performed in a mild-to-moderate degree, even by sedentary pregnant women [2].

The muscle stretching is relevant to Pilates practice because it reduces the pain in the lower back and pelvic regions. It is known that 50% of the pregnant women present symptoms such as back, lower back and pelvic pain. Martin and Silva have found that pregnant women subjected to stretching presented reduced or no lower back discomfort [16-18].

Stretching exercises should be performed in the first pregnancy trimester in order to enable muscle strength gain, mainly in large muscle groups (gluteal, external rotators, transverse abdominal, paravertebral, latissimus dorsi and shoulder girdle muscles), as well as to train the pelvic floor [2].

Barakat et al. have assessed 160 pregnant women. 80 of them performed light muscle resistance training three times a week, and found that women who practiced exercises showed lower gestational weight gain [19].

According to the study by Sihvonen et al. 32 pregnant women have shown direct correlation between pain and activation level in the para spinal muscles of the lumbar spine during the first pregnancy trimester [16].

It is essential performing low-weight exercises, improving body awareness and spine mobility, as well as avoiding eccentric abdominal exercises during this pregnancy period (Figures 1-3) [7].

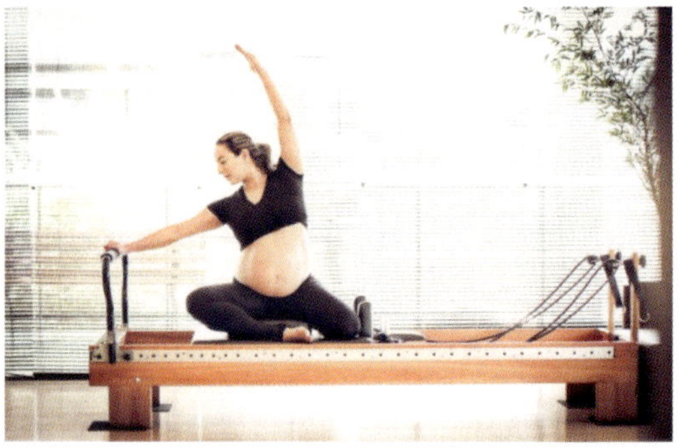

Figure 1: Mermaid on the reformer, stretching and relaxation of the lateral torso muscles; emphasis on the organization of head, neck and shoulders.

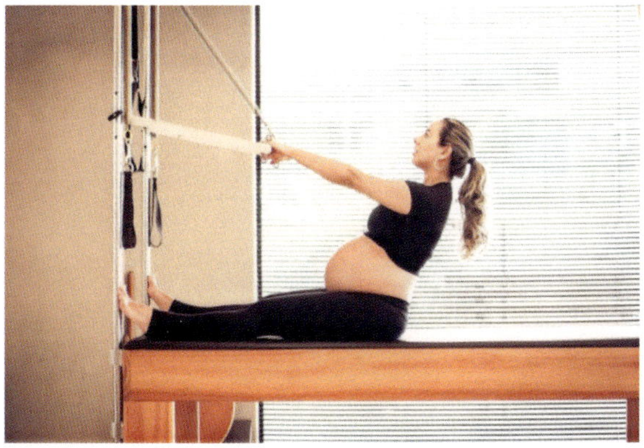

Figure 2: Seated push through, spine alignment and paravertebral muscles strengthening.

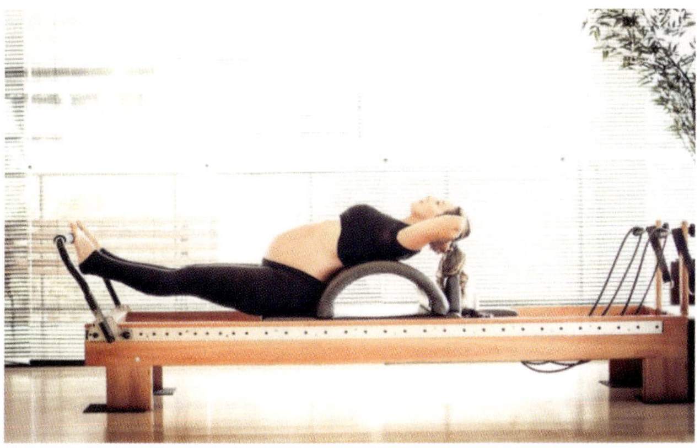

Figure 3: Spine extension on the reformer using flymoon.

Second Trimester

Pregnant women begin to better perceive pregnancy-related changes such as weight gain, as well as bigger breasts and abdomen, during this period. It is worth emphasizing the individuality aspect, since these changes are different from one woman to another [20].

Greater attention should be paid to avoid holding supine positions for a long period from the 20th gestational week on recommendations for physical exercise during pregnancy[2].

The relaxin hormone is released around the 12th gestational week, and it results in joint looseness. Thus, it is necessary being careful at the time to perform stretching exercises, because they may increase the risk of injuries [2].

The enlargement of the pubic symphysis and the exercises may result in pain and stress to this musculature. The relaxin is also responsible for remodeling connective tissues. In addition, it decreases the tensile forces and increases the pressure on the pelvic floor [2,4,5].

The second trimester comes along with possible compensations in the lumbar region during the practice of exercises, thus increasing the lumbar lordosis.

Since, the relaxin hormone level also increases during this period, excessive or forced stretching exercises should be avoided, whereas strengthening exercises should be prioritized.

In addition, exercise adaptations should be done due to changes in the gestational biomechanics. It is worth emphasizing the importance of strengthening the rhomboid, paravertebral, internal and external hip rotator and transverse abdominal muscles, as well as of performing pelvic floor exercises (Figures 4-6) [7].

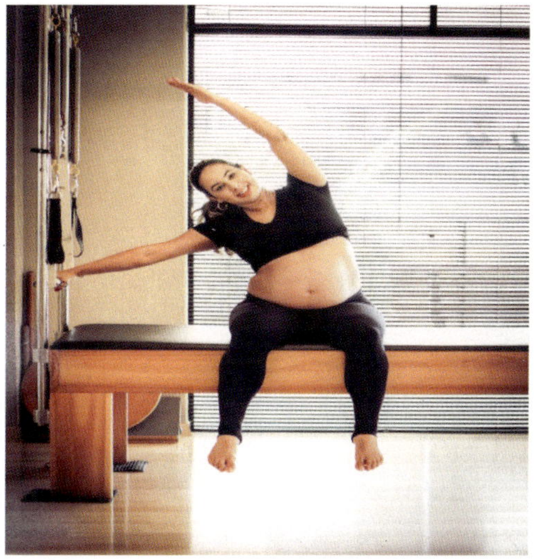

Figure 4: Seated mermaid-torso stretching and mobilization through lateral flexion.

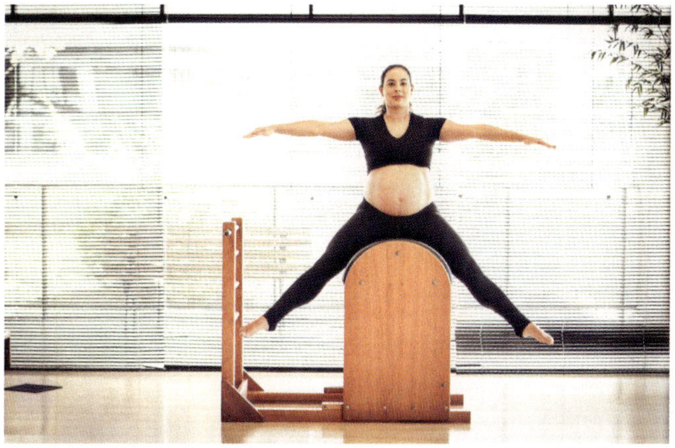

Figure 5: Horse-strengthening of the pelvic floor, adductor and torso stabilizer muscles.

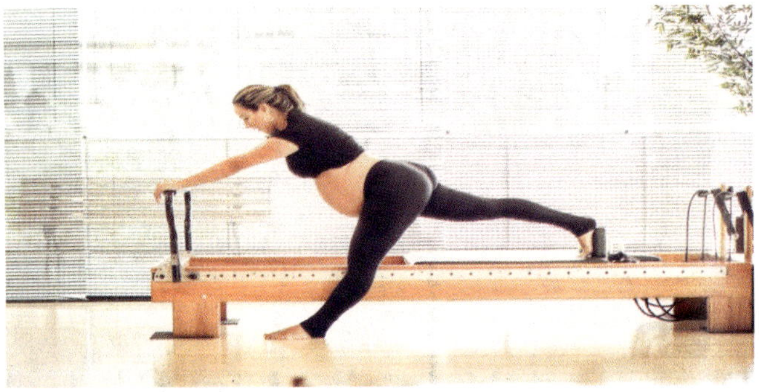

Figure 6: Scooter-stretching of the posterior chain muscles, strengthening of quadriceps and gluteal muscles.

Third Trimester

As the weight gain and the limitations increase, the exercise pace and intensity decrease. The pelvic floor muscles should be continuously trained in order to provide greater awareness about relaxation and flexibility increase [2]. Caromano has analyzed the respiratory pressures in 150 pregnant women divided into first, second and third gestational trimesters and found that the chest mobility and the respiratory pressures decrease in the first trimester and increase throughout pregnancy (Figures 7-9) [23].

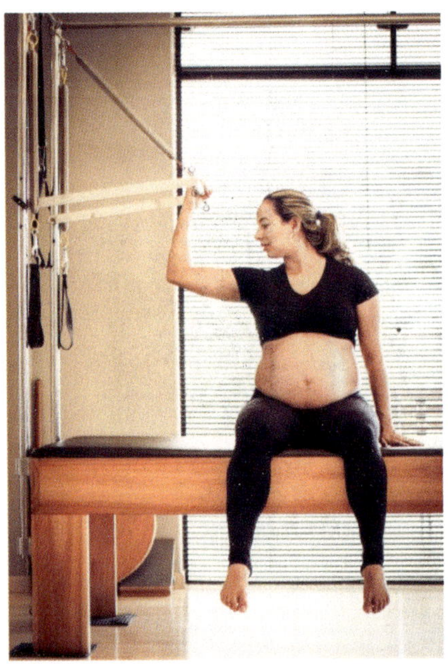

Figure 7: Seated pull down-strengthening of biceps, latissimus dorsi and elbow flexor muscles.

The load in the upper and lower limb exercises, as well as in the pelvic mobilization ones, should be increased in the final gestational stage in order to prepare pregnant women for the postpartum period, when they will take care of their babies. Abdominal contraction associated with pelvic floor contraction is not used if the pregnant woman makes the option for vaginal delivery, because, at the time to deliver the baby, she must perform abdominal contraction and relax the pelvic floor musculature. It is essential continuously monitoring the clinical signs of pregnant women during the practice of exercises at the end of the third trimester, since there may be fluid or blood loss [7].

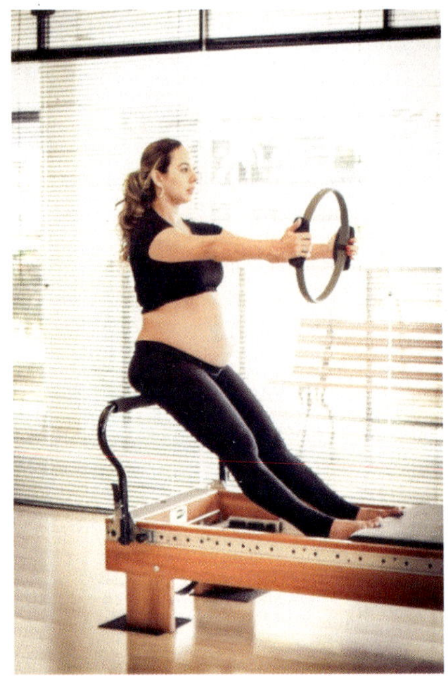

Figure 8: Seated footwork-helps strengthening the legs, as well as controlling the core and the torso stabilizers.

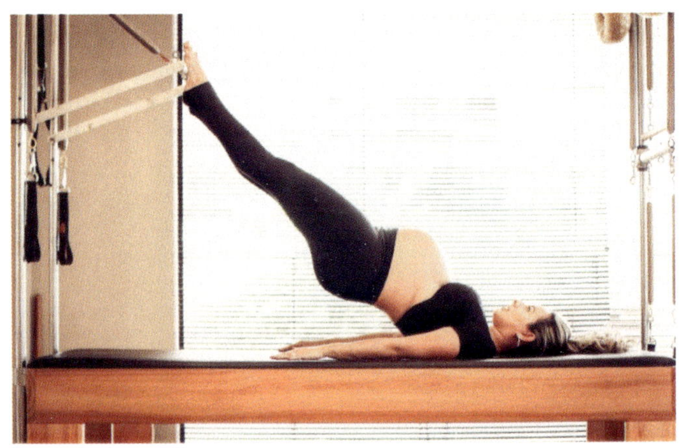

Figure 9: Bridging with extended legs-favors the venous return and helps providing space for the baby to change position.

Conclusion

The knowledge about the physiological and psychological changes affecting pregnant women, in association with the training in Pilate's techniques, may promote and contribute to a gestational period with no complications and to reduce the risk of low-back pain and osteoarticular discomforts. Stabilization, strengthening and stretching exercises should be performed, but the gestational week and the patient's physical and emotional limitations must be respected. It is possible seeing that the physical activity is beneficial to pregnant women. Thus, such practice should be encouraged by health professionals.

References

1. Baciuk EP, Silveira C, Cavalcante SR, Cecatti JG, Pereira RIC, et al. (2006) Evaluation of the physical capacity and its importance for the exercise prescription during pregnancy. Femina 34: 409-416.
2. Nascimento SL, Godoy AC, Surita FG, Silva JLP (2014) Recommendations for physical exercise practice during pregnancy: A critical review. Rev Bras Ginecol Obstet 36: 423-431.
3. Machado CN, Prado AP (2016) Analysis of lower limb strength in the exercise workout of the pilates method. Rev Fisioter Mov 29: 669-675.
4. Midwives RCM (2005) Pilates and pregnancy. J Royal College of Midwives 8: 220-222.
5. Machado CANR (2006) Effects of a physiotherapeutic approach based on the pilates method for patients diagnosed with low back pain during pregnancy. Rev Fisioterapia Brasil 7: 345-350.
6. Leite AC, Araujo KK (2012) Diastasis of the rectus abdominis in postpartum and its relation with obstetric variables. Fisioter Mov 25: 389-397.
7. Kroetz DC, Santos MD (2015) Benefits of the pilates method in the musculoskeletal changes arising from the gestational period. Visão Universitária 36: 72-89.
8. Batista DC, Chiara VL, Gugelmin SA, Martins PD (2003) Physical activity and gestation: Health of pregnant non-athlete and fetal growth. Rev Bras Saúde Matern Infant 3: 151-158.
9. Schmit EFD, Candotti CT, Rodrigues AP, Souza C, Melo MO, et al. (2016) Effects of the pilates method on static body posture of women: A systematic review. Fisioter Pesqui 23: 329-335.
10. Velloso EPP, Reis ZSN, Pereira MLK, Pereira AK (2015) Maternal-fetal response resulting from physical exercise during pregnancy: A systematic review. Rev Med Minas Gerais 25: 93-99.
11. Krawczky B, Mainenti MRM, Pacheco AGF (2016) The impact of pilates exercises on the postural alignment of healthy adults. Rev Bras Med Esporte 22: 485-490.
12. Oliveira NTB, Freitas SMSF, Moura KF, Junior MAL, Cabral CMN (2015) Biomechanical analysis of the trunk and pelvis in exercises of the pilates method: Systematic review. Fisioter Pesq 22: 443-455.
13. Rodrigues WFG, Silva LR, Nascimento MAL, Pernambuco CS, Giani TS, et al. (2011) Prevalence of lower back pain and physical inactivity: The impact of psychosocial factors in pregnant women served by the Family Health Strategy. Einstein 9: 489-493.
14. Moreira LS, Andrade SRS, Soares V, Avelar IS, Amaral WN, et al. (2011) Changes of posture, equilibrium and low back pain during pregnancy. Femina 39: 241-244.
15. Neves C, Medina JL, Delgado JL (2007) Endocrine changes and immunodulation in pregnancy. Arquivos de Medicina 21: 175-182.
16. Sihvonen T, Huttunen M, Makkonen M, Airaksinen O (1998) Functional changes in back muscle activity correlate with pain intensity and prediction of low back pain during pregnancy. Arch Phys Med Rehabil 79: 1210-1222.
17. Dumas GA, Reid JG, Wolfe LA, Griffin MP, MacGrath MJ (1995) Exercise, posture, and back pain during pregnancy. Part 2: exercise and back pain. Clin Biomech 10: 104-109.
18. Martins RF, Silva JLP (2005) An exercise method for the treatment of lumbar and posterior pelvic pain in pregnancy. Rev Bras Ginecol Obstet 27: 275-282.
19. Barakat R, Lucia A, Ruiz JR (2009) Resistance exercise training during pregnancy and newborn´s birth size: A randomised controlled trial. Int J Obes 33: 1048-1057.
20. Costa ES, Pinon GMB, Costa TS, Santos RGA, Nobrega AR, et al. (2010) Physiological alterations from the pespective of women in pregnancy. Rev Rene Fortaleza 11: 86-93.
21. Surita FG, Nascimento SL, Silva JLP (2014) Physical exercise during pregnancy. Revista Brasileira de ginecologia e obstetrícia 36: 531-534.
22. Rett MT, Simoes JA, Herrmann V, Gurgel MSC, Morais SS (2007) Women's life quality after physical therapy treatment for stress urinary incontinence. Rev Bras Ginecol Obstet 29: 134-140.
23. Caromano F, Sayuri E, Cruz CMV, Candeloro JM, Buriti JS, et al. (2006) Thoracic mobility and maximum breathing pressures during the pregnancy. Fisioter Bras 7: 5-7.
24. Ciccone MM, Aquilino A, Cortese F, Scicchitano P, Sassara M, et al. (2010) Feasibility and effectiveness of a disease and care management model in the primary helth care system for patients with heart failure and diabetes. Vasc Health Risk Management 6: 297-305.

Major Correlates of Anemia among Women (Age 15-49) in India and Spatial Variation, Evidence from National Family Health Survey-4

Himani Sharma*, **Singh SK and Shobhit Srivastava**

Department of Mathematical Demography & Statistics, International Institute for Population Sciences, Mumbai, Maharashtra, India

***Corresponding author:** Himani Sharma, Master of Philosophy, International Institute for Population Sciences, Mumbai, Maharashtra, India, E-mail: himani.sharma446@gmail.com

Abstract

Background: In the developing countries like India, Anemia continues to remain a serious nutritional problem. The National Family Health Survey (2015-16) has reported a 53% prevalence of Anemia among women, a sluggish decline from 58% in NFHS-3.

Objective: The study determines the prevalence of anemia among women by several background characteristics. It also tries to examine the socio-economic inequality in anemia among women across Indian states and attempts to analyze the spatial correlation of anemia among women and its co-variates across 640 districts of India.

Methods: The data is taken from the IV round of National Family Health Survey (2015-2016) conducted by the International Institute for Population Sciences, Mumbai. Bivariate analysis and Binary Logistic Regression analysis were used to assess the effects of socio-economic characteristics. Concentration Index and Poor-Rich ratios have been calculated to understand the socio-economic inequality whereas spatial analysis was done to understand the spatial correlation among women and its covariates.

Results: Anemia is highly prevalent among women belonging to rural areas and lowest wealth quantiles. Some behavioral factors of women were found to be positively associated with anemia. The highest inequality is being observed in the north-eastern states like Manipur, Nagaland etc. Moran's I value depicts high auto correlation; the hotspots were found in the Eastern and Western regions of India.

Discussion: Despite slight improvements, hemoglobin concentrations remain low while anemia prevalence remains high in poorest parts of the world. The rich and poor gap seems to be a big matter of concern. Women in India are not only suffering from economic inequalities but also inequalities in terms of food and malnutrition. Wealth is the strongest determinant of anemia among women followed by education and caste.

Keywords: Women; Anemia; Inequalities; Logistic regression; Spatial analysis

Introduction

Nutritional anemia is one of the biggest problems of our country, specifically called as the third pillar of malnutrition. The National Nutritional Anemia Control Programme (NNACP), a centrally sponsored scheme, was launched in India in 1970 with an aim of reducing the prevalence and incidence of anemia in women in reproductive age group, but failed to make any significant impact. In the developing countries like India, anemia continues to remain a serious nutritional problem. The National Family Health Survey (NFHS 2015-16) has reported a 53% prevalence of anemia among women, a sluggish decline from 58% in NFHS-3. When over half of the women in the country suffer due to nutritional anemia, the idea of 'Health for All' seems to be an illusion. Several programmes have been running out in order to provide equal nourishment to each and every individual in the society. Improving the maternal and child health and their survival are central to the achievement of national health goals under the National Rural Health Mission (NRHM) as well as the Millennium Development Goals (MDG) 4 and 5 [1].

Anemia is a result of reduced hemoglobin level in the body. Various intermixed factors cause Anemia but poor intake of nutrients and fibrous food in diet seem to be the ultimate reason behind it. Anemia is known to have disastrous implications on the health of particular groups like children, adolescent girls and women of reproductive age group. Numerous women are living with this problem without even realizing its serious repercussions upon the overall development of wellbeing and its fatal outcomes in future. Anemia can have detrimental effects upon women, i.e. difficult for women to earn income, carry out daily tasks, and care for their families. Conservative estimates suggest anemia is the direct cause of 3% to 7% of maternal deaths worldwide. Other estimates suggest that it is the direct or indirect cause of 20% to 40% of maternal deaths [2]. The steps taken to eradicate malnutrition and anemia have not been accomplishing enough to overcome the pertaining situation.

Review of Literature

The prevalence of anemia as a public health problem is categorized as follows: <5%, no public health problem; 5%-19.9%, mild public health problem; 20%-39.9%, moderate public health problem; 40%, severe public health problem [3].

Literature on effects of anemia on women's health

Females had higher prevalence of anemia than males in virtually all regions, especially Central Asia (43.2% *vs.* 22.8%) and Asia Pacific, high income (19.4% *vs.* 10%) as stated through a study [4]. Deficient iron status or anemia among adolescent girls is a major cause of growth retardation, impaired physical and mental development, delayed menarche, morbidity and future poor reproductive outcomes [5]. The high rates of anemia among Indian women reflect their social and biological vulnerability both within society and the household [6]. A study by [4] revealed that much of the excess anemia in females at other ages was related to iron deficiency including gynecologic conditions that often present as iron deficiency.

Literature on anemia arising from socio-economic inequality

The fact that women are provided an unequal nutrition in the family has been well discussed in many studies. The existing literatures suggest that there is definitely a socio-economic inequality prevalent which proves to be an obstacle for women to obtain a healthy lifestyle. Symptoms of anemia are consistently attributed to a poor quality diet and lack of food due to poverty. Women in India specifically, mention dietary restrictions and 'eating last' or 'eating whatever is leftover' as reasons of inadequate diet [7].

There is evidence that when poorer households gain more money to spend on food, they prefer to buy more expensive, yet not necessarily more nutritious food, such as sugar, salt and processed food [8]. A study conducted in Mumbai by suggests that the problem of under nutrition generally started much earlier in life, with gender discrimination resulting in under nutrition of girls (16-18), which was exacerbated by menstrual iron losses after menarche [9].

NFHS-4 being such a large scale survey provides estimates for several key indicators of health and nutrition. This study tries to undertake the problem of anemia by understanding it through several dimensions, especially focusing upon the socio-economic inequality in the nutritional status of women. Moreover, spatial analysis is important to understand the geographical clustering of anemia among women in India and to understand its spatial variation.

The study determines the prevalence of anemia among women with respect to several background characteristics. It also tries to examine the socio-economic inequality in anemia among women across Indian states and attempts to analyze the spatial correlation of anemia among women and its co-variants across 640 districts of India.

Data and Methodology

The data used in the study has been taken from the IV round of NFHS (2015-2016) conducted by the International Institute for Population Sciences, Mumbai. It provides nationally representative survey data on women's hemoglobin level and other nutritional aspects. The hemoglobin testing was conducted among women age 15-49 using a portable battery operated device called HemoCue Hb 201+ analyzer after the consent was taken.

The analysis is limited to non-pregnant woman age 15-49. Pregnant women have been excluded due to biological reason of them being anemic and hence the sample can get influenced which ultimately affects the results up to a certain extent. The final sample size for women after restricting it only to non-pregnant women was 667,258 cases.

The dependent variable taken for the study is 'anemia among women' which is dichotomous having 0 as "No anemia" and 1 as "yes anemia". For the bivariate analysis, three main levels of anemia were considered, i.e., mild, moderate and severe. Among background characteristics, age of the women, residence, religion, caste, wealth quantile, regions were taken.

Characteristics of women included education of women, Women's nutritional status, parity of women, place of delivery, sanitation facility, tobacco and alcohol consumption food intake categorized as vegetarian food and non-vegetarian food indicating the dietary habits.

Bivariate analysis was used to know the prevalence of anemia among women age 15-49 by some selected background characteristics and Binary Logistic regression analysis was used to assess the effects of socio-economic characteristics. It consists of two models; Model 1 in which only background characteristics were controlled and Model 2, in which background characteristics were controlled along with some peculiar characteristics of women.

Concentration Index and Poor-Rich ratios have been used to understand how socio-economic inequality persists in terms of nutrition of women in society and examine the magnitude of socio-economic inequality in any health outcome. Concentration Index (CI) is employed to study the extent of inequity in anemia across all 37 states of India [10]. The value of concentration index ranges from-1 to +1. When the outcome value is 0, it implies no socio-economic inequality. It is defined as, CI=2 covW (Yi, Ri).

Where Yi is the health status if the 'i'th individual and Ri is the fractional rank of the 'i'th individual (for weighted data) in terms of the value of the household economic status; μ is the (weighted) unconditional mean of the health variable of the sample and 'covW' denoted the weighted covariance.

As the wealth quantile is arranged from the lowest to highest quantile, a negative value indicates the concentration of relevant health variable, e.g. anemia in the lowest wealth quantiles and vice versa for the positive value of +1. The poor-rich ratio, defined as the ratio of the poorest to the richest wealth quintile is used to measure the gap in malnutrition among women in India. The poor-rich ratios are also being calculated for the states of India.

Lastly, the paper intends to analyze the spatial correlation between anemia among women and 640 districts of India. Univariate and bivariate Moran's I statistic was computed with the help of GeoDa, a spatial analysis software. Moran's I is the measure of spatial autocorrelation. It is a generalization of Pearson's correlation coefficient [11].

Spatial autocorrelation indicates the degree to which values are similar or dissimilar to their respective spatial neighbors. Spatial ordinary least square (OLS), the spatial lag model (SLM) and the spatial error model (SEM) have been computed to see the spatial correlation between independent and dependent variables.

Results

Table 1a show that mild anemia was significantly high among women of age 15-24 along with moderate anemia in the same age group. The prevalence of mild, moderate and severe anemia is higher in the rural areas than the urban counterparts. Among castes, scheduled tribes present the highest prevalence of mild, moderate and severe anemia followed by scheduled castes (SCs) and other backward class (OBC).

The people belonging to the lowest wealth quantile (poorest) have the highest prevalence of mild, moderate and severe anemia followed by poorer and middle income groups. The highest prevalence of severe and moderate anemia is found among north, central and southern regions of India whereas mild anemia is more found among eastern, central, northern and southern regions respectively (Tables 1a).

Background characteristics	**Severe**	**Moderate**	**Mild**
Age of women			
15-19	1	11.49	41.65
20-24	0.92	11.85	41.13
25-29	0.83	11.6	40.64
30-34	0.98	11.6	39.49
35 and above	1.2	12.2	39.57
Type of residence			
Urban	0.93	11.19	38.89
Rural	1.08	12.18	41.1
Religion			
Hindu	1.07	12.14	40.58
Muslim	0.88	10.35	39.46
Christian	0.87	11.89	35.24
Others	0.71	10.61	41.83
Caste			
Scheduled caste	1.16	13.24	41.59
Scheduled tribe	1.29	14.1	44.58
Obc	1.08	11.62	39.65
Others	0.76	10.29	39.04
Wealth Quantile			
Poorest	1.17	13.23	44.31
Poorer	1.14	12.33	41.73
Middle	1.14	12.52	39.71
Richer	1.02	11.54	38.64
Richest	0.7	9.82	38.03
Regions			
North	1.06	12.21	38.69
Central	1.02	11.26	39.68
East	0.73	12.21	47.39
North East	0.67	8.17	36.33

West	0.97	10.71	38.45
South	1.4	13.15	37.02
Women characteristics			
Education			
No education	1.59	14.44	42.82
Primary	0.96	11.6	40.64
Secondary	0.62	9.54	36.85
Higher	0.49	9.9	36.77
Women's nutritional status			
Below 18.5 (U-weight)	1.59	14.44	42.82
18.5-24.99(normal)	0.96	11.6	40.64
25- 30+(overweight)	0.59	9.63	36.83
Parity			
1	0.79	11.01	40.63
2 to 3	1.03	12.33	40.26
4 and above	1.1	11.64	40.33
Tobacco consumption			
No	0.99	11.71	40.3
Yes	1.63	13.79	41.02
Alcohol consumption			
Never/occasionally	1.14	12.41	40.06
Daily	0.87	13.81	40.92
Place of delivery			
Home delivery	1.44	14.65	44.69
Institutional delivery	0.79	12.08	42.5
Sanitation facility			
Improved	0.89	11.03	39.19
Unimproved	1.03	12.05	40.08
Open defecation	1.24	13.04	42.16
Food Intake (vegetarian food)			
Daily/occasionally	1.05	12.02	40.46
Never	0.77	9.91	39.19
Food Intake (Non-vegetarian food)			
Never/occasionally	1	11.72	40.17
Daily	1.26	12.96	42.01

Table 1a: Percentage of Women age (15-49) with different levels of Anemia by some selected background Characteristics.

Among the religions, Muslims have 8% while Christians have 33% significantly less likely to get anemia when compared to Hindus. Scheduled tribes (STs) are 22% significantly more likely to have anemia when compared to the SCs. Poorer people are 7% significantly less likely to be anemic; and the prevalence of anemia goes down as the wealth quantile increases.

When compared to north region, central region had 4%; north-eastern region had 41% less likelihood of anemia prevalence. Women with primary education are 5% significantly less likely to be anemic than uneducated ones.

In model 2, background variables are controlled along with some selected characteristics of women. When compared with the underweight, the women with a normal body mass index had 19% lower likelihood of being anemic whereas women who were overweight had 35% lower likelihood of having anemia. The chances of women being anemic grew with the increasing parity, i.e. women with 2 to 3 parities had 1% and 4 and above parities had 11% more likelihood of being anemic. However, both alcohol and tobacco consumption were negatively associated with anemia. Women gone for institutional delivery were 4% less likely to be anemic; women using an unimproved sanitation facility had 12% more likelihood to be anemic. When it comes to food and dietary practices, it was found that women who never consumed vegetarian food had 1% less likely to be anemic whereas women who consumed non-veg food daily had 7% lower likelihood to be anemic (Table 1b).

Women with no or little education have a high prevalence of all levels of anemia in which mild anemia leads the chart. Mild and moderate anemia is more prevalent among women who are underweight or normal whereas it is less prevalent among the overweight women. The highest prevalence of mild, moderate and severe anemia is found among women having one or two parities; which eventually decrease as the parity of women increases.

Among the women who consume alcohol and tobacco, all three levels of anemia have highest prevalence. Highest prevalence of anemia is observed among women who hadn't gone for institutional deliveries as well as in those who do not have an improved source of sanitation. Highest prevalence of anemia is seen among women who consume vegetarian food and non-vegetarian food daily/occasionally.

Multiple logistic regressions have been used in the study consisting of two models-Model 1 controlling only background characteristics and Model 2 controlling both background and peculiar characteristics of women. After controlling for various background variables in model 1, it is evident that age of women, place of residence, religion, caste, wealth quantile, regions and education of women significantly affects the likelihood of suffering from anemia in India. It is clear from the table those women age groups 20-24 have 4% higher likelihood of getting anemic. Rural areas had 2% more likelihood of anemia prevalence than the urban counterparts (Table 1b).

Background characteristics	**Any anemia (%)**	**Model 1**	**Model 2**
Age of women			
15-19®	54.13	1	1
20-24	53.9	1.04*(1.02,1.06)	0.86*(0.81,0.92)
25-29	53.07	0.99(0.98,1.01)	0.79*(0.75,0.85)
30-34	52.06	0.92*(0.9,0.93)	0.77*(0.72,0.83)
35 and above	52.97	0.92*(0.91,0.94)	0.8*(0.75,0.86)
Type of residence			
Urban®	51.02	1	1
Rural	54.36	1.02*(1,1.03)	1(0.97,1.03)
Religion			
Hindu®	53.79	1	1
Muslim	50.68	0.92*(0.91,0.94)	0.93*(0.9,0.96)
Christian	48.01	0.67*(0.66,0.69)	0.67*(0.64,0.7)
Others	53.15	0.99(0.97,1.02)	0.98(0.93,1.03)
Caste			
Scheduled caste®	56	1	1
Scheduled tribe	59.97	1.22*(1.19,1.24)	1.23*(1.19,1.28)
OBC	52.35	0.91*(0.9,0.93)	0.93*(0.9,0.95)
Others	50.09	0.86*(0.85,0.87)	0.87*(0.84,0.9)

Wealth Quantile			
Poorest®	58.72	1	1
Poorer	55.2	0.93*(0.91,0.94)	0.97*(0.94,1)
Middle	53.37	0.89*(0.88,0.91)	0.95*(0.92,0.98)
Richer	51.2	0.87*(0.85,0.89)	0.91*(0.87,0.95)
Richest	48.55	0.85*(0.83,0.87)	0.9*(0.86,0.95)
Regions			
North®	51.96	1	1
Central	51.96	0.96*(0.95,0.98)	0.97*(0.94,1)
East	60.33	1.3*(1.27,1.32)	1.24*(1.2,1.29)
North East	45.16	0.59*(0.57,0.6)	0.59*(0.56,0.61)
West	50.14	0.95*(0.93,0.97)	0.92*(0.88,0.96)
South	51.57	0.99(0.97,1)	0.92*(0.88,0.96)
Women characteristics			
Education			
No education®	56.35	1	1
Primary	54.64	0.95*(0.94,0.97)	0.94*(0.91,0.97)
Secondary	52.34	0.9*(0.89,0.91)	0.91*(0.88,0.93)
Higher	48.09	0.8*(0.78,0.82)	0.85*(0.81,0.89)
Women's nutritional status			
Below 18.5 (U-weight)®	58.85		1
18.5-24.99(normal)	53.2		0.81*(0.79,0.83)
25- 30+(overweight)	47.04		0.65*(0.63,0.67)
Parity			
1®	52.43		1
2 to 3	53.62		1.1*(1.07,1.13)
4 and above	53.07		1.11*(1.07,1.16)
Tobacco consumption			
No®	52.99		1
Yes	56.44		1.03(1,1.07)
Alcohol consumption			
Never/occasionally®	53.61		1
Daily	55.6		0.92(0.76,1.1)
Place of delivery			
Home delivery®	60.78		1
Institutional delivery	55.37		0.96*(0.93,0.99)

Sanitation facility			
Improved®	51.12		1
Unimproved	53.15		1.12*(1.08,1.16)
Open defecation	56.43		0.98(0.95,1.01)
Food Intake (vegetarian food)			
Daily/occasionally®	52.89		1
Never	56.23		0.99(0.96,1.02)
Non-vegetarian food consumption			
Never/occasionally®	53.53		1
Daily	49.87		0.93*(0.9,0.97)
®Reference category; P<0.05*			

Table 1b: Odds ratio of Anemia among women in India by some selected background and Women Characteristics.

Table 2 represents the values of CI regarding anemia among women in India as well as separately for urban and rural areas. The results are depicting a negative value which means there is an unequal distribution of anemia among women in the population. In India, the six major states showing highest negative values for women anemia are Mizoram, Nagaland, Rajasthan, Odisha, Chhattisgarh and Goa respectively. It shows that anemia among women is more concentrated and more robust in the poor population in these states. It is also evident that women anemia is also seen among the urban poor in the states like Nagaland, Mizoram, Rajasthan, Odisha and Chhattisgarh. Whereas, anemia in women is more prevalent among the rural poor in states like Goa, Mizoram, Nagaland, Rajasthan, Odisha and Chhattisgarh.

The poor-rich ratio, defined as the ratio of the poorest to the richest wealth quintile has been calculated for women having anemia. Among women, the highest poor-rich ratios are found in the states like Goa (350), Rajasthan (148 poor/100 rich), Nagaland (198/100 rich), Mizoram (184/100 rich), Meghalaya (159/100 rich), Chhattisgarh (149/100 rich), and Kerala (137/100 rich). Goa has the highest ratio for the urban area also with 357 poor per 100 rich having anemia. For the urban areas, Nagaland and Himachal Pradesh are showing highest poor-rich ratios (Table 2).

State	Total			Rural			Urban		
	C.I.	S.E.	P/R	C.I.	S.E.	P/R	C.I.	S.E.	P/R
Andhra Pradesh	-0.032***	0.005	1.26	-0.027***	0.006	1.21	-0.017*	0.009	1.30
Arunachal Pradesh	-0.036***	0.006	1.02	-0.039***	0.006	1.03	0.006	0.013	1.20
Assam	-0.028***	0.004	1.11	-0.031***	0.004	1.10	0.004	0.011	1.00
Bihar	-0.016***	0.002	1.10	-0.014***	0.002	1.14	-0.021***	0.006	1.14
Chhattisgarh	-0.064***	0.004	1.49	-0.059***	0.005	1.52	-0.060***	0.008	1.45
Goa	-0.067***	0.021	3.50	-0.119***	0.029	3.57	-0.038	0.030	0.00
Gujarat	-0.038***	0.004	1.23	-0.022***	0.004	1.25	-0.028***	0.006	1.19
Haryana	-0.024***	0.003	1.06	-0.019***	0.004	1.04	-0.024***	0.005	1.03
Himachal Pradesh	0.004	0.006	0.98	0.001	0.006	0.97	0.041**	0.021	1.86
Jammu and Kashmir	-0.020***	0.004	1.07	-0.022***	0.004	1.08	-0.045***	0.009	1.36
Jharkhand	-0.039***	0.003	1.25	-0.020***	0.003	1.10	-0.045***	0.006	1.29
Karnataka	-0.039***	0.004	1.23	-0.032***	0.005	1.25	-0.033***	0.007	1.20
Kerala	-0.002	0.008	1.37	-0.013	0.010	1.50	-0.006	0.012	0.91

Madhya Pradesh	-0.042***	0.002	1.24	-0.035***	0.003	1.22	-0.044***	0.004	1.25
Maharashtra	-0.021***	0.004	1.14	-0.026***	0.005	1.13	-0.033***	0.006	1.08
Manipur	-0.023***	0.009	1.25	-0.017*	0.011	1.28	-0.037***	0.014	1.17
Meghalaya	-0.060***	0.005	1.59	-0.032***	0.006	1.27	-0.042***	0.015	1.60
Mizoram	-0.134***	0.009	1.84	-0.112***	0.012	1.73	0.087***	0.014	1.03
Nagaland	-0.110***	0.009	1.98	-0.097***	0.011	1.99	0.124***	0.017	1.89
Delhi	-0.018**	0.007	0.66	0.01	0.037	0.00	-0.019**	0.008	0.67
Odisha	-0.070***	0.003	1.32	-0.069***	0.003	1.44	-0.069***	0.008	1.31
Punjab	-0.033***	0.003	0.95	-0.029***	0.005	1.09	-0.034***	0.007	0.75
Rajasthan	-0.082***	0.003	1.48	-0.073***	0.003	1.44	-0.059***	0.007	1.15
Sikkim	-0.022**	0.011	1.24	-0.036***	0.013	1.21	0.028	0.022	1.41
Tamil Nadu	-0.030***	0.003	1.14	-0.023***	0.004	1.11	-0.029***	0.005	1.18
Tripura	0.014*	0.007	0.89	0.014	0.009	1.02	0.018	0.014	0.89
Uttar Pradesh	0.002	0.001	1.04	0.006***	0.002	0.98	-0.023***	0.003	1.12
Uttarakhand	-0.026***	0.005	0.99	-0.010*	0.006	0.97	-0.043***	0.009	1.38
West Bengal	-0.042***	0.003	1.27	-0.034***	0.004	1.20	-0.030***	0.007	1.23
Telangana	-0.025***	0.006	1.23	-0.025***	0.007	1.12	-0.018*	0.011	1.44
P<0.10 *P<0.05**P<0.01***									

Table 2: Poor-Rich ratio and Concentration Index depicting socio-economic inequality in Anemia among women across Indian states.

Bivariate LISA (Local Indicators of Spatial Association) maps for women

Figure 1 presents a bivariate LISA map which depicts the spatial association between women anemia and selected independent variables. LISA maps help us to understand the spatial correlation at a very local level.

In Map A, younger woman (age 15-19) have a spatial correlation with anemia in 57 districts of eastern, some districts of Orissa, parts of Rajasthan, Gujarat and some districts of north Indian region.

In Map B, the clustering is even high having 83 districts who have a spatial correlated between anemia and Hindu women concentrated in the regions of south-eastern India, eastern India, parts of Madhya Pradesh, Gujarat and Rajasthan and in some parts of upper north India.

In map C, it is evident that 39 districts of eastern, south-eastern and western regions are spatially correlated in terms of women belong to STs Population and their anemic status.

Map D shows a correlation among states having women in the poorest quantile and anemia in the regions of south-eastern, eastern and western part of India.

Map E shows a significant relation between the highest percentage of uneducated women and anemia in 70 districts of eastern, south-eastern, parts of western India and in Jammu and Kashmir region.

Map F shows that women who are underweight are significantly correlated with anemia in 69 districts of western, eastern and south-eastern regions.

About 60 districts of south-eastern India, Eastern India and some parts of north and western India are statistically correlated with high prevalence of home deliveries and women anemia as depicted in Map G.

In Map H, 64 districts of south-eastern, eastern and western part of India are showing spatial association between women going for open defecation and anemia.

In Map I, clustering can be seen among eastern south-eastern, western and northern part is high for women anemia and respondents who never consume non-veg food.

In Map J, clustering can be seen among 24 districts of south-eastern region where there is a high correlation of women consuming any form of tobacco and anemia.

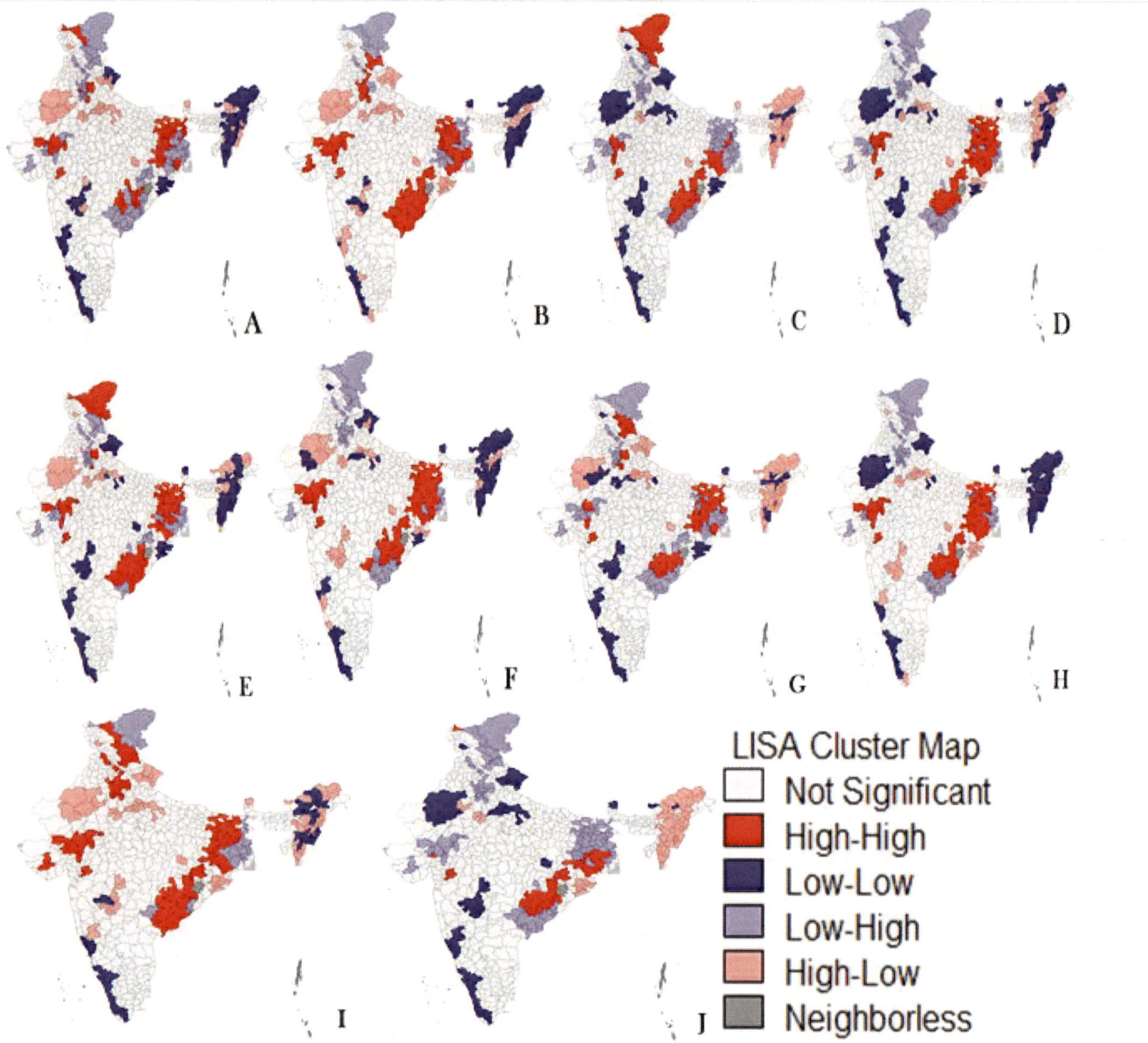

Figure 1: Depicting bivariate LISA maps showing spatial correlation between anemia among women and its co-variates. Note: A: Anemia among women and women aged 15-19 proportion; B: Anemia among women and Hindu women; C: Anemia among women and ST proportion; D: Anemia among women and poorest quantile, E: Anemia among women and no education; F: Anemia among women and under-weight women; G: Anemia among women and home delivery; H: Anemia among women and open defecation; I: Anemia among women and no non-veg. consumption; J: Anemia among women and tobacco consumption [**Note:** The map of India has been altered in the state of Jammu and Kashmir due to unavailability of the data in certain region].

An effort has been made to investigate the regional determinants and influential factors which affect the level of anemia among women in India. After establishing the significant bivariate spatial association between the dependent and independent variables, an OLS model was fitted (Table 3a). After this, SLM and SEM were fitted as per the convenience.

Tables 3a and 3b shows similar patterns observed with reference to regional determinants and drivers of women anemia in India. To carry out spatial analysis, firstly an OLS model was fitted.

Variables	MORAN'S I	P-value	Bi- MORAN'S I	P-value
% Women Anaemia	0.589	0.001	-	-
% Age of women (15-19)	0.699	0.001	0.084	0.001
% Residence (urban)	0.413	0.001	-	-
% Hindu Women	0.753	0.001	0.246	0.001
% Caste (ST)	0.697	0.001	0.164	0.001
% Wealth quantile (poorest)	0.746	0.001	0.218	0.001
% No education	0.714	0.001	0.283	0.001
% Underweight (mother)	0.697	0.001	0.277	0.001
% Place of delivery (Home)	0.66	0.001	0.082	0.001
% Open defecation	0.791	0.001	0.268	0.001
% Tobacco consumption	0.808	0.001	0.293	0.001
% Non-veg Food intake (Never or Occasionally)	0.667	0.001	0.177	0.001

Table 3a: Moran's I statistics showing spatial dependence of Anemia among women and different independent.

Afterwards, spatial lag and error models were computed to know the best fit model for the analysis (Table 3b).

Variables	OLS Model		Spatial Lag Model		Spatial Error Model	
Indicators	Coefficients	Sig. value	Coefficients	Sig. value	Coefficients	Sig. value
% 15-19 aged women	-0.402	0.01	-0.242	0.065	-0.226	0.151
% Hindu women	0.024	0.336	0.014	0.515	0.047	0.106
% St population	0.028	0.228	0.023	0.23	0.046	0.063
% Poorest quantile	0.216	0.001	0.107	0.007	0.007	0.896
% Uneducated women	0.226	0.001	0.143	0.001	0.164	0.008
% Underweight mothers	0.264	0.001	0.177	0.009	0.307	0.001
% Home delivery	-0.189	0.001	-0.123	0.001	-0.081	0.051
% Open defecation	-0.12		-0.066	0.021	-0.073	0.07
% Non-veg consumption daily	0.117	0.002	0.032	0.298	0.124	0.005
% Tobacco consumption	-0.24	0.001	-0.06	0.12	-0.006	0.923
% Alcohol consumption	-0.256	0.421	-0.163	0.541	-0.084	0.723
AIC	4847.05		4676.25		4566.5	
LAMBDA					0.757***	
RHO			0.537			
R-SQUARE	0.275		0.459		0.489	
ADJUSTED R-SQUARE	0.262					

Table 3b: OLS, Spatial Lag & Spatial error model to assess the association between prevalence of Anemia among women and some selected socio-economic factors in India, NFHS- (2015-16).

It was found Akaike Information Criterion (AIC) value was least for the spatial error model which is considered appropriate for the spatial analysis. For the women anemia, the value of lambda is 0.757 which shows the spatial autocorrelation among regions in India.

The spatial error model depicted that women anemia has a higher prevalence among the regions where there is a higher percentage of women who belong to Hindu religion, higher percentage of uneducated women, and higher percentage of women who are underweight, higher percentage of women who never consumed non-veg food.

Discussion

The results suggest that anemia is highly persistent among women of reproductive age group where more than half of the women are suffering from one or the other level of anemia. Eastern regions of India had the highest prevalence of both mild and moderate level of anemia among women. Anemia is highly prevalent among women belonging to rural areas which depict the amount of priority given to health of women in a rural setup. The higher prevalence of anemia in rural areas is likely related to lack of information about adequate nutrition during pregnancy, economic factors and inaccessibility of health care centers [12]. This study focusses on anemia among women with low background status; anemia was significantly associated with diseases like malaria and other plasmodium infections; it is difficult to say that anemia preceded the determining factors or vice-versa. The findings of our study show that women are more prone to be anemic when they are poor which means there is a disparity in the society regarding the type and quality of nutrition given to a woman.

It is also clear that the highest burden of anemia is shared by the poorest people which increase their risk of getting affected to different types of diseases as well. Christians were significantly less likely to have any anemia, in comparison to Hindu's [8]. Though the study is based on repeated cross-sectional surveys, it is unable to differentiate between different types of anemia that may explain the changing pattern of inequalities. Anemia among women seemed to be increasing with number of parities while it started to decline with parity 4 and above. Behavioural factors associated with women anemia e.g. tobacco and alcohol consumption, open defecation was found to be positively associated with anemia. The negative values of CI reflect that inter-state inequality is prevalent in anemia among women in India. It clearly depicts that a disproportionate burden of anemia is being shared by the poor. Many studies reveal that there is a socio-economic inequality in anemia among poor households in India [10]. A study in Ghana reveals that stunting, underweight in under-five children, anemia in women and underweight in women [Body mass index (BMI) <18.5] show inequities that are to the disadvantage of the poorest [13]. Not only the disease risk is more in the poorest society, the benefits of the health care policies are enjoyed by the richest of society more than the poorest the current study reveals that the highest inequality is being observed in the north-eastern states like Manipur, Nagaland etc. Many studies have been done to analyze the prevalent inequality in terms of malnutrition and anemia in north east [14]. The above study clears the fact that the biggest reason of malnutrition among children in north-east is the malnourishment of their mothers. The characteristics of mothers are highly significant in determining the status of malnutrition among children in north-east. Thus, an improvement in only economic sphere will not help until an idea regarding inclusive growth is implemented in north-east. The poor-rich ratios presented in the present study also reveal the gap between rich and poor across north-eastern states; it also suggests the need of proper monitoring and coordination at household and community levels in order to improve the situation of malnutrition in north east. The poor-rich ratios depict the distribution pattern of anemia among poorest and richest category.

Our findings suggest that women belonging to the poorest socio-economic status have higher prevalence of worse anemic status. On contrary, the women belonging from the highest and most well-off households are associated with better nutritional status and were less vulnerable to get anemia. This proves the fact that socio-economic status becomes an important determinant of how anemia and malnutrition is distributed across the states. This socio-economic inequality widens the gap between rich and poor and acts as an important factor of improving or degrading the development of an individual in the society. Spatial analysis reveals a positive autocorrelation between anemia among women and its co-variates among the districts of India. Moran's I value is depicting high auto correlation which means that anemia among women has a spatial clustering across districts of India. The hotspots found in case of anemia among women with its co-variates were in the eastern regions and western regions of India particularly in the states like Andhra Pradesh, Bihar, West Bengal, Odisha, Chhattisgarh and some districts of Rajasthan, Gujarat and Madhya Pradesh.

Conclusion

The results of the study show that women with childbearing experiences are more anemic. A study by [9] also reveals that women without children had higher hemoglobin values than women with living children supports the view that childbirth, lactation, and childbearing tax a woman's nutritional condition; but as it only studied the women from poor backgrounds in Mumbai who probably had inadequate diets, we cannot generalize the results for all concerned women. The argument is furthermore made more valid through another study by [15] which presents that women of childbearing age are at high risk for negative iron balance because of blood loss during menstruation and the substantial iron demands of pregnancy. It suggests that additional research will be important for improving understanding of the distribution of nutritional deficiencies in populations and their risk relations. The standard of living and socio-economic status proved to be the two most important factors in determining anemia among women while the behavioral factors affecting the levels of anemia among women in the third place. It is clear from the spatial analysis that regional heterogeneity has been found in the levels of anemia among women. Bivariate LISA maps help us to understand the clustering of variables included in the study and to identify the districts/regions which need more attention. Despite it, the study cannot explain completely for the outliers existing at the end of the study. The findings of the study suggest more investment towards improving the conditions of women in the regions where anemia among women is high. It also suggests that the childbearing process should be made easier for women. It is a known fact that the nutritional status of women can have serious repercussions for child development and women's health; hence, it is important to develop control and prevention strategies that attend the inequality in terms of socio-economic status in the society. Moreover, all the other essential socioeconomic and demographic factors affecting the nutrition of women should be addressed carefully. Therefore, there is a call for reducing regional disparities and improving the socio-economic status of the poor women. Efforts should also be made to providing equal opportunities of health and nutrition to all, improving women education and reducing higher order births, making childbearing easier and safe for women in order to eradicate the problem of anemia once and for all.

References

1. Ministry of Health and Family Welfare G of I (2013) A strategic approach to reproductive, maternal, newborn, child and adolescent health 1-83.
2. WHO guidance for measuring maternal mortality from a census (2013). World Health Organization 2013.
3. McLean E, Egli I, Cogswell M, Benoist BD, Wojdyla D (2007) Worldwide prevalence of anemia in preschool aged children, pregnant women and non-pregnant women of reproductive age. In Nutritional anemia 12: 444.
4. Kassebaum NJ, Jasrasaria R, Naghavi M, Wulf SK, Johns N, et al. (2014) Plenary Paper red cells, iron, and erythropoiesis. A systematic analysis of global anemia burden from 1990 to 2010. Blood J 123: 615-624.
5. Bharati P, Shome S, Chakrabarty S, Bharati S, Pal M (2009) Burden of anemia and its socioeconomic determinants among adolescent girls in India. Food Nutr Bull 30: 217-226.
6. Bentley ME, Griffiths PL (2003) The burden of anemia among women in India. Eur J Clin Nutr 57: 52-60.
7. Galloway R, Dusch E, Elder L, Achadi E, Grajeda R, et al. (2002) Women's perceptions of iron deficiency and anemia prevention and control in eight developing countries. Soc Sci Med 55: 529-544.
8. Balarajan YS, Fawzi WW, Subramanian SV (2013) Changing patterns of social inequalities in anemia among women in india: Cross-sectional study using nationally representative data. BMJ Open 3: e002233.
9. Brabin L, Nicholas S, Gogate A, Gogate S, Karande A (1998) High prevalence of anemia among women in Mumbai, India. Food Nutr Bull 19: 205-209.
10. Kanjilal B (2017) Nutritional status of children in India⊠: Household socio-economic condition as the contextual determinant. Int J Equity Health 9: 1-20.
11. Chen Y (2013) New approaches for calculating Moran's Index of spatial autocorrelation. PLoS One 8: e68336.
12. Kefiyalew F, Zemene E, Asres Y, Gedefaw L (2015) Anemia among pregnant women in Southeast Ethiopia⊠: Prevalence, severity and associated risk factors Methods Results. BMC research notes 7: 771.
13. Zere E, Kirigia JM, Duale S, Akazili J (2012) Inequities in maternal and child health outcomes and interventions in Ghana. BMC Public Health 12: 252.
14. Ao M (2014) Re-Estimating Malnourishment and Inequality among children in North-east India. Econ Polit Wkly 49: 53-63.
15. Black RE, Allen LH, Bhutta ZA, Caulfi LE, Onis M De, et al. (2008) Maternal and child under nutrition study group. Maternal and child under nutrition⊠: Global and regional 371: 243-260.

Placental Malaria in Newly Delivered Women in the Maternity Hospital of Chud Borgou in 2015

Salifou K[1], Obossou AAA[1*], Noudamadjo A[1], Houkponou F[1], Sidi R[1], Vodounhe M[1], Perrin XR[2] and Alihonou E[2]
[1]Department of Mother and Child, Faculty of Medicine, University of Parakou, Bénin

[2]*Department of Mother and Child, Faculty of Health Sciences of Cotonou, University of Abomey-Calavi, Bénin*

[*]**Corresponding author:** Obossou AAA, Department of Mother and Child, Faculty of Medicine, University of Parakou, Bénin,
E-mail: awadefr2000@yahoo.fr

Abstract

Introduction: Malaria remains a major public health issue in sub-Saharan Africa with high mortality in pregnant women and newborn infants. In the latter, malaria is the consequence of placental transmission of plasmodium. This study aims at identifying the factors associated with placental malaria in CHUD/B in 2015.

Patients and Method: It was a prospective, descriptive and cross-sectional study with an analytical purpose in the CHUD/Borgou Gynecology and Obstetrics department in Parakou. The study population consisted of pregnant women admitted in the Gynecology and Obstetrics department. It was an exhaustive census of all pregnant women admitted in the CHUD/B Gynecology and Obstetrics department.

Results: Placental malaria was diagnosed in 57 pregnant women that is to say a prevalence of 20.28%. The average age of the mothers was 26 ± 6.02 years with extremes of 16 and 51 years. They were housewives in 27% of cases and 33.1% among them were not educated. The factors associated with the occurrence of the infection were the non-use of LLIN (Long Lasting Insecticidal Nets) and fever in the 3rd quarter of pregnancy with respectively p-value of 0.0490 and 0.0388.

Conclusion: Placental malaria, an intermediate step in neonatal infection is common in Parakou and LLIN remains the most effective means of prevention in our context.

Keywords: Placental malaria; Pregnant women; Parakou; Long lasting insecticidal nets

Introduction

Every year, malaria causes about 2,500 deaths of pregnant women and affects around 200,000 to 300,000 newborn infants who suffer from consequences such as death in utero, hypotrophy or congenital malaria [1].

According to the WHO estimates in 2013, fifteen million pregnant women did not receive any dose of preventive intermittent treatment which constitutes one of the vital links of the prevention of this disease during pregnancy [2].

Congenital malaria defined by the presence of asexual forms of the parasite in the newborn infant's peripheral blood in the first seven days of life is secondary to transplacental transmission of plasmodium [3]. Hence, congenital malaria being common in Parakou testifies to the limits of malaria prevention in pregnant women in Benin. Therefore, it was appropriate to start a study on placental malaria whose objective was to identify the factors associated with it.

Method

It was a prospective, descriptive, cross-sectional study with an analytical purpose carried out in the gynecology and obstetrics department of CHUD/Borgou. The study covered the period from April to July 2015. The study population consisted of pregnant women admitted in gynecology and obstetrics department of CHUD/B.

Sampling was exhaustive. All the pregnant women who gave their written informed consent and admitted in the CHUD-Borgou Gynecology and Obstetrics department were involved in the study. All pregnant HIV-infected women were not included in the study. The main variable was placental malaria defined by thick smear and parasite density (TS and PD) or positive Rapid Diagnostic Test (RDT) on the placenta blood.

The independent variables were socio-demographic and clinical variables of the mother. Data collection was carried out with a form drawn up and pre-tested. They were obtained after interviews and at the end of the clinical examination. Data were entered and analyzed with the Epi info version7 software. Qualitative data were expressed as a percentage and quantitative ones as an average with standard deviation. The difference was significant with a p-value less than 5%.

Results

Description of the population

For the 281 newly delivered women surveyed, the average age was 26 ± 6.02 years with extremes of 16 and 51 years. The age group between 20 and 30 years was the most represented. More than 3 newly delivered women out of 4 (76.6%) were under 30 years old. They were housewives in 27% of cases and in 33.1% they were not educated.

Clinical features

During pregnancy, 91.8% had declared that they used the Long-Lasting Insecticidal Net (LLIN) (Table 1).

Incidence of placental malaria

In the study, out of the 281 mothers, 57 were suffering from placental malaria that is to say 20.28%.

Incidence and factors associated with the occurrence of placental malaria

Out of the 281 surveyed during the study period, 57 suffered from placental malaria that is to say 20.28%. The pregnant women's age, the level of education, PNC, the use of SP were the characteristics which were not statistically associated with the occurrence of placental malaria with respectively p-values of 0.6436, 0.3109, 0.7050 and 0.2453.

However, the use of LLIN and fever in the 3rd quarter are (Table 2).

	Number	Percentage (%)
PNC		
0	9	3.2
1-3	87	31
≥ 4	185	65.8
IPT-p/SP		
0	40	14.2
1	72	25.6
≥ 2	169	60.1
Fever in the 3rd quarter		
Yes	67	23.8
No	214	71.3

Table 1: Distribution of the pregnant women according to clinical features in CHUD/B in 2015.

Occurrence Of Placental Malaria	Total	N	Percentage (%)	PR	p
Age					
<20	60	16	26.67	1	0.6436
20-29	140	25	17.86	0.67	
30-39	75	15	20	0.75	
≥ 40	6	1	16.67	0.62	
Level of education					
Not educated	103	25	24.27	1	0 .3109
Primary	75	14	20.59	0.85	
Secondary	82	16	19.51	0.8	
Higher education	21	2	9.52	0.39	
PNC					
No	12	6	50	1	0.705
Yes	269	51	19	0.38	
Use of SP					
No	42	12	28.57	1	0.2453
Yes	239	45	18.83	0.66	

Fever in the 3rd quarter					
No	106	23	21.7	1	0.049
Yes	175	34	19.43	0.89	
Use of LLIN					
No	23	7	30.43	1	0.0388
Yes	258	50	19.38	0.64	

Table 2: Relation between the occurrence of placental malaria in pregnant women and the socio-demographic and clinical features in CHUD/B in 2015.

Discussion

This descriptive, analytical and cross-sectional study was carried out over a short period of the year, which does not permit to have a sufficient population size for a better conclusion. Nevertheless, it was done according to an exhaustive census on a prospective basis to limit selection bias so as to ensure the representativeness of the study sample. It has especially the merit of dealing with a health issue which continues to expand within communities.

In this study, two pregnant women out of ten had placental malaria (20.28%). This incidence is similar to that of a study in Congo in 2006 (21%) [4]. Famanta et al. in Mali in 2011 reported an incidence below ours (1.6%) [5]. This variation in placental malaria can be accounted for the large variation in the climate from a region to another of the African continent and within a region by the distinction of areas of high transmission from those of low transmission. Moreover, the difference in the approaches to malaria prevention in pregnant women is another cause. As a matter of fact if the WHO guidelines regarding malaria prevention in pregnant women are followed in both sides, there are special features in the association of strategies according to countries: preference given to free distribution of mosquito nets rather than sale, 2 courses of chemoprophylaxis with sulfadoxine-pyrimethamine in some countries and more in others. Furthermore, The IEC/BCC aspect more or less neglected can contribute to this large variation of frequencies of placental malaria in Africa. These different considerations can also account for the various factors which determine placental malaria in Parakou. So, the pregnant women's age, the level of education, PNC and the use of SP were not significantly associated with placental malaria in the surveyed.

However, fever in the 3rd quarter was significantly related to the occurrence of the infection. The same is true for the non-use of LLIN. For the latter factor, it should be noted that in 91% of cases, the surveyed had LLINs they were given for nothing during prenatal consultations according to the prevailing national policy to fight malaria in pregnant women in Benin. The positive impact of the use of LLIN by pregnant women was reported in 2011 with a considerable decrease in the proportion of infected parturient women [6]. In addition, a study carried out in Yaoundé in 2016 by Essiben had shown that the non-use of LLIN by pregnant women was a predictive factor of the failure of IPT/SP causing then the occurrence of the infection in the latter [7]. Moreover, it was found that the use of prevention means reduces the risk of the occurrence of the infection by cancelling the parity effect in all the pregnant women [8,9].

In some studies, the improper use of the LLIN could account for the ineffectiveness of this means of prevention [10,11]. The same is true for various strategies to make LLIN accessible: free distribution being made furtively without information base. In Côte d'Ivoire for example, in a study carried out by anthropologists to explain the low use of LLIN, it is mentioned the sizeable gap between the understanding of malaria which underpins the whole policy of mosquito promotion (the linkage mosquito-malaria) and that of populations who seem to give priority to causes such as the sun and fatigue due to work [10]. Furthermore, The LLIN in itself could not be effective if it was not supported by other strategies such as environmental sanitation, chemoprophylaxis and IEC/BCC. In Mali, Dicko found that the combination of IPT and the use of LLIN contribute to malaria prevention in areas of low LLIN coverage for pregnant women and children under 5 years [11]. These outcomes suggest that on the one hand the surveyed in Parakou have a low level of knowledge of PNC and IPT-SP and that promotion for heath is still insufficient in support of our different strategies. Once more there is the issue of the quality of the actions we take. In the current context of neglect of malaria prevention measures by our pregnant women, education for health through IEC/BCC sessions must be the basis of all our strategies. Mentioning negligence both refers to little knowledge of the disease and its etiology, and to a singular perception of the usefulness of the prevention tool and its relation between the disease and its cause [12,13].

Professional Ethics Considerations

This study was conducted after receiving written authorizations from the Director of CHUD-Borgou and the head of the Gynecology and Obstetrics department. We were given the free written informed consent of the pregnant women before their participation. Confidentiality was ensured.

Conclusion

One pregnant woman out of ten had placental malaria during her pregnancy in the CHUD/B Gynecology and Obstetrics department in 2015. It appears that the incidence of placental malaria is lower when LLIN is used. In Benin, the policy of free distribution of LLIN is worth being pursued and its bedrock should be good information on its use.

References

1. World Health Organisation (2008) World malaria report 2008, Geneva.
2. World Health Organization (2014) World Health Statistics.
3. Loke Y (1982) Transmission of parasites across placenta. Adv Parasitol 21: 155-228.

4. Lukuka AK, Fumie OS, Mulumbu MR, Lokombe BJ, Muyembe TJJ (2006) Prevalence of malaria at childbirth in four maternity wards in the city of Kinshasa, Democratic Republic of Congo. Bull Soc Pathol Exot 99: 2-6.

5. Famanta A, Diakité M, Diawara SI, Diakité SA, Doumbia S, et al. (2011) Prevalence of maternal, placental and low birth weight during labor and postpartum in peri-urban areas in Bamako, Mali. Cahiers d'études et de recherches francophones/Health 21: 3-7.

6. Bouyou-Akotet MK, Nzenze-Afène S, Mawili-Mboumba DP, Owono-Medang M, Guiyedi V, et al. (2011) Plasmodial infection and anemia in women parturientes of the Center hospitalier de Libreville between 1995 and 2011. Cahiers d'études et de recherches francophones/Santé 21: 199-203.

7. Essiben F, Foumane P, Tsafack de Nguefack, Eko F, Njotang PN, et al. (2016) Predictors of the failure of intermittent preventive treatment of sulfadoxine-pyrimethamine (TPIp-SP) malaria in pregnant women in Yaoundé. Pan Afr Med J 23: 152.

8. Gies S, Coulibaly SO, Ouattara FT, D'Alessandro U (2009) Individual efficacy of intermittent preventive treatment with sulfadoxine-pyrimethamine in primi- and secundigravidae in rural Burkina Faso: Impact on parasitaemia, anaemia and birth weight. Trop Med Int Health 14: 174-182.

9. Wilson NO, Ceesay FK, Obed SA (2011) Intermittent treatment for the prevention of malaria during pregnancy in Benin: A randomized, open-label equivalence trial comparing sulfadoxine-pyrimethamine with mefloquine. Am J Trop Med Hyg 85: 12-21.

10. Doudou DT, Doannio JMC, Konan LY, Djouaka R, Paré Toé, et al. (2006) Insecticide-treated mosquito nets as a means of fighting malaria: Reasons for a limited adoption in Côte d'Ivoire research report. Natures Sciences Sociétés 4: 431-433.

11. Dicko A, Amadou B, Mohamed D, Abdoulbaki I D, Intimbeye T, et al. (2011) Malaria morbidity in children in the year after they had received intermittent preventive treatment of malaria in Mali: A randomized control trial. PLoS One 6: e23390.

12. Faye SL (2012) Understanding the non-use of long-lasting impregnated bed nets (LLINs) in Niger. Medecine et Sante Tropicales 22: 203-209.

13. Adjétey TAK, Menan EIH, Kassi KF, Yavo W, Barro-kiki PC, et al. (2011) Contribution of mosquito nets impregnated in the prevention of malaria in Ebimpe in Côte d'Ivoire. J Sci Pharm Biol 12: 53-60.

Knowledge, Attitudes, and Practices of Family Planning Among Women of Reproductive Age in Suva, Fiji in 2017

Jay Lincoln[1], **Masoud Mohammadnezhad**[2*] **and Sabiha Khan**[3]

[1]*Master in Public Health, School of Public Health and Primary Care, Fiji National University, Fiji Islands*

[2]*Associate Professor in Public Health, School of Public Health and Primary Care, Fiji National University, Fiji Islands*

[3]*Lecturer in statistics, School of Public Health and Primary Care, Fiji National University, Fiji Islands*

[*]**Corresponding author:** Masoud Mohammadnezhad, Associate Professor in Public health, School of Public Health and Primary Care, Fiji National University, Fiji, Email: masoud.m@hotmail.com

Abstract

Objective: This study aims to identify the level of knowledge, attitudes and practices of family planning among women of reproductive age in Suva, Fiji in 2017.

Methods: A quantitative, cross-sectional study using a self-administered questionnaire among women of reproductive age who attended three designated health clinics around Suva, Fiji from 15th March to 28th April 2017 was used. Using random sampling, those who met the inclusion and exclusion criteria of the study were asked to fill a questionnaire survey. Once the data was collected, it was analyzed with SPSS.

Results: About 325 women participated in the study with the mean age of 31.53(± 7.35). Less than half (148 or 45.5 %) of the participants had a good level of knowledge towards family planning whereas 178 (53.5%) of them had a moderate level of knowledge of family planning. An overwhelming majority of the participants (176 or 54.2%) had high level of attitudes towards family planning. Only 3% of the respondents showed poor level of attitude towards family planning. With regards to practice, the participants showed a poor level of practice of family planning at 80 (24.6%) whereas those with good level of practice of family planning constituted only 31 (9.5%).

Conclusion: This study provides a useful source of empirical information to policy makers to achieve the desired goals in family planning. These findings of the study will help health care providers promote family planning in Fiji.

Keywords: Family planning; Reproductive age; Contraceptive; Pregnancy

Introduction

Family planning refers to couples making informed decisions about having children-that is spacing the pregnancies and number of offspring they will have using contraceptive methods. Over 200 million women in developing countries do not desire pregnancies and they fail to use modern contraceptive methods [1]. This is in spite of the fact that several contraceptive methods, such as condoms, hinder the transmission of sexually transmitted infections (STIs) as well as the risks, pains, and costs associated with abortions [2]. Notably, abortions in developing nations account for a large number of pregnancy-related deaths among mothers and infants [3]. Clearly, irrespective of its considerable benefits, family planning practices are not being carried out by most of the developing countries. The WHO lists several reasons for the lack of motivation in family planning: lack of accessibility to contraceptive methods; fear of side effects and approbation based on social and religion sentiments; the quality of education on the subject that can also be linked to provider bias [4].

Remarkably, all these reasons can be directly linked to the lack of awareness associated with the inability of education to dispel ill-formed ideologies [5]. A study conducted by Sun-Hee Lee in the Pacific Islands showed that the contraceptive prevalence rate (CPR) was below 50 in all the islands including the urbanized ones; the increase in the teenage pregnancy rates by 30% was a matter of concern; and all nations reported high maternal morbidity rates along with the high infant morbidity rates in some nations [6]. In recent times, the problem has possibly aggravated, with the Pacific Islands shown as mostly in deficit in terms of family planning initiatives compared to other developing countries [7,8]. In Fiji, high unplanned pregnancy rates have been found linked with high poverty rates [9].

To explicate the situation, the low fertility and high mortality rates experienced by the nation in the past century was beginning to be overcome by the 2000s. However, since 2009, the level of population growth accompanied by the high number of births had shown that Fiji faces a threat of increased poverty levels because of high birth rates [10]. Clearly, in spite of the considerable efforts toward it in the 1980s, family planning remains a concern for Fiji. The aim of this study is to identify the level of knowledge, attitudes and practices towards of women of reproductive age in Fiji in 2017.

Methods

This quantitative, cross-sectional study was conducted among 325 participants who attended three designated health clinics around Suva, Fiji from 15th March to 28th April 2017. A self-administered questionnaire was used to collect data, which was content and face validated using a pilot study. To do face validity, the questionnaire was given to 10 participants who met the study inclusion and exclusion criteria and were asked to read and let us know about readability and understandability of the questionnaire. We also gave the questionnaire to 3 experts (all academic staff) who were familiar with the study and worked in the relevant field and asked them to check the content of the questionnaire based on is the aim and objective of the study. After collecting their comments we modified the questionnaire. There were seven family planning health clinics which we have chosen three of them randomly including Nuffield Clinic in Tamavua, Wellness Center for Women/Oxfam) at the Colonial War Memorial Hospital (CWMH) in Suva, and Samabula Health Center in Suva. The study population included all Fijian women of reproductive age. The inclusion criteria included women, ages 15-49 that were married and must have attended any one of the three identified family planning clinics under study from 15th March to 28th April, 2017. Furthermore, the study participant must have been a Fijian-anybody in Fiji who possesses Fijian citizenship. The exclusion criteria included men and women under the age of 15 or age 50 and over and those women who are not happy to participate in the study.

Participants who met the inclusion and exclusion criteria who consented to participate in the study were asked to fill a questionnaire survey to identify the level of knowledge, source of knowledge on family planning, and the barriers to their practice of family planning. Section 2 of the questionnaire survey was the knowledge-based section which contained 12 questions where the participant had an option to answer "True, False or Don't Know" or in the first question, "Yes/No and Don't Know". For coding purposes, the correct answer which is "Yes" in the first question, and may be "True or False" for the rest of the questions were recorded as 2. Whereas, the incorrect answer which was "No" in the first question or "True or False" for the rest of the questions was recorded as 0. An answer with "Don't Know" was recorded as 1. Total points to be scored were 24 and the minimum score was 0. The correct answers were quantified as: 0-11 as Poor (low level) knowledge; 12-18 as Moderate (medium level) knowledge; and 19-24 as Good (high level) knowledge. Data collection was done after the researcher received ethical approval from the College of Health Research Ethics Committee (CHREC) of Fiji National University and the Ministry of Health's Fiji National Heath Research Ethics Review Committee (FNHRERC). The data was analyzed with SPSS Version 22 statistical software. The frequency and percentage of KAP are presented in tables and graph.

Results

The mean age of the participants was 31.53 (± 7.35) with a majority of the participants in the age group 25-29 (26.8%). I Taukei women made up a large portion of the sample at 212 (65.2%). A majority of the participants belonged to a Christian denomination, 210 (64.6%). Just over half of the participants were employed (197, 60.6%) with 34.2% (115) of them with an annual income in the income range of $8,000.00 to $14,999.00. A large portion of the participants have a higher level of education (198, 60.9%). Two hundred five or 63.08% of the participants have between 1 and 3 children. In terms of residence, 229 or 70.5% of the participants live in urban area (Table 1).

Variable	Frequency	Percentage
Age	25-39 (87)	26.8
Ethnicity	iTaukei (212)	65.2
Religion	Christian (210)	64.6
Education	Higher (198)	60.9
Employment status	Employed (197)	60.6
Annual Income	8000-14,999 (34.2)	34.2
Number of children	1 to 3 (205)	63.1
Area of residence	Urban (229)	70.5

Table 1: Demographic profile of the participants.

A majority of the participants have heard of some form of contraceptive in their life, 293 (90.2%). Only 74 (22.8%) of the participants correctly answered that birth control pills were not effective if a woman misses taking them for two or three days in a row. A majority, 275 (84.6%) of the participants were aware that sterilization (tying a woman's fallopian tubes) was one way of preventing pregnancy. A large majority, 314 (96.6%) of the participants agreed that health education was important for women who want to use contraception. A majority of participants, 253 (77.8%), agreed that contraceptive pills did not guarantee 100% protection.

A majority of participants, 285 (87.7%), correctly answered that condoms prevented Sexually Transmitted Infections (STIs). A majority, 255 (78.5%) of participants correctly answered that contraceptive pills produced side effects of mood swings and weight gain. Only 74 (22.8%) of participants correctly answered that oral estrogen-containing contraceptive pills had an increased risk of causing breast cancer. A large majority of the participants, 268 (82.5%) answered correctly that a Depo Provera intramuscular injection contraceptive shot must be administered on three monthly basis. A majority of the participants, 275 (69.2%) correctly answered that women who experienced side effects of a contraceptive pill can switch to another form of contraceptive that might have less side effects. A good majority of the participants, 222 (68.3%), correctly answered that using a combination of condom and a contraceptive pill was considered very effective contraception (Table 2).

Questions (n=325)	Responses	N	%
	Yes	293	90.2
	No	26	8
1. Have you ever heard of contraceptive?	Don't know	6	1.8
	Yes	74	22.8
2. Birth control pills are effective even if a woman misses taking them for two or three days in a row.	No	178	54.8

	Don't know	73	22.5
	Yes	275	84.6
	No	10	3.1
3. Female sterilization is one way to avoid pregnancy.	Don't know	40	12.3
	Yes	314	96.6
	No	5	1.5
4. Health education is important for women who want to use contraception.	Don't know	6	1.8
	Yes	253	77.8
	No	26	8
5. Contraceptive pills do not guarantee 100% protection.	Don't know	46	14.2
	Yes	285	87.7
	No	21	6.5
6. Condoms prevent STIs.	Don't know	19	5.8
	Yes	255	78.5
	No	21	6.5
7. Common side effects of contraceptive pills include mood swings and weight gain.	Don't know	49	15.1
	Yes	74	22.8
	No	117	36
8. There is an increased risk of breast cancer in women taking estrogen-containing contraceptives.	Don't know	134	41.2
	Yes	268	82.5
	No	12	3.8
9. Women using the birth control shot (Depo Provera) must get an injection every three months.	Don't know	45	30.8
	Yes	225	69.2
	No	41	12.6
10. If a woman is having side effects of one kind of contraceptive pill, switching to another type might help.	Don't know	59	18.2
	Yes	222	68.3
	No	39	12
11. Using both a condom and the pill is considered to be a very effective contraceptive.	Don't know	64	19.7
	Yes	60	18.5
	No	145	44.6
12. Using the pill increases a woman's risk of ovarian, endometrial or cervical cancer.	Don't know	120	36.9

Table 2: Frequency of responses on knowledge-related questions.

Table 3 displays the results of the participants' attitudes based on a Likert Scale scoring system consisting only of responses of "Strongly Agree/Agree" which are combined to show the total percentage of the responses of the participants to each question.

A majority of the participants, 273 (84%), agreed/strongly agreed that contraceptives should be used to limit a woman's number of children. Likewise, a majority of the participants, 286 (88%) agreed/strongly agreed that contraceptives were necessary to control the spacing of a woman's childbirths. A large majority of the participants, 293 (90.1%), agreed/strongly agreed that spacing allow for healthier children. More than three quarters, 291 (89.5%), agreed/strongly agreed that the ideal age of a woman's child-bearing age is 20-30. About 221 (68%) of the participants agreed/strongly agreed that the ideal number of children is between 3 and 5. A majority of the participants, 289 (88.9%) agreed/strongly agreed that contraceptives provided a sense of safety. For participants on contraceptives, 255 (78.5%), agreed/strongly agreed that the type of contraceptive method they were using was adequate.

Three quarters, 254 (78.2%) agreed/strongly agreed that contraceptives benefited males. Only a small fraction, 82 (25.2%), of the participants agreed/agreed strongly that discussion of contraceptives with their spouses was embarrassing. An even smaller sample of the participants, 66 (20.3%) agreed/strongly agreed that their husbands did not approve of their use of contraceptives. A majority, 291 (89.5%) of the participants, agreed/strongly agreed that contraceptives protected the health of the family and the community. Religion played a big part in a woman's decision to use contraceptives, 271 (83.4%). Likewise, just over three quarters of the participants agreed/strongly agreed that cultural beliefs, 256 (78.8%) played a role into a woman's decision to use contraceptives. A majority of the participants agreed/strongly agreed that husband's objections influenced their spouse's decision to use contraceptives, 269 (82.8%). A majority of the participants, 261 (80.3%), agreed/strongly agreed that a male's attitude about contraceptives play a big role into a woman's decision to use contraceptives.

	Strongly Agree		Agree		Neutral		Disagree		Strongly Disagree		Total
Attitudes (n=325)	n	%	n	%	N	%	n	%	n	%	N (%)
1. Contraceptives should be used to limit my number of children.	110	33.85	163	50.2	29	8.9	19	5.9	4	1.2	273 (84)
2. Contraceptives should be used to increase the time interval between my childbirths.	114	35.1	172	52.9	20	6.2	16	4.9	3	0.9	286 (88)
3. Spacing will allow a child to be healthier.	134	41.2	159	48.9	20	6.2	9	2.8	3	0.9	293 (90.2)
4. The ideal age of having a first child is 20-30.	109	33.5	182	56	25	7.7	7	2.2	2	0.6	291 (89.5)
5. The ideal number of children should be between 3-5.	78	20	143	44	54	16.6	41	12.6	9	2.8	221 (68)
6. Contraceptives provide a sense of safety.	100	30.8	189	58.2	23	7.1	10	3.1	3	0.9	289 (88.9)
7. The method of contraception I am using is adequate.	88	27.1	167	51.4	60	18.5	9	2.8	1	0.3	255 (78.5)
8. Contraceptives benefit males too.	75	23.1	179	55.1	49	15.1	18	5.5	4	1.2	254 (78.2)
9. Discussion about contraception with spouse is embarrassing.	17	5.2	65	20	44	13.5	130	40	69	20.9	82 (25.2)
10. My husband does not approve my use of contraceptives.	16	4.9	50	15.4	54	16.6	151	46.5	54	16.6	66 (20.3)
11. Contraceptive methods can protect the health of family and community.	114	35.1	177	54.5	22	6.8	11	33.9	1	0.3	291 (89.5)
12. Religious beliefs can prevent women from using contraceptives.	99	30.5	172	52.9	22	6.8	23	7.1	9	2.8	271 (83.4)
13. Cultural beliefs can prevent women from using contraceptives.	91	28	165	50.8	30	9.2	31	9.5	8	2.5	256 (78.8)
14. Husband's objections to contraceptives can prevent women from using contraceptives.	84	25.9	185	56.9	23	7.1	28	8.6	5	1.5	269 (82.8)
15. Change in male attitudes on contraceptives may improve contraceptive use.	96	29.5	165	50.8	25	7.7	31	9.5	8	2.5	261 (80.3)

Table 3: Frequency of responses on attitudes- related questions.

Table 4 displays the results of participants' family planning practices. The total frequency and percentage are derived from combing the "Always and Usually" responses to each question.

With regards to a participant's consultation with family planning services, just over half of the participants always or usually consulted with health care professionals in a health center for family planning services, (186 or 57%). Responses of always or usually to the family planning practices, which constitute ideal or positive practices, registered the highest proportion under use of contraceptives for unplanned pregnancy (212, 65%) or roughly two thirds of the participants. Only 2 (0.5%) of the participants have experienced an unplanned pregnancy as a result of lack of family planning. A majority of the participants always or usually practiced family planning every time they did not intend to get pregnant, (196 or 60%). Only 27 (8%) of the participants changed their family planning method from time to time. Similarly, less than 10%, 41 (13%) of the participants practiced a traditional method of family planning (Table 4).

	Always		Usually		Sometimes		Seldom		Never		Total
Practices Questions (n=325)	**N**	**%**	**N**	**%**	**N**	**%**	**N**	**%**	**N**	**%**	**N (%)**
1. How many times a year, do you visit a health centre for family planning services?	123	37.5	64	19.7	59	18.2	27	8.3	52	16	187 (58)
2. Do you use contraceptives to prevent unplanned pregnancy?	157	48.3	55	16.9	40	12.3	9	2.8	64	19.7	212 (65)
3. Have you ever had any unplanned pregnancy due to lack of contraceptive use?	1	0.3	1	0.3	91	8	0	0	232	19.7	2 (0.6)
4. Do you use contraceptives every time when you do not intend to get pregnant?	142	43.7	54	16.6	47	14.5	13	4	69	21.2	196 (60)
5. I use different types of contraceptives.	7	2.2	16	4.9	65	20	53	16.3	184	56.6	23 (7)
6. My current method of contraceptive changes from time to time.	4	1.2	23	7.1	53	16.3	54	16.6	191	58.7	27 (8)
7. Do you practice any traditional contraceptive methods including withdrawal, infertility period, herbal and breast feeding if you were not using any contraceptives?	19	5.9	22	6.2	111	34.2	24	7.4	149	45.6	41 (13)

Table 4: Frequency of responses to practice-related questions.

Discussion

This study addressed the current knowledge, attitudes and the practices among 325 participants. In terms of contraception awareness and the need of health education for women, a high number of the participants answering positively indicated that the United Nations and governmental family planning initiatives from the 1980s to present were potentially successful. This echoes the finding in the Hayes and Robinson study that showed the low fertility rates experienced by women in Fiji resulted in the success of the subsequent family planning initiatives in the 1980s [11]. However, the barriers to knowledge were apparent in the manner in which contraception methods and their use was being perceived. For instance, only 54% of the respondents were aware that missing contraceptive pills for more than 2-3 days in a row can result in pregnancies [12,13]. Similarly, a notable number were unaware of the side effects of taking contraceptive pills, and the potential link between cancer and estrogen-containing contraceptives. Since the latter is still a matter of contention, one can state that the lack of awareness here is not relevant.

However, the fact that many (40%) do not know that such as a contention exists is indicative of the low penetration of the details of family planning among the people in Fiji. This has also been shown in the certainty (68.3%) and uncertainty (19.7%) associated with idea that contraceptive pills are all the same and can be replaced. Another factor shows the lack of detailed awareness among the participants in Fiji. Although a relatively high number of participants (77.8%) were aware that contraceptive pills do not guarantee absolute protection from pregnancy, a lesser number (66.8%) is aware that using a condom and the pill together considerably increases the contraceptive protection. Another possible matter of concern is that female sterilization as a means of avoiding pregnancies was well-established (84.6%). While a corresponding question regarding male sterilization was not asked in this study, the fact that gender disparities have been associated with family planning challenges can be recalled here [14]. A lack of clarity was also observed in the manner in which 30% of the respondents did not know if the birth control shot (Depo Provera) should be taken every three months-owing to the close-ended questionnaires employed here, it was unclear whether this was because they never used the shot as a means of contraception or because they did not know how to use it.

The barriers to the use of contraceptive use among the participants in this study were linked to religious beliefs as well (30.5% strongly agreed/52.9% agreed). Similarly, cultural beliefs were a considerable force in demotivating women from using contraceptives. This finding can be associated with the idea that refusing contraception has been linked to the missionary foundations that enabled colonization [15,16]. The fact that gender disparities are a strong barrier against contraception use has been established by the fact that most of the respondents were of the opinion that contraception use could be better if husbands did not object to contraception and if male attitudes toward contraceptive could be altered. The issue of gender disparity in disabling effective contraception use across developing nations has been established in other studies as well [17]. In addition, the religious beliefs that inhibit women in Fiji from using contraceptives had been linked to the female subservience to males in the Fijian society, especially the large Indo-Fijian population [18].

Clearly, the male control over female sexuality is a thriving problem in Fiji as it is in many developing nations. Greater gender equality is the sign of development, and in resolving this issue [19], Fiji can potentially induce social development as well. Another notable factor here is in the fact that most respondents seem to agree that the ideal number of children should be between 3 and 5. This attitude is possibly an indicator of the fears associated with the reduced rates of fertility Fiji has experienced in the past. However, the fact that poverty is associated with the rapid population expansion needs to be considered here [20]. A family planning program that addresses this issue by describing the number of children in an ideal family unit can be a means of propounding awareness here.

As for the practices associated with family planning in Fiji, a dispersed response to the need for regular visits to the health centers for family planning services was found. This showed that the lack of depth in awareness could be linked to the fact that the health centers were the primary sources of in-depth knowledge and awareness regarding contraceptive use as opposed to advertisements and other such highly influential initiatives. Combining knowledge along with condom social marketing programs can be an effective means of dealing with this problem [21]. Furthermore, changing the contraceptive frequently and using various kinds of contraceptives can be linked to the increased birth rates today. Considering that there is a lack of in-depth awareness regarding contraception use, changing contraceptives is probably not been done effectively, such that it pregnancies can be avoided. Nonetheless, the fact that there have been few unplanned pregnancies when people have been using contraceptives contradicts this fact. Since people do seem to take contraceptive when they do not want pregnancies, it is possible that changing or alternating contraceptive use is not a barrier to family planning in this case.

However, this cross sectional study is the first study was conducted in Fiji, it had some limitations such as using a questionnaire which was not reliable and also lack of generalizing the results of this study to all women in reproductive age in Fiji.

Conclusion

It can be concluded from the facts presented in this paper that the most prominent problem with the knowledge and attitudes regarding family planning was in that several crucial details regarding it were unknown or unclear among the people in Fiji. Other important facts that emerged include the gender disparities and religious beliefs that impact contraceptive use, with gender disparities shown to be a defining factor in negatively impacting contraception use. Some aspects of the study, such as the attitudes toward male sterilization in comparison to female sterilization, also demand further research focus.

References

1. Salisbury P, Hall L, Kulkus S, Paw MK, Tun NW, et al. (2016) Family planning knowledge, attitudes and practices in refugee on migrant pregnant and post-partum women on the Thailand-Myanmar border: A mixed methods study. Reprod Health 13: 94.
2. Thorsteinson K, Lund SL, Storgaard M, Ronsholt FF, Johansen IS, et al. (2016) Sexually transmitted infections and use of contraceptives in women living with HIV in Denmark: The SHADE cohort. BMC Infect Dis 16: 81.
3. Family planning can reduce high infant mortality levels (2002) The Alan Guttmacher Institute pp: 1-4.
4. http://www.who.int/mediacentre/factsheets/fs351/en/
5. Mustafa R, Afreen U, Hashmi HA (2008) Contraceptive knowledge, attitude and practice among rural women. J Coll Physicians Surg Pak 18: 542-545.
6. Lee SH (1995) Discussion paper 14: Reproductive health and family planning in the Pacific: Current situation and the Way Forward.
7. Dix E, Nathan SA, Rawstorne P (2015) Informing the introduction of contraceptive implants in the Pacific: A mixed methods study of contraceptive beliefs and behaviors in Tonga. Aust N Z J Public Health 40: 115-119.
8. Kennedy EC, Buckley SM, Subramaniam S, Demmke A, Latu R (2013) The case for investing in family planning in the Pacific: Costs and benefits of reducing unmet need for contraception in Vanuatu and the Solomon Islands. Reprod Health 10: 30.
9. http://www.pacificpolicy.network/2014/04/pacifics-high-teen-pregnancy-rates/
10. Naidu SL, Heller GZ, Koroi Z, Dearkin L, Gyaneshwar R (2017) Knowledge, attitude, practice and barriers regarding safe sex and contraceptive use in rural women in Fiji. Pac J Reprod Health 1: 223-231.
11. Hayes G, Robertson A (2010) Family planning in Asia and the Pacific: Addressing the Challenges. In UNFPA-ICOMP Regional Consultation. Bangkok, Thailand.
12. Cammock R (2015) I taukei family planning behavior in Fiji's central division. Pac J Reprod Health pp: 34-46.
13. Davies C, Dubie M, Mesibov GB (2012) Intimate relationships and sexual health: A curriculum for teaching adolescents/adults with high-functioning autism spectrum disorders and other social challenges. Shawnee Mission, Kan: AAPC Publishing.
14. Chattier P (2014) Measuring poverty as if gender matters: Perspectives from fieldwork in Fiji. SSGM Discussion Paper P: 10.
15. Hodges S (2008) Contraception, colonialism and commerce: Birth control in South India, 1920-1940. Aldershot. Ashgate, England.
16. Bullough VL (2001) Encyclopedia of birth control. Santa Barbara, Calif: ABC-CLIO.
17. Vasilenko SA, Kreager DA, Lefkowitz ES (2015) Gender, contraceptive attitudes, and condom use in adolescent romantic relationships: A dyadic approach. J Res Adolesc 25: 51-62.
18. Chandra D, Lewai V (2005) Women and men of Fiji Islands: Gender statistics and trends. Suva: Population studies programme. Univ of the South Pacific.
19. Gill K (2010) Indian women in Fiji: Their health strategies. Vancouver: Webzines of Vancouver.
20. Frankel J, Firth S (2007) From election to coup in Fiji: The 2006 campaign and its aftermath. ANU E Press, Canberra, Australia.
21. Sewak A, Singh G (2012) Assessment of the Fiji-based condom social marketing (CSM) program. Sex & Cult 16: 389-407.

Gynecological Morbidity among Women in Reproductive Age: A Systematic Review and Meta-Analysis

Merga Dheresa[1*], Nega Assefa[1], Yemane Berhane[2], Alelmayhu Worku[2], Bizatu Mingiste[1] and Yadeta Dessie[1]

[1]*Department of Health and Medical Sciences, Haramaya University, Harar, Ethiopia*

[2]*Addis Continental Institutes of Public Health, Addis Ababa, Ethiopia*

[*]**Corresponding author:** Dheresa M, Department of Health and Medical Sciences, Haramaya University, Harar, Ethiopia, E-mail: mderesa@yahoo.com

Abstract

Background: Prevention against infection and dysfunction of reproductive organ including sexually transmitted disease is one of the three dimensions of reproductive health. Gynecological morbidities affect women's physical health, sexual function, social role, psychological life and religious life. For accurate estimation of gynecological morbidity, population based data are considered to be gold standard. There are no global wide population studies on gynecological morbidities. In this paper, we aimed to determine the prevalence of gynecological morbidity among the reproductive age women in the world.

Methods: Using various key words, electronics databases were searched systematically to identify observational studies published so far in English. Meta-analysis was made to summarize the prevalence of gynecological morbidity. A random-effects model was used to calculate pooled prevalence. Publication bias was evaluated by testing for funnel plot asymmetry, Begg's rank correlation test and Egger's linear regression test. All statistical calculations were made using STATA Version 12.0 software.

Result: Eighteen studies, at least with one outcome variable were included in the final analysis. Ten studies were eligible for pelvic organ prolapse, 8 were eligible for infertility, 11 for menstrual disorder, and 15 for reproductive tract infection. The summarized random effect prevalence of pelvic organ prolapse was 13%, infertility was 8%, reproductive tract infection was 38%, and menstrual disorders were 28%. The overall pooled random effect prevalence of gynecological morbidity was 22% (95% CI=17%-27%, I2=99.38%, p=000). The potential publication bias was suggested by funnel plot asymmetry.

Conclusion: The polled prevalence of overall gynecological morbidity was high. This pooled prevalence enabled us to conclude that the effect of gynecological morbidities is high to hamper the productivity of reproductive age women in the world particularly in a developing nation.

Keywords: Gynecological morbidity; Systematic review; Meta-analysis; Women

Introduction

Maternal health has been given due attention since 1978 Alma-Ata declaration and it is considered as one component of the basic primary health care. Even though priority has been given to maternal mortality prevention, little attention is given to non-pregnant women [1].

However, in the 1994 International conference on Population and Development held in Cairo and in the 1995 World Congress on women which held in Beijing, general attention has been given to comprehensive women's health. This shifts orientation of fertility reduction and population policies to reproductive health [2]. Reproductive health is a state of complete physical, mental and social wellbeing; it is not merely the absence of disease or infirmity in all matters relating to the reproductive system and its functions and processes [3].

Protecting against infections and dysfunctions of the reproductive tract including sexually transmitted infections, avoiding of unwanted pregnancies, and keeping safe motherhood are the broad dimension of reproductive health among adult women [4].

Obstetrics, Gynecological, and Contraceptive morbidities are the three broad categories of reproductive morbidities [5]. Gynecological morbidity is structural and functional disorder of the reproductive tract (genital tract). Though gynecological morbidity is not related to pregnancy, delivery and puerperum, it may be related to sexual behavior [6,7].

Gynecological morbidities have negative impact on women health-related quality of life, in terms of marital disharmony excluding them from social and religious life [8]. The untreated conditions can cause pregnancy related complications, congenital infections, and chronic pain which significantly increase the risk of acquiring Pelvic Inflammatory Disease and HIV [9]. Gynecological disorders have a substantial impact on female reproductive ability, and mental health ability which perform routine physical activities [10].

Community based gynecological morbidity has served as important tool for epidemiological surveillance, health service planning, and policy advocacy; thus, it is considered to be the gold standard for research on gynecological morbidity among women [11,12]. There is a paucity of population based research on gynecological morbidities with the prevalence ranges of 24.4% to 79.4% [4,13-15].

There are no global wide studies on the magnitude of gynecological morbidities that can be used for policy advocacy. Therefore, summarizing the prevalence of gynecological morbidity among reproductive age women is provided to develop research priorities. We performed a systematic review and meta-analysis on studies conducted on gynecological morbidities which aimed at exploring the prevalence of gynecological morbidities among reproductive age women in the world.

Methods

Literature search strategy

This systematic review was conducted based on PRISMA guidelines [16]. We searched all published articles on the prevalence of gynecological morbidity. Electronic data bases such as PubMed were searched to identify observational studies on the subject.

Papers were also identified by searching references from all included studies. No date restriction was applied in the search. The authors first screened the title, and abstracts. Then reviewed the full-text of the eligible articles.

Criteria for inclusion and exclusion

We included all epidemiologic studies which reported the prevalence of gynecological morbidity among 15-49 years old women all over the world. Only studies which used random sampling or census data to find participants were included.

All source studies were original cross-sectional study or a baseline survey of longitudinal study which is written in English and contained the minimum information necessary to calculate pooled analysis of prevalence (number of the subjects and number of gynecological morbidity events).

Studies were included if they explicitly defined gynecological morbidity which in turn may include at least one types of gynecological morbidity (i.e. Reproductive tract infection, menstrual dysfunction, pelvic organ prolapse and infertility).

We excluded studies if the participants were not in the age range of 15-49, pregnant women, if the study reported only the overall prevalence of gynecological morbidity without mentioning the morbidity types. We also excluded studies not only with qualitative study but also studies that utilized non-random sampling.

Data extraction

The standardized data abstraction form was designed to capture and code all relevant studies level information required for analysis. Authors selected the studies and extracted the data. For all included studies, we recorded the following information:

- Author
- Year of publication
- Countries
- Sampling method
- Data collection method
- Number of subjects
- Number of people with gynecological morbidity

Quality assessment of included studies

We used the Joanna Briggs Institute (JBI) Prevalence Critical Appraisal Tool [17] to assess quality of individual paper (Table 1).

S. No	Author (year)	JBI Quality Items										
		1	2	3	4	5	6	7	8	9	10	Score
1	Abraham A et al. (2014)	Y	Y	Y	Y	Y	Y	Y	Y	Y	Y	10
2	Verma A et al. (2015)	Y	Y	Y	Y	Y	N	U	Y	Y	N	7
3	Fahimeh et al. (2011)	Y	Y	Y	Y	Y	Y	Y	Y	Y	Y	10
4	Filippi V et al. (1997)	Y	Y	Y	N	Y	Y	Y	Y	Y	Y	9
5	Inamdar IF et al. (2013)	Y	Y	Y	Y	Y	Y	N	Y	Y	Y	9
6	Masterson A et al.(2014)	Y	Y	Y	Y	Y	U	U	Y	Y	Y	8
7	Gokler M et al. (2014)	Y	Y	Y	Y	N	Y	Y	Y	Y	Y	9
8	Miteshkumar N (2010)	Y	Y	Y	Y	Y	Y	Y	Y	Y	Y	10
9	Bhatnagar N et al. (2013)	Y	Y	Y	Y	Y	U	U	Y	Y	Y	8
10	Philippov O et al. (1998)	Y	Y	Y	Y	N	Y	Y	U	N	N	6
11	Chellan R (2004)	N	N	N	N	N	N	N	N	N	N	10
12	Riyami et al. (2004)	Y	Y	Y	Y	Y	Y	Y	Y	Y	Y	10
13	Garg S et al. (2002)	U	Y	U	Y	Y	Y	U	Y	N	N	5
14	Poornima S et al. (2013)	Y	Y	Y	Y	Y	Y	Y	N	N	Y	8

15	Kaur S et al. (2013)	Y	N	U	N	Y	Y	Y	Y	Y	Y	7
16	Kumari S et al. (2000)	Y	U	U	N	Y	Y	Y	Y	Y	N	6
17	Siae M et al. (2002)	Y	Y	Y	Y	Y	Y	Y	Y	Y	Y	10
18	Gosalia VV et al. (2012)	Y	Y	Y	Y	Y	N	N	N	N	N	5

Table 1: Quality assessment of the 18 paper used for the meta-analysis [Y= yes, N=No, U=unclear].

Statistical analysis

To include proportion close to 0 and 1, we enabled the Freeman-Tukey double arcsine transformation option (ftt) [18]; otherwise, studies with estimated proportion at 1 and 0 would be excluded from the analysis leading to a biased pooled estimate. The transformed prevalence is weighted very slightly towards 50% and, thus, studies with prevalence of 0 can be included in the analysis [19].

Meta-analyses were conducted using the metaprop [18] command for prevalence and metainf for influence of single study. Meta-analyses were conducted summarizing the prevalence of gynecological morbidity among women of reproductive age. First, the prevalence of each type of gynecological morbidity (pelvic organ prolapse, infertility, reproductive tract infection and menstrual disorder) was analyzed separately.

Then overall gynecological morbidity prevalence was assessed by stratifying by types of gynecological morbidities. According to the expected heterogeneity across studies, a random-effects model was used to calculate pooled prevalence. In all cases 95% confidence intervals were calculated using the binomial exact method to calculate. Statistical heterogeneity was evaluated with the Cochran chi-square (χ^2) and quantified with the I2 statistic (low is 25%, moderate 25-50%, high 50%) [20,21].

Publication bias was evaluated by testing for funnel plot asymmetry, Begg's rank correlation test and Egger's linear regression test. Significance was set at a P value of less than 0.05. Sensitivity analyses include investigation of the influence of a single study on the combined association by omitting one study in the pooled analysis. All statistical calculations were made using the Stata Statistical Software Package, Version 12.0. Ancillary analyses were performed using comprehensive meta-analysis software.

Result

Systematic review

The literature search returned 222 publications from Medline/PMC. Additional 60 studies were included from other sources (Google Scholar and reference lists of relevant publications).

Two hundred forty-two studies were remained after removing duplicates. While screening relevant titles, 102 studies were excluded. This means a total of 140 full texts were assessed. The outcome variable for this study was gynecological morbidity (reproductive tract infection, menstrual disorder, pelvic organ prolapse and infertility).

Studies which report at least one types of the gynecological morbidity were accepted for meta-analysis. After applying the quality criteria, 122 studies were further excluded (some of the studies were systematic review, several were studied among women out of reproductive age, and others were qualitative study which did not provide numerical estimates on incidence and/or prevalence of gynecological morbidity.

Still other studies were not mentioned which types of gynecological morbidity they studied). Finally, 18 studies were retained for the review and meta-analysis (Figure 1).

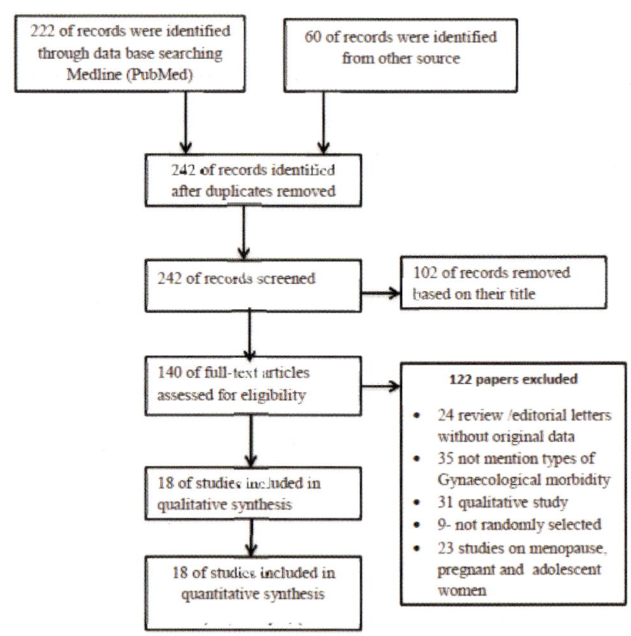

Figure 1: The Flow diagram of inclusion and exclusion identified was studied for the meta-analysis of overall prevalence.

Study characteristics

The retained 18 studies [10,13,15,22-36] were conducted in different parts of the globe. Almost 33.3% of studies were conducted in urban area [15,24,26,30,33,36], 11% were conducted in both urban and rural areas [27,31].

In addition, 5.5% in rural area and the rest, places where studies are conducted is not mentioned as urban or rural areas (Table 2).

Categories	Q (heterogeneity statistics)	*df	*I^2 (Heterogeneity test)	p	Publication bias	
					P (Begg's test)	P (Egger's test)
*POP	1123.11	9	99.20%	<0.001	0.283	0.004
Infertility	353.79	7	98.02%	<0.001	0.266	0.038
*RTI	1360.3	14	98.97%	<0.001	0.138	0.4
Menstrual disorder	537.72	10	98.14%	<0.001	0.533	0.142
Overall	6975.99	43	99.38%	<0.001	0.56	0.235
B/n sub group	47.37	3	-	<0.001	-	-

Table 2: Heterogeneity and publication bias test in four types and overall gynecological morbidities among reproductive age women [*I^2 =the variation in ES attributable to heterogeneity, *df =degree of freedom, *POP =pelvic organ prolapse; *RTI=reproductive organ prolapse].

From the retained 18 studies, 2 papers contain two outcome variable (one study reports menstrual disorder and reproductive organ prolapse while the other reports reproductive tract infection and pelvic organ prolapse) [23,31]. Six studies contain three outcome variables (4 of them contain menstrual disorder, reproductive organ prolapse and reproductive tract infection. The rest 2 studies report menstrual disorder, reproductive tract infection and infertility) [10,15, 25,30,33,35,36]. Four studies contain four outcome variables (menstrual disorder, pelvic organ prolapse, reproductive tract infection and infertility) [13,22,26,32].

Six papers reported only one outcome variables (3 of them report only reproductive infection, 2 of them report infertility and the rest 1 report pelvic organ prolapse) [24,27-30,34] (Table 2). Ten studies were eligible for pelvic organ prolapse [10,13,15,22,26,29,31,32,35,36] and contain 8,703 sample size. The prevalence of the pelvic organ prolapse ranges from 0.4%-41%. Eight studies were eligible for infertility [13,22,25,26,28,30,32,33] and contain 6,436 sample size. The prevalence of infertility among the paper was ranging from 1%-16%.

For menstrual disorder, 11 studies were identified [10,13,15,22,23,25,26,32,33,35,36], the total sample population were 7,247 and prevalence of menstrual disorder was ranging from 11%-53%. Among the identified paper, 15 studies were eligible for reproductive tract infection [10,13,15,22-27,31-37] and contain 26,248 sample sizes.

The prevalence of reproductive tract infection ranges from 7-70%. The sample size of individual studies ranged from 200-18,040 (Table 3).

S. No	Author (year)	Country	Age	Sample size	Outcome Variable			
					Menstrual disorder	RTI*	POP*	Infertility
1	Abraham A et al. (2014)	India	15-45	540	135	39	2	17
2	Verma A et al. (2015)	India	15-44	215	-	91	-	-
3	Fahimeh et al. (2011)	Iran	18-45	1117	336	420	462	-
4	Filippi V et al. (1997)	Turkey	15-49	862	103	345	147	-
5	Inamdar IF et al. (2013)	India	15-49	750	351	189	114	87
6	Masterson A et al. (2014)	Lebanon	18-45	452	242	241	-	-
7	Gokler M et al. (2014)	Turkey	18-49	570	-	-	-	73
8	Miteshkumar N (2010)	India	15-49	1046	403	587	-	12
9	Bhatnagar N et al. (2013)	India	15-49	750	115	82	27	26
10	Philippov O et al. (1998)	Siberia	18-45	2000	-	-	-	333
11	Chellan R (2004)	India	15-44	18040	-	5827	-	-
12	Riyami et al. (2004)	Oman	15-49	364	-	81	64	-
13	Garg S et al. (2002)	India	15-45	380	98	216	60	31
14	Poornima S et al. (2013)	India	15-49	400	83	282	-	27

15	Kaur S et al. (2013)	India	15-49	200	36	49	16	-
16	Kumari S et al. (2000)	India	15-49	2990	-	-	227	-
17	Siae M et al. (2002)	Tanzania	15-49	382	-	244	-	-
18	Gosalia VV et al. (2012)	India	15-49	750	195	198	3	-

Table 3: Summary of overall characteristics of studies retained for systemic review and meta-analysis [*pop=pelvic organ prolapse, *RTI=Reproductive Tract Infection].

Age of study participant was between 15-49 years. 51% of them were in the age ranges of 35-49 years. Regarding their marital status, 86.5% of women were currently married and 5% were never married. Among those currently married women 33% of them were married before the reach 18 years old. 87% of study participants were multiparous; 39% of the study participants were illiterate, 17.5% were attended primary education, and 43% were attended secondary education and above [10,13,15,22-36].

Pooled analysis in different outcome categories

Pelvic organ prolapse: The point prevalence of pelvic organ prolapse with 10 individual study populations ranges between 0% and 41%, with an overall summarized random effect meta-analysis prevalence of 13% (95% CI=8- 12, I2=99.31% p=0.000) (Figure 2).

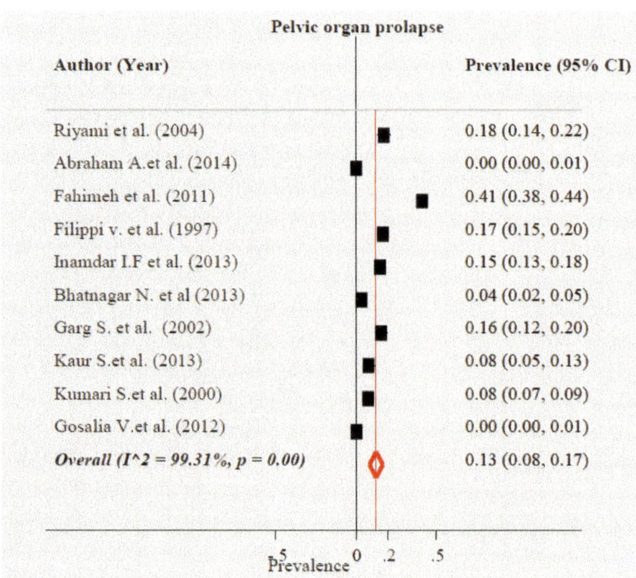

Figure 2: Random model meta-analysis of prevalence of pelvic organ prolapses among women.

Infertility: The prevalence point of infertility with 8 individual study populations ranged between 1% and 17%. The pooled meta-analysis prevalence of infertility was 8% (95%=4-12, I2=98.26%, p=000) (Figure 3).

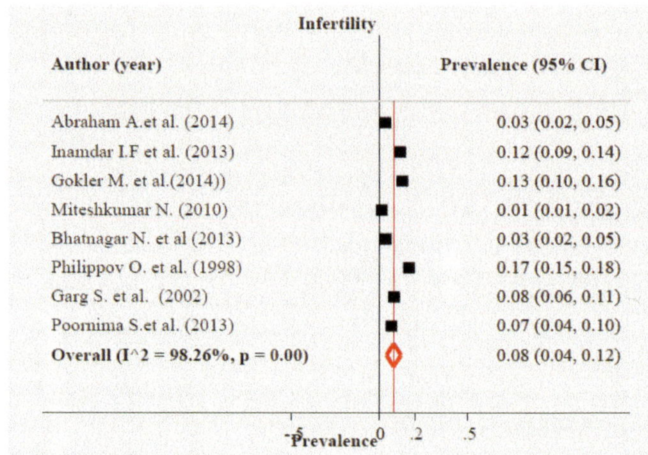

Figure 3: Random model Meta-Analysis of prevalence of infertility among women.

Reproductive tract infection: The prevalence point of reproductive tract infections among 15 individual studies ranged from 7% to 70% and an overall pooled meta-analysis prevalence was 38% (95% CI=30%-46%, I2=99.23%) (Figure 4).

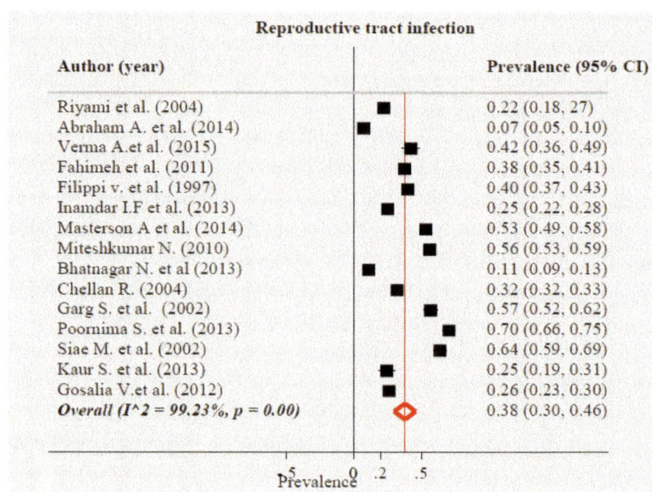

Figure 4: Random effect model meta-analysis of prevalence of RTI among women.

Menstrual disorder: Menstrual disorders' point prevalence ranged from 12% to 54% with 11 individual study population and the pooled meta-analysis prevalence of 28% (95% CI=30%-46%, I2=98.30%) (Figure 5).

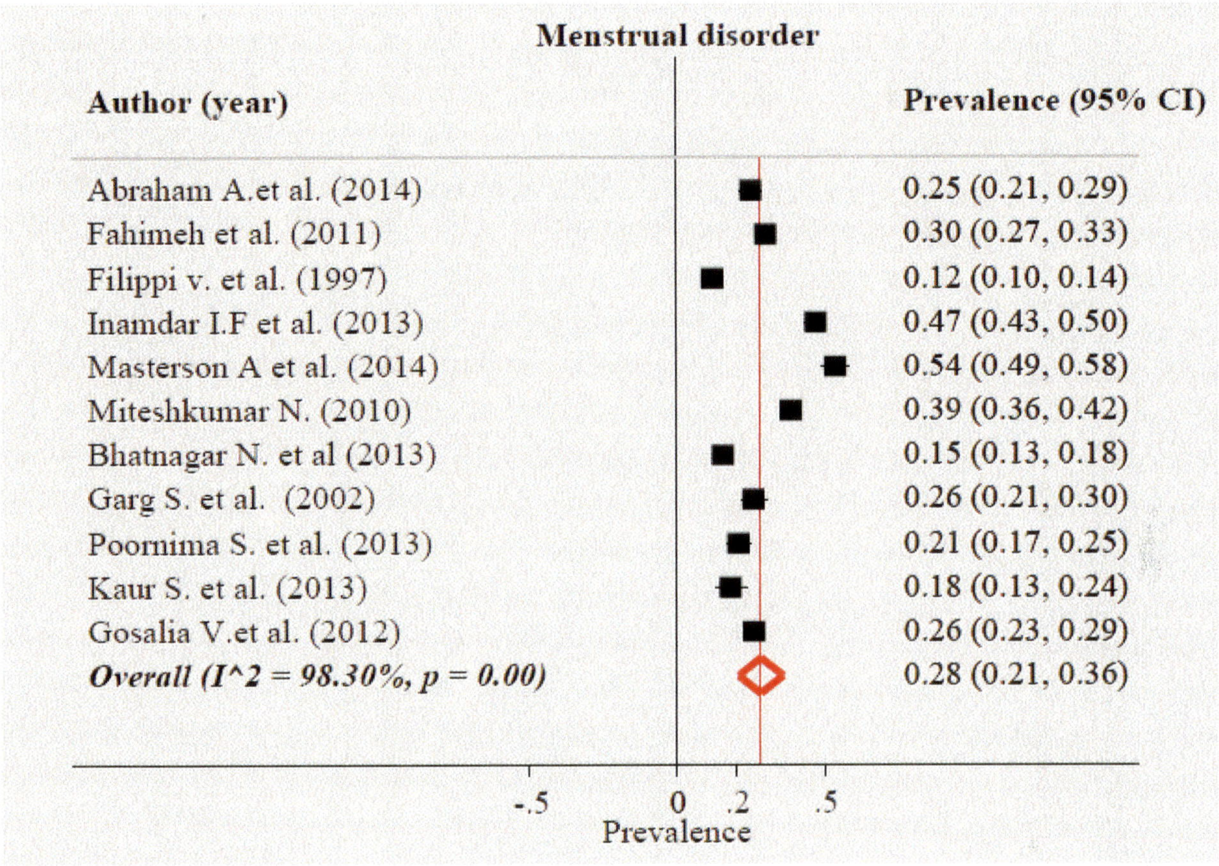

Figure 5: Random effect model meta-analysis of prevalence of menstrual disorder among women.

High level of heterogeneity (I2=98.30%-99.31%) was noted within the studies in each type of gynecological morbidities (Figures 2-5).

High level heterogeneity was noted within the studies and among groups of studies (I2=98.02%-99.20%, p=00) (Table 2).

Overall gynecological morbidity prevalence

Overall gynecological morbidity prevalence was assessed all types of gynecological morbidities by stratifying. Pelvic organ prolapse with 11 studies, infertility with 8 studies, reproductive tract infection with 15 studies, menstrual disorder with 11 studies, totally 44(some individual studies have more than one outcome variable) studies with 48,634 study population were included in the overall pooled summary of meta-analysis prevalence.

The point prevalence of gynecological morbidity with 44 individual study populations ranges from 0% (in pelvic organ prolapse) to 70% (in reproductive tract infection).

The overall pooled random effect meta-analysis prevalence of gynecological morbidity was 22% (95% CI=17%-27%, I2=99.38%, p=000) (Figure 6).

Publication Bias

Publication bias was evaluated by testing for funnel plot asymmetry, Begg's rank correlation test and Egger's linear regression test. Egger's regression test indicated evidence of publication bias for gynecological morbidity (p=0.004 for pelvic organ prolapse and p=0.03 for infertility). However, there was no evidence of publication bias for reproductive tract infection (p=0.40), menstrual disorder (p=14) and overall gynecological morbidity (p=23).

Begg's test indicated that there was no evidence of publication bias of all types of gynecological morbidities (Table 2). Each funnel plot appears asymmetry that suggested the presence of a potential publication bias of all types of gynecological morbidities (Figures 7 and 8).

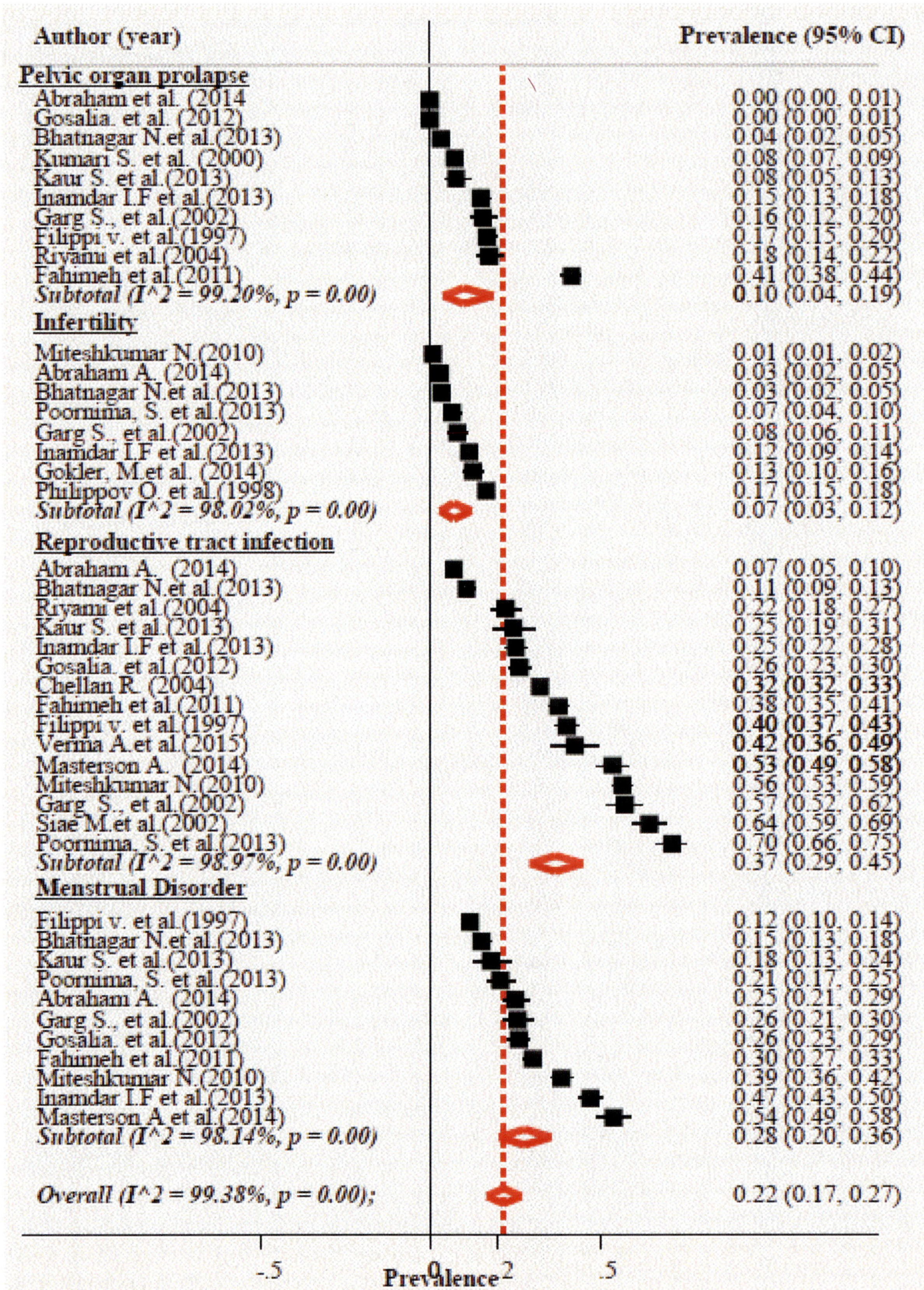

Figure 6: Meta-analysis of prevalence of GM stratified by types among women.

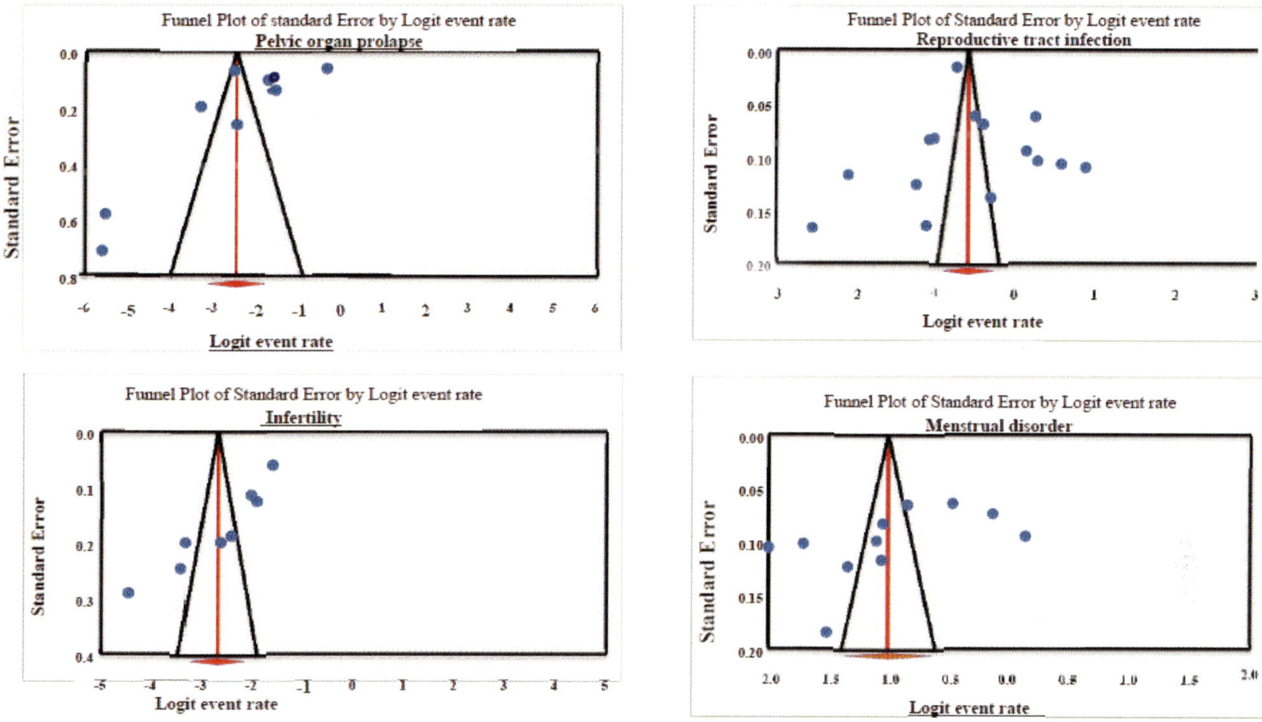

Figure 7: Funnel plot to assess publication bias depending on the symmetry of the funnel plot.

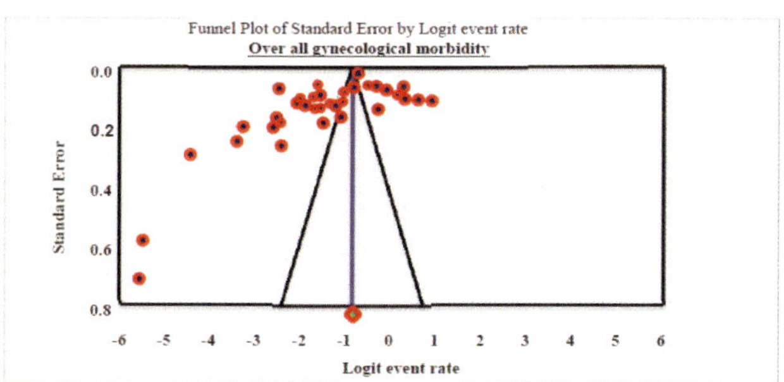

Figure 8: Funnel plot to assess publication bias using asymmetry of the plot.

Sensitivity analysis

To test the robustness of meta-analysis results, we performed graph of individual studies influence on the pooled meta-analysis prevalence using STATA command option (matainf). The pooled meta-analysis was influenced only by original study (Chellan R), so omissions of other studies make little or no difference. When (Chellan R) excluded from the pooled analysis, pooled prevalence of gynecological morbidity reduced from 22% (95% CI=17-27) to 21% (95% CI=16-27) but statistically not significant.

Discussion

This is a comprehensive report attempting to sensitize the prevalence estimation of gynecological morbidity among reproductive age women by using meta-analysis. This comprehensive systematic review with meta-analysis of observational studies conducted in the world included 18 reports and 31,808 women population. Thus, it was possible to provide a reliable estimate of prevalence.

Our comprehensive systematic review and meta-analysis found that 10% of women have had pelvic organ prolapse, 7% of them were infertile; reproductive tract infection is the most 37% followed by menstrual disorder 28%. The pooled random model meta-analysis of overall gynecological morbidity is 22% (95% CI=17%-27%). The average number of complaints of gynecological morbidity ranges from (1.2-1.5); different types of gynecological morbidities may appear concurrently on individual women. The existence of some types may favor condition for the occurrence of the other [13,38,39].

The studies included in this analysis were conducted among reproductive age women at house hold level and health facility among women seeking care for other than gynecological problem. All the studies were observational epidemiological cross-sectional studies drawing sample population by random sampling method.

The response of clients on gynecological morbidity varies by place where interview is conducted and the profession of the interviewer. Respondents complained many types of problem when they were interviewed in a health facility and by health workers [4,13,35]. The proportion of women reporting symptoms were the higher when they were interviewed by physician at health facility than when they were interviewed by lay person at household level [35]. This result strongly suggests that anticipation of treatment influences responses, either by overcoming silence or inviting exaggeration [40]. The result of the prospective study also suggests that repeated interview may elicit greater reporting symptoms than a single interview. Such a trend may reflect the development of closer rapport between respondent and interviewer over successive round or improved proficiency on the part of interviews. Therefore, the results of cross-sectional studies did not compared with prospective studies [40].

Addressing gynecological morbidity is a complex process as women either don't consider it as a significant health problem or hesitate to talk on it. Even though, women with gynecological morbidity face serious social consequences in terms of marital disharmony, exclusion from social and religious life [41]. Gynecological morbidity has a great impact on life of women, their child and family as well. Women with gynecological morbidity may be challenged with multifaceted health, psychological and social problem. According to WHO, reproductive ill health accounts for 36.6% of the total disease burden among women aged 15 to 45 years at a global level [13]. It result in 250 million years of reproductive life loss each year in worldwide and reduce the overall productivity of women as much as 20% [36].

Majority of women do not seek health care until it becomes an emergency. Women were associated with causes of this morbidity with curse, evil eye, watch craft, excessive body heat, and sterilization. Some women accept the problem as normal health ill of women; as a result, they do not seek care [42,43]. Certain untreated conditions can cause pregnancy related complications, congenital infections, infertility, chronic pain and significantly increase the risk of acquiring Pelvic Inflammatory Disease and HIV [41].

Gynecological morbidity was associated with illiteracy, ignorance, gender discrimination and poor social status, lack of decision making power and inability to afford seeking health care, parity, early mirage and age [13,27,44-47].

Cultural sensitive prevention, care and treatment are needed to alleviate the burden of this problem. Educating and empowering women are the magic bullet to maximize women's health and quality of life. In turn, healthy women contribute a lot for countries development.

High levels heterogeneity exhibited within the studies and among groups of studies the (I2=98.02%-99.20%, p=00). Egger's regression test indicated evidence of publication bias for gynecological morbidity (p=0.004 for pelvic organ prolapse and p=0.03 for infertility). But, there was no evidence of publication bias for reproductive tract infection (p=0.40), menstrual disorder (p=14) and overall gynecological morbidity (p=23). Begg's test indicated no evidence of publication bias of all types of gynecological morbidities.

Studies included in this analysis were conducted in different setup, geographic location, among participants of different cultural background and economic difference with different methodology. This variation leads to heterogeneity of the studies. In addition to this, the bias may be introduced into each study. Some of the paper asked whether participants have problem at any time in the life, in the past 6 month, in the past 3 month and other asked whether they are currently experiencing it. Recall periods of more than 2-4 weeks for closed question, or few days for open-ended questions, they appear to introduce bias from under reporting and misclassification [11].

Measurement and definition variation also affect the results of the same studies. This problem is more observed on menstrual disorder variable. The common recorded types of menstrual disorder include volume (heavy, normal or light), regularity (irregular, regular or absent), frequency (frequent, normal or infrequent), and duration (prolonged, normal or shortened) of menstrual episodes. Each term could be interpreted differently across the globe. To avoid this confusion, the Federation of International Gynecological and Obstetrics (FIGO) introduced a new classification called the PALM-COEIN system of abnormal uterine bleeding (AUB). The basic system comprises four categories that are defined by visually objective structural criteria (PALM: Polyp, Adenomyosis, Leiomyoma, and Malignancy or Hyperplasia); five (COEIN: Coagulopathy, Ovulatory disorders, Endometrium, iatrogenic and not yet classified) [48,49].

The pooled meta-analysis was influenced only by original study (Chellan R) [27]. When (Chellan R) [27] excluded from the pooled analysis, pooled prevalence of gynecological morbidity reduced from 22% (95% CI=17-27) to 21% (95% CI=16-27) but statistically it is not significant. In our study, the individual studies did not influence the pooled estimated prevalence of gynecological morbidities.

Limitation

This systematic review is not free of limitation: majority of the papers used in this analysis were studied in South East Asia. The prevalence of gynecological morbidity from this analysis couldn't be inferred to other developing countries. Unpublished data did not include in this analysis and thus publication biased likely may occur. The other limitation was the papers included in this study were only papers that were written in English language. This may also introduce language bias.

Conclusion

The polled prevalence of overall gynecological morbidity was 22%. This prevalence is not an over estimated prevalence instead it may be underestimated because of silence of women in reporting the problem due to cultural influences, ignorance and embarrassment to talk about the problem. This study showed tips of the ice-berg of gynecological morbidities, and the magnitude of the problem is more than the reported one. From this prevalence, we can conclude that the effect of gynecological morbidity is high to hamper the productivity of reproductive age of women in the world particularly in developing regions.

The common reported gynecological morbidities were reproductive tract infection and menstrual disorders. Theses might be more prevalent among reproductive age women than other. Pelvic organ prolapse is common among menopause women than reproductive age women. Heterogeneity was noted in this analysis for the studies were drawn all over the world with different back ground and methodology. The burden of gynecological morbidity was higher among economically and culturally disadvantageous women.

Authors' Contributions

MD, NA, YB, AW, BM and YD, conceived and designed the paper, performed the statistical analysis, and wrote the paper. All authors read and approved the final manuscript.

References

1. WHO (1978) Declaration of Alma-Ata.
2. AbouZahr C (2003) Safe motherhood: a brief history of the global movement 1947-2002. Br Med Bull 67: 13-25.
3. WHO (1999) Interpreting reproductive health: ICPD Plus 5 Forum. The Hague 4: 28.
4. Bhatia JC, Cleland J, Leela B, Rao NSN (1997) Levels and determinants of gynecological morbidity in a District of South India. Studies in Family Planning 28: 95-103.
5. Zurayk H, Hind K, Nabil Y, Mawaheb El-M, Mohamed F (1993) Concepts and measures of reproductive morbidity. Health Transition Review 3: 17-39.
6. Antrobus P, Adrienne G, Antrobus SN (1994) Challenging the culture of silence: Building alliances to end reproductive tract infections. International Women's Health Coalition, New York, USA.
7. Jejeebhoy S, Koenig M, Elias C (2003) Investigating reproductive tract infection and other gynecological disorders: A multidisciplinary research approach, Cambridge University Press p: 11-29.
8. Ware JE Jr (1995) The status of health assessment 1994. Annu Rev Public Health 16: 327-354.
9. Faundes A (1994) Reproductive tract infections. Int J Gynaecol Obstet 46: 181-187.
10. Kaur S, Jairus R, Samuel G (2013) An exploratory study to assess reproductive morbidities and treatment seeking behavior among married women in a selected community, Ludhiana, Punjab. Nursing and Midwifery Research Journal 9: 3.
11. Sadana R (2000) Measuring reproductive health: review of community-based approaches to assessing morbidity. Bull World Health Organ 78: 640-654.
12. Koenig M, Shepherd M (2001) Alternative study designs for research on women's gynecological morbidity in developing countries. Reprod Health Matters 9: 166-175.
13. Inamdar IF, Sahu P, Doibale MK (2013) Gynecological morbidities among ever married women: A community based study in Nanded city, India. IOSR-JDMS 7: 5-11.
14. Sajan F, Fikree FF (1999) Perceived gynecological morbidity among young ever-married women living in squatter settlements of Karachi, Pakistan. J Pak Med Assoc 49: 92-97.
15. Tehrani FR, Simbar M, Abedini M (2011) Reproductive morbidity among Iranian women; issues often inappropriately addressed in health seeking behaviors. BMC Public Health 11: 863.
16. Moher D, Liberati A, Tetzlaff J, Altman DG (2009) The preferred reporting items for systematic reviews and meta-analyses: The PRISMA statement. J Clin Epidemiol 62: 1006-1012.
17. Zachary M, Sandeep M, Dagmara R, Karolina L (2014) The development of a critical appraisal tool for use in systematic reviews addressing questions of prevalence. Int J Health Policy Manag 3: 1-6.
18. Nyaga VN, Arbyn M, Aerts M (2014) Metaprop: A stata command to perform meta-analysis of binomial data. Arch Public Health 72: 39.
19. Simonian RD, Laird N (1986) Meta-analysis in clinical trials. Control Clin Trials 7: 177-188.
20. Higgins JP, Thompson SG (2002) Quantifying heterogeneity in a meta-analysis. Stat Med 21: 1539-1558.
21. Li ZZ, Li YM, Lei XY, Zhang D, Liu L, et al. (2014) Prevalence of suicidal ideation in Chinese college students: A meta-analysis. PLoS One 9: e104368.
22. Anitha A, Sara V, Mini S, Krishnapillai V, Soumya G, et al. (2014) Pattern of gynecological morbidity, its factors and health seeking behavior among reproductive age group women in a rural community of Thiruvananthapuram district, South Kerala. Indian J Community Health 26: 230-237.
23. Masterson AR, Usta J, Gupta J, Ettinger AS (2014) Assessment of reproductive health and violence against women among displaced Syrians in Lebanon. BMC Womens Health 14: 25.
24. Anjana V, Jitendra K, Bratati B (2015) A comparative study of prevalence of RTI/STI symptoms and treatment seeking behavior among the married women in urban and rural areas of Delhi. Int J Reprod Med p: 563031.
25. Bhanderi MN, Kannan SJ (2010) Untreated reproductive morbidities among ever married women of slums of Rajkot City, Gujarat: The role of class, distance, provider attitudes, and perceived quality of care. J Urban Health 87: 254-263.
26. Bhatnagar N, Khandekar J, Singh A, Saxena S (2013) The silent epidemic of reproductive morbidity among ever married women (15-49 years) in an urban area of Delhi. J Community Health 38: 250-256.
27. Chellan R (2004) Gynecological morbidity and treatment seeking behavior in South India: Evidence from the reproductive and child health survey 1998-1999. J Health Popul Dev Ctries p: 15.
28. Gokler ME, Unsal A, Arslantas D (2014) The prevalence of infertility and loneliness among women aged 18-49 years who are living in semi-rural areas in western turkey women aged 18-49 years who are living in semi-rural areas in western Turkey. Int J Fertility Sterility 8: 155-162.
29. Kumari S, Walia I, Singh A (2000) Self-reported uterine prolapse in a resettlement colony of north India. J Midwifery Womens Health 45: 343-350.
30. Philippov OS, Radionchenko AA, Bolotova VP, Voronovskaya NI, Potemkina TV (1998) Estimation of the prevalence and causes of infertility in western Siberia. Bull World Health Organ 76: 183-187.
31. Asya R, Afifi M, Fathalla MM (2004) Gynecological and related morbidities among ever-married Omani women. Afr J Reprod Health 8: 188-197.
32. Garg S, Sharma N, Bhalla P, Sahay R, Saha R, et al. (2002) Reproductive morbidity in an Indian urban slum: Need for health action. Sex Transm Infect 78: 68-69.
33. Poornima S, Katti SM, Mallapur MD, Vinay M (2013) Gynecological problems of married women in the reproductive age group of urban Belgaum, Karnataka. Al Ameen J Med Sci 6: 226-230.
34. Msuya SE, Mbizvo E, Pedersen BS, Sundby J, Sam NE, et al. (2002) Reproductive tract infections and the risk of HIV among women in Moshi, Tanzania. Acta Obstet Gynecol Scand 81: 886-893.
35. Veronique F, Tom M, Aysen B, Wendy G, Nuray Y (1997) Asking questions about women's reproductive health: validity and reliability of survey findings from Istanbul. Tropical Medicine and International Health 2: 47-56.
36. Vibha VG, Pramodkumar BV, Vikas GD, Manindrapratap S, Sanat KR, et al. (2012) Gynecological morbidities in women of reproductive age group in urban slums of Bhavnagar City. NJCM 3: 557-660.
37. Kaur S, Jairus R, Samuel G (2013) An exploratory study to assess reproductive morbidities and treatment seeking behavior among married women in a selected community, Ludhiana, Punjab. Nurs Midwifery Res J 9: 3.
38. Jayanti MP, Shilpa K, Shobha S, Pratibha M, Vinita S (2012) Current Chlamydia trachomatis infection: A major cause of infertility. J Reprod Infertil 13: 204-210.
39. Gogate A, Gogate S, Karande A, Khanna R, Dollimore N, et al. (1998) Reproductive tract infections, gynecological morbidity and HIV seroprevalence among women in Mumbai, India. Bull World Health Organ 76: 277-287.
40. Bhatia J, Cleland J (2000) Methodological issues in community-based studies of gynecological morbidity. Stud Fam Plann 31: 267-273.
41. Faúndes A (1994) Reproductive tract infections. Int J Gynaecol Obstet 46: 181-187.
42. Rangaiyan G, Sureender S (2000) Women perception of gynecological morbidity in south India; Cause and remedies in cultural context. J Family welfare 46: 31-38.

43. Hemachandra DK, Manderson L (2009) Menstrual problems and health seeking in Sri Lanka. Women Health 49: 405-421.
44. Gaash B, Kausar R, Bashir S (2005) Reproductive tract infections in Kargil: A community based study. Health and Population-perspectives and issues 28: 1-8.
45. Jejeebhoy S, Koeing M (2003) Social context of gynecological morbidity: correlates, consequences and health seeking behavior. London: Cambridge University Press 3: 30.
46. Bonetti TR, Erpelding A, Pathak LR (2002) Reproductive morbidity: A neglected issue? Report of a clinic based study in Far-western Nepal, Kathmandu, Nepal p: 2.
47. Indra PK, Dhillon BS, Padam S, Saxena BN, Saxena NC (2003) Self-reported gynecological problems from twenty three districts of India (An ICMR Task Force Study). Indian J Community Med XXVIII: 2.
48. Munro MG, Critchley HO, Fraser IS, FIGO Menstrual Disorders Working Group (2011) The FIGO classification of causes of abnormal uterine bleeding in the reproductive years. Fertil Steril 95: 2204-2208.
49. Bahamondes L, Ali M (2015) Recent advances in managing and understanding menstrual disorders. F1000 Prime Rep 7: 33.

Postpartum Family Planning Utilization among Postpartum Women in Public Health Institutions of Debre Berhan Town, Ethiopia

Takele Gezahegn Demie[1*], Tigist Demissew[2], Tufa Kolola Huluka[1], Derara Workineh[3] and Helen G Libanos[1]

[1]*Department of Public Health, College of Health Sciences, Debre Berhan University, Debre Berhan, Ethiopia*

[2]*Department of Surgical, College of Health Sciences, Debre Berhan University, Debre Berhan, Ethiopia*

[3]*Dawe Serer District Health Office, Bale Zone, Oromia Regional State, Ethiopia*

[*]**Corresponding author:** Takele Gezahegn Demie, Department of Public Health, College of Health Sciences, Debre Berhan University, Debre Berhan, Ethiopia, E-mail: takele.gez44@gmail.com

Abstract

Background: A mother's health has become one of the important agendas in the development of a nation. Family Planning (FP) use during post-partum has the potential to significantly reduce unintended pregnancies and ensure adequate birth spacing.

Objectives: The aim of this study was to assess Family Planning (FP) use among postpartum women and factors associated with it in public health institutions of Debre Berhan town, Ethiopia.

Method: A facility-based cross-sectional study was conducted among 248 women in Debre Berhan town. Simple random sampling technique was used for sample selection. An interviewer-administered structured and pre-tested questionnaire was used to collect data. Data entry and cleaning were done using Epi Info version 3.5.4, and analyzed using SPSS version 20.0 software. Multivariate binary logistic regression analysis was employed to identify factors associated with Postpartum Family Planning (PPFP) use. Variables significantly associated with Postpartum Family Planning (PPFP) use in bivariate analysis were selected for multivariate analysis.

Result: Among total study subjects, about 238 (96%) women had information about Family Planning (FP). Sixty three (25.4%) postpartum mothers were reported resumption of sexual intercourse. In total, 82 (41.6%) women started using contraceptive during postpartum period. Resumption of sexual intercourse [(AOR=2.01; 95% CI: (1.906-5.402)], resuming of sex before six month [(AOR=1.89; 95% CI: (1.906-5.402)] and return of menses [(AOR=1.907; 95% CI: (5.01-20.174)] were significantly associated with utilization of Postpartum Family Planning (PPFP).

Conclusion: Postpartum Family Planning (PPFP) use is still low. Therefore, strengthening health education, sexual and Family Planning (FP) counseling, integrating with other service delivery and promoting PPFP should be recommended.

Keywords: Antenatal care; Amenorrhea; Family Planning (FP); Postpartum women; Public health

Abbreviations: AOR: Adjusted Odds Ratio; ANC: Antenatal Care; COR: Crude Odds Ratio; ETB: Ethiopian Birr; FP: Family Planning (FP); HCs: Health Centers; IUCD: Intra Uterine Contraceptive Device; LAM: Lactation Amenorrhea Method; PNC: Postnatal Care; PPFP: Postpartum Family Planning (FP); SRS: Simple Random Sampling; SPSS: Statistical Software for Social Sciences; WHO: World Health Organization

Background

A mother's health has become one of the important agendas in the development of a nation. The postnatal period is especially critical for mothers as most deaths of mothers occur within this period. This time is an ideal time to deliver interventions that improve the health and survival of mothers. An important element that has been identified in women's health care is sexual practice and Family Planning (FP) during the postpartum period [1,2]. In developing countries, the rapid population growth is attributed to high levels of fertility. Modern contraception has been proven as the most effective method for fertility reduction. Effective contraception also prevents unintended pregnancy and ensures adequate birth spacing. Pregnancy and child birth changes a woman's priorities, attitudes, lifestyle, sexual behaviors, the decision for contraceptive uptake, and the preferred contraceptive method [3-7]. Postpartum Family Planning (PPFP) is defined as the prevention of unintended pregnancy and closely spaced pregnancies through the first 12 months following childbirth [5,6,8]. It is the initiation and use of contraceptives during the first year after delivery [9]. During postpartum period, Family Planning (FP) can prevent about 30% of maternal mortality and 10% of child mortality if couples space their pregnancies more than 2 years apart. In contrary, closely spaced pregnancies within the first year postpartum increase the risks of preterm birth, low birth weight and small-for-gestational-age babies. The risk of child mortality is highest for very short birth-to-pregnancy intervals (i.e. less than 12 months). The timing of the return of fertility after childbirth is variable and unpredictable. Women can get pregnant before the return of menstruation [3,5,8,10,11]. Global and national policies have refocused attention on PPFP as an important intervention to ensure healthy outcomes for women and infants [12]. Uptake of PPFP remains low in sub-Saharan Africa and very little is known about how pregnant women arrive at their decisions to adopt PPFP [11]. The postpartum period is an important intervention for improving access to Family Planning (FP) service. Postpartum women are among those with the greatest unmet need for Family Planning (FP). Significant factors influencing the uptake of Family Planning (FP) are likely to be: level of education, antenatal and postnatal Family Planning (FP) counseling, menses return, breastfeeding status, and return of sexual activity [13-18]. Modern contraceptive use by currently married Ethiopian women has steadily increased over the last 15 years, jumping from 6% of women using modern contraceptive method in 2000 to 35% in 2016 [19]. In Addis Ababa and Dire Dewa, 55% and 21% of childbearing women adopted modern postpartum Family Planning (FP) (PPFP) respectively [20]. About 86% of the women in Ethiopia have an unmet need during their first year postpartum, but only 8% are using any method of Family Planning (FP). Only 5% of women during the 12-month postpartum period desire another birth within two years [6,14,21-23]. Though the World Health Organization (WHO) recommends that pregnancies be spaced by at least 24 months, nearly half (47%) of postpartum women have short (<23 months) birth-to-pregnancy intervals in Ethiopia [6]. Resumption of sex exposes postpartum mothers to risk of unintended pregnancy even before return of menstruation after delivery. Nearly half, (47%), of women use contraceptive during the extended postpartum period. Among those, 10 (2.4%) women adopted Family Planning (FP) in the first 42 days after delivery, 76 (18%) during the first three months and 156 (37%) during the first six months after delivery. Injectable, accounts to 77%. Discussion with husband, knowledge of Family Planning (FP) and use of antenatal care (ANC), postnatal care (PNC) and child immunization services was positively correlated with likelihood of using PPFP [24]. Many of the studies focus on the socio-economic, cultural and physical barriers which women need to overcome in order to adopt a method of contraception. However, less attention has been paid to Family Planning (FP) uptake among postpartum women. Therefore, this study aimed to assess the prevalence and determinant factors of utilization of contraceptive methods among postpartum women in public health institutions Debre Berhan town, Ethiopia. The result of the study can be used to develop educational programs and effective PNC strategies on Postpartum Family Planning (PPFP).

Methods and Materials

Study setting and participants

A facility-based cross-sectional study was conducted in public health institutions of Debre Berhan town from March 1-15, 2016. Debre Berhan town is a capital of North Shewa Zone of Amhara regional state, Ethiopia. The town is situated 130 kilometers to the Northeast of Addis Ababa, on the main route of the country's corridor which connects the capital city of Ethiopia, Addis Ababa, with Tigray Regional State. There are one public referral hospital and three Health Centers (HCs) in this town. Around 250, 200, 70 and 30 mothers' accessed service from Debre Berhan referral hospital, Kebele 04 HC, Kebele 07 HC and Kebele 08 HC respectively within 14 weeks postpartum since the previous year. The study participants were postpartum women who came for postnatal care (after six weeks postpartum) or brought their babies for immunization and/or come for Family Planning (FP) (within 14 weeks of postpartum). Critically ill women and those who didn't consent for participation were excluded from the study.

Sample size and sampling technique

This study was done on 248 postpartum women. Sample size was determined using the single population proportion formula considering 95% confidence level, an expected proportion of women who resumed sexual intercourse within six weeks postpartum of 57.8% [1] and marginal error of 5%. Study participants were selected from all public health institutions in the town with proportional allocation to population size (i.e. client flow) using simple random sampling (SRS) techniques.

Data collection and study variables

Pre-tested interviewer-administered questionnaire was used to collect data. The questionnaire comprise of socio-demographic characteristics of the participant, maternal medical and obstetric history, postpartum sexual history, and Postpartum Family Planning (PPFP) utilization. Questionnaire was adapted from previous literatures [1,25-27], and prepared in English and translated to Amharic. Completeness and consistency of data was checked on daily basis. The dependent variable was Postpartum Family Planning (PPFP). In this study postpartum is the period beginning immediately after the child birth and extending for about six weeks. Modern Family Planning (FP) includes male/female sterilization, pills, Intra Uterine Contraceptive Device (IUCD), Injectable, Implants, male/female condom, Lactation Amenorrhea Method (LAM), Emergency Contraception (EC).

Data management and analysis

Data was entered and cleaned using EpiInfo version 3.5.4 and analyzed by SPSS software version 20. Descriptive statistics were used to summarize findings: means and standard deviations for numerical variables, and frequencies along with percentages for categorical variables. The prevalence of early resumption of sexual intercourse was computed as the proportion of participants who resumed sexual intercourse before end of six weeks postpartum. Binary logistic regression was performed to determine the factors associated with PPFP. A crude odds ratio with 95% confidence interval was calculated for all variables included in the bivariate model. All variables found significantly associated at p-value<0.05 with Postpartum Family Planning (PPFP) use in the bivariate analysis were selected for multivariate analysis. A 95% confidence interval that excludes the null value, 1, indicates statistical significance.

Result

Participants socio-demographic characteristics

A total of 248 postpartum mothers were interviewed giving 100% response rate. Majority of the mothers (41.5%) belongs to 25-29 years age group with mean age of 27.40 (± 4.96 SD). Majority of the women, 209 (84.3%), were follower of Orthodox Christian by religion, and about 225 (90.7%) of the study participants were from Amhara by ethnicity. Of the study participants, 100 (40.3%) were housewife; 78 (31.5%) had attained elementary level of education; and 226 (91.1%) were married and in-union. About 184 (49.3%) had delivered their second child; and 243 (65%) of their spouses had attained secondary level of education (Table 1).

Item	Response	Frequency	Percentage (%)
Age	15-19	3	1.2
	20-24	66	26.6
	25-29	103	41.5
	30-34	51	20.6
	35-39	20	8.1
	40+	5	2
Residence	Urban	189	23.8
	Semi-urban	59	76.2
Religion	Orthodox	209	84.3
	Protestant	15	6
	Muslim	23	9.3
	Catholic	1	0.4
Ethnicity	Amhara	225	90.7
	Oromo	12	4.8
	Tigre	4	1.6
	Gurage	5	2
	Agaw	2	0.8
Current marital status	Married and in-union	226	91.1
	Engaged (Illegally)	9	3.6
	With boy friend	6	2.4
	Divorced	6	2.4
	Widowed	1	0.4
Maternal educational status	Illiterate	23	9.3
	Informal education attendant	13	5.2
	Elementary attendant	78	31.5
	High school/prep.	67	27
	College/university	67	27
Occupation of mother	House wife	100	40.3
	Governmental employed	57	23
	Private employee	17	6.9
	Self-employed	34	13.7
	Farmer	26	10.5
	Student	11	4.4
	Other	3	1.2

Monthly income (in ETB)	0-585	13	5.2
	586-1650	31	12.5
	1651-3145	108	43.5
	3146-5195	68	27.4
	5196-7758	21	8.5
	7759+	7	2.8

Table 1: Socio-demographic characteristics of the postpartum women in Debre Berhan town public health institutions, Ethiopia, May 2016.

Postpartum sexual characteristics of study participants

Overall, 63 (25.4%) postpartum mothers were reported resumption of sexual intercourse during the first six weeks after childbirth. The earliest time was within the first week of postpartum. Majority of the women (92.3%) did not receive any advice about postpartum sexual intercourse (Table 2).

Items	Response	Frequency	Percentage (%)
Resumed sexual intercourse	Yes	88	35.5
	No	160	64.5
Timing of resumption	Before 6 weeks	63	55.44
	After 6 weeks	25	44.56
Got advice/information about postpartum sexual intercourse	Yes	19	7.7
	No	229	92.3

Table 2: Postpartum sexual characteristics of postpartum women in Debre Berhan town, public health institutions, Ethiopia, May 2016.

Postpartum Family Planning (FP) utilization

Out of 248 interviewed, 238 (96%) women had information (awareness) about Family Planning (FP). But, only 82 (41.6%) women of those who had awareness started using contraceptive. Partners feeling towards the using of contraceptive method during postpartum period was found positive (Table 3).

Items	Response	Frequency	Percentage (%)
Use Family Planning (FP)	Ever user	196	82.7
	Current user	82	41.6
Contraceptive methods used (for current user)	Condom	3	3.7
	Pills	3	3.7
	Injectable	34	41.5
	Implant	20	24.4
	IUCD	22	26.8
Attitude of sexual partner towards contraceptive use by the women	Positive	185	75.5
	Indifferent	19	7.8
	Has no feeling	11	4.5
	Against	6	2.4

	Don't know	24	9.8

Table 3: Postpartum Family Planning (PPFP) utilization by postpartum women in Debre Berhan town public health institutions, Ethiopia, May 2016.

The reasons why the women do not use postpartum contraceptive

Among the women who do not use contraceptive during postpartum period, most of them [197 (54.6%)] reason out using contraceptive is not necessary as they were not started sexual activity (Figure 1).

Also only 21(8.7%) women have information about safe contraceptive method for lactating mothers.

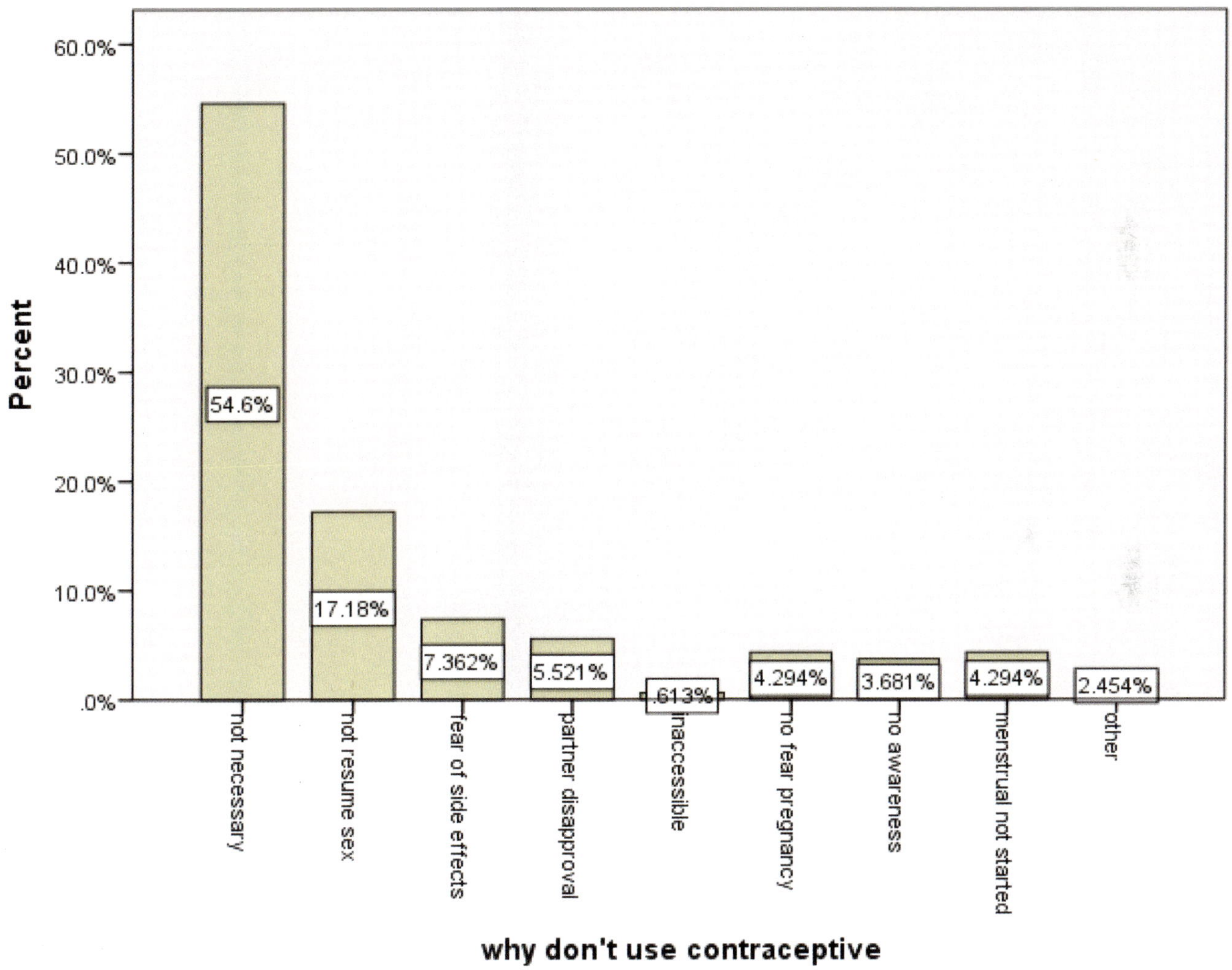

Figure 1: Reasons for why postpartum women do not use contraceptive methods in Debre Berhan town public health institutions, Ethiopia, May 2016.

Association between participants characteristics and contraceptive utilization during postpartum period

Starting sexual intercourse during the first six weeks postpartum was associated with the utilization of Family Planning (FP) during postpartum period.

Those women who resumed sexual intercourse during the first 6 weeks postpartum were used contraceptive methods two times than those who did not resume sexual activity.

Also the timing of resumption of sexual intercourse and return of menses were found to be associated with Postpartum Family Planning (PPFP) utilization.

Women who had saw menses and started sexual intercourse during postpartum period were two times more likely to use Postpartum Family Planning (PPFP) within the first six weeks than those who didn`t see menses and initiated sexual intercourse (Table 4 and Figure 2).

Women who had saw menses and started sexual intercourse during postpartum period were two times more likely to use Postpartum Family Planning (PPFP) within the first six weeks than those who didn`t see menses and initiated sexual intercourse (Table 4 and Figure 2).

Variables	Postpartum Family Planning (PPFP) Use		P-value	OR with 95% CI	
	Yes	No		COR	AOR
	N (%)	N (%)			
Start Sex			0		
Yes	44(53.7%)	38(46.3)	0	3.5(1.96, 6.6)	2.01(1.906, 5.402)***
No	28(24.3%)	87(75.7%)		0.5(1)	
Time of Resuming Sex			0.008		
During first 6 weeks	29(65.9%)	20(71.4%)	0.008	2.5(1.27, 4.78)	1.89(1.906, 5.402)**
Since 45 days	15(34.1%)	8(28.6%)	0.042	0.29(1)	
Menses			0.047		
Resumed	59(72%)	96(83.5)	0.047	0.5(0.26, 1)	1.907(5.01, 20.174)*
Not resumed	23(28%)	19(16.5%)	0.019	1.6(1)	
Religion			0.435		
Others	61(74.4%)	91(79.1%)	0.435	0.77(0.39, 1.5)	
Orthodox	21(25.6%)	24(20.9%)	0.135	1.95(1)	
Parity			0.567		
1-2	63(76.8%)	83(72.2%)	0.326	0.33(0.36, 3)	
3-4	18(22%)	28(24.3%)	0.415	0.39(0.04, 3.76)	
	1(1.2%)	4(3.5%)	0.215	4(1)	
Age of Women			0.292		
15-24	18(22%)	33(28.7%)	0.771	0.85(0.275, 2.6)	
25-35	58(70.7%)	69(60%)	0.253	0.55(0.196, 1.536)	
	6(7.3%)	13(11.3)	0.117	2.17(1)	
Husband Education Status			0.111		
Illiterate	1(1.2%)	3(2.6%)	0.373	2.85(0.285, 28.61)	
Informal school attendant	5(6.1%)	10(8.7%)	0.277	1.9(0.597, 6.07)	
Primary school	21(25.6%)	21(18.3%)	0.896	0.95(0.45, 2)	
High school/preparatory	16(19.5)	40(34.8%)	0.019	2.38(1.15, 4.92)	
College/university	39(47.6%)	41(35.7%)	0.823	1.05(1)	
Maternal Education Status			0.344		
Illiterate	2(2.4)	8(7%)	0.088	4.13(0.81, 21)	
Informal school attendant	3(3.7%)	6(5.2%)	0.334	2.07(0.47, 9)	
Primary school	21(25.6%)	30(26.1%)	0.3	1.5(0.697, 3.13)	

High school/preparatory	25(30.5%)	41(35.7%)	0.143	1.7(0.84, 3.44)	
College/University	31(37.8%)	30(26.1%)	0.898	0.97(1)	

Table 4: Determinants of Postpartum Family Planning (PPFP) utilization among postpartum women of Debre Berhan town, Ethiopia, May 2016.

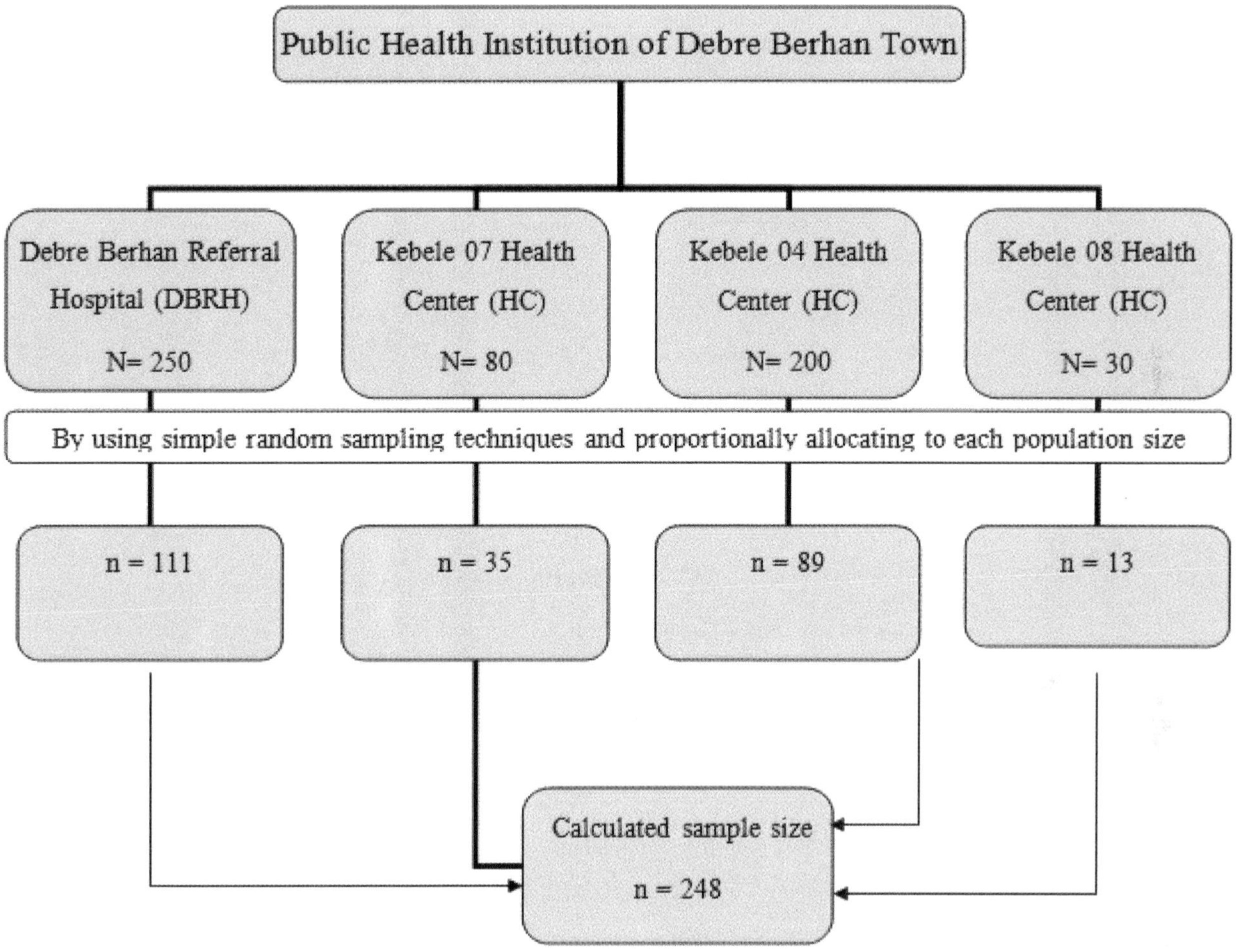

Figure 2: Flow chart indicating sample processes of postpartum women among Debre Berhan town public health institutions, Ethiopia, May 2016.

Discussion

This is a facility based cross sectional study in an attempt to assess Postpartum Family Planning (PPFP) use during the first 6 weeks after child birth. The mean age of study subjects was 27.40 (± 4.96) with the youngest mother is 18 years and oldest being 42 years which almost similar with the study conducted in 6 Addis Ababa. Majority of study participants were Orthodox (84.3%) by religion and Amhara (90.7%) by ethnicity. Likewise, research conducted in Addis Ababa revealed similar findings [1]. Among 248 study participants, only 63 (25.4%) had resumed sexual intercourse during postpartum period within the first six weeks, which is lower compared to the result of the study done in Ethiopia [1] and Nigeria [25]. This may be attributed to over dominance of Orthodox religion followers of study participants and their strong adherence to their religion. But regarding the time of resumption of sexual intercourse, earliest time was within the first week which was similar with study done in Addis Ababa [1] but shorter compared to study conducted in Uganda [27] and Nigeria [25]. This difference may be attributed to cultural difference.

Women stated many reasons as to why they resumed sexual intercourse within 6 weeks of postpartum period. The demand by husbands (85.2%) was an important factor as reported by the women. It is so far higher than similar study conducted in Ethiopia [1] which was indicated to be 31.6%. The other reason for sexual resumption includes: feeling comfortable (54.5%), fulfilling cultural demands (28.4%). This is comparable with the result of the study done in Ethiopia [1] but higher than the result of the study conducted in Uganda [27]. This may be due to cultural differences. In this study significant number (21.0%) of mothers experienced some sort of health related morbidity including. This was similar to that study conducted in Ethiopia [1] and in Uganda [27] which was 21.1% and 22.2% respectively. Other studies conducted where also indicated similar finding [21,26,28]. On the other hand, the reasons stated for not resuming sex included: husband was away, religion expectation, no interest, poor self-image, not feeling good secondary to stitch or Cesarean section done, health profession advices, cultural prohibition, not start to see menstruation. These are similar reason listed in the study conducted in Ethiopia [1] and Uganda [27]. Religion expectation is the major reason why the women do not resume sexual intercourse during puerperium.

Only 7.7% ever received an advice from a health care provider about postpartum sexual activity which is lower compared to study conducted in Ethiopia [1]. Among study participants 41.6% were currently started using contraceptive methods. This result is comparable with the result of the study conducted in three African countries [29] but slight lower than the result of the study done in Ethiopia [1]. Resumption of sexual intercourse, time of initiation of sexual intercourse and return of menses were found to be significantly associated with Postpartum Family Planning (FP) utilization by postpartum women. This association also shown in the study conducted in different African countries [21] and in Addis Ababa [1].

Conclusion

Only 25.4% of the study participants resume sexual intercourse within 6 weeks of postpartum. Postpartum Family Planning (PPFP) utilization is low in the study area. Injectable contraceptive methods were the most preferred choice among respondents in the study. Those who resumed sexual intercourse before 6 weeks and who had seen menses were more likely used postpartum contraceptive methods. Resumption of sexual intercourse, time of initiation of sexual intercourse and return of menses were found to be significantly associated with Postpartum Family Planning (PPFP) utilization by postpartum women.

Family Planning (FP) service providers and all health care providers should focus specifically on immediate postpartum contraception by providing health education on fertility return behaviors, benefits of breastfeeding in preventing unintended pregnancies within the first six months postpartum and initiation of contraception before the return of menses or resumption of sexual activity as conception could precede return of menses after delivery. Strengthening Family Planning (FP) counseling, integrating PPFP with maternal and child health service delivery and promoting PPFP should be recommended.

Author Contributions

Derara Workineh and Takele Gezahegn conceived and designed the study. Derara Workineh, Takele Gezahegn, Tufa Kolola, Tigist Demissew, and Helen G Libanos were involved in the conduct, analysis, data interpretation, and report writing. Takele Gezahegn drafted the manuscript and reviewed, edited and finalized the manuscript. All authors have read and agreed to the final manuscript.

Acknowledgments

We are thankful to Debre Berhan University for material support and to Debre Berhan town public health institutions for their cooperation. We are also thankful to the study participants for their voluntary participation.

Ethics and Consent

Ethical clearance was obtained from the Ethical Review Committee of Debre Berhan University, Institute of Medicine and Health Sciences. A formal letter was obtained from the department of Public Health, Debre Berhan University and Health Department of North Shewa Zone. All participants were given detail information about the purpose of the study, no names were used to report findings and informed verbal consent was obtained from all participants for their willingness to participate in the study.

Paper Context

There is limited literature about PPFP utilization. Also most of them are reports and reviews. This paper presents primary data about the utilization of PPFP. Postpartum Family Planning (PPFP) utilization is low. This indicates that much has to be done in the future to increase utilization and integration of PPFP with other services. Health education should be provided on fertility return behaviors, and initiation of contraception before the return of menses or resumption of sexual activity.

References

1. Tesfay F, Mesfin E (2014) Assessment of sexual activity in post-partum in union women in Addis Ababa, Ethiopia: A prospective cross sectional descriptive study in six immunization clinics.
2. Alum AC, Kizza IB, Osingada CP, Katende G, Kaye DK (2015) Factors associated with early resumption of sexual intercourse among postnatal women in Uganda. Reprod Health 12: 1-8.
3. Wuni C (2015) Contraceptive uptake among postpartum women attending child welfare clinics in Sunyani Municipality, Ghana.
4. Singh S, Darroch JE (2012) Adding it up: Costs and benefits of contraceptive services: Guttmacher Institute and UNFPA.
5. World Health Organization (2013) Programming strategies for Postpartum Family Planning: 9-56.
6. International Pathfinder (2016) Expanding contraceptive options for postpartum women in Ethiopia: Introducing the postpartum IUD.
7. Cleland J, Conde-agudelo A, Peterson H, Ross J, Tsui A (2012) Family Planning, contraception and health. Res Gate 380: 149-156.
8. USAID, Australian AID, Jhpiego, IPPF, Save the Children, et al. Statement for collective action for postpartum Family Planning: 1-2.
9. Sarvamangala K, Taranum A (2013) Menstrual pattern, sexual behavior and contraceptive use among postpartum women in a tertiary care hospital in Davangere. Medica Innov 2: 61-66.
10. Welsh A (2015) Best practice in postpartum Family Planning. Royal College of Obstetricians and Gynaecologists 1: 1-12.
11. Eliason S, Baiden F, Quansah-asare G, Graham-hayfron Y, Bonsu D, et al. (2013) Factors influencing the intention of women in rural Ghana to adopt postpartum Family Planning. Reprod Health 10: 1-8.
12. Rao SR, Clark H, Rajamani D, Ishaku S, Mane B, et al. (2015) Progesterone vaginal ring: Results of a three-country acceptability study. New York.
13. Verma S, Singh KK, Tanti S (2015) Timing of initiation of contraceptives in extended postpartum period among Indian women.

14. USAID AFPI (2009) Family Planning needs during the extended postpartum period in Ethiopia 27: 1-4.
15. USAID, Foundation B & MG (2011) Counseling for postpartum Family Planning and postpartum IUCD.
16. USAID (2009) Family Planning needs during the extended postpartum period in Mali.
17. USAID (2008) Family Planning needs during the extended postpartum period in Uttar Pradesh, India. Access Fam Plan Initiat pp: 13-15.
18. Report M (2011) Postpartum Family Planning: Building a global movement meeting report pp: 1-12.
19. Central Statistical Agency (CSA) and ICF International. Ethiopia Demographic and Health Survey (2016).
20. Central Statistical Agency, ICF International. Ethiopia demographic and health survey 2011 (2012).
21. Borda M, Winfrey W (2010) Postpartum fertility and contraception: An analysis of findings from 17 Countries pp: 11-50.
22. Central Statistical Agency (CSA) and ICF International. Ethiopian demographic and health survey: Key indicators report (2016).
23. Central Statistical Agency (CSA) Ethiopia mini demographic and health survey. FMoH (2014).
24. Mahilet ASF (2015) Assessment of postpartum contraceptive adoption and associated factors in Butajira Health and Demographic Surveillance Site (HDSS), in Southern Ethiopia.
25. Anzaku A, Mikah S (2014) Postpartum resumption of sexual activity, sexual morbidity and use of modern contraceptives among Nigerian women in jobs. Ann Med Health Sci Res 4: 210-216.
26. Barber SL (2007) Family Planning advice and postpartum contraceptive use among low-income women in Mexico. Int Fam Plan Perspect 33: 6-12.
27. Alum AC, Kizza IB, Osingada CP, Katende G, Kaye DK (2015) Factors associated with early resumption of sexual intercourse among postnatal women in Uganda. Reprod Health 12: 107.
28. Sileo KM (2014) Determinants of Family Planning service uptake and use of contraceptives among postpartum women in Rural Uganda. Master's Theses P: 602.
29. Hounton S, Winfrey W, Barros AJD, Askew I (2015) Patterns and trends of postpartum Family Planning in Ethiopia, Malawi, and Nigeria: Evidence of missed opportunities for integration. Glob Health Action 8: 1-10.

Magnitude of Postpartum Hemorrhage among Women Delivered at Dessie Referral Hospital, South Woll, Amhara Region, Ethiopia

Mastewal Arefaynie Temesgen*

Public Health Department, College of Medicine and Health Sciences, Wollo University, Ethiopia

***Corresponding author:** Mastewal Arefaynie Temesgen, Public Health Department, College of Medicine and Health Sciences, Wollo University, Dessie, Ethiopia; E-mail: marefaynie@yahoo.com

Abstract

Background: Postpartum hemorrhage refers loss of more than 500 and/or 1000 ml of blood within 24 hour following vaginal, caesarean delivery respectively. It is significant public health problem both in developed and developing countries, causing considerable maternal mortality and morbidity. It is highly fatal if diagnosis and treatment is not provided early. In Ethiopia, the government launches different strategies to prevent postpartum hemorrhage. But still more than half of the maternal mortalities occurred after delivery due to hemorrhage. Even though postpartum hemorrhage is one of the major direct causes of maternal death in Ethiopia, there are only few studies done in the country. Therefore, determining magnitude and associated factors that causes postpartum hemorrhage is important to make different interventions.

Objective: The aim of this study is to assess magnitude and factors associated with postpartum hemorrhage in Dessie referral hospital.

Methods and materials: Institutional based cross-sectional study was conducted in Dessie referral hospital from 5th January 2017 to 10th January 2017. A one year document review (8th July 2015-7th July, 2016) was conducted. Data was collected using structured data extraction format from patient cards, admission and discharge summary registrations, operation registration log books and delivery registration log books. Descriptive statistics were done to characterize the study population using different variables. Bivariate and multiple logistic regression models were fitted to control confounding factors. Odds ratios with 95% confidence intervals were computed to identify determinants of preeclampsia.

Result: In this study, the overall magnitude of postpartum hemorrhage was 5.8%. Delivering women who have not ANC follow-up were about eleven (AOR, 11.3, 95% CI, 4.2-30.2) times more risk of developing PPH than those who have ANC follow-up. Delivering women who had 24 hour and more duration of labor were eight (3.0, 23.0) (AOR, 8.3, 95% CI, 3.0-23.0) times more risk of PPH development as compared to these who had less than 24 hour duration of labor.

Conclusion and Recommendation: The overall magnitude of postpartum hemorrhage is low in this study when compared with previous studies. But still it needs the attention of the government to reduce maternal and child mortality and morbidity. Non utilization of ANC, cesarean section, prolonged duration of labor and multiparty are predictors of postpartum hemorrhage. Health care providers should give high attention to initiate ANC, women who give birth by cesarean section.

Keywords: Magnitude; Postpartum hemorrhage; Hepatic dysfunction; Delivery; Cesarean section

Abbreviations: ANC: Antenatal Care; AOR: Adjusted Odds Ratio; CI: Confidence Interval; COR: Crude Odds Ratio; DHS: Demographic and Health Survey; EDHS: Ethiopia Demographic and Health Survey; PNC: Postnatal Care; PPH: Postpartum Hemorrhage

Introduction

Postpartum hemorrhage (PPH) refers loss of more than 500 and/or 1000 ml of blood within 24 hour following vaginal, caesarean delivery respectively. It is also defined as blood loss sufficient to cause hypovolemia, a 10% drop in the hematocrit or requiring transfusion of blood products regardless of the route of delivery [1-4]. PPH is the leading cause of maternal mortality in developing countries (25-43%), but pulmonary embolism is the leading cause of the maternal mortality in case of developed countries. It is a frequent complication of deliveries and its incidence is 2-4%, after vaginal deliveries and 6% after caesarean sections (C/S) [3-7]. Uterine atony, retained products of conception, trauma in genital tract and coagulation abnormalities are important causes of PPH [4,5,8-11]. PPH has long and short term impacts like, chronic illness, disability, increased risk of death and/or poor growth and development of their children, hepatic dysfunction, adult respiratory distress syndrome and renal failure [2,4,12-14]. Reducing maternal mortality is one of the hot agendas, globally and nationally. The government of Ethiopia provides free maternal and pre delivery waiting services regardless of social and economic status of the women. But with this effort, still maternal mortality ratio is high at the national level [15]. PPH is one of the leading direct causes of maternal morbidity and mortality in Ethiopia [16]. But there are only few studies done in the country and particularly in Amhara region.

Therefore, the findings of this study would contribute to the existing knowledge, to explore more about the magnitude and associated factors for PPH and help on the provision of emergency obstetric and gynecological care and functioning health facility based on evidence. Additionally, the finding would be used as baseline data for improving obstetric care in South Wollo by providing base line data for programs implementers and non-governmental organizations (NGOs). It also helps as an input for future planning and intervention for appropriate strategies to prevent maternal morbidity and mortality associated PPH and it would also use as a base line for the scientific community. So the objective of the study is to assess the magnitude and associated factors of PPH in Dessie Referral Hospital from 8th July 2015 to 7th June, 2016.

Methods and Materials

Study setting

The study was conducted at Dessie referral hospital which is located in Dessie town, 401 km away from Addis Ababa, Ethiopia and 482 km from Bahirdar. The catchment total population is estimated to be 8,000,000 of which females are 49.5% and reproductive age women are estimated to be 23.47%. Obstetric ward is the one that serves around 1500 clients per year. The ward is staffed with 3 gynecologist and 31 midwives who provides different maternal health services with a total of 31 beds. One year (8th July 2015 to 7th July, 2016) document review was done for this study.

Sample size determination and procedure

All mothers who were gave birth in Dessie referral hospital were the source and study population. The sample size was determined by using single population proportion, by considering the following assumptions. P=17% [4], Confidence level of 95%, Margin of error 4%. Therefore with this formula, and considering 10% non-response rate, the total sample size was 380 women's chart. All unique medical registration numbers of clients who have gave delivery from 8th July 2015 to 7th July, 2016 was selected from the delivery registration log book, sorted based on their unique medical registration number starting from least and was coded (1,2,3,4,...). Then, by using systematic sampling technique charts was selected. The selected charts were taken from the card room. Then, the trained BSc nurses were filled the required data from the selected charts. The required data which missed from clients chart was searched and filled in to the data extraction format from delivery and operation registration log books.

Study variables and measurement

Postpartum hemorrhage is the outcome variable of this study whereas, age, parity, ANC follow-up, mode of delivery, uterine atony, retained placenta, genital tract trauma, prolonged labor, types of pregnancy, Polyhydraminous were the independent variables that affects PPH. PPH is measured in this study with diagnosis of gynecologist (care provider) who gave deliver services in the hospital and recorded as PPH or not. The data was collected using structured data extracting format developed by using different literatures and client registration book. The data was collected by 4 trained BSc nurses. To assure the quality of data, detail training was given for one day. The data extraction format was pretested at Dessie referral hospital on women's chart not included one the sampling frame before the actual data collection has begun on 30 client card. Day today activities was supervised and corrected by principal investigator.

Data analysis

The completed questionnaire was checked for completeness and consistency by the principal investigator and the coordinators each day and code was given to the completed questionnaire. The data were entered using Epi Info version 3.5.1 and transferred to SPSS 20.0 statistical package for analysis. Data cleaning was performed to check for accuracy, consistencies, and values. Then errors were identified and corrected. Univariate analysis using frequency technique was used to describe the data according to some important characteristics of the study subjects. Then the data were expressed in percentage, means, medians and standard deviations. Then bivariate logistic regression was used to see the crude association between the independent variables and the dependent variable and the strength of association was expressed in Odds Ratio (OR). Variables with ($p<0.25$) were analyzed by using multivariate logistic regression to control confounding effects. For all statistical tests P-value ≤ 0.05 was used as a cut-off point for statistical significance.

Result

Reproductive history of women who give delivery in Dessie referral hospital

A total of 380 women charts were reviewed in this study. But 3 women's charts were not included in the analysis due to incompleteness. The mean age of women's was 28 years (SD 4). About 355 (94.2%) were married and about 61% were from rural dwellers. One 198 (52.5%) of participants were multipara and 50 (13.3%) had no ANC visit. Abnormalities detected during ANC follow-up were twin pregnancy 27 (7.2%) followed by APH 17 (4.5%). 50 (13.33%) deliveries were cesarean sections (Table 1).

Variables		Frequency	Percent
Age of mother	15-19	20	5.3%
	20-24	127	33.70%
	25-29	147	39%
	30-34	63	16.70%

	≥ 35	20	5.30%
Residence of the women	Urban	148	39.30%
	Rural	222	60.70%
Marital status	Single	22	5.80%
	married	355	94.20%
Parity	Primi Para	101	26.79%
	Multi Para	198	40.05%
ANC visit during the current pregnancy	No	50	13.30%
	Yes	327	86.70%
Gestational age during delivery in weeks	32-37 weeks	20	5.30%
	37-42 weeks	317	84.10%
	>42 weeks	40	10.60%
Place of delivery	Home	47	12.50%
	Institutional	330	87.50%
Mode of delivery	SVD	327	86.70%
	C/S	50	13.33%
Duration of labor	<24 hours	330	87.50%
	>24 hours	47	12.50%
Rapture of membrane before onset of labor	<12 hours	63	57.80%
	>12 hours	46	42.20%

Table 1: Reproductive history of women who give delivery at Dessie Referral Hospital, July 2015-2016 (n=377).

Proportion and causes of postpartum hemorrhage

About 22 cases of PPH were registered which makes the magnitude of PPH is 5.8% during one year period. The causes of PPH identified during the study period were uterine atony (45%) followed by retained placenta (40%) and genital tear (14%) (Figure 1).

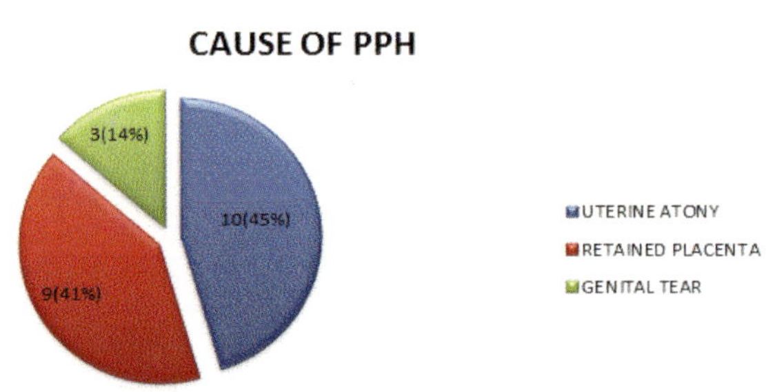

Figure 1: Causes of PPH in women who give delivery at Dessie Referral Hospital, 8th July 2015 to 7th July, 2016.

Factors associated with PPH

Different factors were analyzed for their independent effect on PPH. Delivering women who have not ANC follow-up were about eleven (AOR, 11.3, (30.2), 95% CI, 4.2-30.2) times more risk of developing PPH than those who have at least one ANC follow-up. Delivering women who had 24 hour and more duration of labor were eight (AOR, 8.3, 95% CI, 3.0-23.0) times more risk of PPH development as compared to these who had less than 24 hour duration of labor. Delivering women who had given delivery by cesarean section were about five (AOR, 5.3, 95% CI, 1.8-15.8) times more risk of developing PPH as compared to these who had given spontaneous vaginal delivery (Table 2).

Variables	Postpartum hemorrhage		COR	AOR
	Yes	No		
ANC				
No	12 (24%)	38 (76%)	10.0 (4.1, 24.7)	11.3 (4.2, 30.2)
Yes	10 (3.05%)	317 (96.8%)		
Duration of labor				
<24 hours	12 (3.6%)	318 (96.3%)		

≥ 24 hours	10 (21.2%)	37 (78.7%)	7.2 (2.9, 17.7)	8.3 (3.0, 23.0)
Mode of Delivery				
SVD	14 (4.3%	313 (96.3%)		
C/S	8 (16%)	42 (78.7%)	4.3 (1.7,10.8)	5.3 (1.8, 15.8)
Parity				
Primi Para	1 (0.99%)	100 (99%)		
Multi Para	7 (4.6%)	144 (95.36%)	4.9 (0.6, 40.1)	4.3 (0.6, 36.0)
Grand multi Para	14 (11.2%)	111 (88.8%)	12.6 (1.6, 97.6)	12.4 (1.6, 97.2)

Table 2: Factors associated with PPH among women who give delivery at Dessie Referral Hospital, July 2015-2016 (n=377).

Discussion

In a one year period the overall magnitude of PPH was 5.8% (22 of 377). The magnitude is relatively lower than previous studies. In Pakistan hospital [7.1%] and prospective study done at Gonder town (18%), Uganda (9%), Cameron (23%) [1,4,8,14]. The difference could be due to coverage differences of the study subjects and study design. Improvement of ANC services through time would contribute for the discrepancy. ANC is an important maternal health interventional area which reduces the occurrence of PPH by providing early diagnosis and treatment of preexisting disease, complications and health promotion and disease prevention actions like, feeding practice, personal hygiene which are essential services to decrease pregnancy related complications like PPH. Other justification would be, in Ethiopia institutional delivery utilization is increased from time to time which prevents PPH by removal of retained products, giving oxytocin for contraction of uterus. In our study the blood loss is estimated based on provider's observation and judgment. But other studies use standard blood loss measurements. In line with other findings, the commonest causes of PPH in this study are uterine atony (45%) and retained placenta (41%) [8,14].

ANC follow-up reduces occurrence of PPH. In Ethiopia Now a days, the government provides focused ANC for pregnant women based on evidence. Therefore pregnant women get interventions based on their problem. During ANC follow-up, potential risk factors for pregnancy related complications including PPH are predicted and interventions like, iron-follet supplementation, nutritional interventions are important actions to reduce PPH. During ANC service providers encourage institutional delivery, family planning utilization reduces high risk pregnancies (too many, narrow and late) which are potential risk factor for PPH. Prolonged labor increases the risk of PPH by eight folds. The result is supported by other literatures. As the duration of labor increases the risk of developing PPH also increases. Prolonged labor will also cause uterine atony [12,14].

Parity of the women had increase development of PPH. The finding is supported by other researches [1,8,13]. As the number of pregnancies and live birth increases the risk of PPH is high. Parity increases both the occurrence of secondary and primary PPH. Advanced age would increase the risk of anemia and blood coagulation problem which are responsible factors for PPH. Cesarean section increases the risk of PPH than vaginal delivery. The finding is supported by other researches [8-11]. Cesarean section increases the vasodilatation and most emergency cesarean section is performed to relief abnormal labor condition that that increases uterine atony.

Limitations

It mainly focuses on individual level factors and factors related to the health system and the service providers did not included, the socio cultural factors and related misconception on maternal health services feeding practices. So the study would not representative of the catchment area since women who were give delivery at home were not assessed. The data is secondary which makes us from detail analysis of different factors.

Conclusion and Recommendations

The overall magnitude of postpartum hemorrhage is low in this study when compared with previous studies. But still it needs the attention of the government to reduce maternal and child mortality and morbidity. Non utilization of ANC, cesarean section, prolonged duration of labor and multiparty are predictors of postpartum hemorrhage. Based on the findings the following recommendations were given. As maternal health services (ANC, institutional delivery and PNC) are potential times for counseling of mothers about post-partum FP, counseling about modern family planning should get more focus. There is great need to prioritize education of girls to empower them to use postpartum FP and policies need to encourage women to be supported by their spouses and to promote postpartum family planning. In addition there is need to improve the quality of knowledge on the recommended postpartum contraceptives to enable extended post-partum mothers make informed choices, which can be facilitated by strengthening client-provider interaction especially through maternal and child health services.

Ethical Consideration

Letter of ethical clearance was obtained from Wollo University collage of medical and health sciences, institutional health research ethics review committee about the importance of the research for the community and the harms that would be occurred during data collection. Official letter was written to Dessie referral hospital. Collection of clinical data from hospital registers and medical records is authorized by the hospital administrative and does not require women consent. Confidentiality of information was maintained by giving codes for women's chart rather than recording their name.

Authors' Contributions

MA was the principal investigator (conception and design of the study, acquisition of data, analysis of data, interpretation of data, and revising the paper), and also involved in data analysis, revising the paper and manuscript write-up.

Acknowledgements

We would like to thank all contributors those who made the finalization of this research.

Competing interests

The author declares that he has no competing interest.

Funding

The funding for this study was self.

References

1. Gani N, Ali TS (2013) Prevalence and factors associated with maternal postpartum hemorrhage in Khyber agency, Pakistan. J Ayub Med Coll Abbottabad 25: 81-85.
2. Goonewardene M, Silva C, Medawala M, Karunarathana S (2012) The occurrence, management and outcomes of postpartum hemorrhage in teaching hospital in Srilanka. J Obstet Gynaecol 34: 144-154.
3. Gebeyehu R, Woyessa A (2012) Prevention of postpartum hemorrhage in rural Ethiopia p: 13.
4. Abate T, Kebede B, Feleke A, Misganaw E, Rogers N (2014) Prospective study on birth outcome and prevalence of postpartum morbidity among pregnant women who attended for care in Gonder Town, North West Ethiopia. J Androl 3: 125.
5. Chohan A, Butt F, Mansoor H, Falak T (2006) Primary postpartum hemorrhage: Outcome of different treatment measures Willingdone hospital, Lahore 22: 16-20.
6. Aslam M, Ahmed SR, Rajaba MT (2012) Primary postpartum hemorrhage, still a big challenge in developing world. Annals of King Edward Medical University 18: 17-24.
7. Deshmukh U, Vardhan M (2015) A retrospective study of postpartum hemorrhage at BRIMS 13: 668-670.
8. Ononge S, Mirembe F, Wandabwa J, Campbell OM (2016) Incidence and risk factors for postpartum hemorrhage in Uganda. Reprod Health 13: 38.
9. Sheldon WR, Blum J, Vogel JP, Souza JP, Gülmezoglu AM, et al. (2014) Postpartum hemorrhage management, risks, and maternal outcomes: Findings from the World Health Organization multicounty survey on maternal and newborn health. Int J Gynaecol Obstet Title 1: 5-13.
10. Lutomski JE, Byrne BM, Devane D, Greene RA (2012) Increasing trends in atonic postpartum hemorrhage in Ireland: An 11-year population-based cohort Study 119: 306-314.
11. Kramer MS, Berg C, Abenhaim H, Dahhou M, Rouleau J, et al. (2013) Incidence, risk factors, and temporal trends in severe postpartum hemorrhage. Am J Obstet Gynecol 209: 449e1-e7.
12. Tort J, Rozenberg P, Traoré M, Fournier P, Dumont A (2015) Factors associated with postpartum hemorrhage maternal death in referral hospitals in Senegal and Mali: A cross-sectional epidemiological survey. BMC pregnancy and childbirth 15: 235.
13. Halle GE, Emade FK, Bechem NN, Palle JN, Fongaing D, et al. (2016) Prevalence and risk factors of primary postpartum hemorrhage after vaginal deliveries in the Bonassama district hospital, Cameroon 13: 1-12.
14. Bhavana G, Abhishek MV, Mitta S (2016) A study of risk factor of postpartum hemorrhage and indications for caesarean section. Int J Reprod Contracept Obstet Gynecol 5: 2017-2021.
15. Lisonkova S (2016) Atonic postpartum hemorrhage: Blood loss, risk factors and third stage management. J Obstet Gynaecol Can 38: 1081-1090.
16. CSA (2016) Ethiopia demographic and health survey: Central Statistical Agency Addis Ababa and Calverton.

Identification and Characterization of *Candida* on CHROMAgar™ in Pregnant Women of Multan, Pakistan

Sidra Manzoor[1], Mubashar Aziz[2] and Ahsan Sattar Sheikh[3*]

[1]*Department of Molecular Biology and Biotechnology, University of Veterinary and Animal Sciences, Lahore, Pakistan*

[2]*Department of Pathobiology, Faculty of Veterinary Sciences, Bahauddin Zakariya University, Multan, Pakistan*

[3]*Institute of Food Science and Nutrition, Bahauddin Zakariya University, Multan, Pakistan*

[*]**Corresponding author:** Ahsan Sattar Sheikh, Institute of Food Science and Nutrition, Bahauddin Zakariya University, Multan, Pakistan, E-mail: assheikh@bzu.edu.pk

Abstract

Introduction: Infections to vagina with fungi/yeast are ten times more common during pregnancy because of hormonal and biochemical fluctuations. Increased use of antibiotics and presence of high levels of reproductive hormones during pregnancy also stimulate yeast colonization with *Candida* species. These two contributes significantly to be an important risk factor in Vulvovaginal Candidiasis (VVC) and Urinary Tract Infections (UTI), a complication during pregnancies. Overall occurrence of UTI/vaginal yeast infections increases with progression of pregnancy and maximizes by third trimester worldwide.

Study parameters: In the current study, pregnant women were look for presence of UTI by *Candida* species in different trimesters within the city of Multan. The total of 70 women with different gestational stages, attending gynecologists, aged 18-39 years were included in the investigation. A clean catch urine samples were cultured on CHROMAgar™ *Candida*, a selective medium, for the isolation and presumptive identification of yeast species. Of all samples, 25 women (36%) were positive for *Candida* yeast infection (symptomatically and asymptomatically). Colonies were identified as *C. albicans* (48%), *C. krusei* (16%), *C. tropicalis* (16%) along with some mixed infections with *C. parapsilosis* and *C. krusei*. Two of the mixed cultures (8%) were isolated with *C. albicans* and *C. tropicalis*, one (4%) with *C. albicans* and *C. krusei*, one (4%) with *C. tropicalis* and *C. krusei*.

Results: The highest incidence, 36% (n=9/25), of candiduria was recorded in the age group of 30-35 years. The colony counts in urine were also studied in different gestational stages and age. Total of 23% isolations share high counts (>1000 CFU/mL). While other 33% have intermediate (<600 CFU/mL) and 30% isolates were with low colony counts (<150 CFU/mL). The species distribution in these positive specimens reveals increased percentages of non-albicans species with increasing gestational stage.

Conclusion: From these findings it is concluded that incidence of candiduria in pregnant women were higher in 2nd and 3rd trimester of pregnancy with an increase in mixed *Candida* infections in young women. It is recommended to educate the group so that less young individuals are affected.

Keywords: Pregnancy; Infection; *Candida albicans*; Non-albicans species

Introduction

Vaginosis in pregnancy is most commonly linked to infection by *Candida* species [1]. In female, *Candida* is also part of normal flora and become opportunistic pathogen. In these women with Vulvovaginal candidiasis (VVC), most common problem and affects women two or more episodes yearly [2-4], can also involve urinary tract [5,6]. The infection accounts for 40-50% of all women cases within their childbearing age [7]. Accurate prevalence of these infections are quite difficult to assess as one third to three quarter of affected women 'feel' asymptomatic [7,8]. Recent randomized screening in pregnant women indicates complications like candidiasis, bacterial vaginitis, and/or trichomonasis, are on the increase that could result in spontaneous preterm birth in 46% of pregnancies by 15-19 weeks of gestation [9]. It has been reported that about 75% females develop it at least once in their lifetime [10]. *Candida albicans* is most frequently (90%) isolated form compared to other non albicans species [11]. Recent reports on *Candida* infections suggests that there is a shift in colonization pattern by *C. galabrata* [12] and other non-albicans species within developed countries [13]. From data, it is estimated that *Candida galabrata* account for 4-5% in these country individuals. While other non albicans species appear to be still less common that includes *Candida tropicalis* and *Candida parapsilosis* [14].

It is very difficult to ascertain the involvement of *Candida* species in vaginosis and later with candiduria. During vaginosis more than 50% of these individuals are asymptomatic and harbor endogenous vaginal microbiota [15]. This asymptomatic vaginosis very efficiently gets into urinary tract that could result without tissue invasion [16,17]. Milder signs and symptoms in urinary *Candida* infection don't permit proper diagnosis [18]. Factors like socio-economic variables, maternal smoking, other genital infections and short cervix contributes to increase colonization by *Candida* species [19]. These UTIs are also associated to number of gynecological and obstetric complications, such as preterm birth [20], premature rupture of the membranes, chorioamnionitis [18], postpartum endometritis, inflammatory pelvic disease, intrauterine growth retardation [21], and low birth weight of the new born [1]. There are reports of transfer of *Candida* species from vaginal infection to new born also [5,22]. Increased UTI colonization and candiduria are believed to be due to higher incidences of vaginosis resulting from high estrogen levels, high glycogen content, and use of antifungal agents in treatment of VVC [21,23]. Identification of shared similar drug resistance markers in *Candida* and its species, from urine and vaginal, demonstrates their common ancestral origin [19]. Pregnancy is typically broken into three periods, or trimesters [20]. It has been elucidated with good conviction that *Candida* species can be cultured from the urine or vagina in more than >25% of pregnant women who are approaching term [24]. Prevalence survey in 228 hospitals from 29 European countries determined that just 9.4% of nosocomial UTIs were caused by *Candida* species [11]. During this period considerable high rates are observed with non albicans species. This isolation frequency of non-albicans species especially in some countries, are unclear and dubious of its selection [20]. This scenario is further compounded with presence of antifungal resistance in non-albicans *Candida* species that is a worry for future [25].

Material and Methods

Sample area and collection

Total of 70 randomly collected urine samples from pregnant women in different pregnancy trimesters was included in the study. The subjects were between 18 to 39 years. Sampling was done in local winter-spring season (more marriages in winter months). Urine was collected from antenatal patients' vising medical centers, maternity homes of Multan, Pakistan. Patients were inquired to complete a detailed questionnaire. The questionnaire includes demographic data (age, age at marriage, cousin marriage), number of pregnancies/deliveries, trimester, signs and symptoms related to *Candida* infection. The midstream urine was collected in sterile urine containers (China) and transferred to Micro/Molecular Biology Laboratory (MMBL) at IPAB, Bahauddin Zakariya University, Multan 60800 in a cooler packed with ice packs for further processing.

Media preparation and sample processing

CHROMAgar™ *Candida* was provided by CHROMAgar™, Paris, France. Media plates with antibiotics were made according to the manufacturer instructions. Prepared plates were stored in dark at 4°C till further use. Individual sample (1 mL) was centrifuged in sterile 1.7 mL microfuge tube (China) at 1400 g for 1 minute (Heareus, Germany). Samples having more than 10 WBC/HPF were selected for inoculation on to CHROMAgar™ *Candida* plates (0.1 mL of neat urine) with a pasture glass spreader in a clean bench surface (Dalton, UK). Plates were incubated (Memmert, Germany) at 36 ± 0.5°C for 48 hours. Colonies were identified according to manufacturer's instruction or described by Odds and Bernaerts.

Statistical analysis

Data was formulated from the questionnaire for all parameters and were analyzed for ANOVA and correlation of significance by SPSS 17 (SPSS Inc., USA).

Results

Isolation and identification

Direct presumptive identification of yeast species is a challenging task. Several brands of chromogenic media are available for rapid identification of yeast. This also includes CHROMAgar™ *Candida* [26,27]. This media provides straight forward advantage in time over conventional identification methods in mixed yeast infections. This is also important in significant clinical bearing [28]. In a total of 70 samples, only 25 samples (36%) turned positive for *Candida species* (Table 1).

The chromogenic substances in media help to identify *C. albicans*, *C. krusei*, *C. tropicalis*, and *C. parapsilosis*. The *C. albicans* colonies were identified as green, *C. tropicalis* as steel blue, and *C. krusei* as fuzzy rose colored colonies. *C. parapsilosis* appears with pink to pale yellow colonies [29]. Other groups have also reported further success in differentiation of *C. dubliniensis* from *C. albicans* on CHROMAgar™ *Candida* medium which our group did not performed. From the total positive cultures, *C. albicans* (48%) share the maximum load (Table 1).

Non albicans *Candida* share just 32% in pure culture category. Mixed culture infections of *C. albicans* with either *C. krusei* or *C. tropicalis* (12% and 8% respectively) as non albicans were also recorded in the study.

	Pure culture				Mixed culture			
Age Group	*C. albicans*	*C. krusei*	*C. tropicalis*	*C. parapsilosis*	*C. albicans* *C. krusei*	*C. albicans* *C. tropicalis*	*C. krusei* *C. tropicalis*	*C. krusei* *C. parapsilosis*
18-23 Y (n=21)	2 (10%)	2 (10%)	1 (5%)	-	-	1 (5%)	1 (5%)	1 (5%)
24-29 Y (n=29)	4 (13%)	1 (3%)	-	-	2 (7%)	-	-	-
30-35 Y (n=19)	6 (32%)	1 (5%)	2 (11(%)	-	-	-	-	-
36-41 Y (n=1)	-	-	1 (100%)	-	-	-	-	-
	n=20				n=5			

Table 1: Relationship between age and *Candida* species infection in pregnant women.

Pregnancy trimester and *Candida* species

Breakup of pregnancy into trimester showed that most positive yeast infection occurred in the 3rd trimester (36%) (Table 1). Out of 15 positive cultures only 2 had mixed culture outcome (Table 2). In the 2nd trimester, highest number of specimens collected turned positive (47%). The species isolated and identified in all trimester specimens showed that 80% have single organism (Table 1).

CFU/mL	Age groups (Years)			
	18-23	24-29	30-35	36-41
<150 (n=9)	4	3	1	1
<300 (n=4)	2	-	2	-
<600 (n=10)	4	3	3	-
>1000 (n=7)	1	3	3	-

Table 2: Relationship between age and vaginal *candida* burden in pregnant women.

Interestingly, 60% of positive colorizations were within 3rd trimester (Table 2). Presence of *C. krusei C. albicans* or *C. tropicalis* or *C. parapsilosis* were identified in 4 cultures (20%) and 4 mixed cultures respectively (Table 2).

Age, *Candida* species and yeast burden

There were 15 *Candida albicans* cultures (60%) isolated that were either pure or mix with *C. krusei* or *C. tropicalis*. All mixed infections (20%) were, interestingly, present in all young age groups (18-23 years) and (24-29 years). In the middle age group, only single organism infection (predominantly *C. albicans*- 67%) occurred (Tables 2 and 3).

Talking about the yeast burden, most infections (>600 CFU/mL) were identified in middle age groups (24-29) years and 30-35 years) (Table 3). This group also is dominated by pure cultures by 2/3 positivity with *C. albicans*. Low yeast counts were predominantly noticed in only younger age groups (Table 3).

Pregnancy (trimester)	Infected n=25	Pure Culture				Mixed Culture			
		C. albicans	C. krusei	C. tropicalis	C. parapilosis	C. albicans C. krusei	C. albicans C. tropicalis	C. krusei C. tropicalis	C. krusei C. parapilosis
1st (n=11)	2 (18%)	-	-	1	-	1	-	-	-
2nd (n=17)	8 (47%)	4	2	-	-	1	1	-	-
3rd (n=42)	15 (36%)	8	2	3	-	-	-	1	1
Total=70	25	12	4	4	-	2	1	1	1

Table 3: Distribution of positive culture with trimesters of pregnancies.

Statistical analysis

ANOVA and correlation analysis on various factors indicated that yeast infections were highly significant (p=0.000 at 95% CI) to the pregnancy in this study. Analysis also correlates to *Candida* cell counts which is highly significant to pregnancy month (Pearson's Correlation 0.872 and significance of 0.000 at 0.01% CL) and trimester (Pearson's Correlation 0.447 and significance of 0.000 at 0.01% CL).

Data also specify that numbers of pregnancies are also significantly placed to the age and symptoms (Tables 4 and 5).

Pearson's Correlations (n=70)						
Variables		Age	CFU/mL	Deliveries	Pregnancies	Candida Sp.
Age	Pearson Correlation					
	Sig (2-tailed)					
CFU/mL	Pearson Correlation	1		-	-	-
	Sig (2-tailed)					
Deliveries	Pearson Correlation	0.422**	1	1	-	-

	Sig (2-tailed)	0	-			
	Pearson Correlation	0.506**	-	0.784**		-
Pregnancies	Sig (2-tailed)					
	Pearson Correlation	0	0.557**	0	1	
Candida Sp.	Sig (2-tailed)	-	0	-	-	1

Table 4: Pearson's correlation of *Candida* species.

Interestingly, as the age of patient increases, chance of symptomatic rather asymptomatic infection also increases. This criterion of positively relate to number of pregnancies and deliveries (Table 5). Correlation dissection showed that in 1st and 2nd trimesters yeast burden is highly significant to pregnancy month and infecting *Candida* species (Tables 4 and 5). Comparison of same parameters in 2nd and 3rd trimester (most positive cultures) indicates that pregnancies correlates highly to symptoms and the month of pregnancy. *Candida* counts, however, were highly negatively rerated to *Candida* species and deliveries (Tables 5 and 6).

Pearson's Correlations (2 tailed)									
Variables	**Age**	**Symptoms**	**Trimester**	**Month**	**Hospital**	**Pregnancies**	**Deliveries**	**Candida Sp.**	**CFU/mL**
Age	1								
Symptoms	0.354**	1							
	0.001								
Trimester			1						
Pregnancy month	0.346**		0.811**	1					
	0.001		0						
Hospital				0.251*	1				
				0.021					
Pregnancies	0.615**	0.466**			0.307**	1			
	0	0			0.004				
Deliveries	0.372**	0.340**				0.823**	1		
	0	0.002				0			
Candida Species						-0.333**	-0.300**	1	
						0.002	0.006		
CFU/mL			0.398**	0.301**			-0.230*	-0.245*	1
			0	0.005			0.035	0.025	

Table 5: Pearson's correlations of trimester 2 and 3 (n=59).

ANOVA		
	Between groups	
Candida Species	Within groups	0.792
CFU/mL	Between groups	0.991

	Within groups	
Deliveries	Between groups	0.004*
	Within groups	
Pregnancies	Between groups	0.000**
	Within groups	

Table 6: Analysis of variance with age.

Discussion

During pregnancy, vagina is more susceptible to many infections because of its proximity, results in higher incidences of lower urinary tract colonization [16,17]. In a literature citation, candiduria indicates an asymptomatic presentation in patients, yet presence of yeast is noted in the urine as a serendipitous in routine urinalysis or urine culture [16]. These infections have lower cure rates [25] with more resistant species [20]. It has been demonstrated further that micro biota of vagina is of similar patterns as observed in urine [30]. Recent literature also highlights yeast drug resistance in non albicans yeast strains than in any other [4,22]. Thus, rapid identification of these yeast strains provides valuable information concerning treatment regimens in clinical settings [27,31]. Rein and colleagues [32] provided an outlined for infections in 60-90% women. In our study, total of 70 patients, 17 women were placed in 2nd trimester of pregnancy out of which 8(47%) were positive for *Candida* species (Table 2).

In 3rd trimester, one third (36%) specimens were positive. Jointly together, they share two third of women get candiduria during their antenatal days which is statistically important (Table 5). This is contradictory to recent finding where trimester doesn't have any adage [33]. In number of other studies, however, demonstrated that from the conception day till it reaches 2nd and 3rd trimester, *Candida* infections were recorded highest [5,25,34]. Similar conclusion was drawn from study of Rein et al. [32] where 10% of infections were in 1st trimester as compared to 36-55% in the 3rd trimester. Some other studies provide some controversies on rates of candiduria. These studies show that 3rd trimester has similar rates to that of 23-26 (2nd trimester) weeks of gestation [35]. This provides a positive backing to our study (Table 3).

CHROMAgar™ *Candida* has previously been reported to provide valuable results in identifying *Candida* species [2,26,27]. The accurate identification of *Candida* species on colony color and morphology provide fast and decisive offering for clinical treatment regimens [2,28]. Use of such culture medium also addresses the important issue of non albicans species which are emerging all around and is a matter of grave concern around the world [3,12,22]. In our hands, results conclude that all major pathogenic *Candida* species were conveniently identified on CHROMAgar™ *Candida*. This advantage of early identification is an essential step for clinician to use specific treatment protocols in lowering yeast burden in pregnant women. This provides lowering of complication during pregnancies [19,25]. In our study, *Candida albicans* was isolated in all cultures (either pure or mixed). The non albicans group shares; *Candida krusei* (28%), *Candida tropicalis* (20%), and *Candida parapsilosis* (4%) (Table 2). In a large multicenter study from Spain, *Candida albicans* were recovered as high as 68%, followed by *Candida galabrata* (8%) and *Candida tropicalis* (4%) [18]. The occurrence of such numbers has also been reported by da Silva et al. [17] from Brazil. Another large sample study from Iran, provided similar results as of our study results [16].

However, lower incidences of *Candida albicans* are reported from Tanzanian pregnant women [36-38] where hygienic and socio-economic conditions may have played the differences. In North America, Europe and Latin American studies with CHROMAgar™ show that *Candida albicans* share the burden 51.5%, 47.8%, and 36.5%, respectively [18,23]. Taken together, in our study in this part of the world, we observed similar isolation rate as indicated in above mentioned studies. In Mexican study, on the contrary, other isolated species includes were *Candida parapsilosis*, *Candida tropicalis*, *Candida krusei*, and *Saccharomyces cerevisiae* [18,19,23]. In many other studies on specifically candiduria, *Candida albicans* is shown to share 50-70% burden followed by *C. galabrata*, and *C. tropicalis*, which is the third most common species [39,40]. Similar findings were recorded in this study also except presence of *C. galabrata* which we did not follow because of antibiotic resistance [19,38].

In present study, we also looked at the nature of asymptomatic and symptomatic yeast infection as per reported worldwide for *Candida* species. We find little lower symptomatic reporting of candiduria that is reported in other parts of the world. This may be linked to less education in the females. Significance of trimesters of pregnancy were also ascertained in the investigation. Our data show that 36% of the collected samples were positive with non albicans species (Table 2). Importantly of these, most common non albicans species, was *Candida tropicalis* in our case study (n=9/25) (Table 1). Similar patterns were seen in other studies [3,5,39,40]. Portuguese data from Negri et al. [39] provide good support to the notion that non albicans strains are becoming more important day by day.

The age distribution data in the study show that *Candida* infection is predominantly present in middle age (30-35 years) group. Majority of these isolates were pure infection of *Candida albicans* (55.6%) (Table 1). This is in agreement with the results of American and Brazilian studies [13,40]. On the contrary, Venezuelan study provided similar good support to age groups for other *Candida* infections [41]. Our data also signifies to the fact that more non albicans species and mixed infections were isolated in 18-23-year group (Table 1). We also incline to infer from our data that non albicans species are on rise [2,10,17]. In this study, *C. tropicalis* is next most prevalent species after *C. albicans*. Repentigny and co-workers [42] suggested that higher cases of this species tend to be a result of patients being neutropenic which isn't been convincible address in literature. This high level of colonization of non albicans were observed in older subjects which is not seen in our study (Table 1). It is also documented that occurrence of nonalbicans species (up to 20-30% in some cases) are associated to recurrent candidiasis [12]. Quantification of viable yeast cell indicates that 23% of the isolates have higher than >1000 CFU/mL of urine. Other studies have also provided similar results [43-45]. Of these 1/3 of positive specimens had intermediate numbers and 30% had low counts (<150 CFU/mL) (Table 3). Interestingly low yeast counts were detected in younger subjects with more non-albicans species.

Over and above, worldwide and our data indicates that infections with *C. krusei*, *C. tropicalis* and other non-albicans species have gone up [18,44]. Occurrence of this high rate is quite disquieting. Recent literature highlights the notion that *C. krusei* along with *C. tropicalis* are involved in invasive fungal infections [18,19]. Other studies demonstrate that these organisms also show resistance to ttariazoles with high mortality [4]. Presence of these species in relatively high number of young pregnant women from Punjab, Pakistan is alarming. Possible explanation to the scenario may be due to malnutrition, lower immunity levels and use of antifungal agents that needs to be further investigated like other workers have done in other parts of the world (Tables 1 and 2) [19,45].

Conclusion

This study, first of its kind in south Punjab, concludes finally that candidiasis in Pakistani women is at the same rate, same species distribution as per seen in other parts of the developing world [43]. A larger future project would provide more insight into *Candida* species infections in non-pregnant and pregnant (different trimesters) women would provide discernment in resident microbiota that could contribute to this pathological conditions.

Acknowledgement

Thanks to Céline Picard, CHROMAgar™ Microbiology, Paris, France, (http://www.CHROMAgar.com) for providing sample of CHROMAgar *Candida* medium to conduct this research work which would not been possible otherwise.

References

1. Aslam M, Hafeez R, Ijaz S, Tahir M (2008) Vulvovaginal candidiasis in pregnancy. Biomedica 24: 54-56.
2. Guzel AB, Ilkit M, Akar T, Burgut R, Demir SC (2011) Evaluation of risk factors in patients with vulvovaginal candidiasis and the value of ChromID Candida agar versus CHROMAgar Candida for recovery and presumptive identification of vaginal yeast species. Med Mycol 49: 16-25.
3. Sobel J (2011) Genital candidiasis. Medicine 38: 286-290.
4. Mendling W, Brasch J (2012) Guideline vulvovaginal candidasis (2010) of the German Society for gynecology and obstetrics, the working group for infections and infect immunology in gynecology and obstetrics, the German Society of dermatology, the board of German dermatologists and the German speaking mycological society mycoses 55: S1-S13.
5. Kauffman CA, Fisher JF, Sobel JD, Newman CA (2011) Candida urinary tract infections-diagnosis. Clin Infect Dis 52: S452-S456.
6. Sobel JD, Vazquez JA (1999) Fungal infections of the urinary tract. World J Urol 17: 410-414.
7. Fidal PF, Cutright J, Steele C (2000) Effects of reproductive hormones on experimental vaginal candidiasis. Infect Immun 68: 651-657.
8. Halbreich U (2009) Women's reproduction related disorders. J Affect Disord 1: 24-26.
9. Mann PA, McNicholas PM, Chau AS, Patel P, Mendrick C, et al. (2009) Impact of antifungal prophylaxis on colonization and Azole susceptibility of Candida species. Antimicrob Agents Chemother 53: 125026-5034.
10. Achkar JM, Fries BC (2010) Candida infections of the genitourinary. Clin Microbiol Rev 23: 253.
11. Babić M, Hukić M (2010) Candida albicans and non albicans species as etiological agent of vaginitis in pregnant and non-pregnant women. Bosnian J Basic Med Sci 10: 90-97.
12. Vermitsky JP, Self MJ, Chadwick SG, Trama JP, Adelson ME, et al. (2008) Survey of vaginal-flora candida species isolates from women of different age groups by use of species-specific PCR detection. J Clin Microbiol 46: 1501-1503.
13. Tortorano AM, Rigoni AL, Biraghi E (2003) The European confederation of medical mycology (ECMM) survey of candidaemia in Italy: Antifungal susceptibility pattern of 261 non albicans Candida isolates from blood. J Antimicrobiol Chemother 52: 679-682.
14. Szilagyi J, Foldi R, Gesztelyi R, Bayegan S (2012) Comparison of the kidney fungal burden in experimental disseminated candidiasis by species of the Candida parapsilosis complex treated with fluconazole, amphotericin B and caspofungin in a temporarily neutropenic murine model. Chemother 58: 159-164.
15. Watson CJ, Fairley CK, Grando D, Garland SM, Myers SP, et al. (2013) Associations with asymptomatic colonization with Candida in women reporting past vaginal candidiasis: An observational study. Eur J Obstet Gynaecol Reprod Biol 169: 376-379.
16. Mahmoudabadi A, Zarrin M, Ghanatir F, Vazirianzadeh (2012) Candiduria in hospitalized patients in teaching hospitals of Ahvaz, Iran. J Microbiol 4: 198-203.
17. Da Silva EH, Ruiz LS, Matsumoto FE, Auler ME, Giudice MC, et al. (2007) Candiduria in a public hospital of Sao Paulo (1999-2004): Characteristics of the yeast isolates. Rev Inst Med Trop Sao Paulo 49: 349-353.
18. Miceli MH, Diaz JA, Lee SA (2011) Emerging opportunistic yeast infections. Lancet Infect Dis 142: 142-151.
19. Badiee P, Hashemizadeh Z (2014) Opportunistic invasive fungal infections: Diagnosis & clinical management. Indian J Med Res 139: 195-204.
20. Kalkanci A, Guzel, AB, Khalil IIJ, Aydin M, Ilkit M, et al. (2012) Yeast vaginitis during pregnancy: Susceptibility testing of 13 antifungal drugs and boric acid and the detection of four virulence factors. Med Mycol 50: 585-593.
21. Roberts CL, Rickard K, Kotsiou G, Morris JM (2011) Treatment of asymptomatic vaginal candidiasis in pregnancy to prevent preterm birth: An open-label pilot randomized controlled trial. BMC Pregnancy and Childbirth 11: 18.
22. Kazi YF, Saleem S, Kazi N (2012) Investigation of vaginal microbiota in sexually active women using hormonal contraceptives in Pakistan. BMC Urology 12: 22.
23. Dias LB, Melhem MDC, Szeszs MW, Filho JM, Hahn RC (2011) Vulvovaginal Candidiasis in Mato Grosso, Brazil: Pregnancy status, causative species and drugs tests. Brazilian J Microbiol 42: 1300-1307.
24. Trofa D, Gacser A, Nosanchuk JD (2008) Candida parapsilosis, an emerging fungal pathogen. Clin Microbiol Rev 21: 606-625.
25. Fisher JF, Sobel JD, Kauffman CA, Newman CA (2011) Candida urinary tract infections--treatment. Clin Infect Dis 52: S457-S466.
26. Bouchara JP, Declerck P, Cimon B, Planchenault C, Gentile L, et al. (1996) Routine use of CHROMAgar Candida medium for presumptive identification of Candida yeast species and detection of mixed fungal populations. Clin Microbiol Infect 2:202-208.
27. Madhavan P, Jamal F, Chong PP, Ng KP (2011) Identification of local clinical Candida isolates using CHROMAgar Candida as a primary identification method for various Candida species. Trop Biomed 28: 269-274.
28. Odds FC and Bernaerts R (1994) CHROMAgar Candida, a new differential isolation medium for presumptive identification of clinically important Candida species. J Clin Microbiol 32: 1923-1929.
29. Fraisse T, Lachaud L, Sotto A, Lavigne JP (2011) Recommendations of the infectious disease committee of the French association of urology diagnosis, treatment and monitoring candiduria. Prog Urol 21: 314-321.

30. Zahra S, Seifi Z, Mahmoudabadi A (2012) Sensitivity of vaginal isolates of Candida to eight antifungal drugs isolated from Ahvaz, Iran. Jundishapur J Microbiol 5: 574-577.

31. Nadeem SG, Hakim ST, Kazmi SU (2010) Use of CHROMAgar Candida for the presumptive identification of Candida species directly from clinical specimens in resource-limited settings. Libyan J Med 5: 2144.

32. Rein MF, Holmes KK (1983) Non-specific vaginitis Vulvovaginal candidiasis and trichomonasis. J Infec Dis 4: 281.

33. Parveen R, Azmi MA, Tariq RM, Mahmood SM, Hijazi M, et al. (2008) Determination of antifungal activity of Cedrus deodara root oil and its compounds against Candida albicans and Aspergillus fumigates. Pak J Bot 42: 3645-3649.

34. Moharram AM, Ati MG, Othman EOM (2013) Vaginal yeast infection in patients admitted to Al-Azhar University Hospital, Assiut, Egypt. J Basic App Mycol (Egypt) 4: 21-32.

35. Cotch MF, Hillier SL, Gibbs RS, Eschenbach DA (1998) Epidemiology and outcomes associated with moderate to heavy Candida colonization during pregnancy Vaginal Infection Prematurity Study Group. Amer J Obstet Gynaecol 178: 374-380.

36. Namkinga LA, Matee MIN, Kivaisi, K, Kullaya A (2005) Identification of Candida strains isolated from Tanzanian pregnant women with vaginal candidiasis. East African Medical Journal 82: 226-234.

37. Mujica MT, Finquelievich JL, Jewtuchowicz V, Iovannitti CA (2004) Prevalence of Candida albicans and Candida non-albicans in clinical samples during 1999-2001. Rev Argent Microbiol 36: 107-112.

38. Oliveira R, Azeredo J, Henriques M, Silva SC, Negri M, et al. (2010) Effect of itraconazole on Candida glabrata biofilm matrix CEB- abstracts in Proceedings 4th International Conference Biofilms IV: Communities bridging disciplines pp: 32.

39. Negri M, Martins M, Henriques M, Svidzinski T (2010) Examination of potential virulence factors of Candida tropicalis clinical isolates from hospitalized patients. Mycopathologia 169: 175-182.

40. Okungbowa FI, Isikhuemhen OS, Dede APO (2003) The distribution frequency of Candida species in the genitourinary tract among symptomatic individuals in Nigerian cities. Rev Iberoam Micol 20: 60-63.

41. Passos XS, Sales WS, Maciel PJ, Costa CR, Miranda KC, et al. (2005) Candida colonization in intensive care unit patients' urine. Mem Inst Oswaldo Cruz 100: 925-928.

42. Repentigny L (1992) Serodiagnosis of Candidiasis, Aspergillosis, and Cryptococcosis. Clin Infect Dis 14: S11-S22.

43. Carricajo A, Boiste S, Thore J, Aubert G, Gille Y, et al. (1999) Comparative evaluation of five chromogenic media for detection, enumeration and identification of urinary tract pathogens. Eur J Clin Microbiol Infect Dis 18: 796-803.

44. Nelson M, Wanjiru WM, Muturi W (2013) Prevalence of vaginal candidiasis and determination of the occurrence of Candida species in pregnant women attending the antenatal clinic of Thika District Hospital, Kenya. Open J Med Microbiol 3: 264-272.

45. Vidal C, Viasus D, Carratalà J (2013) Pathogenesis of invasive fungal infections. Cur Opin Infect Dis 26: 270-276.

Management of Obstetric Emergencies at the Maternity Center of the University Hospital Center of Oueme-Plateau (CHUD O/P) in Benin

Bagnan-Tonato JA[1], Lokossou MSHS[1], Ogoudjobi OM[1], Tognifode V[1], Obossou AAA[2*], Aboubacar M[1], Adisso S[1], Ali ARORS[1], Lokossou A[1] and Perrin RX[1]

[1]*Department of Mother and Child, Faculty of Health Sciences of Cotonou, University of Abomey-Calavi, Bénin*

[2]*Department of Mother and Child, Faculty of Medicine, University of Parakou, Bénin*

[*]**Corresponding author:** Obossou AAA, Department of Mother and Child, Faculty of Medicine, University of Parakou, Bénin, E-mail: awadefr2000@yahoo.fr

Abstract

Introduction: Obstetric emergencies constitute public health problems in our countries.

Objective: To analyze how obstetric emergencies are managed from the clinical, therapeutic, and prognosis point of view in the gynecology and obstetrics department of the Centre Hospitalier Universitaire Départemental of Ouémé-Plateau.

Patients and methods: It was a cross-sectional, descriptive and analytical study carried out at the maternity CHUD-OP over a period of 06 months from February 2016 to August 2016. It was conducted on an exhaustive sample of all patients admitted to the CHUD-OP maternity and treated for complications of gravido-puerperium. Non-obstetric emergencies were not included. Statistical analysis and testing were performed on CS PRO 6.2 and SPSS software by comparing averages and deviations, using the Pearson chi-square for the dichotomous variables, accepting a significant probability $p \leq 0.05$. The principles of confidentiality were respected.

Results: The frequency of admission of obstetric emergencies was 34.9%. Epidemiologically, the mean age was 27.35 ± 5.71 years. 31.4% were nulliparous, and 69.3% had low-paid occupational activities. Clinically, the reference was in 70.4% of cases the mode of admission, non-medical (95.1%) and without venous access (59.1%). The causes were: dystocia (30.7%); hemorrhagic emergencies (25.9%); hypertensive emergencies (21.5%); fetal hypoxia (17.8%) and infections (4.0%). Therapeutically, the average duration of a treatment was 4.1 ± 1.3 hours and was performed in 67.5% of cases by a caesarean. At the prognostic level, the sequences of layers were complicated in 10.1% of the cases, marked mainly by anemia (38.1%) and arterial hypertension (28.6%). Maternal and neonatal lethality cases represented 3.8% and 11.5%, respectively.

Conclusion: The maternal and fetal mortality rate associated with obstetric emergencies is still high at CHUD-OP. The reductionof morbidity and mortality requires the improvement of the quality of care and the reference system.

Keywords: Obstetric emergency; Morbidity; Mortality; Pregnancy; Delivery

Introduction

The obstetric emergency, the first circumstance of maternal mortality, is a real public health issue. Despite the implementation of multiple programs to combat maternal mortality, about 830 women worldwide die from preventable causes linked to their pregnancy and childbirth with 99% of all maternal deaths occurring in developing countries particularly in sub-Saharan Africa. The maternal mortality ratio in Sub-Saharan Africa is 510 maternal deaths per 100,000 live births, compared to 12 per 100,000 live births in developed countries [1]. In Benin in 2015, out of 100,000 live births, 405 women died from complications of childbirth [2]. Apart from the main causes of maternal deaths, delays in decision-making, access to health facilities and care occupy a no less important place in the worsening of the maternal and perinatal prognosis.

Objective

To analyze the clinical, therapeutic and prognostic aspects of obstetric emergencies in the gynecology and obstetrics department of the Centre Hospitalier Universitaire Départemental of Ouémé-Plateau (CHUD O/P).

Patients and Methods

This was a cross-sectional, descriptive and analytical study conducted at CHUD O/P maternity over a period of 06 months from February 2016 to August 2016. The source population consisted of all pregnant or post-partum patients (0 to 42 days) admitted to the emergency department of the obstetric gynecology department of the CHUD O/P during the study period. The target population was those patients with complications of gravido-puerperality.

The obstetric emergency is defined as any pathological situation occurring during pregnancy, during delivery or within 42 days of the sequelae and in which a diagnosis and treatment must be made very quickly to preserve the maternal and/or fetal vital prognosis. In operational terms, it is the woman whose life is threatened immediately within 24 to 48 hours by an obstetric pathology [3].

- Inclusion criteria: All patients admitted to CHUD O/P maternity and treated forcomplications of gravoderma-puerperium.
- Criteria for non-inclusion: Non-obstetric emergencies were not included.
- Sampling: It was exhaustive and the sample size was 622 cases of obstetric emergencies. The variables studied were socio-demographic, diagnostic, therapeutic and prognostic. Statistical analysis and testing was performed on CS PRO 6.2 and SPSS software by comparing means and standard deviations, using the Pearson chi-square for the dichotomous variables, accepting a significant probability p 0.05. For ethical considerations, confidentiality and anonymity were respected.

Results

Epidemiological aspects

- Frequency: During the study period, 622 obstetric emergencies were collected on 1784 admissions, a 34.9% prevalence of admissions. 1549 childbirth were performed.
- The average age of patients was 27.3 years old with extremes of 15 and 48 years old. The most represented age group is that of patients aged between 20 and 34 years old (80%). They were primigest and paucigest in 26.5% and 38.7% of cases respectively and had never given birth in 31.4% of cases. The mean gesture was 3.04 ± 1.94 with extremes of 1 and 12 and the mean parity was 1.91 ± 1.92 with extremes of 0 and 10.
- The most represented occupational groups consisted: of salespeople, artisans respectively 42.1%, 27.2%. The majority (63.2%) were enrolled up to primary level in 30.7% (191/622).
- Medical and surgical history: High blood pressure (HTA), blood transfusion, viral hepatitis was found in 14.5%, 6.3% and 2.3% of cases, respectively. A uterine scar was noted in 19.5% of cases.

Diagnostic aspects

- Pregnancy monitoring: Pregnancy monitoring was done 9 times out of 10 by a trained agent. The mean prenatal consultation was 4.38 ± 2.39 with extremes of 0 and 12. Nearly 6 out of 10 pregnancies (62.4%) had at least 4 prenatal visits. The prenatal assessment was partially completed; HIV testing (91.3%); obstetric ultrasound (83.3%); blood grouping (28.4%).
- The reference of a peripheral structure was the admission mode in 70.4% of the cases (438/622). Transportation was unmonitored in 95.2% of cases (417/438), without an ad hoc injection system in 42.2% of cases (185/438). The reference period was 1 to 2 hours in 38.5% of cases.
- Obstetric emergencies involved 87.6% of pregnant women. They occurred at an average gestational age of 35.69 WA ± 7.89 with extremes of 5 and 43 weeks of amenorrhea (WA). The majority occurred in the third trimester of pregnancy (91.9%) (Table 1).

	Number (N=622)	Frequency in Percentage (%)
Pregnant women	545	87.6
1st trimester (<15 WA)	33	6.1
2nd trimester (15-28 WA)	11	2.0
3rd trimester	501	91.9
Term pregnant women [28-37 WA]	101	18.5
Before term pregnant women [37-41 WA]	347	63.7
Post term pregnant women (>41 WA)	53	9.7
Women in postpartum	77	12.4

Table 1: Distribution of patients according to the period (gravido-puerpéralité) of occurrence of emergencies.

Main signs of severity were: palpebral mucosa (19.9%), severe hypertensive (15.1%), meconium amniotic fluid (8.5%), shock (6, 4%), convulsive seizures (4.5%), hyperthermia (4.2%), hemorrhage with high abundance (3.2) and coma (0.2%).

The biological assessments noted severe anemia in 8.8%; leukocytosis in 38.1% and thrombocytopenia in 7.1% of cases.

From the highest to the lowest frequency, there were:

Dystocia (30.7%); hemorrhagic emergencies (25.9%); hypertensive emergencies (21.5%); fetal hypoxia (17.8%) and infections (4.0%).

Dystocia was mechanical in about ¾th of the cases (74.8%) (Table 2).

	Number (N=199)	Frequency in Percentage (%)
Mechanical dystocia	95	47.74
Bone dystocia	55	27.64

Ovular dysfocia	40	20.10
Dynamic dystocia	50	25.12
Other		
Fetal-pelvic disproportion	33	17.2
Pre-rupture syndrome	20	10.4
Failure to commit	1	0.5

Table 2: Distribution of patients by dystocia Distribution of patients according to dystocia.

Hemorrhage in the 2nd and 3rd trimester (43.5%) and postpartum haemorrhage (32.3%) accounted for a significant proportion of hemorrhagic emergencies. Severe preeclampsia dominated hypertensive emergencies with 43.3% of patients (Table 3).

Funicular causes have been the most frequent etiologies in cases of fetal hypoxia; 15 out of 25 had an ovular infection; 9 endometritis and 1 sepsis (Tables 4 and 5).

	Number (N=161)	Frequency in Percentage (%)
1st Trimester	39	24.2
Haemorrhagic Abortion	25	15.53
Ectopic pregnancy	13	8.1
Molecular Pregnancy	1	0.6
2nd and 3rd Trimesters		43.5
Placenta previa hemorrhagic	33	20.5
Retro-placental hematoma	28	17.4
Uterine rupture	9	5.6
Postpartum hemorrhage		32.3
Hemorrhage of the deliverance	25	15.5
Contemporary hemorrhage of the deliverance	22	13.7
Postpartum Postpartum Hemorrhage	5	3.1

Table 3: Distribution of patients according to hemorrhagic emergencies.

	Number (N=134)	Frequency in Percentage (%)
Pre-eclampsia		
Severe	58	43.3
Moderate	12	9.0
Gestational hypertension	24	17.9
Eclampsia pre and per partum	22	16.4
Postpartum eclampsia	17	12.7
Hypertensive encephalopathy	1	0.7

Table 4: Distribution of patients according to hypertensive emergencies.

	Number (N=63)	Frequency in Percentage (%)
Anemia	24	38.1
High Blood Pressure	18	28.6
Hemorrhage	8	12.7
Infection of the surgical wound	6	9.5
Postpartum eclampsia	4	6.3
Fistule	1	1.6
Sequelae of ophthalmology of hypertension (Blindness)	1	1.6
Motor and neurological sequelae of hypertension	1	1.6

Table 5: Distribution of patients according to the nature of the complications.

Therapeutic aspects

Blood transfusion was required for 118 patients (18.9%) due to severe anemia. The management of hypertensive emergencies was carried out by magnesium sulphate for cases of severe preeclampsia in 95.9% of cases (93/97) and by Clonidine and/or Nicardipine for hypertensive outbreaks according to the protocol.

The delivery was performed by Caesarean section in 83.8% of cases (420/501). The indications were: fetal hypoxia 97.1% (99/102); dystocia 95.4% (187/196); infectious emergencies 93.8% (15/16); hypertensive emergencies 65.5% (76/116); haemorrhagic emergencies 58.9% (43/73).

Furthermore, we performed: 3 hysterectomies of haemostasis (0.5%); 13 salpingectomies (2.9%) for ectopic pregnancy; 25 Manual aspiration intrauterine (4.0%) and 101 uterine revision (16.2%). The rachi-anesthesia was the mode of anesthesia practiced in 61.3% of the cases. The average duration of patient care was 4.18 ± 1.33 hours with extremes of 0.25 (15 min) and 191.30 min.

Prognostic aspects

Maternal prognosis

- Morbidity: The sequels were complicated for 63 patients, representing a rate of 10.1%. Complications were dominated by anemia (38.1%), hypertension (28.6%), hemorrhage (12.7%) and surgical wound infections (9.5%). The duration of hospitalization was 2-7 days in 77% (479/622) of the cases.
- Mortality: We recorded 24 maternal deaths, i.e. a maternal mortality rate of 24/62=0.8%. They were mostly referred (21/24). The causes were from the higher to the lower frequency: hemorrhages (50%), postpartum infections (20.7%) and anemia (12.5%).

Fetal prognosis

- Morbidity: 475 live births out of 537 were recorded (88.4%) with 25.8% having poor adaptation to ectopic life, requiring neonatal resuscitation and neonatal transfer. Neonatal distress (41.6%) and neonatal infection (23.4%), neonatal distress (10.4%) and prematurity (16.9%) accounted for most of the reasons for transfer.
- Mortality: Fetal mortality was 11.5%.

Discussion

Epidemiological aspects

Obstetric emergencies accounted for more than one-third of admissions in our service. A study carried out in 2013 by Tchaou et al. at Parakou University Hospital reported a similar frequency of 31.8% (1,231 obstetric cases including 507 emergencies) [4]. Lower frequencies have been reported by other authors including Kadima et al. [5] in Mali in 2013 (6.03%), Steven et al. in 2012 in America (0.6%), Oliveira et al. (2006) in Brazil (2.1%) [6,7]. These disparate frequencies show that obstetric emergencies remain a public health problem, affecting mainly the developing countries and testify to the level of development of the health system.

According to the WHO, Girard et al. these are preventable causes in the majority of cases [2,8].

Clinical aspects

The reference was the mode of admission in 70.4% of the cases. Our rates are much higher than those of Tshabu at the CUGO and Cissé in Senegal which were respectively 23.3% and 46.7% [9,10].

The Ouémé-Plateau Departmental University Hospital Center is the only public reference center in the Ouémé-Plateau area in southern Benin. It covers an area of 1,676 km^2 and includes a population estimated at 1,100,404 inhabitants in 2013.

This was a non-medical reference (95.1%) and without venous access (59.1%). The reference period was 1 to 2 hours in 38.5%. Tshabu et al. reported to the CUGO that 80.5% of the patients referred were not provided with medical assistance during their transport and without venous access (37.9%) [9]. These poor discharge conditions aggravate the maternal and fetal prognosis and reveal a poor organization of the referral system for obstetric emergencies. These transfers were responsible for 87.5% (21/24) of deaths in our study.

The causes of obstetric emergencies are the same from one study to another, but their ranking differs from one country to another. By 2015, 85% of global obstetric emergencies according to WHO [2] are due to hemorrhages, postpartum infections, high blood pressure and abortions.

In our study, classified by decreasing frequency are: dystocia, hemorrhagic emergencies, hypertensive emergencies, fetal hypoxia of unidentified causes and infectious emergencies with 30.7%, 25.9%, 21.5%, 17.9% and 4.0% respectively.

Dystocias

The frequency of dystocia was 30.7%. They were dynamic and mechanical with a predominance of mechanical dystocia (74.8%). These were pelvic abnormalities (28.6%), fetal pelvic disproportions (17.2%) and dystocia presentations (23.8%). Tchaou et al. [4] also found a predominance of dystocia (32.0%) over a period of 6 months.

These women should have been referenced before any work started if the basin abnormalities were detected.

Haemorrhagic emergencies

They are dominated by hemorrhages in the second and third trimesters of pregnancy (43.5%). They aggravate morbidity and perinatal mortality by induced prematurity and postpartum hemorrhage.

Hypertensive emergencies

Data from the literature show that the prevalence of hypertension during pregnancy varies between 10 and 15% [11]. It is a risk factor for mortality during pregnancy. The prevalence rate of hypertension in our series is 21.5% much higher than the rates found by Hounkponou et al. in Parakou (6.2%) [12].

The hypertension was complicated by eclampsia for 4 patients (6.3%) with 2 deaths rising, the problem of the follow-up of the pregnancies by qualified agents in our countries.

Foetal hypoxia

Perinatal hypoxia involves the vital prognosis of the fetus within hours or even minutes after its installation. It requires fast and adequate care. Philopoulos demonstrates that the use of Fetal Electrical Monitoring is associated with a significant reduction in neonatal and infant mortality [13].

In our series, the prevalence was 17.8%. Caesarean delivery was the mode of delivery in 98% of cases (101/103).

Infectious emergencies

The frequency of infectious emergencies was 4.0% dominated by ovular infection (60%). Higher rates were found by Tchaou in Parakou (12.4%) and Ngbale in Bangui (10.7%) [3,14]. Advances in antibiotic medicine have greatly improved the prognosis of these emergencies. Antibiotic therapy was performed in more than 9 out of 10 women in our study.

Therapeutic aspects

Emergency management met the recommendations in most cases with a surgical penalty in 67.5% of cases.

Pronostic aspects

24 maternal deaths were recorded, i.e. a maternal case fatality rate of 3.8%. This rate is way above the 0.4% reported by Tchaou in 2013 in Parakou [4]. Hemorrhage was the leading cause of death (50%) followed by infections (20.7%). The same finding was made by Chelli et al. in Tunisia, where hemorrhage was implicated in 35.5% of cases in maternal death followed by hypertension (19.3%) [15]. Foumane in Yaoundé found high blood pressure as the leading cause of maternal death (22.4%) followed by HIV/AIDS (19.2%) and septic abortions (17.2%) [16].

The obstetric hemorrhagic emergency constitutes a specific situation which imposes an immediate multidisciplinary management where obstetrician, anesthetist-resuscitator and interventional radiologist are involved.

We have recorded 62 perinatal deaths, 46 of which are per-partum. Neonatal mortality is one of the major contingents of infant mortality in developing countries. Garba et al. in Niger finds a hospital neonatal mortality rate of 85.7% [17].

Conclusion

Our study shows that emergency obstetric care deserves consolidation in our regions with the need to improve the referral system and the ongoing retraining of health workers on emergency obstetric and neonatal care.

References

1. http://www.un.org/fr/millenniumgoals/reports/2015/pdf/rapport_2015.pdf
2. Larousse Medical (2009) The essential reference for understanding medical terms and treatments, from the most classic to the most modern. (5th edn.), Illustrated Dictionary Larousse, France.
3. Tchaou BA, Hounkponou NF, Salifou K, Zoumènou E, Chobli M (2015) Obstetric emergencies at the university hospital of Parakou in Benin: Clinical, therapeutic and evolutive aspects. Eur Sci J 11: 1857-7881.
4. http://www.malimedical.org/2015/65d.pdf
5. Clark SL, Meyers JA, Frye DR, Mcmanus K, Perlin JB (2012) A systematic approach to the identification and classification of near-miss eventsonlabor and delivery in a large, national health care system. Am J Obstet Gynecol 207: 441-445.
6. De Oliveira FC, Costa ML, Cecatti JG, Pinto Silva JL, Surita FG (2013) Maternal morbidity and near miss associated with maternal age: The innovative approach of the 2006 Brazilian demographic health survey. Clinics 68: 922-927.
7. World Health Organization (2015). World Health Statistics 2015.
8. Girard F (2001) The severe complications of pregnancy: State of play in Lorraine in the framework of the European survey. J Gynecol Obstet Reprod Biol 30: 2S10-2S17.
9. Tshabu-Aguèmon C, Denakpo J, Adisso S, Mampassi E, de Souza J (2012) Maternal and perinatal mortality related to obstetric referrals at the U.G.O. of the CNHU-HKM of Cotonou. Ramur 17: 1.
10. Cissé ML, Raad B, Diouf A, Wade F, Moreau JV (2010) Assessment of obstetric evacuations at the hospital of Kolda. Med Black Afr 57: 37-43.
11. Sananes N, Gaudineau A, Akladios C, Lecointre L, Langer B (2016) Hypertension and pregnancy.EMC Obs 1: 1-15.
12. Hounkponou NFM, Codjo LH, Sidi R, Dohou SH, Djoh Ndiang KI (2017) Prevalence and risk factors for vasculo-renal syndromes in hospitals in Parakou (Benin) in 2015. Med d'Afrique Noire 64: 237-242.
13. Philopoulos G (2015) Fetal electronic monitoring and its association with neonatal and infant mortality in a database: A sensitivity analysis. J Gynecol Obstet Reprod Biol 44: 451-462.
14. Ngbale RN, Goddot-Nangouma MJC, Gaunefet CE, Songo-Kette T, Koirokpi A (2012) The motherhood of the community hospital of Bangui: About 84 cases of "escapees beautiful". Med Black Afr 59: 322-326.

15. Chelli D, Dimassi K, Zouaoui B, Sfar E, Chelli H (2009) Evolution of maternal mortality in a Tunisian maternity level 3 between 1998 and 2007. J Gynecol Obstet Reprod Biol 38: 655-661.
16. Foumane P, Dohbit JS, Meka ENU, Nkada MN, Ze Minkande ET (2015) Etiologies of maternal mortality in the gynecological-obstetric and pediatric hospital of Yaounde: A series of 58 deaths. J Med Health Sci 16.
17. Garba M, Kamaye M, Alido S, Zoubeirou H, Oumarou Z, et al. (2017) The determinants of early neonatal mortality at Issa-Gazobi maternity in Niamey. J Pediatr Child Care.

Inhibin B as a Marker for Detection of Ovarian Activity in Premature Ovarian Failure

Maysoon Sharief*, **Dhamya Salih Alharoon and Hutham Tariq Mohammed**

Department of Gynecology and Obstetrics, College of Medicine, University of Basrah, Basrah Health Directorate, Basrah, Iraq

***Corresponding author:** Maysoon Sharief, Department of Gynecology and Obstetrics, College of Medicine, University of Basrah, Basrah Health Directorate, Basrah, Iraq, E-mail: maysoonsharief60@yahoo.com

Abstract

Objective: To evaluate Inhibin B in women with premature ovarian failure POF and its role as a marker for ovarian reserve in comparison to FSH.

Methodology: This study was conducted in the infertility center in Basra Maternity and Child Hospital. About 75 women were divided into 3 groups, each of 25 women, group (A) with premature ovarian failure, Group (B) menopause women and group (C) normally fertile cycling women. Inhibin B and FSH were measured and comparison were made between the three groups, then Inhibin B and FSH level were studied in group (A) before and after (4-6 months) of hormonal replacement therapy.

Results: The mean FSH was (81.4 ± 28.4 IU/ml) in group A, (97.7 ± 25.5 IU/ml) in group B and (4.87 ± 2.3 IU/ml) in group C. Inhibin B was (1.8 ± 2.8 pg/ml) in group A, (1 ± 0.9 pg/ml) in group B and (53.1 ± 17.1 pg/ml) in group C. After hormonal replacement therapy in group A, mean FSH was (56.3 ± 13.4 IU/ml) and mean Inhibin B was (1.4 ± 12.4 pg/ml). There was significant decrease in FSH level but no significant changes in Inhibin B among group A women.

Conclusion: Inhibin B level in women with premature ovarian failure is so low when compared to normal cycling women and close to the levels in the menopause women, it was not affected by exogenous estrogen intake as seen with FSH. Because it's main source in the female body is the preantral follicles, all this indicates Inhibin B is a good marker for ovarian reserve in women with premature ovarian failure.

Keywords: Inhibin B; Premature ovarian failure; Menopause; Chemotherapy

Introduction

Premature ovarian failure (POF) is defined as ovarian defect characterized by premature depletion of ovarian follicles (arrested folliculogenesis) before the age of 40 years [1-3]. The end of a woman`s reproductive lifespan is marked by the beginning of menopause, which is defined as the last menstruation the woman had, which is caused by the depletion in the ovarian reserve [4,5]. In the general population and in many ethnicities in the recent human history the average age of natural menopause was not changed and remained at 50-52 years [6,7]. Premature ovarian failure considered a common condition as it affects 1% of all women under the age of 40 years, and 0.1% in women aged less than 30 years [8]. The causes of (POF) include idiopathic, genetic, autoimmune, latrogenic, toxins and occupational chemicals and infections [9-16]. Most of women with (POF) present with menstrual irregularity, 10% with amenorrhea. Additionally, affected women have very low levels of circulation estradiol. So clinical symptoms observed are similar to those observed with the onset of menopause, such as hot flushes, vaginal dryness, dyspareunia, insomnia, vaginitis and mood swings [17]. Inhibin is a protein secreted by granulosa (female) and Sertoli (male) cells in response to FSH [18]. It is found in blood, and in great quantities in seminal fluid and follicular fluid. Gonadal inhibin is the main peptide hormone that regulates FSH synthesis and secretion during folliculogenisis and spermatogenesis, the main role of inhibin is to selectively suppress the production of FSH by the pituitary.

Inhibin enhances LH stimulation of androgen synthesis in the theca cells to serve as substrate for aromatization to estrogen in the granulosa cells, whereas activin suppresses androgen synthesis. This important paracrine regulation of androgen as substrate for aromatization to estrogen in the granulosa cells, whereas activin production in thecal cells by inhibin and activin is exerted primarily through modification of the expression of steroidogenic enzymes [19]. The anterior pituitary gland secretes FSH and LH from a specialized cells call the gonadotrops, GnRH from the hypothalamus, testosterone from the testes in male and estradiol, progesterone from the ovaries in female as well as gonadal inhibin, activin and follistatin regulate the synthesis and secretion of gonadotropins from the pituitary gland [19]. FSH stimulates the sertoli cells in testes and the granulosa cells in ovary to produce inhibin. In females, the granulose cells of the ovary produce inhibin, and inhibin production by each follicle increases as the granulosa cell population expands during normal follicle growth and maturation [20,21]. Due to the postnatal activation of the gonadotropin secretion, Inhibin B level is sustained till 18-24 months. Then serum Inhibin B has a positive relationship with age. several years prior to the onset of puberty due to the increase in the follicular activity in the pre-puberty phase, after that Inhibin B levels increase progressively with the stages of puberty indicating high follicular activity prior to the development of ovulatory menstrual cycle [22].

During the follicular phase of menstrual cycle the major form of Inhibin secreted from the ovary is Inhibin B in which it rises sharply in early follicular phase with the peak following the FSH rise and then progressively fall during the rest of the follicular phase, another peak is on day 2 mid cycle LH peak then a rapid decline and constant low levels during the luteal phase [22].

Material and Methods

This study was conducted in the infertility center at Basra Maternity and Child Hospital during a period from October 2015 till September 2016. Written consent was taken from all women who participated in this study. The participants in this study were divided in to 3 groups.

Group A: About 25 women with premature ovarian failure POF, with age less than 40 years, amenorrhea more than 6 months, no history of medical diseases like diabetes mellitus, hypertension, thyroid disorder, no exogenous estrogen intake in the preceding 3 months, no history of chemotherapy, with serum FSH more than 40 IU/ml.

Group B: About 25 menopausal women aged more than 45 years with amenorrhea more than one year, with no history of medical diseases like diabetes mellitus or thyroid disorder, no hormonal replacement therapy, and serum FSH levels 6 months apart more than 40 IU/ml.

Group C: About 25 normal women were proven fertile with regular menstrual cycle, with no history of hormonal contraception since one year.

All participating women were interviewed in detail for medical, surgical and treatment (especially cytotoxic chemotherapy and exogenous estrogen) history and thorough physical examination was done for exclusion of any gross underlying disease. No one of the participants had any history of auto immune disease or radiotherapy or chemotherapy treatment or history of surgical removal of gonads. Blood samples from group C (normally fertile women) were taken at day 3 of menstrual cycle, blood samples from group A (women with POF) and group B (menopause women) were taken randomly and FSH and Inhibin B levels were measured in all 3 groups.

Participant in group A (women with POF) started oral hormonal replacement therapy. They were given estrogens and Progestogen in the form of tablet Proglyuton (estradiol valerate 2 mg, Norgestrel 0.5 mg) once daily for at least 12 weeks then blood samples were collected and serum FSH and Inhibin B were measured. Serum was collected after centrifugation and stored at -80°C until assayed. Serum concentration of FSH was measured by using highly specific micro particle enzyme assay (MILA). Inhibin B was measured in duplicate using a solid phase sandwich ELISA (Oxford Bio-Innovation, Oxford, UK). Data were analyzed using SPSS statistical software. Descriptive statistics are given as the Mean and SD, independent sample t-test was used to see the mean significance difference between groups.

Results

In this study, 75 women were included who were divided into 3 groups as mentioned in the methodology. Table 1 shows the characteristic features of all 3 groups regarding age, BMI and menstrual cycle. The mean (± SD) age of group A (women with POF) was (30.16 ± 5.05 years) with a range of (19-39 years), while group B (menopaused women) with mean age of (48.04 ± 1.6 years) with a range of (45-50 years), and the last group C (normal menstruating women) its mean was (29.33 ± 4.9 years) with a range of (21-40 years). Age differences were not significant between group A and C. No statistical significance regarding the age of menarche between the three groups. But, there was significant difference between the three groups especially A, C and B, C regarding BMI. And a significance difference between the three groups especially A, C and A, B regarding the duration of amenorrhea.

Baseline Characteristics	Group A	Group B	Group C	P-value (A/B)	P-value (B/C)	P value (A/C)
Age Mean (years) ± SD	30.16 ± 50.05	48.04 ± 1.6	29.33 ± 4.9	<0.0001	<0.0001	0.017
(Range)	(19-39)	(45-50)	(21-40)	Significant	Significant	No Significance
BMI Mean (kg/m^2) ± SD	26.1 ± 2.3	27.4 ± 2.4	23.6 ± 1.5	0.73	<0.0001	<0.0001
(Range)	(24-30)	(23-30)	(22-26)	No Significance	Significant	Significant
Age of Menarche (Years)	14.2	13.1	13.4	0.024	0.042	0.029
(Range)	(12-15)	(12-15)	(12-15)	No Significance	No Significance	No Significance
Duration of Amenorrhea						
Last mense <35 days	0	0	23			
Last Mense 35-120 days	3	0	2			
Last mense >120 days	22	25	0			

Table 1: The base line characteristics of the entire studied group.

A Table 2 shows the mean (± SD) of the plasma levels of FSH and Inhibin B in all the three groups, the mean FSH level in group A was (81.4 ± 28.4 IU/ml) and ranged (37-150 IU/ml), in group B the mean level of FSH was (97.7 ± 25.5 IU/ml) with a range of (65-150 IU/ml), and the last group C the mean FSH level was (5.87 ± 2.3 IU/ml) with a range of (3.2-12 IU/ml). Plasma level of FSH was elevated in group A, B in contrast to group C, which was highly significant.

Mean Inhibin B level in group A was (1.8 ± 2.8 pg/ml) with a range of (0-15 pg/ml), Inhibin B level in group B was (1 ± 0.9 pg/ml) with a range of (0-4 pg/ml), while in group C the mean Inhibin B was (53 ± 17.1 pg/ml) and a range of (30-80 pg/ml).

This table showed that serum Inhibin B level was high in group C in comparison to group A and B which is statistically significant.

Parameter	Group A	Group B	Group C	Significance P-value
FSH mean ± SD (IU/ml)	81.4 ± 28.4	97.7 ± 25.5	4.87 ± 2.3	(A/B) 0.065
Range	(37-150)	(65-150)	(4.2-12)	(A/C)<0.0001
				(B/C)<0.0001
Inhibin B Mean ± SD (pg/ml)	1.8 ± 2.8	1 ± 0.9	53.1 ± 17.1	(A/B) 0.19
Range	(0-15)	(0-4)	(30-80)	(A/C)<0.0001
				(B/C)<0.0001

Table 2: Relationship between FSH and Inhibin B in all three groups.

Table 3 shows the relationship between Inhibin B levels with different levels of serum FSH in group A (women with POF), the higher level of Inhibin B was ≤ 15 pg/ml in 23 cases with FSH level >40 IU/ml, and two cases with FSH level between 13 and 39 IU/ml. The table presents a reverse relationship between Inhibin B level and FSH level.

Inhibin Level	FSH >40 IU/ml	FSH 13-39 IU/ml	FSH <12 IU/ml	Total
Inhibin <15 pg/ml	23	2	0	25
Inhibin 16-25 pg/ml	0	0	0	0
Inhibin >25 pg/ml	0	0	0	0
Total	23	2#	0*	25

Table 3: The relationship between Inhibin B level with different levels of FSH in group A before treatment (n=25).

Table 4 shows the relationship between the level of Inhibin B and FSH level in women with POF after 4-6 months of hormone replacement therapy, there was a decline in FSH level in 17 cases from >40 IU/ml to <12 IU/ml, in contrast to an increase in the level of Inhibin B in one case only from <15 pg/ml to between (16-25 pg/ml).

Inhibin Level	FSH >40 IU/ml	FSH 13-39 IU/ml	FSH <12 IU/ml	Total
Inhibin <15 pg/ml	3	4	17	24
Inhibin 16-25 pg/ml	0	1	0	1
Inhibin >25 pg/ml	0	0	0	0
Total	3	5	17	25

Table 4: The relationship between FSH and Inhibin B after 4 to 6 months of treatment with hormonal replacement therapy (n=25).

Table 5 shows the levels of FSH and Inhibin B after hormonal replacement therapy in group A, in which the mean FSH was (17.16 ± 13.4 IU/ml) with a range of (15-69 IU/ml), mean Inhibin B was (1.8 ± 2.9 pg/ml) and a range of (0-16 pg/ml). There was a significant decrease in FSH (P ≤ 0.0001) while no significant change in Inhibin B.

Group	Inhibin B Mean ± SD Range (pg/ml)	FSH B Mean ± SD Range (IU/ml)
POF prior to treatment	1.8 ± 2.8 (0-15)	81.4 ± 28.4 (37-150)
POF after Treatment	1.8 ± 2.9 (0-16)	17.16 ± 13.4 (16-69)

Table 5: FSH and Inhibin B levels after HRT in group A.

Discussion

Premature ovarian failure is common condition and had led to increase the concern in general population because in the current society there is a trend towards delaying pregnancy to later life and this had led to increase the infertility issues related to old age. Also the use of hormonal contraception might conceal this condition until the woman decides to discontinue the hormonal contraception and get pregnant. Diagnosis usually delayed due to the wide variety of symptoms for patient with premature ovarian failure. Also, there are no predictive factors for idiopathic POF and for the largest portion of the causes. All these issues together with the health and emotional impact of being menopaused at young age urge the need for finding and researching markers for early detection and even prediction of the condition. The term ovarian reserve have been based on the remaining follicular pool that's left in the ovary, when the process of ovarian aging occur usually the first marker to decrease is the anti mullarian hormone (AMH) followed by a decline in Inhibin B levels and lastly increasing in the FSH all these with the decrease in the antral follicular count. Therefore, ovarian reserve can be screened by variety of tests as FSH, estradiol, ovarian volume, clomiphene challenge stress test or antral follicles count [23-26].

The clomiphene citrate challenge test (CCCT) is a an accepted test for evaluating ovarian reserve but it requires days and multiple blood samples to be collected, the gonadotropins analogue stimulation test is based on FSH, E2, LH before and after GnRh administration. This test is expensive, need multiple injections, multiple blood samples and with limited value. Another tests for ovarian reserve is ultrasound and antral follicular count, and ovarian biopsy [27,28]. Hence, the need for a direct and precise marker for measuring ovarian reserve that can distinguish between complete absence of germ cells in ovary and lesser abnormality in ova production. Inhibin B is produced by granulosa cells so it might be more accurate in this regard. Inhibin B can be used as a marker for ovarian aging as it decreases with increasing age due to the decrease in number of follicles. This study was conducted to find the rule of Inhibin B in the assessment of ovarian function in women with premature ovarian failure in comparison with FSH.

The increase in FSH in old women is well documented, and it is commonly used to measure the ovarian reserve. FSH values are above 40 IU/ml at two occasions 4-6 months apart is indicative for ovarian failure. In this study, all women in group A and B (POF and menopaused) had high FSH results above 40 IU/ml. In group A there was no case reached the normal threshold of Inhibin B 25 pg/ml which goes with Corson et al. [25] but disagreed with what is reported by Seifer et al. [29]. The explanation probable for this disco-ordination with Seifer et al. [29] is due to the assay methodology, because till now there are no international assay standards for Inhibin B [30]. We found undetectable levels of Inhibin B <15 pg/ml in both group A (POF) and group B (menopaused), whereas among group C all women were found to have above the detectable levels of Inhibin B (15 pg/ml). It has been clarify that there is cyclical variation of Inhibin B throughout the menstrual cycle; beside low day 3 serum Inhibin B concentration was predictive of poor response to ovulation induction [29].

Hofman et al. [30] correlates Inhibin B in 19 women with normal ovarian reserve and 15 women with abnormal clomiphene citrate challenge test, Inhibin B was low at day 3 in women with abnormal CCCT and was higher in women with normal reserve In addition there was a negative correlation between day 3 FSH and Inhibin B. In our study among group A there were undetectable Inhibin B levels and a negative correlation between FSH and Inhibin B. The hormonal patterns of POF patients also implicate Inhibin as being causative in the disease mechanism. A defect in Inhibin secretion has been reported in women with POF [31] and Inhibin concentrations were lower in women with ovarian failure during both ovulatory and anovulatory cycles compared with infertile women with normal ovulatory cycle [32]. It has also noted that women with impending POF had lower follicular and luteal phase Inhibin concentration [33].

In this study women age above 45 years had lower serum Inhibin B concentration in comparison with younger women this is an agreement with Klein et al. study [34] who found that women aged 40-45 years compared with younger women had lower serum Inhibin B concentration in the early follicular phase. Previous studies demonstrated that women with POF and amenorrhea for less than 3 months are more likely to ovulate than women with longer period of amenorrhea and these ovulatory cycles are associated with lower FSH levels, although they remain elevated compared with FSH levels in regularly cycling women [35].

In this study after 4-6 months of hormonal replacement therapy (HRT), there was an increase in Inhibin B levels in one case only in contrast to decline in serum FSH levels in 17 cases. The significant limitations of the FSH assay derives from exogenous oestrogen intake, the fluctuation in FSH level as commonly seen with exogenous estrogen intake which is frequent in ovarian failure following chemotherapy or radiotherapy may be reasonable [36] and may cause fluctuation in FSH level as well as resumption of ovulation. Furthermore, FSH is an indirect marker, its rises takes long time and mildly elevated FSH may be seen in women with reduces ovarian reserve. Recent years have witnessed Inhibin B as a predictor of ovarian reserve, it is produced mainly in granulosa cells and it's undetectable in menopaused women [37]. Approximately, 40% of premenopausal women starting 2 years before final menstruation have undetectable Inhibin B level [38].

A study was done by Halder A et al. [39] who found that undetectable or less than 18 pg/ml Inhibin B levels in all POF cases as well in all menopausal women. Its level did not influenced by exogenous oestrogen intake 3 months prior to test. Thus, Inhibin B might offer an enhanced test for distinguishing women with POF [39]. In case of surgical menopause caused by oophorectomy, the rise in FSH is caused by the fall in inhibin, estradiol and progesterone after oophorectomy in which Inhibin B is cleared from circulation within 12 h of bilateral oophorectomy, confirming the ovary as the predominant source for these circulatory proteins in women [40].

In the present study we did not find any case of POF with normal FSH and Inhibin B and both are good markers for oogenesis. However, it appears that Inhibin B level is superior because it was not influenced by previous exogenous oestrogen intake. In conclusion, Inhibin B is not affected by exogenous oestrogen intake in comparison to FSH; it can be used as a non-invasive method in determining the ovarian reserve in women with premature ovarian failure seeking fertility.

References

1. Santoro N (2003) Mechanisms of premature ovarian failure. Ann Endocrinol 64: 87-92.
2. Timmreck LS, Reindollar RH (2003) Contemporary issues in primary amenorrhea. Obstet Gynecol Clin North Am 30: 287-302.
3. Nick P (2012) Menopause and post-menopausal women. Obstet Gynecol 8: 553-563.

4. Perry JR, Corre T, Esko T (2013) A genome-wide association study of early menopause and the combined impact of identified variants. Hum Mol Genet 22: 1465-1472.
5. Chevy C, Lynsey C, Andrew NS (2015) The genetics of premature ovarian failure: current perspectives. Int J Women's Health 7: 799-810.
6. Gold EB, Bromberger J, Crawford S, Samuels S, Greendale GA, et al. (2001) Factors associated with age at natural menopause in a multiethnic sample of midlife women. Am J Epidemiol 153: 865-874.
7. McKinlay SM (1996) The normal menopause transition: An overview. Maturitas 26: 137-145.
8. Coulam CB, Adamson SC, Annegers JF (1986) Incidence of premature ovarian failure. Obstet Gynecol 67: 604-606.
9. Bachelot A, Rouxel A, Massin N (2009) Phenotyping and genetic Studies of 357 consecutive patients presenting with premature ovarian failure. Eur J Endocrinol 161: 179-187.
10. Murabito JM, Yang Q, Fox C (2005) Heritability of age at natural menopause in the Framingham heart study. J Clin Endocrinol Metab 90: 3427-3434.
11. Conway GS, Kaltsas G, Patel A, Davies MC, Jacobs HS (1996) Characterizations of idiopathic premature ovarian failure. Fertil Steril 65: 337-341.
12. De Bruin ML, Huisbrink J, Hauptmann M (2008) Treatment related risk factors for premature menopause following Hodgkin lymphoma. Blood 111: 101-108.
13. Jin M, Yiqi Y, Huang H (2012) An update on primary ovarian insufficiency. Sci China Life Sci 55: 677-686.
14. Kappeler CJ, Hoyer PB (2012) 4-vinylcyclohexene diepoxide: A model chemical for ovotoxicity. Syst Biol Reprod Med 58: 57-62.
15. Morrison JC, Givens JR, Wiser WL (1975) Mumps oophoritis: A cause of premature menopause. Fertil Steril 26: 655-659.
16. Kate M, Nick P (2011) Premature ovarian failure. J Fam Plann Reprod Health Care 37: 35-42.
17. Kalantaridou SN, Davis SR, Nelson LM (1998) Premature ovarian failure. Endocrinol Metab Clin North Am 27: 989-1006.
18. Ying SY (1988) Inhibins, activins, and follistatins: Gonadal proteins modulating the secretion of follicle-stimulating hormone. Endocrine Reviews 9: 267-293.
19. Yogeshwar M, Jie Z, Rama M, Chris H, Winifred PS (2014) Inhibin at 90: From discovery to clinical application: A historical review. Endocrinol soci 35: 234-276.
20. Hillier SG, Wickings EJ, Illingworth PI (1991) Control of immunoactive inhibin production by human granulosa cells. Clin Endocrinol (Oxf) 35: 71-78.
21. Welt CK (2004) Regulation and function of inhibins in the normal menstrual cycle. Semin Reprod Med 22: 187-193.
22. Groome NP, Illingworth PJ, O'Brien M, Pai R, Rodger FE, et al. (1996) Measurement of dimeric Inhibin B throughout the human menstrual cycle. J Clin Endocrinol Metab 81: 1401-1405.
23. Hansen LM, Batzer FR, Gutmann JN, Corson SL, Kelly MP, et al. (1999) Evaluating ovarian reserve follicle stimulating hormone and estrodiol variability during cycle days 2-5. Hum Reprod 11: 486-489.
24. Hofmann GE, Sosnowiski J, Scott RT, Thie J (1996) Efficacy of selection criteria for ovarian reserve screening using the clomphine citrate challenge test in tertiary fertility center population. Fertile Steril 66: 49-53.
25. Corson SL, Gutmann J, Batzer FR, Wallace H, Klein N, et al. (1999) Inhibin B as a test of ovarian reserve for infertile women. Hum Reprod 14: 2818-2821.
26. Padma RJ (2011) Ovarian reserve tests. J Hum Reprod Sci 4: 108-113.
27. Hendriks DJ, Mol BW, Bancsi LF, TeVelde ER, Broekmans FJ (2005) Antral follicle count in the prediction of poor ovarian response and pregnancy after in vitro fertilization: A meta-analysis and comparison with basal follicle-stimulating hormone level. Fertil Steril 83: 291-301.
28. Vital VS, Tellez S, Alvaarado I (2000) Clinical histologic correlation in reproductive pathology. Obstet Gynecol 95: S83.
29. Seifer DB, Messerlian GL, Hogan JW (1997) Day 3 serum Inhibin B is predictive of assisted reproductive technologies outcome. Fertil Steril 67: 110-114.
30. Helen L, shanthi M, Marko H, Nigel P (2008) Development of new antibody to the human Inhibin/Activin B subunit and its application to improve Inhibin B ELISAs. Immun Meth 329: 102-111.
31. Buckler HM, Evans CA, Mamtora H, Burger HG, Andersone DC (1991) Gonadotropin, Steroid, and Inhibin levels in women with incipient ovarian failure during anovulatory and ovulatory rebound cycles. Clin Endocrinol Metab72: 116-124.
32. Kwee J, Schats R, McDonnell J, Lambalk CB, Schoemaker J (2004) Intercycle variability of ovarian reserve tests: Results of a prospective randomized study. Hum Reprod 19: 590-595.
33. Klein NA, Illingorth PJ, Groome NP, McNeilly AS, Battaglia DE, et al. (1996) Decreased Inhibin B secretion is associated with the monotropic FSH rise in older, ovulatory women: A study of serum and follicular fluid levels of dimeric inhibin A and B in spontaneous menstrual cycles. Clin Endocrinol Metabol 81: 2742-2745.
34. Welt CK, Hall JE, Adams JM, Taylor AE (2005) Relationship of estradiol and inhibin to the follicle-stimulating hormone variability in hypergonadotropic hypogonadism or premature ovarian failure. Clin Endocrinol Metab 90: 862-830.
35. Howell S, Shalet S (1998) Gonadal damage from chemotherapy and radiotherapy. Endocrinol Metab North Clinic 17: 927-943.
36. Burger HG, Dudley EC, Hopper JL, Groome N, Guthrie JR, et al. (1999) Prospectively measured levels of serum follicle-stimulating hormone, estradiol, and the dimeric inhibins during the menopausal transition in a population-based cohort of women. Clinic Endocrinol Metab 84: 4025-4032.
37. Burger HG, Dudley EC, Hopper JL, Shelley JM, Green A, et al. (1995) The endocrinology of the menopausal transition: A cross-sectional study of a population based sample. Clin Endocrinol Metab 80: 4035-4037.
38. Burger HG, Dudley EC, Hopper JL, Groome N, Guthrie JR, et al. (1999) Prospectively measured levels of serum follicle-stimulating hormone, estradiol, and the dimeric inhibins during the menopausal transition in a population-based cohort of women. Clinic Endocrinol Metab 84: 4025-4032.
39. Halder A, Fauzdar A, Ghosh M, Kumau A (2003) Serum Inhibin B: A direct and persies marker of ovarian function. Clinic Diagnos Res 1: 131-137.
40. Muttukrishna S, Sharma S, Barlow DH, Ledger W, Groome N, et al. (2002) Serum inhibins, estradiol, progesterone and FSH in surgical menopause: A demonstration of ovarian pituitary feedback loop in women. Hum Reprod 17: 2535-2539.

Practice of Menstrual Hygiene and Associated Factors among Female High School Students in Adama Town

Haile Anchebi T[1], **Zeleke Shiferaw B**[2*], **Olana Fite R**[3] **and Garoma Abeya S**[4]

[1]*Department of public Health, College of Health Sciences, Adama General Hospital and Medical College, Adama, Ethiopia*

[2]*Department of Nursing, Wolkite University, College of Medicine and Health Sciences, Wolkite, Ethiopia*

[3]*Department of Nursing, College of Medicine and Health sciences, Woliata Sodo University, Woliata Sodo, Ethiopia*

[4]*Department of Social and Population Health, Adama Hospital Medical College, Adama, Ethiopia*

***Corresponding author:** Zeleke Shiferaw B, Department of Nursing, Wolkite University, College of Medicine and Health Sciences, Wolkite, Ethiopia, E-mail: basfendaz@gmail.com

Abstract

Background: Good menstrual hygienic practices are essential during menstruation period. Young women especially in developing countries often lack information about good menstrual hygiene practices. The objective of this study was to assess the level of menstrual hygienic practice and the associated factors among female high school students in Adama town.

Methods: A cross-sectional, institution based study was conducted from April 11th-25th, 2016. Multistage sampling technique was used to select the participants. Data was cleaned, coded and entered in to Epi-data 3.1 and analyzed using SPSS version 20:00. Binary and multiple logistic regression analysis were done to determine the association between the menstrual hygienic practice and the predicator variables. A p-value of less than 0.05 was taken as significant association.

Result: A total of 398 female students were involved in the study giving a response rate of 94.3%. Of the total respondents about 57% had good level of menstrual hygiene practice. Mothers education status [AOR=0.608; 95% CI=0.374-0.990], source of money for sanitary materials [AOR=2.267; 95% CI=1.076, 4.772], respondents feeling on comfort ability of the school [AOR=0.557; 95% CI=0.366-0.846] were significantly associated with level of knowledge about menstrual hygienic practice.

Conclusion: The study showed that more than half of the respondents had good level of menstrual hygiene practice. Mothers' educational status, source of money for sanitary materials and respondents feeling on comfort ability of the school were found to be predictors of menstrual hygiene practice among the students. Thus, designing health information and communication programs on awareness about menstruation and menstrual hygiene practice is implicated.

Keywords: Menstruation; Hygiene practice; Adama town

Abbreviations: COR: Crude Odds Ratio; AOR: Adjusted Odds Ratio; CI: Confidence Interval; SPSS: Statistical Package for Social Sciences

Background

Good menstrual hygienic practices such as use of sanitary pads and adequate washing of the genital areas are essential during menstruation period. Having a good menstrual hygienic practice will enhance the confidence of females in many aspects. On the other hand, Poor menstrual hygienic practices will increase susceptibility to reproductive health related problems [1,2].

Menstrual hygiene practice is influenced by many factors including female's knowledge about menstruation [3,4]. In relation to cultural taboos females are often deprived of utilizing the main resources in the community. Furthermore, academic performance and involvement is highly affected by different conditions associated with menstruation [5].

Although the period of adolescence is a healthy part of life, many adolescents are often less informed, less experienced and less comfortable with accessing reproductive health information and services than adults [6,7].

Assessing the menstrual hygiene practice level of females and addressing the gap is essential to reinforce safe and hygienic practice during menstruation [8]. The practical challenges of menstrual hygiene practice are made even more difficult by socio-cultural factors and millions of girls continue to be denied their rights to have sufficient information about menstrual hygiene, water and sanitary health, education, dignity and gender equity. This may result to incorrect and unhealthy behavior during their menstrual period [9,10].

Many schools do not support adolescent girls or female teachers in managing menstrual hygiene with dignity. Inadequate water and sanitation facilities make managing menstruation very difficult, and poor sanitary protection materials can result in blood-stained clothes causing stress and embarrassment. Even at the household level, they generally have little control over access to a private latrine or money for sanitary materials [10,11].

Females of reproductive age group need to have access to clean and soft absorbent sanitary products which in the long run protect their health from various infections [12].

Failure to provide appropriate menstrual hygiene facilities at home or at school level also decrease the level of having good menstrual hygiene practice among female students [11]. Thus, it is important to assess and address the problems related with the menstrual hygiene practice of female students; which in turn is crucial in improving female student's confidence, academic performance and sexual and reproductive health.

Therefore, this study was conducted to assess the level of menstrual hygiene practice and associated factors among female high school students found in Adama town. The finding of this study will be helpful for school related health policy makers in understanding predictors of menstrual hygiene practice among high school female students and in designing the possible interventions.

Methods

Study area and period

The study was conducted in Adama town from April 11-25, 2016. In the study area, there are a total of 9 governmental high schools. According to the data from Adama town education affairs office a total of 15,691 students were enrolled during the academic year of 2015/16 in these schools.

Study design

A cross-sectional descriptive study was conducted.

Source population

The source population was all female governmental secondary schools students in Adama town.

Study population

The study population was selected female governmental secondary schools students in Adama town.

Inclusion and exclusion criteria

All regular female students were included into the study. Female students who were sick and unable to respond were excluded from the study.

Sample size determination

Single population proportion formula was used to calculate the required sample size. Proportion of level of knowledge towards menstruation of 50% [p], margin of error of 5% [d], and 95% confidence level [1.96] and adding non-response rate of 10%, the sample size was determined to be 422.

Sampling procedure

As to the sampling technique, a multistage stratified sampling technique was used; where first, 6 schools were selected among the 9 governmental high schools by lottery method, then, the respective sample was allocated to each high schools proportionally based on the female students population in each high schools.

Finally, the study units were selected from each year of study (grade) using simple random sampling technique considering the list of female students as a sample frame.

Variables

Dependent variable: Menstrual hygiene practice

Independent variable: Socio-demographic characteristics (Age, grade level, ethnic group, religion, mothers educational level, fathers educational level, monthly income of the family) and Students experience (school comfort to keep hygiene, comfort at school time, comfort around male students, feeling unclean and missing class).

Operational Definition

Menstrual hygiene practice: To measure the respondent's menstrual hygiene practice. 10 closed ended menstrual hygiene practice related questions were presented and for each correct answer 1 point and 0 for incorrect ones given.

Respondents who scored 6 and above were considered as having good menstrual hygiene practice and a score of less than 6 was considering as having poor menstrual hygiene practice.

Data collection

Data collection instrument

Data was collected using pre-tested structured self-administered questionnaires. It is composed of 'closed-end' questions assessing different variables like the respondents socio-demographic characteristics, menstrual hygiene practice and experience. To ensure its consistency it was translated to 'Amharic' and 'Afan Oromo' language and back translated to English by language professionals.

Data collection procedure

The questionnaire was distributed to the students by three data collectors with past experience on data collection, the data was collected while students were in class rooms and the instructors cooperated with data facilitators in disseminating the questionnaire.

Finally, the filled questionnaire was checked for completeness and consistency of the data by the data collector's supervisor on daily basis.

Data quality assurance

To ensure the quality of the data; training was given for the data collectors and supervisors two days ahead of the actual data collection date, the questionnaire were translated by language professionals, pretest were conducted on 5% of the sample and relevant corrections were made.

During data collection supportive supervision were made and data were checked for the completeness.

Data entry and analysis

The collected quantitative data was cleaned, coded and entered in to Epi-data 3.1 software, and then exported to Statistical package for social sciences(SPSS) version 20:00 for analysis.

First descriptive analysis was carried out for each variable. Next, bivariate analysis was done to identify the association between the independent and the dependent variables. Those variables with a p-value<0.25 in bivariate analysis were selected for multivariate logistic regression, and then those variables with a p-value<0.05 were considered to be statistically significant in multivariate analysis.

Result

Socio-demographic characteristics

In this study a total of 398 female students were participated giving a response rate of 94.3%. Of these 200 [50.3%] were in the age group 14-16 years and 198 [49.7%] were in 17-19 age groups.

Most of the respondents 139[34.9%] were from Oromo ethnic group, concerning their religion. More than half 233[58.5%] of them are followers of Orthodox religion [Table 1].

Variables	Response category	Frequency	Percentage (%)
Age	14-16 years old	200	50.3
	17-19 years old	198	49.7
Grade	Grade 9	199	50
	Grade 10	199	50
Ethnic group	Oromo	139	34.9
	Amhara	98	24.6
	Woliata	94	23.6
	Tigre	23	5.8
	Other	44	11.1
Religion	Orthodox	233	58.5
	Muslim	81	20.4
	Protestant	76	19.1
	Other	8	2.1
Mother educational status	Below and Primary	276	69.3
	Secondary and above	122	30.7
Father educational status	Below and Primary	228	57.3
	Secondary and above	170	42.7
Parents' monthly income	700-1500 Birr	72	18.1
	1600-2400 Birr	84	21.1
	2500-3300 Birr	124	31.2
	>3300 Birr	118	29.6

Table 1: Socio-demographic characteristics of female high school students in Adama town, April 2016(n=398).

Experience during menstruation

From the respondents, more than two-third 278(69.80%) of them reported that they are not feeling comfortable on classroom (school time), about 188(47.20%) of them reported that their school is uncomfortable to keep their hygiene during menstruation and 186(46.70%) of them missed class during menstruation time [Figure 1].

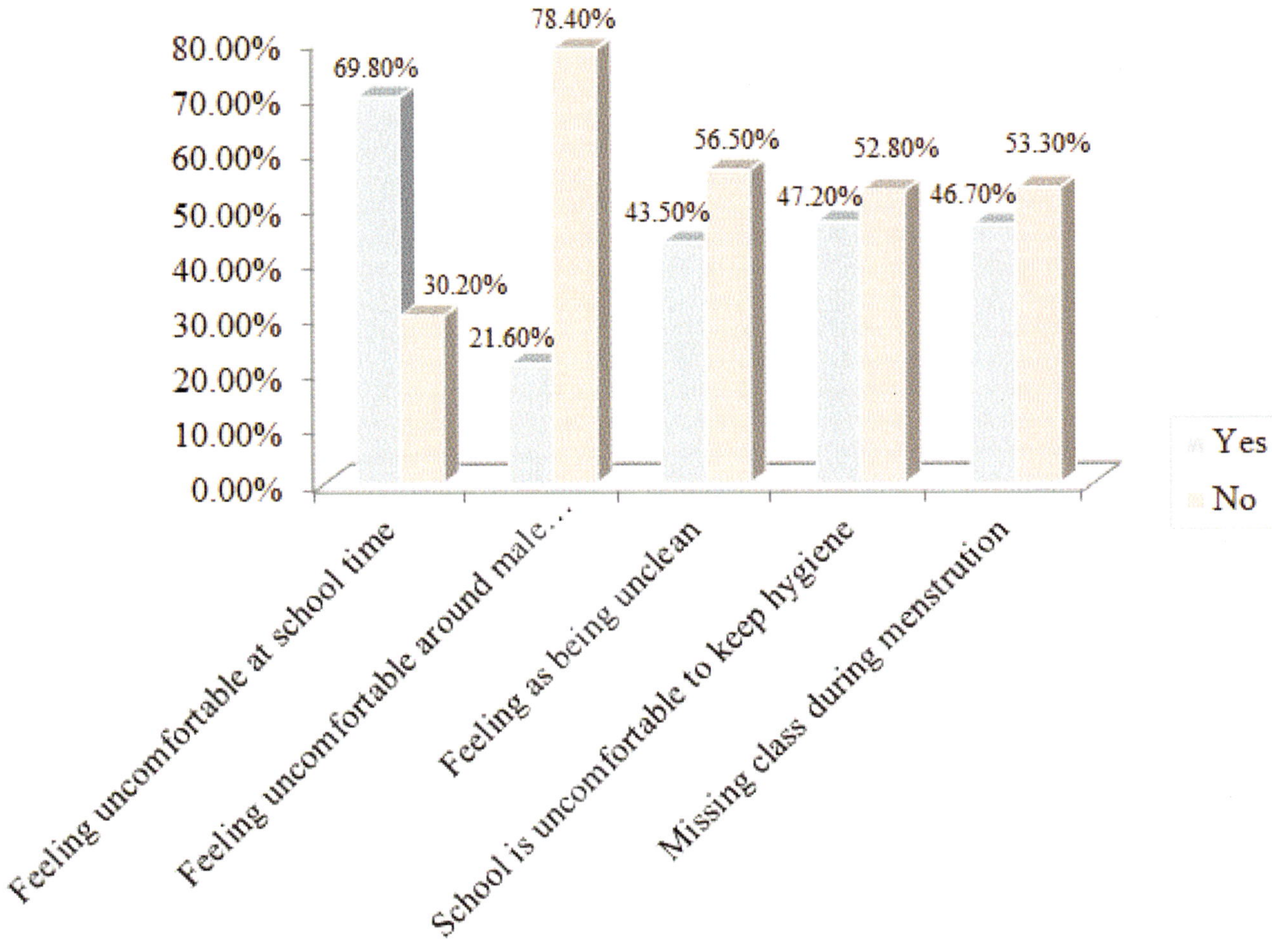

Figure 1: Experience during menstruation of female high school students in Adama town, April 2016(n=398).

Menstrual hygiene practice

Based on the finding of this study, 387(97.2%) of the respondents used absorbent during menstruation and from those 21(5.3%) used sanitary pads. The source of money for 360(90.5%) of the students were their parents.

For 204(51.3%) of the students the source of information were their mothers. About 327(82.2%) disposed the used material as protection into latrine. Of the total respondents 211(53.0%) took daily bath during menstruation [Table 2].

Variables		Frequency	Percentage (%)
Uses absorbent	Yes	387	97.2
	No	11	2.8
Material used	Rag made	12	3
	Sanitary pad	21	5.3
	Tampon	339	85.2
	Other	26	6.5
Money source to buy materials	Parents	360	90.5
	Earn it	38	9.5

Source of information on menstrual hygiene	Mother	204	51.3
	Friends	67	16.8
	Mass media	62	15.6
	Teachers	52	13.1
	Other	13	3.3
Disposal place	Open field	17	4.3
	Latrine	327	82.2
	In waste bins	41	10.3
	Other	13	3.3
Clean clothes with soap and water	Yes	210	52.8
	No	188	47.2
Clean external genitalia	Yes	385	96.7
	No	13	3.3
Cleaning material used	Water	156	39.2
	Water and soap	229	57.5
	Not washing	13	3.3
Daily bath	Yes	211	53
	No	187	47
Drying place for cloth	Outside the house	249	62.6
	Inside the house	149	37.4
Use paper to dispose Sanitary materials by wrapping	Yes	219	55
	No	179	45
Changing absorbents	<3 times	51	12.8
	≥ 3 times	347	87.2

Table 2: Menstrual hygiene practice of female high school students in Adama town, April 2016(n=398).

Level of menstrual hygiene practice

Concerning the respondents level of menstrual hygiene practice about 171(43.0%) of them had poor level of menstrual hygiene practice, while 227(57.0%) of them had good menstrual hygiene practice [Figure 2].

Factors associated with practice of menstrual hygiene practice

As shown in the Table 3 below those factors found associated on bivariate analysis with p-value ≤ 0.25 were entered to multivariable analysis. Accordingly, mothers education status, money source to buy sanitary materials, feeling the school as being uncomfortable were found significant predictors of good menstrual hygiene practice.

Accordingly, students who doesn't felt the school was comfortable 43.3% less likely to had good menstrual hygiene practice than students who felt school was comfortable (AOR=0.557; 95%CI=0.366-0.846).

Furthermore, students whose source of money was their parents were 2.3 times more likely to had a good menstrual hygiene practice as compared to those students who earn the money by themselves (AOR=2.267; 95% CI=1.076, 4.772).

Regarding mothers educational status, students whose mother attended secondary and above level of education were 39.2% less likely to had good menstrual hygiene practice than students whose mother attended below and primary level of education (AOR=0.608; 95% CI=0.374-0.990) [Table 3].

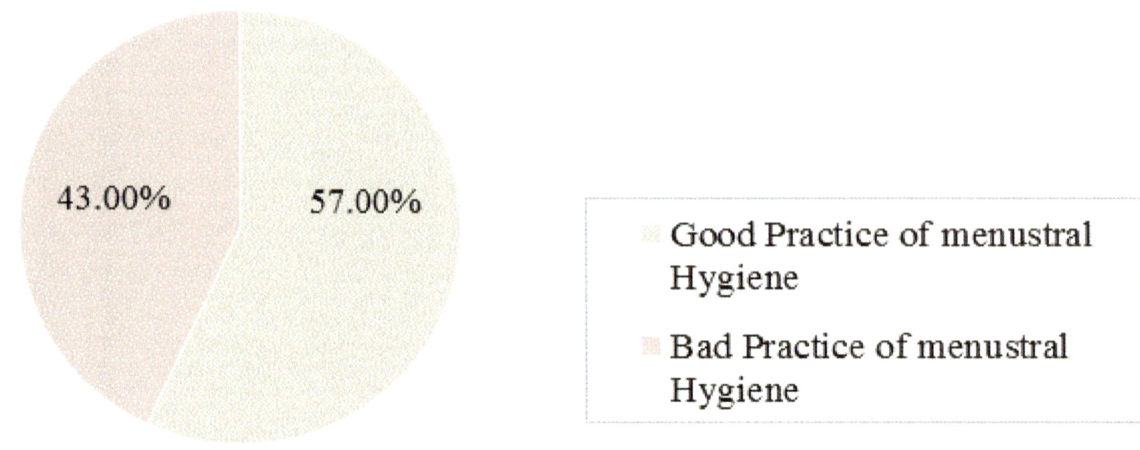

Figure 2: Level of menstrual hygiene practice of female high school students in Adama town, April 2016(n=398).

Variables		Menstrual Hygiene Practice		COR(95% CI)	AOR(95% CI)
		Good	Poor		
Age	14-16 years old†	121	79	1	1
	17-19 years old	106	92	0.752(0.505,1.120)	0.784(0.520,1.183)
Mother educational level	Primary and below†	170	106	1	1
	Secondary and above	57	65	0.547(0.356,0.841)*	0.608(0.374,0.990)*
Father educational level	Primary and below†	138	90	1	1
	Secondary and above	89	81	0.717(0.480,1.070)	0.829(0.524,1.311)
School uncomfortable to keep hygiene	Yes†	120	68	1	1
	No	107	103	0.589(0.394,0.880)*	0.557(0.366,0.846)*
Source of money to buy sanitary materials	Parents†	201	159	1	1
	Earn it	26	12	1.714(0.838,3.503)	2.267(1.076,4.772)*

Table 3: Factors associated with menstrual hygiene practice of female high school students in Adama town, April 2016(n=398) [†: Reference category, *: Significant association].

Discussion

This study assessed the menstrual hygiene practice of high school students and associated factors. Concerning the menstrual hygiene practice, more than 40% of the respondents had good menstrual hygiene practice. Presence of gap in educating female students about techniques of keeping sexual health might be the possible explanation for this. Therefore, provision of special education at high school level is required for female students including safe menstrual hygiene practice [13,14].

In this study 57% of the respondents had good practice of menstrual hygiene. This is higher than a finding from a study conducted in western Ethiopia [15] and India in which only 39.9% and 1.82%. This might be due to the difference in the study area in which most of the study participants of participants in this study from urban area. This in its turn will increase the access of getting health information and communication related to menstrual hygiene practice from several medias.

The difference in the study period could also be another possible explanation. Similarly, a research done in Nepal [16] and Lebanon [17] showed that about 46.7% and 50.6% of the students had good menstrual hygiene practices respectively.

Students who don't felt comfortable in their school environment were found to be 43.3% less likely to had good menstrual hygiene practice than their counterparts. Consequently, their lower level of practice could be related to their felling about the school environment [18].

In this study for about 51.3% of the respondents, mothers were the main source of information about menstrual hygiene. This is in contrast with the study finding from Amhara regional state of Ethiopia [19], in which mothers were the second source of information which accounts about 22.96%. This might be related due to cultural differences in the study areas.

Conclusion

In this study majority of the respondents had good menstrual hygiene practice. According to the findings of this study, source of information about menstrual hygiene practice was their mothers. Majority of the respondents felt uncomfortable during school time while experiencing menstruation. As finding showed that mothers education status, source of money for buying sanitary materials, feeling the school as being uncomfortable were significant predictors of good menstrual hygiene practice.

Therefore, it is recommended that strategy and policy makers should develop appropriate evidence-based strategies and curricula in high schools concerning female's reproductive health and specifically about menstruation and menstrual hygiene practice. Thus, designing strategies towards awareness creation and attitude changing activities about menstruation and menstrual hygiene practice through provision of different regular health information and communication programs is implicated.

Declarations

Ethics approval and consent to participate

The study was conducted after obtaining ethical clearance from Adama General Hospital and Medical College. An official letter was obtained from each school. Verbal informed consent was obtained from the participants age 18 and above and for study participants whose age were less than 18 years parental informed consent was obtained.

Personal identification data like respondents name were not included in the questionnaires. Students were informed they have full right either not to participate or terminate their participation at any stage from the study. All the data obtained in due course were confidentially kept.

Competing interest

The authors declared no conflict of interest.

Funding

Adama Hospital and Medical College has covered the required fund for the research project.

Authors' contributions

Haile T conceptualized and designed the study. Haile T, Zeleke B, Olana R and Garoma S analyzed and interpreted the data, drafted the manuscript and critically reviewed the manuscript. All the authors read and approved the manuscript.

Acknowledgements

We would like to thank Adama General Hospital and Medical College for funding this research project. Our gratitude goes to Adama special zone education office, the respective high schools, supervisors, data collectors, respondent who participated on this study. Finally, we thank for language editing Mr. Mark Demos (Former American peas corps volunteer, in Ethiopia) and Mr. Sefu Bogale (English language teacher in Wolkite university).

References

1. Prajapati D, Shah JP, Kedia G (2015) Menstrual hygiene: Knowledge and practice among adolescent girls of rural Kheda district. NJCM 6: 349-353.
2. Ali TS, Rizvi SN (2010) Menstrual knowledge and practices of female adolescents in urban Karachi, Pakistan. J Adolesc 33: 531-541.
3. Karout N (2015) Knowledge and beliefs regarding menstruation among Saudi nursing Students. J Nurs Educ Pract 6: 23-30.
4. Dasgupta A, Sarkar M (2008) Menstrual hygiene: How hygienic is the adolescent girl? Indian J Comm Med 33: 77-80.
5. Sudheshna R, Dasgupta A (2012) Determinants of menstrual hygiene among adolescent girls. A multivariate analysis. National J Comm Med 3: 294-301.
6. Ramachandra K, Gilyaru S, Eregowda A, Yathiraja S (2016) A study on knowledge and practices regarding menstrual hygiene among urban adolescent girls. Int J Contemporary Peadiatrics 3: 142-145.
7. Shalaby NS, Elsabour MA, Abd Allah IM (2012) Effect of a health education program about reproductive health on the knowledge and attitude of adolescent female, Port Said University students. J American Science 8: 541-548.
8. Verma P, Ahmad S, Srivastava RK (2013) Knowledge and practices bout menstrual hygiene among higher secondary school girls. Indian J Comm Health 25: 265-271.
9. Ninama R, Dund JV (2015) Knowledge and practice regarding menstrual hygiene among adolescent girls. SJAMS 3: 2704-2709.
10. Vidiya VP, Rekha U (2016) Menstrual hygienic practices among adolescent girls of rural North Karnataka region, India. Int J Community Med Public Health 3: 1872-1876.
11. Dasgupta A, Sarkar M (2008) Menstrual hygiene: How hygienic is the adolescent girl? Indian J Community Med 33: 77-80.
12. Narayan KA, Srinivasa DK, Pelto PJ, Veerammal S (2001) Puberty rituals, reproductive knowledge and health of adolescent school girls in South India. Asia-Pac Popul J. 2: 225-238.
13. Gultie TK (2014) Practice of menstrual hygiene and associated factors among female Mehalmeda high school students in Amhara regional state, Ethiopia. Sci J Public Health 2: 189-195.
14. Lawan UM, Nafisa WY, Aisha BM (2010) Menstruation and menstrual hygiene amongst adolescent school girls in Kano, Northwestern Nigeria. Afr J Reprod Health 14: 201-208.
15. Upashe SP, Tekelab T, Mekonnen J (2015) Assessment of knowledge and practice of menstrual hygiene among high school girls in Western Ethiopia. BMC Women's Health 15: 1-8.
16. Auemaneekul N, Bhandari S, Kerdmongkol P (2013) Menstrual hygiene practices among adolescents in a Rural District of Nepal. Asia J Public Health 4: 8-15.

17. Santina T, Wehbe N, Ziade FM, Nehme M (2013) Assessment of beliefs and practices relating to menustral hygiene of adolescent girls in Lebanon. Int J Health Sci Res 3: 75-88.

18. Shanbhag D, Shilpa R, D'Souza N, Josephine P, Singh J, et al. (2012) Perceptions regarding menstruation and practices during menstrual cycles among high school going adolescent girls in resource limited settings around Bangalore city, Karnataka, India. Int J Collab Res Intern Med Public Health 4: 1353-1362.

19. Gultie TK, Hailu D, Workineh Y (2014) Age of menarche and knowledge about menstrual hygiene management among adolescent school girls in Amhara Province, Ethiopia: Implication to Health Care Workers & School Teachers. PLOS ONE 9: 1-9.

The Preventive Practice of and Associated Factors of HIV/AIDS among Female Sex Workers in Dessie Town, Northeast Ethiopia, 2017

Abay Woday[1*], **Yonatan Menber**[2], **Fuad Yimam**[2], **Negesse Melese**[2] **and Samuel Dagne**[3]

[1]*Department of Public Health, College of Medical and Health Science, Samara University, Ethiopia*

[2]*Department of Public Health, College of Health Science, Alkan University, Ethiopia*

[3]*Department of Public Health, College of Health Science, Woldia University, Ethiopia*

***Corresponding author:** Abay Woday Tadesse, Department of Public Health, College of Medical and Health Science, Samara University, Afrar, Ethiopia E-mail: abaywoday@yahoo.com

Abstract

Background: Commercial sex workers have been recognized as the high risk segment of the population since the last three decades. Though few studies have been conducted to dates in Ethiopia, all of them are focusing on the knowledge of female sex workers towards HIV/AIDS. However, no study has been done to assess the preventive practices of HIV/AIDS among female sex workers in Ethiopia as well in the study area. Therefore, this study aims to assess comprehensive knowledge and preventive practice of HIV/AIDS among female sex workers in Dessie town, North West Ethiopia, 2017.

Methods: A quantitative community based cross-sectional study triangulated with qualitative methods was employed among 592 female sex workers from 15th April 2017 to 25th May 2017 in Dessie town. A standardized, pretested and structured interviewer administered questionnaire, in-depth interview and observation were used to collect the data. The study participants were selected by employing multistage cluster sampling technique. Bivariate and multivariable logistic regression was employed to determine the association between dependent and explanatory variables. Statistically significant level was declared at P-value less than 0.05. Transcription and narration was done for the qualitative section.

Result: About 54.8% of female sex workers had good preventive practice of HIV/AIDS. After adjustment; alcohol consumption (AOR=0.25; 95% CI=0.11, 0.39) and khat chewing (AOR=0.28; 95% CI=0.15,0.62] were found the hindering factors of preventive practice but being membership with organizations those working on HIV/AIDS (AOR=2.55,95% CI=1.52-4.27) was found significantly associated with preventive practice of HIV/AIDS among FSWs.

Conclusion: The preventive practice of HIV/AIDS among female sex workers was found suboptimal. Therefore, the government, stakeholders and the community should give high attention to the high risk segment of population. Further analytic studies should be done on this area to explore more information on the determinant factors of knowledge and preventive practice of HIV/AIDS among female sex workers and other high risk groups.

Keywords: Preventive practice; Female sex workers; Community; Chronic illness

Introduction

Acquired Immunodeficiency Syndrome (AIDS) is a chronic illness caused by Human Immunodeficiency Virus (HIV) that damages a person's ability to fight the disease and leaving the body vulnerable to ordinarily innocuous infections [1]. Sex workers have been among the populations most affected by HIV since the beginning of the epidemic for more than three decades. In both concentration and generalization of the epidemics, HIV prevalence is considerably 12 times higher among commercial sex workers than in the general population. Sex workers often have little control over these factors because of social marginalization and the criminalization of sex work [2].

The global HIV prevalence among female sex workers (FSWs) has been estimated at 11.8%. Of these, the highest prevalence (36%) found concentrated in sub-Saharan Africa thus leading to the classification of the group as a higher-risk [3]. In Ethiopia, discrepancies in socio-economic status have forced an increasing number of people to seek any source of income, including female sex selling. The survey conducted by PSI in collaboration with Dessie Town Bureau of Labor and Social Affairs (BoLSA) in 2016 has estimated that there are nearly a half thousand (4655) female sex workers found in Dessie Town, Amhara Regional state [4]. The hotspot survey result showed that the town has the third highest number of female sex workers (FSWs) next to Bahir Dar and Gondar town.

According to 2012 progress report of Ethiopia, only 42.3% of Female sex workers reached by HIV prevention program. In the same year, from 44.8% FSWs tested for HIV 25% were found Positive [5]. The study conducted in Gondar town on street FSWs on condom utilization practice revealed that 57.4% of female sex workers were consistently condom use during any sexual practices [6]. Studies conducted across Africa found that sex workers in many places are highly vulnerable to HIV and other sexually transmitted infections due to multiple factors. The identified factors were; having many sex partners, hazardous working environment, alcohol consumption, smoking, drug use, physical violence and barriers in the negotiation of consistent condom use [7,8].

Different strategies, policies, programs have been tried in the past to reduced transmission and the incidence of new cases of HIV at global, regional and national levels. In particular, HIV prevention and care strategies were focusing on the already affected part of population [9-11]. As a result, much has changed in the response to HIV over the last three decades, especially in the areas of prevention, testing and treatment. What remains in missing is a respectful and inclusive response to marginalized and vulnerable populations including sex workers were given little attention across the globe especially in Sub-Saharan countries including Ethiopia [2]. Moreover, to the best of the researchers' knowledge no study has been conducted in the district to assess the preventive practice and associated factors of HIV/AIDS among FSWs. Therefore, this study will generate more evidence to close this information gap in the study area.

Methods and Materials

Study setting and participants

Community-based cross-sectional study design triangulated with qualitative method was employed from 15th April 2017 to 25th May 2017 among female sex workers resided in Dessie Town, North-Eastern Ethiopia. Dessie Town is located 401 Kms away from the capital city, Addis Ababa. The city has a total population of 301, 241. Of these, 4655 are female sex workers those are making their business by selling sex in Bars, Red-lights, hotels and home based establishments [4]. It has also different levels of hotels, night clubs, 06 public health facilities (01 referral hospital and 05 health centers). It has also different lower level of private health facilities and 04 private general hospitals.

To determine the required sample size, both single population proportion and double population proportion formals were used for the two specific objectives but the larger sample size was obtained by using single population proportion formula. Therefore, the sample size 592 was calculated by using a single population proportion formula with assumptions: 5% type I error, 95% CI, 57.4% of level of preventive practice of HIV/AIDS among Female Sex Workers (FSWs) resided in Northwest Ethiopia was taken as population proportion [6], Design effect of 1.5 and an estimated non-response rate of 5%.

$n= (Za/z)^2 (P) (1-P)/d^2$

Where; n=required sample size, $Z\alpha/2$=critical value for normal distribution at 95% confidence level (1.96), p=The level of preventive practice of HIV/AIDS among FSWs, DEFF=Design effect of intra cluster homogeneity and d=Type I error). Based on the above assumptions, the final required sample size required for the study was 592. The study participants included in the study were FSWs resided in Dessie town for at least six months, were at least 15 years of age, able to hear, mentally oriented, and not seriously sick were included in this study.

From the total 10 lower administrative units (Kebeles) found in Dessie town, 5 were identified as Hotspot Kebeles then 3 kebeles were selected randomly and all of the female sex workers resided in the selected three kebeles (lower administrative unit) were studied by using cluster sampling technique (Figure 1).

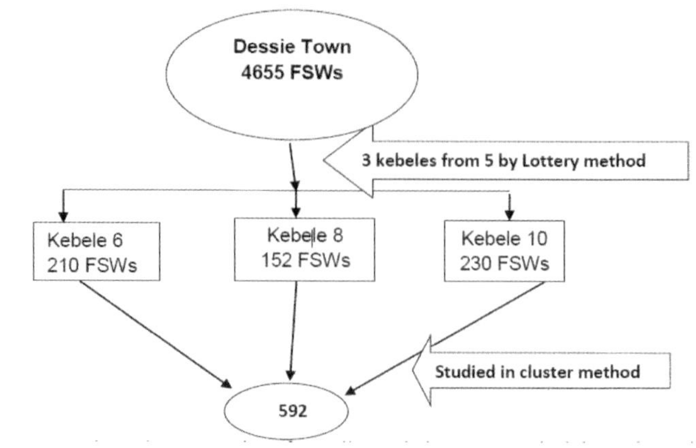

Figure 1: Schematic presentation of sampling techniques to recruit the study participants in Dessie town, 2017.

The qualitative data collection was conducted by observation of condom demonstration using penile model among five (05) participants and nine (09) in-depth interview among the three types of FSW (Hotel based, Home based and street based) until the required data was saturated by using observation and in-depth interview guiding tools.

Data processing and analysis

The standardized, pretested and semi structured interviewer administered questionnaire was used to assess the preventive practice of HIV/AIDS and associated factors among FSWs by including important variables for the study and was organized by sections for socio-demographic, behavioral factors, knowledge of condom use, practice of consistent condom use, and other life style related factors.

The tool was also checked for clarity and consistency; it was pretested in two Lower administrative units (Kebeles) of Dessie town on 5% of FSWs to address any unclear or misunderstood questions and corrections were made based on the pretest findings. The data was collected by six trained B.Sc. nurses. The questionnaire was translated from English version to the local language (Amharic) and again back to English version.

The qualitative part was collected by using observation of condom demonstration and in-depth interview by using tape recorder with participation of all type of female sex workers. The data were collected at convenient time to study participants which was at night and day time.

The preventive practice was measured by asking:

- Do you consistently use condom for any sexual intercourse even with your constant partner?
- Do you share any sharpen materials with any on else around you?

FSWs who answered both questions were defined as having adequate level of preventive practice of HIV/AIDS.

The data was cleaned, coded and entered in to Epi data version 3.1 software and exported into SPSS version 20.0 for analysis. The descriptive analysis was done and the results were displayed in the form of texts, tables, and figures. Then binary logistic analysis was conducted to measure the association between the dependent variable with each independent variable: Socio-demographic, socio-economic, and behavioral factors, condom utilization related factors were among included factors using odds ratio with 95% confidence interval.

Finally, multivariable logistic regression analysis was done in order to control possible potential confounders and to identify predictors of comprehensive knowledge and practice of condom utilization among FSWs. Statistical significance was declared at P-value<0.05.

The qualitative data was transcribed, translated, transferred in to open code software version 3.6, read repeatedly, coded and categorized thematically. Finally, it was interpreted with thematic analysis.

Results

Participants' socio-demographic characters

A total of 584 female sex workers were interviewed with the response rate of 98.6%. Six condom demonstration observations by using penile model and seven in-depth interviews were conducted.

Of the total respondents; 46.7% were in the age group above 25 years, the mean age was 24.6 ± 5.3 SD (16-47 years), 31.5% of FSWs were unable to read and write, 53.4% were single, 33.7% were divorced and 62.5% of respondents had history migration from rural areas (Table 1).

Variables	Category	Number of FSWs	Percentage (%)
Age (in years)	15-19	101	17.3
	20-24	211	36
	≥ 25	272	46.7
Completed educational level	Can't read and write	184	31.5
	Only read and write	128	21.9
	Attend elementary school	170	29.1
	Attend Secondary school and above	111	19
Religion	Orthodox	523	89.6
	Muslim	32	5.5
	Protestant	16	2.7
	Catholic	13	2.2
Current marital status	Single	312	53.4
	Married	29	5
	Divorced	190	32.5
	Widowed	53	9.1
Residence before joining FSW	Urban	219	37.5
	Rural	365	62.5

Table 1: Socio-demographic characteristics of FSWs resided in Dessie Town, North-Eastern Ethiopia, 2017.

Classification and participation of female sex workers

Based the establishment, near to half (48%) of the participants were categorized as Hotel based FSWs, 40% were Home based FSWs and 12% were Street based female sex workers (Table 2).

HIV/AIDS knowledge of FSWs

Almost all of the participants (98.2%) have ever heard about HIV/AIDS from different information sources but only 377 (64.7%) of FSWs had adequate knowledge towards HIV/AIDS.

Regarding the HIV related knowledge; 89% of the participants know that consistent condom use can reduce HIV transmission, 82% know healthy looking persons can be HIV carriers, 19.7% of the FSWs belief that HIV can be transmitted through insect bites and 18.5% of the participants perceived that HIV can be transmitted via eating together with infected persons.

Of the total respondents; 60.5% of participants knew that Female sex workers are most at risk for HIV infection (Table 3). The qualitative findings also support that FSWs correctly identified that HIV/AIDS is not curable disease, unsafe sex is the major way of HIV mode of transmission and condom can prevent the transmission.

A 20 years old street based FSW said that "I know all HIV/AIDS transmission and prevention methods that is why I did not had sex without condom and did not share sharp material with anyone else around me even with my children".

Variables	Category of variables	Frequency	Percentage (%)
	Hotel based	280	48
	Home based	234	40
Type of female sex workers	Street based	70	12
	Yes	337	57.7
Membership with HIV/AIDS related associations	No	247	42.3
	Yes	365	62.5
Took any HIV related trainings	No	219	37.5
	Yes	206	35.3
Ever worked as peer educator	No	378	64.7

Table 2: Classification of FSWs based on their establishment in Dessie Town, North-Eastern Ethiopia, 2017.

	Number of FSWs	
Knowledge related questions	Yes	No
Is using condom consistently can reduce the chance of HIV infection?	521 (89.2%)	63 (10.8%)
Does healthy looking person may have HIV/AIDS in blood?	480 (82.2%)	104 (17.8%)
Does HIV/AIDS can be transmitted by mosquito bite?	115(19.7%)	469 (80.3%)
Does HIV/AIDS can be transmitted by eating together?	108 (18.5%)	476 (81.5%)
Does having uninfected faithful partner can reduce the chance of getting HIV infection?	220 (37.7%)	364 (62.3%)
Are Female Sex Workers at risk of HIV/AIDS?	353 (60.5%)	231 (39.5%)
Had adequate knowledge about HIV/AIDS*	377 (64.6%)	207 (35.4%)

Table 3: Knowledge of FSWs towards HIV/AIDS of FSWs in Dessie Town, North-Eastern Ethiopia, 2017 [*Yes=If answered correctly all of the five questions].

Behavioral factors and HIV/AIDS among FSWs

Of the total respondents, 320 (54.8%) had HIV/AIDS preventive practice and 65.6% of them use condom always and consistently. The study also revealed that 66.3% of the study participants use any substance. Of those substance users; 43.1% use alcohol, 38.6% use khat and the rest 18.3% use both alcohol and khat together (Table 4).

In the qualitative methods, most FSW demonstrated condom properly starting from checking the expiry date by presence of air or reading the expiry date to proper removal of condom after utilization. This showed proper condom utilization of FSWs.

The in-depth interview and condom demonstration also supported that most of FSWs used condom always and properly. 28 years old home based FSW said that "I did not drink more and I did not agree even when customer need sex without condom to pay more money above the agreement."

Variables	Category	Number of FSWs	Percentage (%)
	Unknown person	290	49.3
	Any person who can pay	117	20
	Tourist	108	18.5
	Student	115	19.7
	Merchant	118	20.2
Type of sexual clients	Others	66	11.3

Condom use during last sex?	Yes	521	89.2
	No	63	10.8
Frequency of condom use	Never use	32	5.5
	Sometimes	60	10.3
	Most of the time	109	18.7
	Always	383	65.6
	Refusal by partner	80	39.8
Reason for not consistently use condom? (n=201)	got drunk	52	25.8
	trust my partner	47	23.4
	Others	20	10
Type of substance used	Alcohol	165	43.1
	Khat	148	38.6
	Other	70	18.3
Preventive practice of FSWs towards HIV/AIDS	Consistently use condom	384	65.7
	Not sharing sharpen materials	471	80.7
Had adequate level of HIV/AIDS preventive practice		320	54.8

Table 4: Behavioral factors and HIV/AIDS preventive practice of FSWs in Dessie Town, North-Eastern Ethiopia, 2017.

Factors associated with preventive practice

Regarding HIV/AIDS preventive practice; alcohol consumption (AOR=0.25; 95%CI=0.11,0.39) and khat chewing (AOR=0.28; 95% CI=0.15,0.62) were found hindering factors of preventive practice but being membership with organizations those working on HIV/AIDS (AOR=2.55,95% CI=1.52-4.27) was found significantly associated with preventive practice of HIV/AIDS among FSWs (Table 5).

Independent variables		Preventive Practice of HIV/AIDS		COR (95%CI)	AOR (95% CI)
		Yes	No		
Age	15-19	50	51	1	1
	20-24	129	82	1.61(1.00,2.61)	0.98(0.51,1.89)
	≥ 25	160	112	1.46(0.92,2.32)	0.93(0.47,1.83)
Residence of FSWs	Urban	117	102	0.73(0.52,1.02)	0.96(0.59,1.55)
	Rural	223	142	1	1
Adequate Knowledge on HIV/AIDS	No	85	122	1	1
	Yes	112	265	0.61 (0.53,1.07)	1.02(0.64,1.65)
Kind of substance use	Alcohol	67	98	0.38 (0.36, 0.68)	0.25 (0.17,0.49)*
	Khat	50	98	0.29 (0.16,0.53)	0.21 (0.13,0.52)**
	Other	45	25	1	1
Membership of an association	No	111	136	1	1
	Yes	229	108	2.59(1.85,3.64)	2.55(1.52,4.27)**

Gotten any training related to HIV/AIDS	No	112	107	1	1
	Yes	228	137	1.59(1.13,2.23)	1.36(0.81,2.31)
Work as peer promoter	No	202	176	1	1
	Yes	138	68	1.76(1.24,2.51)	1.66(0.96,2.86)

Table 5: Factors associated with preventive practice of FSWs for HIV/AIDS in Dessie Town, North-Eastern Ethiopia, 2017 [*=P-value less than 0.05 and **=p-value less than or equal to 0.001].

Discussion

Studies conducted in Africa revealed that female sex workers had adequate knowledge and awareness regarding to HIV/AIDS compared to the other segment of population. However, FSWs had suboptimal level of preventive practice of HIV/AIDS. Therefore, this study aims to assess the level of preventive practice of HIV/AIDS and associated factors among female sex workers in Dessie Town, North-Eastern Ethiopia, 2017.

The study revealed that 64.7% of Female sex workers (FSWs) had adequate knowledge of HIV/AIDS in Dessie town. This result is higher than the study done in Gondar town street sex workers (31.4%) [12], study done in Northern Uganda youth (29%) [13], the 2014 Ethiopian progress report on the HIV/AIDS response for female general population (18%) [14], the study done in Wayu Tuka district, western Ethiopia (25%) [15] and the EDHS 2011 female 15-49 years (19%) [16]. This might be due to the current better involvement of governmental interventions after the priority setting of HIV/AIDS high risk segment of population. On top of this, the study population variability (in terms of socio-economic and demographic characters), the study participants resided in urban can have more access of information about HIV/AIDS via social medias like radio and television, and study period variability.

The qualitative findings also support that, a 23 years old hotel based FSW said "HIV transmit by unsafe sex, mother to child, using sharp material together and by blood. Using condom always and not sharing sharp materials together are the preventive methods. And also HIV cannot transmit by eating together, by mosquito bite and using toilet together".

The study revealed that 54.8% of the study participants had adequate level of preventive practice of HIV/AIDS and 65.7% of them were consistently used condom in every sexual intercourse even with their constant partners. The level of HIV/AIDS preventive practice among FSWs in this study was found lower than the study done in Ecuador (56.9%) [17], study done in Eastern Ethiopia (54.7%) [18], study conducted in Nepalian FSWs (82.2%) [19], Study done in china (59.6%) [20] and study done among Chili FSWs (93.4%) [21]. The discrepancy might be due to higher cut off point in this study, geographical, time, socio-economic and community awareness variations across the study areas.

The study found that alcohol consumption (AOR=0.25; 95% CI=0.11,0.39) and khat chewing (AOR=0.28; 95% CI=0.15,0.62) were found hindering factors of preventive practice compared with the non-users. This finding is line with study done in India among FSWs [22]. This shows using either combined or separated substance may lead to forgetting of consistent condom use and increased the risk of acquisition of HIV and other sexually transmitted infection among risky groups and the larger population.

The study found that FSWs who were member of organizations working on HIV/AIDS program had 2.55 times (AOR=2.55; 95% CI=1.52,4.27) more likely to have HIV/AIDS preventive practice compared with FSWs who were not working as members. This indicates that as there is exposure on HIV/AIDS related program the preventive practice will increase simultaneously.

The in-depth interview also showed that the exposure of MARPs program increased their knowledge and preventive practice gradually. The program capacitates the skill to negotiate condom use with clients. The study could have the following limitations. Firstly, it was difficult to establish a cause-effect relationship and the study also shares the limitation of cross-sectional study design. However, the study was supplemented with qualitative study method and due attention was given to the study procedures, including the process of training, and close supervision throughout the field activities.

Conclusion

Female sex workers in in Dessie Town have below median comprehensive knowledge on HIV/AIDS. Comprehensive knowledge of FSWs on HIV/AIDS was found associated with young age group, higher educational level and working as peer promoters. The in-depth interview and condom demonstration observation also supported hat FSWs' comprehensive knowledge and preventive practice improved with exposure to MARPs program. The predictors of preventive practice of fsws were substance use and being membership with organizations working on HIV/AIDS program. Therefore, the government should give high attention for the female sex workers regarding awareness creation to build good comprehensive knowledge to reduce the transmission of new HIV infection among high risk groups including FSWs and in the larger population too. Further, qualitative researches are highly demanding to explore the knowledge, attitude and practice of FSWs towards HIV/AIDS.

Ethical Issues

Ethical clearance was obtained from the Alkan College of Health Science, Department of Public Health. The participants recruited into this study were resident of Dessie town; were involved in the study after confidentiality, benefits, risks to participating, justice, rights to deny well explained. Finally, those who were willing to participate in the study and gave verbal informed consent were included. Moreover, the results were disseminated to the responsible bodies who were involved in the health care activities of FSWs.

Competing Interests

The authors declare that they have no competing interests.

Authors' Contributions

All authors conceived and designed the study. FY, AW and NM supervised the data collection. YM, NM and AW performed the data analysis, interpretation of data and drafted the manuscript. AW, NM, YM and FY had interpreted and critically reviewed the manuscript. All authors read and approved the final manuscript.

Acknowledgments

Authors thank Alkan University, School of Public Health for its ethical review process and funding. Authors also thank supervisors, data collectors, study subjects and all other individuals for their contributions.

References

1. Pinsky L, Douglas PH (2009) Handbook on HIV and AIDS. Columbia University.
2. WHO (2013) Implementing comprehensive HIV/STI programmes with sex workers. Geneva, Switzerland.
3. World Health Organization (2012) Prevention and treatment of HIV and other sexually transmitted infections for sex workers in low and middle-income countries: Recommendations for a public health approach. Geneva, Switzerland.
4. PSI and Dessie Town bureau of labor and social affairs (BoLSA) (2016) Hotspot town level mapping and female sex worker size estimation in Dessie town.
5. Federal HIV/AIDS prevention and control office (2012) Country progress report on HIV/AIDS Response. Addis Ababa, Ethiopia.
6. Tamene MM, Tessema GA, Beyera GK (2015) Condom utilization and sexual behavior of female sex workers in Northwest Ethiopia: A cross-sectional study. The Pan African medical journal 21: 50.
7. WHO (2014) Global update on the health sector response to HIV. Geneva, Switzerland.
8. Office FHAPaC (2011) HIV behaviour change communication frame work (Ethiopia). Addis Ababa, Ethiopia: Federal HIV/AIDS Prevention and Comntrol Office.
9. Soliman C, Taher Z, Sattar A, Shawky S, Feyisetan B, et al. (2008) Key findings of Bio-BSS among high risk groups in the Middle East, Egypt case study. XVII International AIDS Conference.
10. USAID, PSI (2014) An effective model for the integration of modern family planning services into community-level HIV programming for female sex workers in Ethiopia.
11. Most at risk populations sex workers and HIV/AIDS in Uganda: Synthesis of information and evidence to inform response. KMCC, Uganda (2014).
12. Megabiw BA (2013) Comprehensive knowledge, attitude and practice of street adults towards human immunodeficiency virus/acquired immune deficiency syndrome (HIV/AIDS) in Northwest Ethiopia. J AIDS HIV Res 5: 181-187.
13. Ciccio L, sera D (2009) Assessing the knowledge and behavior towards HIV/AIDS among youth in Northern Uganda: A cross-sectional survey. Italian Newspaper of Tropical Medicine 15: 1-4.
14. Federal Democratic Republic of Ethiopia (2014) Country progress report on the HIV response.
15. Kejela LO, Dessie Y, Misker D (2015) Comprehensive HIV/AIDS knowledge level among out-of-school youths in Wayu Tuka district, Western Ethiopia. Eur J Prev Med 3: 11-16.
16. CSA (2011) Ethiopian demographic and health survey.
17. Cabezas MC, Fornasini M, Dardenne N, Borja T, Albert A (2013) A cross-sectional study to assess knowledge about HIV/AIDS transmission and prevention measures in company workers in Ecuador. BMC public health 13: 139.
18. Oljira L, Berhane Y, Worku A (2013) Assessment of comprehensive HIV/AIDS knowledge level among in-school adolescents in eastern Ethiopia. J Int AIDS Soc 16: 17349.
19. Barrientos JE, Bozon M, Ortiz E, Arredondo A (2007) HIV prevalence, AIDS knowledge, and condom use among female sex workers in Santiago, Chile. Cadernos de saude publica 23: 1777-1784.
20. Shi Y, Guo S, Bo F, Zhang X, Cao Z, et al. (2012) Impact evaluation of a sexually transmitted disease preventive intervention among female sex workers in Hohhot, China. Int J Infect Dis pp: e59-e64.
21. Lall SB (2014) Knowledge and attitude on HIV-AIDS and practice of sexual behavior among female sex workers: a pilot study in Jhapa, Nepal. IOSR J Dent Med Sci 13: 46-52.
22. Medhi GK, Mahanta J, Kermode M, Paranjape RS, Adhikary R, et al. (2012) Factors associated with history of drug use among female sex workers (FSW) in a high HIV prevalence state of India. BMC public health 12: 273.

Prevalence of Symptomatic Pelvic Floor Disorders among Japanese Women

Takeshi Hasuda[1], **Atsushi Ueda**[2] **and Chang-Nian Wei**[2*]

[1]*Department of Obstetrics and Gynecology, Jikei Hospital, Kumamoto, Japan*

[2]*Department of Public Health, Faculty of Life Sciences, Kumamoto University, Kumamoto, Japan*

[*]**Corresponding author:** Chang-Nian Wei, Department of Public Health, Faculty of Life Sciences, Kumamoto University, Honjo 1-1-1, Chou-ku, Kumamoto, 860-8556, Japan, E-mail: cnwei@kumamoto-u.ac.jp

Abstract

Objective: There is little epidemiological data regarding pelvic organ prolapse (POP) in Japan, despite it being recognized as a disease can be treated in the outpatient or inpatient settings. Our aim was to estimate the prevalence of symptomatic POP among Japanese women.

Methods: This cross-sectional study evaluated 8,407 randomly selected women (20-90 years old) who were employed at the Japanese Agriculture Group. Trained research assistants distributed a Japanese self-administered questionnaire that was specifically designed for this study. The participants were asked to provide information regarding their demographic characteristics and symptoms of POP or urinary incontinence (UI). The potential risk factors included age, body mass index, self-reported conditions or comorbid diseases, parity, heavy lifting at work, perceived health status, and occupation.

Results: The weighted prevalence of POP was 5.64% (95% CI: 5.15-6.13%), the prevalence of UI was 44.25% (95% CI: 43.19-45.31%), and at least one pelvic floor disorder was reported by 46.15% of the women (95% CI: 45.09-47.22%). The proportion of women who reported having symptomatic POP generally increased with age and peaked at the age of 70-79 years (20-29 years old: 0.86%, 30-39 years old: 3.45%, 40-49 years old: 3.59%, 50-59 years old: 5.79%, 60-69 years old: 6.12%, 70-79 years old: 6.27%, and ≥80 years old: 5.37%; $p<0.001$).

Conclusion: The present study provided the first population-based estimate of the prevalence of POP among Japanese women. The prevalence of symptomatic POP increased with age and peaked at 70–79 years. Approximately half of adult Japanese women reported experiencing symptoms of at least one pelvic floor disorder (POP and/or UI).

Keywords: Pelvic organ prolapse; Prevalence; Japanese women; Pelvic floor disorder; Urinary incontinence

Introduction

Pelvic organ prolapse (POP) a symptomatic pelvic floor disorder that involves the downward descent of the pelvic organs and can result in protrusion from the vagina [1]. POP typically affects some combination of the anterior vagina wall, posterior wall, and/or the uterus or apex of the vagina [2]. POP does not directly cause severe morbidity or mortality [3], although pelvic floor disorders (POP, urinary and fecal incontinence, voiding, and sexual dysfunction) has adverse effects on daily life [4], health status [5], and quality of life [3,4,6]. POP has numerous risk factors, including parity [7-9], older age [7,10,11], obesity [12,13], hysterectomy [14], chronic medical conditions [7], heavy lifting [15], constipation [5], smoking status [16,17], employment [18], and race/ethnicity [7,19]. Furthermore, >200,000 surgeries are performed each year in the US to treat POP, which is the most common indication for hysterectomy among middle-aged women [5,20], and the annual economic burden of POP is >$1 billion in the US [5,10]. POP is also the most common non-cancer indication for hysterectomy among American menopausal women [21]. There is little epidemiological data regarding POP in Japan, despite it being recognized as a disease can be treated in the outpatient or inpatient settings. Moreover, only a few studies have evaluated the distributions of POP according to racial, geographical, and socioeconomic status in the American [7,10,22], British [17], Italian [23], French [24], Turkish [25], Australian [26], and Swedish populations [27]. Therefore, this study aimed to identify the risk factors and prevalence of symptomatic POP among Japanese women.

Methods

The present study evaluated 20,900 women who were Japanese Agriculture Group (JA) employees between August 2014 and July 2015. The JA is a cooperative agricultural association that employs individuals to perform agricultural, industrial, managerial, medical, and educational functions. The population for the present study included JA office staff, service women, teachers, nurses, part-time workers, sales women, part-time agricultural workers, and full-time agricultural workers. Six JA medical centers served the JA employees: the Kumamoto and Oita centers (Kyushu, South Japan), the Yamaguchi and Aichi centers (middle Japan), and the Chiba and Iwate centers (North Japan). These centers were chosen through the Kumamoto University community health network. This study used a cross-sectional design, which was approved by the ethics committee of the

Kumamoto University Faculty of Life Sciences (approval number: 839). All participants provided their informed consent, and the study was performed in accordance with the tenets of the Declaration of Helsinki. Women were considered eligible to participate if they were >20 years old and were not currently pregnant. Trained research assistants distributed self-administered questionnaires that were designed for this study. To ensure anonymity, the participants were not required to provide their name on the questionnaire, and were asked to return the completed questionnaire to the researchers, a designated collection box, or directly to the participating centers within two weeks (Table 1).

Age (years): Height (cm): Weight (kg):	
Q1: Please indicate if you have any of the following symptoms (multiple answers are allowed).	1: Do you experience bulging near your vagina or something protruding (falling out) of your vagina? Yes/No
	2: Has your vagina bulged? Yes/No
	3: Can you see or feel your uterus? Yes/No
	4: Can you see something that has dropped from your pelvis? Yes/No
Q2: If you answered "yes" to the previous questions, were you ever examined in a hospital for your symptoms?	1: Was not examined
	2: Was examined and treated
	3: Was examined but not treated
	4: Was examined and did not need treatment
Q3: Please check the following boxes if you have any of these symptoms (multiple answers are allowed).	1: Urine leaks when you sneeze or cough
	2: Urine leaks when you do heavy lifting
	3: Urine leaks when you need to go to the toilet
	4: Difficulty emptying bladder
	5: Frequently need to urinate: During the day (>8 times) or At night (>3 times)
Q4: Do you feel constipated?	Yes/No
Q5: Please indicate the number of times you have delivered a child in the following methods.	1: Vaginal delivery-time(s): 2: Caesarean section-time(s): 3: Dystocia-time(s):
Q6: Please identify any conditions that you have (multiple answers are allowed)	a) Hypertension, b) hyperlipidaemia, c) diabetes mellitus, d) intracerebral haemorrhage, e) subarachnoid haemorrhage, f) stroke, g) myocardial infarction, h) angina pectoris, i) cardiac failure, j) arrhythmia, k) cystitis, and l) pyelonephritis
Q7: Would you describe your health as	1) Poor 2) fair 3) good 4) excellent
Q8: Are you employed as a	1) JA office staff 2) Part-time agricultural worker 3) Full-time agricultural worker 4) Other (please describe your role)
Q9: Do you routinely perform work-related tasks that exert force on your stomach?	1) Never 2) A few times each month 3) A few times each week 4) Every day

Table 1: Questionnaire representing the study.

When the present study was initiated, there was no validated tool for assessing POP and the related symptoms among Japanese women. The questionnaire was constructed with expert's group works and was modeled on the lot of previously validated questionnaires [18,22,25,27,28] and tools that are used to evaluate outpatients during gynecological visits in Japan. Based on these findings, we developed a nine-question self-reported questionnaire to identify patients with symptomatic POP (Table 1). The participants recorded their age (years), height (cm), and weight (kg), and then answered several questions regarding the symptoms of POP:

1) Do you experience bulging near your vagina or something protruding? 2) Has your vagina bulged? 3) Can you see or feel your uterus? and 4) Can you see something that has dropped in your pelvis? Women who answered any of the questions using "yes" were defined as having symptomatic POP. Urinary incontinence was defined as the self-reported presence of any of the following symptoms: 1) urine leaking during sneezing or coughing, 2) urine leaking during heavy lifting, 3) urine leaking during the urge to toilet, 4) difficulty emptying the bladder, or 5) frequent urination (>8 times during the day or >3 times at night). The presence of one or more pelvic floor disorders was assessed based on the participants' responses regarding POP symptoms

and urinary incontinence. Responses were assigned scores of 0 for "no" and 1 for "yes".

Body mass index was calculated as weight divided by height squared (kg/m^2), and the participants were categorized as being underweight (<18.5 kg/m^2), normal weight (18.5-24.9 kg/m^2), overweight (25.0-29.9 kg/m^2), or obese (≥ 30.0 kg/m^2). Participants were asked to self-report their parity as the total number of vaginal and cesarean deliveries. Participants were also asked to report their existing medical conditions, and the responses were categorized based on the total number of positive responses: zero, one, two, and three or more. Ages were categorized in 10-year increments (20-29 years old to ≥ 80 years old). The internal consistency of the questionnaire was good (Cronbach's alpha=0.87). The test-retest reliability was tested, 50 subjects were randomly selected from expectation assessment group, who filled in the questionnaire twice, two weeks days apart (r=0.84).

Weighted prevalence estimates and 95% confidence intervals (CI) were calculated using SPSS software (version 20.0; SPSS Inc., Chicago, IL). Pearson's χ^2 test was used to assess the association between pelvic floor disorders and the participants' demographic characteristics. Differences were considered statistically significant at a P-value of <0.05.

Results

Among the 20,900 selected women, 12,383 women did not respond. Eight thousand five hundred seventeen (40.8%) questionnaires were returned. One hundred ten of these women were missing age or POP data and were excluded. Thus, our final study sample included 8,407 women. The mean participant age was 61.1 ± 11.5 years (range: 20-90 years) and the median parity was 2 (range: 0-8).

Women with and without pelvic floor disorders exhibited similar distributions for most age categories (p>0.05), with the exception of the 20-29 year old group and the ≥ 80 year old group. Symptoms of least one pelvic floor disorder were reported by 46.15% of the women (95% CI: 45.09-47.22%). Symptomatic POP was reported by 5.64% of the women (95% CI: 5.15-6.13%), and urinary incontinence was reported by 44.25% of the women (95% CI: 43.19-45.31%). The proportion of symptomatic POP generally increased with age (Table 2) and peaked at the age of 70-79 years (20-29 years old: 0.86%, 30-39 years old: 3.45%, 40-49 years old: 3.59%, 50-59 years old: 5.79%, 60-69 years old: 6.12%, 70-79 years old: 6.27%, and ≥ 80 years old: 5.37%; p<0.001) (Table 2).

Variables	No. of Women	Weighted prevalence (%)		
		POP	UI	One or more pelvic Floor disorder
		(n=474)	(n=3,720)	(n=3,880)
Overall	8,407	5.64 (5.15-6.13)	44.25 (43.19-45.31)	46.15 (45.09-47.22)
Age (years)				
20-29	116	0.86 (0.82-2.54)	7.76 (2.89-12.63)	8.62 (3.15-13.73)
30-39	290	3.45 (1.35-5.55)	22.76 (17.93-27.58)	23.45 (18.57-28.32)
40-49	808	3.59 (2.31-4.87)	40.35 (36.96-43.73)	41.21 (37.82-44.61)
50-59	2,123	5.79 (4.80-6.79)	49.69 (47.57-51.82)	51.25 (49.12-53.37)
60-69	3,057	6.12 (5.27-6.97)	46.29 (44.52-48.05)	48.64 (46.87-50.41)
70-79	1,771	6.27 (5.14-7.40)	42.69 (40.38-44.99)	44.95 (42.63-47.26)
≥ 80	242	5.37 (2.53-8.21)	38.43 (32.30-44.56)	40.50 (34.31-46.68)
P-value		0.01	<0.001	<0.001
BMI (kg/m^2)				
<18.5	415	3.89 (2.22-5.56)	26.26 (22.46-30.07)	27.04 (23.20-30.88)
18.5-24.9	6,216	5.34 (4.78-5.90)	41.63 (40.41-42.86)	43.52 (42.28-44.75)
25.0-29.9	1,553	6.70 (5.45-7.94)	55.38 (52.90-57.85)	57.57 (55.11-60.02)
≥ 30.0	223	8.07 (4.50-11.65)	61.43 (55.05-67.82)	63.76 (57.36-69.99)
P-value		0.063	<0.001	<0.001
Self-reported conditions or comorbidities (cumulative count)				
0	4,478	4.53(3.92-5.14)	39.08 (37.65-40.51)	40.62 (39.18-42.06)
1	2,710	5.79(4.91-6.67)	46.83 (44.95-48.71)	48.75 (46.86-50.63)

2	913	8.65 (6.83-10.48)	54.98 (51.76-58.21)	58.05 (54.85-61.25)
≥ 3	306	11.44 (7.87-15.00)	65.03 (59.69-70.38)	68.63 (63.43-73.83)
P-value		<0.001	<0.001	<0.001
Parity				
0	1,228	2.36 (1.51-3.21)	31.27 (28.68-33.86)	31.76 (29.16-34.36)
1	525	4.00 (2.32-5.68)	38.10 (33.94-42.25)	40.00 (35.81-44.19)
2	2,901	5.76 (4.91-6.60)	44.92 (43.11-46.73)	47.26 (45.44-49.08)
≥ 3	3,753	6.85 (6.04-7.66)	48.84 (47.24-50.44)	50.87 (49.27-52.47)
P-value		<0.001	<0.001	<0.001
Heavy lifting at work				
Never (0)	4,223	4.05 (3.45-4.64)	37.18 (35.72-38.63)	38.50 (37.04-39.97)
A few times-Each month (1)	1,707	5.67(4.48-6.65)	49.85 (47.48-52.23)	51.73 (49.36-54.10)
A few times-Each week (2)	1,253	8.70 (7.14-10.26)	53.07 (50.31-55.84)	56.50 (53.76-59.25)
A few times-Every day (3)	1,224	8.09 (6.56-9.62)	51.80 (49.00-54.60)	54.17 (51.38-56.96)
P-value		<0.001	<0.001	<0.001
Perceived health status				
Poor (0)	605	8.10 (5.93-10.27)	44.63 (40.67-48.59)	46.45 (42.47-50.42)
Fair (1)	2,108	8.25 (7.08-9.43)	54.08 (51.95-56.21)	56.97 (54.86-59.09)
Good (2)	5,061	4.35 (3.79-4.91)	41.95 (40.59-43.31)	43.41 (42.04-44.78)
Excellent (3)	633	4.90 (3.22-6.58)	29.54 (25.99-33.10)	31.75 (28.13-35.38)
P-value		<0.001	<0.001	<0.001
Occupation				
JA office staff (0)	572	4.90 (3.13-6.66)	32.52 (28.68-36.36)	33.74 (29.87-37.62)
Others (1)*	4,225	5.09 (4.43-5.75)	47.62 (44.36-50.88)	42.25 (40.76-43.74)
Part-time				
Agrarian (2)	903	6.42 (4.82-8.02)	51.46 (49.58-53.34)	50.17 (46.90-53.43)
Agrarian (3)	2,707	6.39 (5.47-7.31)	40.50 (39.02-41.98)	53.53 (51.65-55.41)
P-value		0.075	<0.001	<0.001

Table 2: Weighted prevalence of pelvic floor disorders according to demographic characteristics among Japanese women. [POP: Pelvic Organ Prolapse; UI: Urinary Incontinence; BMI: Body Mass Index; JA: Japanese Agriculture. Data are in % (95% Confidence Interval), and p-values were calculated using Pearson's χ^2 test with appropriate sampling weights; *Others included teacher, nurse, housewife, part-time worker, and sales women].

The prevalence of symptomatic POP was associated with the following demographic factors: self-reported medical conditions (no conditions: 4.53%, one condition: 5.79%, two conditions: 8.65%, three or more conditions: 11.44%; p<0.001), parity (nulliparous: 2.36%, 1 delivery: 4.00% 2 deliveries: 5.76%, and ≥ 3 deliveries: 6.85%; p<0.001), heavy lifting at work (never: 4.05%, a few times each month: 5.67%, a few times each week: 8.70%, every day: 8.09%; p<0.001), and perceived health status (poor: 8.10%, fair: 8.25%, good: 4.35%, excellent: 4.90%; p<0.001). Similar patterns were observed among participants with urinary incontinence or more than one pelvic floor disorder. The prevalence of POP exhibited marginal associations with body mass index (p=0.063) and occupation (p=0.075). The prevalence of constipation decreased with age (20-29 years old: 41.38%, 30-39 years old: 40.69%, 40-49 years old: 35.40%, 50-59 years old: 28.64%, 60-69 years old: 21.49%, 70-79 years old: 22.36%, ≥ 80 years old: 21.07%; p<0.001). We found the 46.0% of the women did not undergo evaluations for their symptoms, 21.1% of the women were examined, 10.5% of the women were examined but did not need treatment, 1.9%

of the women needed treatment but were not examined, and 20.5% of the women had missing data.

Discussion

In Japan, treatment for POP in the outpatient or inpatient setting is typically covered by national health insurance. However, Japanese epidemiological data are rare, despite POP being the common indication for gynecological surgery. The present study provided the first population-based estimates of the prevalence of symptomatic POP among Japanese women. Our data indicate that approximately 5.64% of Japanese women experience symptoms that are consistent with POP, and that the prevalence of POP increased with age and peak at the age of 70-79 years (6.3%).

Several previous studies have reported that older age was associated with higher prevalence for POP in different countries [4,5]. For example, Jennifer et al. reported that the prevalence peaked at 5.1% among 60-69 year old American women [7]. In 2015, >29.65% of Japanese women were ≥ 65 years old [29], compared to only 16.32% of American women being ≥ 65 years old [30]. Therefore, the minor differences in the peak prevalence of POP may be related to the different age distributions of the Japanese and American populations.

According to the 2015 Japanese census, the total Japanese population is expected to decline from 126.6 million in 2015 to 97.1 million in 2050 [29]. In contrast, the total American population is expected to grow from 312.3 million in 2015 to 403. 7 million in 2050 [30]. Our findings agree with findings from previously studies, which revealed that the prevalence of POP increases with age [7,10,11,22]. Thus, patient age is an important risk factor to consider, especially based on the changing demographics of older Japanese women. For example, 33.95 million (26.82%) Japanese individuals were ≥ 65 years old in 2015, and this population is expected to grow to 37.68 million (38.81%) by 2050 [29]. Similarly, the ≥ 70 year old population is expected to increase from 24.24 million in 2015 to 31.04 million in 2050. In addition, women greatly outnumber men in the ≥ 65 year old age group, with Japan having 4.65 million more elderly women in 2015, compared to the population of elderly men [29]. This disparity increases with age, as women account for 51% of 65-69 year old Japanese individuals, 65% of 85-89 year old Japanese individuals, and 82% of 95-99 year old individuals [29]. Given the aging Japanese population, and the increasing proportion of women in older age groups, it is expected that the prevalence of POP will exhibit substantial increases during the next several decades. Although many observers have casually made this claim, there have been no reliable data to justify this claim. Therefore, our findings provide valuable information that may be used to model the future need for healthcare and medical services among Japanese women. Furthermore, this information may help policy makers predict the future public health burden of pelvic floor disorders, and highlight the importance of funding research to study the etiology, prevention, and treatment of these conditions [1,10].

The present study also aimed to establish a system for predicting the prevalence of POP, similar to the system that is used by the Pelvic Floor Disorder Network. Our data indicate that the prevalence of POP and/or urinary incontinence may be affected by several risk factors, such as obesity, comorbid medical conditions, heavy lifting, constipation, and parity. However, further studies are needed to evaluation these associations in greater detail. Our questionnaire also evaluated whether women sought care when they experienced symptoms of POP (question 2), and we found that approximately one-half of the women did not seek an evaluation or treatment when they developed symptoms of POP. This result may be related to a lack of knowledge regarding normal and abnormal support for pelvic organs among Japanese women.

The limitations of our study include the high non-response rate, which may have resulted in overestimation or underestimation of the actual prevalence of POP and urinary incontinence. However, the large sample size may help to decrease any error that is related to overestimation or underestimation. Furthermore, we compared the age distributions between our study population and the general Japanese population, which revealed that our participants were significantly older, compared to the general Japanese population.

Conclusion

Our results clearly indicate that the epidemiological characteristics of POP among Japanese predict an increase in the prevalence of symptomatic POP. Therefore, these data should be seen as a call to action for the Japanese healthcare community, which must prepare for the rapidly growing segment of ≥ 65 year old women who may require health support and treatment for POP.

Acknowledgements

The authors thank the Japanese Agriculture Group for supporting this study, as well as Ms. Yoko Matsuyama and Tajiri Sakamoto for data collection and clerical support.

References

1. Hunskaar S, Burgio K, Clark A, Lapitan MC, Nelson R, et al. (2005) Epidemiology of urinary and fecal incontinence and pelvic organ prolapse. In: Abrams P, Cordozo L, Koury S, Wein A, eds. Third international consultation on incontinence (1st edn.) Health Publication: Paris.
2. Abrams P, Cardozo L, Fall M, Griffiths D, Rosier P, et al. (2002) The standardization of terminology of lower urinary tract function: report from the standardization Sub-committee of the International Continence Society. Neurourol Urodyn 21: 167-178.
3. Jelovsek JE, Barber MD (2006) Women seeking treatment for advanced pelvic organ prolapse have decreased body image and quality of life. Am J Obstet Gynecol 194: 1455-1461.
4. Barber MD, Maher C (2013) Epidemiology and outcome assessment of pelvic organ prolapse. Int Urogynecol J 24: 1783-1790.
5. Rortveil G, Brown JS, Thom DH, Eeden SK, Creasman JM, et al. (2007) Symptomatic pelvic organ prolapse prevalence and risk factors in a population-based, racially diverse cohort. Obstet Gynecol 109: 1396-1403.
6. Barber MD, Kuchibhatla MN, Pieper CF, Bump RC (2001) Psychometric evaluation of 2 comprehensive condition-specific quality of life instruments for women with pelvic floor disorders. Am J Obstet Gynecol 185: 1388-1395.
7. Wu JM, Vaughan CP, Goode PS, Redden DT, Burgio KL, et al. (2014) Prevalence and trends of symptomatic pelvic floor disorders in U.S. women. Obstet Gynecol 123: 141-148.
8. Sze EH, Sherard GB, Dolezal JM (2002) Pregnancy, labor, delivery, and pelvic organ prolapse. Obstet Gynecol 100: 981-986.
9. Patel DA, Xu X, Thomason AD, Ransom SB, Ivy JS, et al. (2006) Childbirth and pelvic floor dysfunction: An epidemiologic approach to the assessment of prevention opportunities at delivery. Am J Obstet Gynecol 195: 23-28.

10. Wu JM, Hundley AF, Fulton RG, Myers ER (2009) Forecasting the prevalence of pelvic floor disorders in U.S. Women: 2010 to 2050. Obstet Gynecol 114: 1278-1283.
11. Tinelli A, Malvasi A, Rahimi S, Negro R, Vergara D, et al. (2010) Age-related pelvic floor modifications and prolapse risk factors in postmenopausal women. Menopause 17: 204-212.
12. Kudish BI, Iglesia CB, Sokol RJ, Cochrane B, Richter HE, et al. (2009) Effect of weight change on natural history of pelvic organ prolapse. Obstet Gynecol 113: 81-88.
13. Greer WJ, Richter HE, Bartolucci AA, Burgio KL (2008) Obesity and pelvic floor disorders: A systematic review. Obstet Gynecol 112: 341-349.
14. Kesharvarz H, Hillis SD, Kieke BA, Marchbanks PA (2002) Hysterectomy surveillance-United States 1994-1999. MMWR Surveill Summ 51: 1-8.
15. Jorgensen S, Hein HO, Gyntelberg F (1994) Heavy lifting at work and risk of genital prolapse and herniated lumbar disc in assistant nurses. Occup Med 44: 47-49.
16. Hendrix SL, Clark A, Nygaard I, Aragaki A, Barnabei V, et al. (2002) Pelvic organ prolapse in the women's health initiative: Gravity and gravidity. Am J Obstet Gynecol 186: 1160-1166.
17. Mant J, Painter R, Vessey M (1997) Epidemiology of genital prolapse: Observations from the Oxford family planning association study. Br J Obstet Gynaecol 104: 579-585.
18. Swift S, Woodman P, O'Boyle A, Kahn M, Valley M, et al. (2005) Pelvic organ support study (POSST): The distribution, clinical definition, and epidemiologic condition of pelvic organ support defects. Am J Obstet Gynecol 192: 795-806.
19. Whitcomb EL, Rortveit G, Brown JS, Creasman JM, Thom DH, et al. (2009) Racial differences in pelvic organ prolapse. Obstet Gynecol 114: 1271-1277.
20. Subak LL, Waejen LE, Eeden S, Thom DH, Vittinghoff E, et al. (2001) Cost of pelvic organ prolapse surgery in the United States. Obstet Gynecol 98: 646-651.
21. Wilcox LS, Koonin LM, Pokras R, Strauss LT, Xia Z, et al. (1994) Hysterectomy in the United States, 1988-1990. Obstet Gynecol 83: 549-555.
22. Nygaard I, Barber MD, Burgio KL, Kenton K, Meikle S, et al. (2008) Prevalence of symptomatic pelvic floor disorders in US women. JAMA 300: 1311-1316.
23. Progetto Menopausa Italia Study Group (2000) Risk factors for genital prolapse in non-hysterectomized women around menopause results from a large cross-sectional study in menopausal clinics in Italy. Europ J Obs Gyn Reprod Biol 93: 135-140.
24. Fritel X, Varnoux N, Zins M, Breart G, Ringa V (2009) Symptomatic pelvic organ prolapse at midlife, quality of life, and risk factors. Obstet Gynecol 113: 609-616.
25. Cam C, Sakalli M, Ay P, Aran T, Cam M, et al. (2007) Validation of the prolapse quality of life questionnaire (P-QOL) in a Turkish population. Eur J Obstet Gynecol Reprod Biol 135: 132-135.
26. Hunt FJ, Holman AJ, Einarsdottir K, Moorin RE, Tsokos N (2013) Pelvic organ prolapse surgery in Western Australia: A population-based analysis of trends and peri-operative complications. Int Urogynecol J 24: 2031-2038.
27. Tegerstedt G, Maehle-Schmidt M, Nyren O, Hammarström M (2005) Prevalence of symptomatic pelvic organ prolapse in a Swedish population. Int Urogynecol J Pelvic Floor Dysfunct 16: 497-503.
28. Fukumoto Y, Uesaka Y, Yamamoto K, Ito S, Yamanaka M, et al. (2008) Assessment of quality of life in women with pelvic organ prolapse: Condition translation and trial of P-QOL for use in Japan. Jpn J Urol 99: 531-542.
29. National Institute of Population and Social Security Research (2012) Population projections for Japan: 2011-2060.
30. U.S. Census Bureau (2000) Projections of the resident population by Age, Sex, Race, and Hispanic Origin: 1999-2100.

Social Support among Pregnant Adolescent and Young Adults during Prenatal Ultrasound Study in A Single Tertiary Level Hospital

Sara Lee[1], **Noam Lazebnik**[2*], **Krystel Tossone**[3], **Matthew Bauer**[4] **and Rina Lazebnik**[1]

[1]*Department of Pediatrics, University Hospitals Cleveland Medical Center, Cleveland, Ohio, USA*

[2]*Department of Obstetrics and Gynecology, University Hospitals Cleveland Medical Center, Cleveland, Ohio, USA*

[3]*Begun Center for Violence Prevention Research and Education, Case Western Reserve University, Cleveland, Ohio, USA*

[4]*School of Medicine, Case Western Reserve University, Cleveland, Ohio, USA*

***Corresponding author:** Noam Lazebnik, Department of Obstetrics and Gynecology, University Hospitals Cleveland Medical Center, Cleveland, Ohio-44106, USA, E-mail: noam.lazebnik@uhhospitals.org

Abstract

Introduction: Prenatal care and support is essential to improving birth outcomes for teen pregnancy. Pregnant teens and young adults have access to a variety of support people. The study evaluated the identity of personal social support of pregnant adolescents and young adults (AYA) during prenatal ultrasound study.

Methods: We conducted a descriptive retrospective observational study from a tertiary OBGYN referral center from August 2010 to April 2013; participants were pregnant women 21 years of age or younger referred for ultrasound study. The main outcome measure was documentation of social support person(s) accompanying the patient.

Results: A total of 517 patients with an age range of 13 to 21 (mean 17.75) underwent 1,058 ultrasound studies. The father of the baby was the most frequent person accompanying the patient (33.4%), followed by the patient's mother (25.2%). Age was significantly associated with type of support person, with older AYA more likely to present with the father of the baby. Finding an abnormality on ultrasound did not result in increased follow-up or a change in support person.

Discussion: The majority of adolescents and young adults will show to an ultrasound study accompanied by one or more individuals as social support. Patient's age is the strongest variable affecting who will be the social support person.

Keywords: Adolescent health; Preconception care; Patient education; Pregnancy

Introduction

Teen birth rates in the United States have declined almost continuously since the early 1990s, largely due to the widespread use of contraception. Nevertheless, the teen birth rate in the United States is higher than that of many developed countries, and the social and economic consequences of teen pregnancy remain significant [1-4]. Adolescents and young adults (AYA) who experience pregnancy are less likely to finish high school, more likely to rely on public assistance, and more likely to be incarcerated [4]. Additionally, the estimated cost of teen pregnancy to American taxpayers is about. About 4 billion dollars per year in lost productivity, tax revenue, and medical costs [5]. Furthermore, AYA who become pregnant are at risk for numerous health-related complications, including low birth weight infants, preterm labor and delivery, and postpartum depression [6].

Lack of prenatal care in adolescents significantly increases the risk of preterm delivery and low birth weight (LBW) infants independently of the risk associated with their age [7,8] Teens are less likely to seek prenatal care for a variety of reasons, including fear of repercussions, the presence of an undesired pregnancy, or lack of access to appropriate resources [7,9].

Pregnant teens and young adults have access to a number of support systems, including family, friends, partner and institutional sources, e.g. school, church [10]. Increased social support during pregnancy has been shown to be associated with improved birth outcomes. A recent study from our own institution supports this view by noting that pregnant AYA experienced improved birth outcomes, as measured by length of gestation and birth weight, when the father of the baby (FOB) was present at the patient's first ultrasound study appointment [11,12]. Prenatal ultrasound study appointment is a standardized procedure with definable results and is an experience in pregnancy during which the pregnant mother may want to bring support person(s). Even though it has been shown that social support during teen pregnancy improves outcomes, very little research has been done to delineate the types of support that teens have access to during their ultrasound study while pregnant.

In this study, we sought to elucidate the differences among pregnant adolescent patients in terms of who they brought to their ultrasound study appointments based upon their age, the trimester in which they first presented for prenatal care and compliance with follow-up ultrasound study. In addition, we noted whether there has been a change in social support once fetal or maternal problems were identified. The purpose of this study was to evaluate the identity of personal social support of pregnant adolescents and young adults during prenatal ultrasound study.

Methods

This is a retrospective observational study from a tertiary OBGYN referral center. The computerized archiving and reporting system of the Fetal Imaging Unit at University Hospitals Cleveland, Ohio, over a period of 30 months from August 2010 to April 2013, was searched using maternal age between 12 to 21 years to identify pregnant AYA patients. Approval for this retrospective chart review study was obtained from the Institutional Review Board (IRB) of University Hospitals Cleveland Medical Center.

Patients included in the study were all seen at a single tertiary academic medical center in Cleveland, Ohio. Data collected included gestational age at each ultrasound study visit, support person(s) present, sonographic detection of definitive fetal anomalies and abnormalities related to fetal growth, amniotic fluid volume, placental disorders, and uterine, cervical and ovarian abnormalities.

Ultrasound studies included studies in any trimester, biophysical profile studies, and limited studies in which only the cervical length was checked. The ultrasound studies were performed by Maternal-Fetal Medicine trained physicians. The studies were performed in accordance with guidelines published by the American Institute of Ultrasound in Medicine (AIUM) for studies in the first, second, and third trimesters.

For inclusion in this study, the requirements were: singleton pregnancy with maternal age between 12 and 21, attendance at one or more ultrasound appointments, known gestational age at the time of appointment either by a known last menstrual period (LMP) and/or confirmed by an ultrasound study, documented presence and identity of a support person(s) at these visits, availability of complete ultrasound reports, and delivery records.

Cases of intra-uterine fetal death or early trimester miscarriage (n=22), ultrasound study prior to elective abortion (n=9), and cases accompanied by female prison guard [13] were excluded. Cases in which the patient presented with both the father of the baby and other individuals, with the mother of the patient and other individuals, or both the father of the baby and the patient's mother or father, were classified into the group of "more than one support person" in some but not all statistical calculations, tables and figures. Foster family members and social workers were included in the "other" group of social support.

Subgroup analysis by AYA age groups was conducted in order to analyze the relationship between maternal age and social support. Potentially confounding factors (such as insurance status, income, education, etc.) were not included as the available stored data in the ultrasound unit does not include such data.

Data Analysis

To answer the first research question, "is there an association between different support types and a patient's age at the first ultrasound visit", we employed a Kruskal-Wallis test, due to the violation of normal assumption between age group and support type (Shapiro Wilk's Test $p<0.0001$). Following this, depending on statistical significance of the Kruskal-Wallis test, post-hoc Mann Whitney U tests are performed on each support pair with a Bonferroni correction ($\alpha=0.05/7=0.007$) to determine where the statistically significant differences may lie.

To answer "is there an association between the patient's gestational age (according to trimester) at first ultrasound and who accompanies her"; we conducted a chi-square test of association due to the nominal nature of both natures.

We performed a chi-square test to determine whether there was a change in the support type that the patient from first to second appointment depending on detection of fetal anomaly.

We employed a Kruskal-Wallis test (due to violation of normal assumption-Shapiro Wilk's Test $p<0.0001$) to answer the question "what is the association between type of support a patient brings at first appointment and gestational age (in weeks) at delivery?" Following this, depending on statistical significance of the Kruskal-Wallis test, post-hoc Mann Whitney U tests are performed on each support pair with a Bonferroni correction ($\alpha=0.05/7=0.007$) to determine where the statistically significant differences may lie.

Finally, we performed a multinomial logistic regression to determine which variables of interest-patient age, trimester of first appointment, number of visits, fetal anomaly in first ultrasound, and known LMP-were associated with the odds of type of support at first appointment.

Results

A total of 517 patients met the inclusion criteria and underwent 1,058 ultrasound studies. Of these, 62 patients (12%) had only a single ultrasound visit, 169 (32.7%) had 2 studies, 152 (29.4%) had 3 studies and 134 (25.9%) patients had 4 or more studies. 352 (68%) patients were pregnant for the first time; for 113 (21.7%) this was the second pregnancy, and 52 (10.3%) had been pregnant three times or more. Maternal age ranged between 13 and 21, with a mean and median age of 17.75 and 18.0 respectively, and a standard deviation of 1.56 years.

Table 1 details the identity and nature of the relationship to the patient of the support person(s) present during the ultrasound study. The father of the baby most often accompanied the patient (33.4%), followed by the patient's mother (25.2%). The father of the pregnant patient (0.7%) and either parent of the father of the baby were the least likely to be present. The father of the male partner (father of the baby) was never present (Table 1).

Support Type	Number of all visits	Percentage of all visits
Biological father of the baby	353	33.40%
Mother of the patient	267	25.20%
Patient only	183	17.30%
Family members other than parents	163	15.40%
Friends (Males and Females)	59	5.40%
Other	26	2.50%
Father of the patient	7	0.70%

Table 1: Support person(s) accompanying the patient on any one of the 1,058 ultrasound studies.

Table 2 shows median patient age differences between support types and accompanying Bonferroni-corrected Mann Whitney U Tests. The Kruskal Wallis test indicated statistically significant difference between patient age and support type at first appointment $\chi^2=52.49$, $p<0.0001$). Because $\alpha=0.007$, the statistically significant differences in patient age and support type were among FOB *vs.* mother of patient ($p<0.0001$), mother of patient versus other support type ($p<0.0001$), FOB versus more than one support type ($p<0.0001$), mother of patient versus more than one support type ($p=0.005$), and mother of patient *vs.* alone ($p<0.0001$) (Table 2).

Comparison	Median Age Difference	Z-Score	Mann-Whitney U	p-value[a]
Alone *vs.* Fob[b] (n=190)	-1.00 year	-1.82	3847	0.07
Fob *vs.* Mother of patient (n=192)	2.00 years	-6.55	2136.5	<0.0001
Mother of patient *vs.* Other (n=219)	-1.00 year	-3.52	4271.5	<0.0001
Other *vs.* More than one support type (n=232)	0 years	-0.6	6387	0.54
Alone *vs.* More than one support type (n=199)	0 years	-2.41	3969	0.02
Fob *vs.* More than one support type (n=205)	1.00 year	-4.2	3508.5	<0.0001
Mother of patient *vs.* More than one support type (n=201)	-1.00 year	-2.78	3902.5	0.005
Mother of patient *vs.* Alone (n=186)	-1.00 year	-4.93	2545	<0.0001

Table 2: Kruskal Wallis mean age differences and Mann Whitney U tests between patient age and support type at first appointment (n=516) [[a]Bonferonni-corrected $\alpha=0.007$; [b]FOB=Father of baby].

The chi-square test of association between gestational age at first ultrasound and support type indicated no statistically significant difference in gestational age and type of support ($\chi^2=8.74$, $p=0.07$). Of those in the first trimester, 24.14% were accompanied by the FOB. This is higher than 16.18% of those in the second/third trimester who were accompanied by the FOB. Of those in the first trimester, 27.35% were accompanied by another person, compared to only 18.39% in the second/third trimester.

The chi-square test of association between detection of fetal anomaly at first ultrasound and a change in support type at second appointment found no statistically significant difference ($\chi^2=0.01$, $p=0.92$). About the same amount that had a problem detected (40.43%) changed their support type as those who did not have a problem detected (41.18%).

The Kruskal-Wallis Test of difference in mean ranks between support type at first appointment and gestational age in weeks at delivery indicated no statistically significant difference ($\chi^2=2.66$, df=3, $p=0.45$). Therefore, no accompanying Bonferroni-corrected Mann-Whitney U tests was employed.

The multinomial logistic regression modeling the odds of support type at first appointment according to variables of interest is reported in Table 3. Overall, patient's age had the only statistically significant association with increased odds of support type ($p<0.0001$), although number of visits for Other versus Alone was also statistically significant ($p=0.03$). Older patients had 2.05 times the odds of having the FOB at the first ultrasound than their mother (95%CI=1.63-2.57, $p<0.0001$) (Table 3).

Variables	β	SE	OR (95% CI)	p-value
Outcome: FOB[a] *vs.* Alone				
1st Trimester *vs.* 2nd/3rd trimester first visit	0.19	0.2	1.47 (0.75-2.91)	0.27
Knows LMP at first visit	0.24	0.2	1.61 (0.87-2.99)	0.13
Fetal anomaly at first ultrasound	0.1	0.2	1.21 (0.55-2.69)	0.64
Patient age	0.15	0.1	1.16 (0.92-1.46)	0.21
Number of visits	-0.1	0.2	0.89 (0.65-1.22)	0.47
Outcome: Mother of patient *vs.* alone				
1st Trimester *vs.* 2nd/3rd Trimester first visit	0.16	0.2	1.37 (0.67-2.81)	0.39
Knows LMP at first visit	0.15	0.2	1.36 (0.72-2.57)	0.35
Fetal anomaly at first ultrasound	-0.3	0.2	0.59 (0.28-1.24)	0.16

Patient age	-0.6	0.1	0.57 (0.46-0.70)	<0.0001
Number of visits	-0.1	0.2	0.95 (0.69-1.22)	0.77
Outcome: More than one support *vs.* alone				
1st Trimester *vs.* 2nd/3rd Trimester first visit	0.06	0.2	1.12 (0.57-2.19)	0.74
Knows LMP at first visit	0.01	0.2	1.01 (0.56-1.82)	0.97
Fetal anomaly at first ultrasound	-0.1	0.2	0.81 (0.39-1.65)	0.55
Patient age	-0.3	0.1	0.73 (0.60-0.90)	0.003
Number of visits	-0.3	0.2	0.76 (0.55-1.05)	0.09
Outcome: Other *vs.* Alone				
1st Trimester *vs.* 2nd/3rd Trimester first visit	-0.1	0.2	0.90 (0.47-1.75)	0.76
Knows LMP at first visit	0.1	0.2	1.22 (0.69-2.16)	0.5
Fetal anomaly at first ultrasound	-0	0.2	0.96 (0.48-1.94)	0.91
Patient age	-0.2	0.1	0.83 (0.58-1.02)	0.08
Number of visits	-0.4	0.2	0.70 (0.51-0.97)	0.03
Outcome: FOB *vs.* Mother of patient				
1st Trimester *vs.* 2nd/3rd Trimester first visit	0.03	0.2	1.07 (0.52-2.20)	0.85
Knows LMP at first visit	0.09	0.2	1.18 (0.62-2.29)	0.61
Fetal anomaly at first ultrasound	0.36	0.2	2.05 (0.94-4.49)	0.07
Patient age	0.72	0.1	2.05 (1.63-2.57)	<0.0001
Number of visits	-0.1	0.2	0.93 (0.67-1.30)	0.69

Table 3: Multinomial logistic regression modeling odds of support type at first appointment given variables of interest (n=493) [aFOB = Father of Baby].

Discussion

Adolescent pregnancy is a priority health issue in the Unites States due to increased economic and societal costs. Social support refers to the people or resources that an individual can turn to in times of life changes and stressors [13]. We chose ultrasound study appointments as our 'prenatal care visits' because it is a standardized procedure with definable results that allows for the presence of a support person. Our study shows that the majority of pregnant AYA (83%) come to ultrasound study accompanied by social support. The father of the baby was the most likely person to accompany the patient to an ultrasound study followed by the patient's mother. The father of the pregnant patient was present the least. No parent of the father of the baby was present.

We found a difference in support person according to patient age. When compared to patients who came with their mothers alone or with the mother and the father of the baby together, patients who presented with only the FOB were older. For younger teens, the mother is likely still the primary caregiver. Older patients may have more independence or have a developed relationship with a male partner. They may also be more likely to seek support from friends and more distant relatives once they are no longer under the care of their own parents.

We sought to identify differences in gestational age at which the first ultrasound study was conducted according to the patient's support type. While there was no statistically significant difference between groups, some trends were noted that might warrant further investigation. For example, 24% of patients who presented in the first trimester came with the father of the child as compared to 16% of patients who presented in the second or third trimesters. Additionally, 27% of patients who came with "another person" presented in the first trimester compared to 18% who presented later. This indicates the possibility that patients who come with the father of the baby or another person are more likely to present earlier when compared to other groups. This finding correlates with that already described in which older patients are more likely to come with the father of the baby or "another person." It might suggest that older teens are more inclined to seek care earlier, and they may be more likely to have specific social support. One might speculate that older patients who present with the father of the baby have desired pregnancy when compared to younger patients, and are therefore more likely to be proactive in seeking care.

Follow-up ultrasound study when ordered by the care provider is an important part of prenatal care. We questioned if patients who had abnormal finding on an ultrasound study were more likely to show to a follow-up study in comparison to AYA who were scheduled for follow-up study to confirm normal fetal growth without confirmed abnormality. In addition, we questioned whether or not there was a change in the person serving as social support in comparison to the initial ultrasound study. After controlling for patient age and gestational age, we found that patients who had a detected fetal, uterine, or cervical anomaly on the initial ultrasound visit were no more likely to return for a second visit than patients with normal prior ultrasound study. In fact, 73% of those with detected problems returned compared to 77% of those with normal studies. Additionally, detection of an anomaly had no effect on the rate at which patients changed who they brought as their support person to the next appointment. These results are surprising for two reasons: first, we expected patients with abnormal ultrasound study findings to return for follow-up appointments at a higher rate than those with normal study; and second, we hypothesized that if these women appeared unaccompanied or with no parental presence at their first study visit, that they would bring the father of the child or a parent to the follow-up appointment. One possible explanation for this apparent dissonance is that abnormal findings on ultrasound are a deterrent to follow-up. Much like patients who are diagnosed with gestational diabetes and then fail to return for follow-up, perhaps these women fear additional bad news. Future research should focus on trying to identify which factors are most important in determining the likelihood of follow-up.

We reviewed available literature in order to compare our findings with those reported by other researchers. Unfortunately we were unable to find similar studies. Despite numerous publications detailing various findings among AYA population no study has previously sought to elucidate the differences among pregnant adolescent patients in terms of who they brought to their ultrasound study appointments based upon their age, the trimester in which they first presented for prenatal care and compliance with follow-up ultrasound study. As such we can't comment on any commonalities or lack of between our study and others.

The strength of this study is that the support person has been verbally identified directly at each visit by the care provider and did not rely on any proxy measures of support. In addition, all ultrasound studies were performed by the same physicians at a single institution allowing for greater consistency in findings. The study analyzed AYA patients in a single tertiary level medical center, our results might reflect only the local population and not necessarily the entire AYA population.

The study did not have the statistical power to study social support among Caucasian and Hispanic adolescents as the great majority of patients were African American. This study was also limited by information regarding social, education background, and family status of AYA included. The identity of the support person(s) was self-reported and not verified. Future directions should focus on further stratifying AYA into more nuanced groups to identify if there are other factors that may be playing a role in how they determine their support type, other than their age. Additionally, it will be useful to ascertain whether there is a difference in support type based upon whether or not the pregnancy was planned and/or desired, a factor that was not examined in this study.

We conclude that among the AYA population the father of the baby is the most commonly self-identified person accompanying the adolescent or young adult pregnant patient to an ultrasound study. Either parent of the father of the baby is the least likely to participate in social support. The patient's age is the strongest variable affecting who will be the social support person.

Quick Points

- The majority of adolescents and young adults choose to have a social support person for their prenatal ultrasound visit.
- The father of the baby is the most common social support person, followed by the patient's mother.
- Choice of social support and rates of follow-up are not affected by the abnormal ultrasound findings.

References

1. Martin JA, Hamilton BE, Ventura SJ (2013) Births: Final data for 2011. Natl Vital Stat Rep 62:1-69.
2. Lindberg L, Santelli J, Desai S (2016) Understanding the decline in adolescent fertility in the United States 2007-2012. J Adolesc Health 59: 577.
3. Kost K, Maddow-Zimet I (2016) US teenage pregnancies, births and abortions, 2011: National trends by age, race and ethnicity. Guttmacher Institute.
4. Hoffman SD, Maynard RA (2008) Kids having kids: Economic costs and social consequences of teen pregnancy (2nd edn), Urban Institute Press, Washington, DC.
5. Hoffman SD (2013) By the numbers: The public costs of adolescent childbearing, 2006. Washington, DC: The national campaign to prevent teen pregnancy.
6. Chen XK, Wen SW, Fleming N (2007) Teenage pregnancy and adverse birth outcomes in large population based retrospective cohort study. Int J Epidemiol 36: 368.
7. Debiec KE, Paul KJ, Mitchell CM (2010) Inadequate prenatal care and risk of preterm delivery among adolescents: a retrospective study over 10 years. Am J Obstet Gynecol 203: 122.
8. Shah MK, Gee RE, Theall KP (2014) Partner support and impact on birth outcomes among teen pregnancies in the United States. J Pediatr Adolesc Gynecol 27: 14.
9. Vieir CL, Coeli CM, Pinheiro RS (2012) Modifying effect of prenatal care on the association between young maternal age and adverse birth outcomes. J Pediatr Adolesc Gynecol 25: 185.
10. Lee SH, Lazebnik R, Kuper-Sassé M (2016) Is the presence of the father of the baby during first prenatal ultrasound study visit associated with improved pregnancy outcomes in adolescents and young adults? Int J Pediatrics p: 4632628.
11. Alio AP, Mbah AK, Grunsten RA (2011) Teenage pregnancy and the influence of paternal involvement on fetal outcomes. J Pediatr Adolesc Gynecol 24: 404.
12. Harville EW, Madkour AS, Xie YJ (2014) Parent-child relationships, parental attitudes towards sex, and birth outcomes among adolescents. Pediatr Adolesc Gynecol 27: 287.
13. Ozbay F, Johnson DC, Dimoulas E, Morgan CA, Charney D (2007) Social support and resilience to stress. Psychiatry 4: 35-40.

The Impact of Incarceration on Greek Female Prisoners' Self-reported Health Status

Stella-Olga Milioni* and Mary Geitona

Department of Social and Educational Policy, University of Peloponnese, Damaskinou & Kolokotroni Str, 20100, Corinth, Greece

***Corresponding author**: Stella-Olga Milioni, Department of Social and Educational Policy, University of Peloponnese, Damaskinou & Kolokotroni Str, 20100, Corinth, Greece, E-mail: elinamil1@yahoo.gr

Abstract

Objective: Studies attempting to investigate issues around detainees' health status is limited in Greece and it is mainly focusing on specific prisons. The scope of this research was to investigate the impact of incarceration on health status of the Greek female prisoners' population.

Methods: A cross-sectional survey was conducted to both female correctional institutions existing in Greece during the years 2014 and 2015. A semi-structured questionnaire was given to incarcerated women who voluntarily accepted to take part. Data were collected via personal interviews and were anonymized. Statistical analysis was performed through descriptive statistics, bivariate analysis and multiple regression analysis with the use of SPSS 20.

Results: Out of 524 female prisoners, 397 met the inclusion criteria and participated in the study. 66.3% reported a moderate or poor health status, while the respective rate before detainment was 23.4%. Health status deterioration and poor mental health were referred by more than half of the participants. The access to health services and the quality of provided healthcare during imprisonment were considered as poor/very poor by 44.8% and 46.1% respectively. Almost half of the respondents expressed their dissatisfaction with the accommodation, the cleanliness, the nutrition as well as with the overall prison environment. Furthermore, the access to health services, the quality of provided healthcare and the experienced detention conditions affect female prisoners' self-reported general and mental health status.

Conclusion: Female imprisonment impacts negatively prisoners' self-reported health status. Our findings give a cue for additional explore with the specific end goal to meet the health needs of this vulnerable population as well as to improve everyday life in prison and life after release.

Keywords: Prisoners; Women health; Risk factors; Health services; Health care

Introduction

Prison population has increased by almost 20% in the last 15 years [1]. In 2015, more than 10.35 million people were incarcerated throughout the world, either as pre-trial prisoners or having been sentenced [1]. The female inmates have grown by 50% the same period, while the respective rate for the male prison population was 18% [1,2]. The expanding detainment rates directly affect inmates' overall health status [3]. The high commonness of prisoners' health related problems seems to be ascribed to various socio-economic characteristics for example destitution, low wage and low training level [4-7].

Additionally, previous studies uncover that inmates have difficulty in the access to health services and do not receive the appropriate care like people in the community [8-10]. The jail conditions are described by seclusion, mutual life, viciousness, uncertainty and congestion [10-12]. Imprisonment is for the most part connected with unhealthy lifestyle such as smoking, lack of physical activity and inappropriate nutrition that prompt the expanding rates of physical and mental ailments [10-12]. Health status is also worsening by unhealthy conditions of incarceration such as absence of clean facilities or means of personal hygiene [13]. Gender is considered to be an important factor in assessing the health status of the prison population [14-16].

Incarcerated women often come from an economically and socially disadvantaged environment, experience greater physical and mental health problems and have more needs in contrast to male detainees as well as to the general population [17-23]. Furthermore, women in prison have been found to be mostly dependent on alcohol or drugs [24], 10 times at greater risk of harming themselves than men [25] and three times more likely to have suffered physical or sexual abuse before their detainment in comparison with people in the community [26-29]. As far as sex and gender as a variable in healthcare utilization, it has been found that female prisoners report higher rates of demand health services than incarcerated men [30].

In Greece, research in the field of evaluating prisoners' self-reported health status is limited with few existing studies focusing on male prison population and on male detention facilities [31-38]. Only three studies focusing on female incarceration conditions and self-reported health status have been published recently from the female prison in Attica that highlighted this issue in the country [39-41]. Against this background, a study focusing on the whole Greek female prison population was necessary, given that imprisonment effect prisoners' overall health status, everyday life, as well as their future after release. Thus, the purpose of this study was to explore the influence of incarceration on Greek female prisoners' self-reported health status in relation to the provided healthcare and the experienced detention conditions during incarceration.

Methodology

Study design and sample selection

Given that women in Greek penal institutions reach approximately 4.9% of the total prison population [2], there are only two female prisons in the country, one in the prefecture of Attica and one in Central Greece. A cross-sectional survey was conducted to both female detention centers between January 2014 and December 2015 by the University of Peloponnese which was given an entry permit by the Ministry of Justice [40,41]. The study was also approved by School of Social Sciences Ethics Committee [40,41].

Out of a total of 524 incarcerated women in the two female prisons existing in Greece, 397 met the inclusion criteria and accepted to participate in the study. Being in solitary confinement, suffering from serious psychiatric problems and inability to understand the Greek language constituted the exclusion criteria. Analytical information on the sampling design is presented in Figure 1.

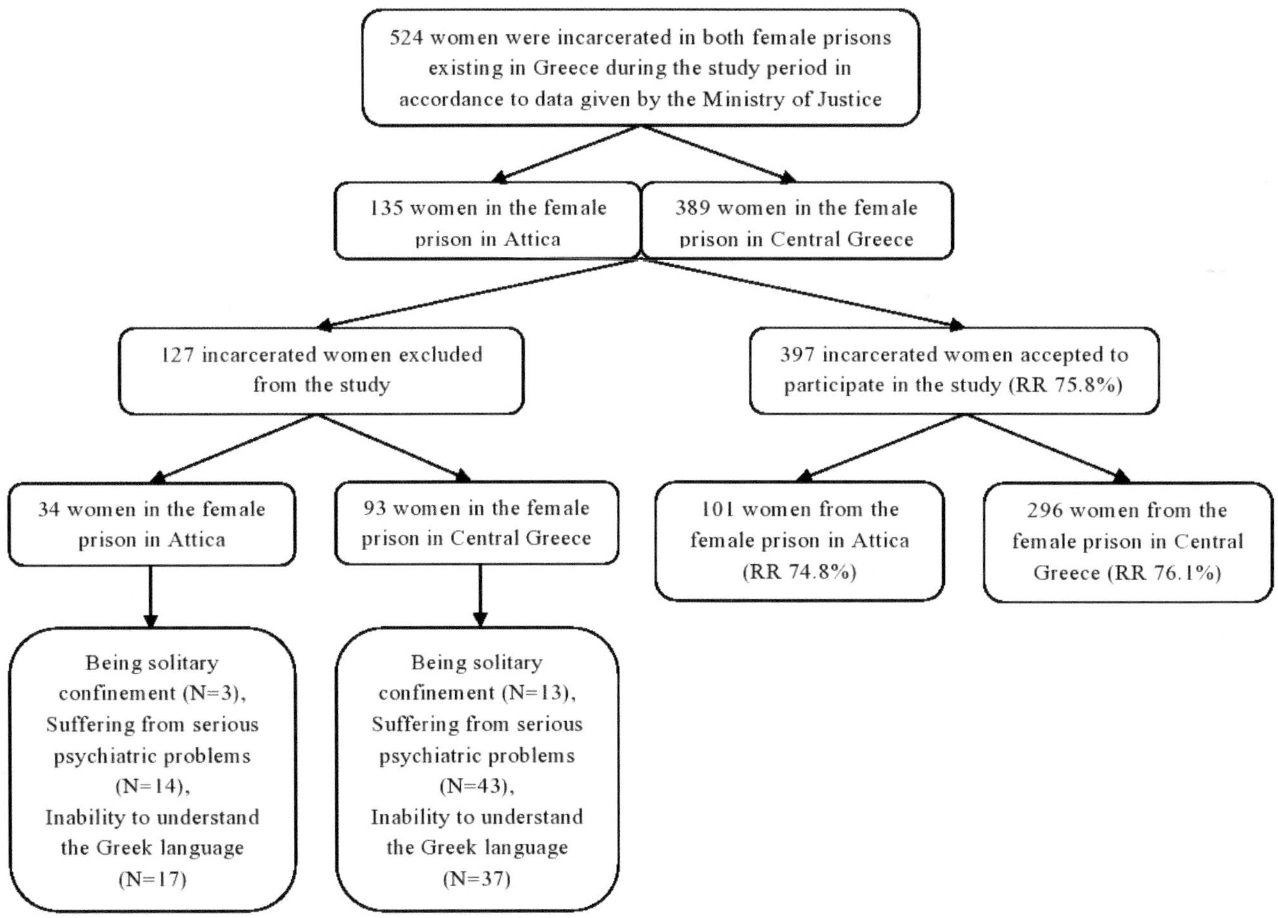

Figure 1: Flowchart of the sampling design.

The recruitment process was undertaken by prison's social workers, specially trained for the purpose of the study by the university research team. The prisoners were informed on the study objectives and scope and asked if they wanted to take part after a verbal consent. The list of participants was subsequently given to the University research team and the interviews were scheduled.

Study instrument

A questionnaire was developed based on international literature review [42-44]. A pilot research was carried out in January 2014 on a convenience sample of 20 female prisoners from the target population in order to evaluate its clarity, comprehensiveness and content validity [45] and feedback was incorporated into the final version which included four sections. The first section consisted of questions regarding prisoners' socio-demographic and detention characteristics. Self-reported health status and health risk behavior related questions were investigated in the second section. The third section included questions with regard to the access and utilization of health services as well as with the quality of the provided healthcare.

Questions relevant to the incarceration conditions such as accommodation, cleanliness, nutrition and the overall satisfaction with the prison environment were referred to the forth section. The questionnaire included several close-ended questions with a five-point scale, where responses ranged from "very poor" to "very good" in order to evaluate female prisoners' general/ mental health status, their access to health services, the quality of provided healthcare and their satisfaction on the experienced detention conditions.

The rates of expressed negative feelings such as sadness, anxiety or discomfort and their affect in inmates' everyday life were also investigated with a five-point scale from "very little" to "very much". Closed-ended questions were also included to explore the use of tobacco and drugs. Data collected via face to face interviews with the inmates in Greek language by a researcher of the University of Peloponnese, with more than five years' experience in managing vulnerable population groups, without the prison's personnel presence. All information received was anonymized to ensure confidentiality.

Statistical Analysis

Statistical analysis was performed through descriptive statistics and bivariate analysis. The results are presented as absolute (n) and relative (%) frequencies for the nominal and ordinal variables and as mean values for the quantitative variables. The proportions of answers poor/ very poor or good/very good were presented as a cumulative result. When variables were not normally distributed, nonparametric tests were performed. In particular, in order to investigate the difference between general health status before and during detention, the Wilcoxon test was used.

Multiple regression analysis with backward method was also used to determine the factors which effect on self-reported general and mental health status, and then the proportion of total variation for general and mental health status were explained with the selected independent variables. The statistical analyses were conducted on S.P.S.S. 20 (Statistical Package for Social Sciences).

Results

Out of a total of 524 incarcerated women in Greece, 397 were met the inclusion criteria and accepted to participate in the survey, reaching a 75.8% response rate. The majority (76.1%) of the study population was Greek with a mean age of 44.3 years (Table 1). 33.8% was unmarried and 68.8% reported having children. 36.8% had secondary education and 68.5% was employed before their incarceration. The main reasons of imprisonment were financial reasons (33.3%), drug trafficking (31.7%) and theft/robbery (19.4%). The rates were lower for murders (7.6%) and other reasons (8%). It should also be noted that only 29.2% of the participants were pre-trial prisoners. For the vast majority (82.4%) of the respondents, this was the first time being in prison (Table 1).

Variables	N	%
Mean Age=44.3 (SD. 12.5)		
Citizenship		
Greek	302	76.1
Other	95	23.9
Marital status		
Unmarried	134	33.8
Married	116	29.2
Divorced	96	24.2
Widow	51	12.8
Children		
Yes	273	68.8
Occupation before detention		
Employee	272	68.5
Student	6	1.5
Unemployed	56	14.1
Pensioner	22	5.6
Housework	33	8.3
Other	8	2
Education level		
Compulsory	125	31.5
Secondary	146	36.8

Tertiary	79	19.9
Postgraduate	47	11.8

Table 1: Socio-demographic characteristics of the sample.

Health status and high risk behavior

Health deterioration during imprisonment was reported by 68.3% of the participants. More specifically, female prisoners were asked about their general health as well as their mental health status (Table 2). About 66.3% described their current general health as moderate or poor/very poor, in contrast to the 23.4% before incarceration. 50.7% rated their mental health as poor/very poor. The latter is further supported by the fact that 74.1% reported that they have been feeling "much/very much" sadness, anxiety or discomfort during the detention. About 73.8% also mentioned that these feelings affected negatively their everyday life in prison (Table 2).

Health status	General health	Mental health
Good/very good	33.70%	20.60%
Moderate	37.30%	28.70%
Poor/very poor	29.00%	50.70%

Table 2: Self-reported general and mental health status during incarceration.

With regard to high risk behavior prior to and during their detention, 68.3% of the participants were smokers. 36.4% used to smoke more than 21 cigarettes per day before, whereas this percentage increased to 57.2% during detention. 27% and 10.6% of the participants admitted that they had used drugs or injected drugs before the entrance to prison. These rates decreased to 13.9% and 1% respectively during detention.

Access to and utilization of health services

Female prisoners were asked to assess their access to health services as well as the quality of the health care provided during their imprisonment. The access to health services both inside and outside the prison, as well as the quality of provided healthcare in prison were described as poor/ very poor by 44.8% and 46.1% of the sample, respectively (Figure 2). Furthermore, 45.5% stated that it was easy to reach a hospital in an emergency, 34.6% answered negatively, while 19.9% said that they did not know.

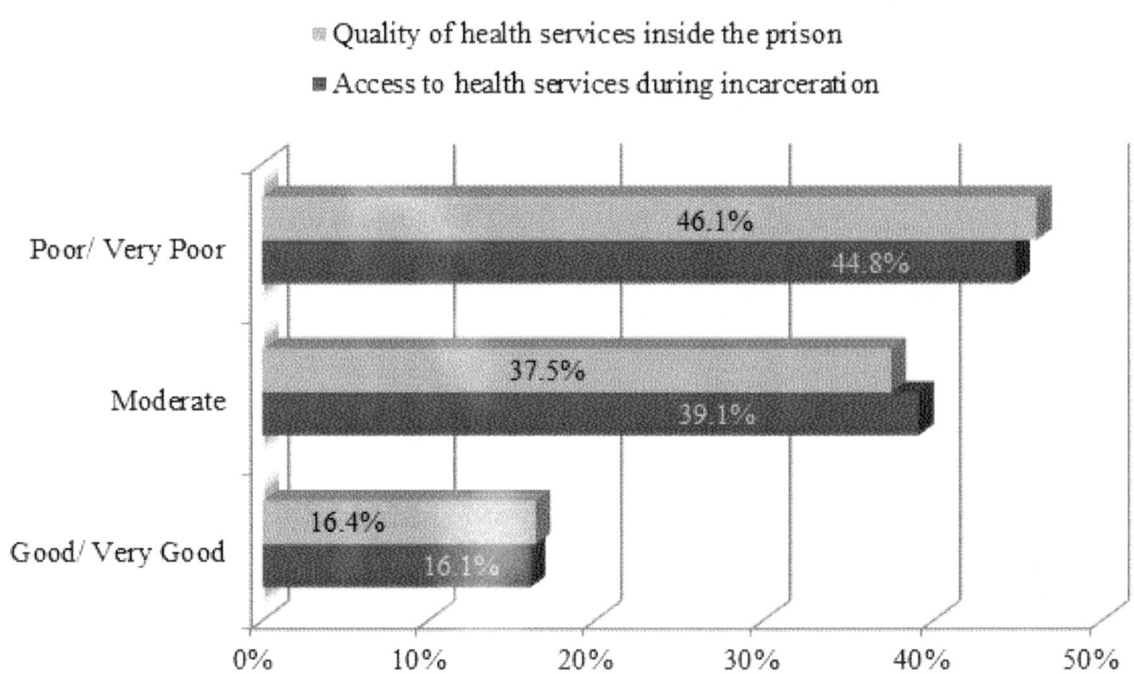

Figure 2: Access to and Quality of health services during incarceration.

Detention conditions

As far as prison conditions, 48.6% and 47.1% reported the accommodation and nutrition during the detention was bad/ very bad respectively. Similar were the results about cleanliness in sanitary areas and cleanliness in communal areas and in cell, where 47.1% and 44.4% of the sample respectively was dissatisfied. The overall prison environment was described as bad/very bad (49.9%), moderate (37.3%) and only 12.8% of prisoners rated it as good/very good.

Multiple regression analysis

In order to determine which factors affect the self-reported general health status of female prisoners, a multiple linear regression analysis was performed (Table 3).

The model showed that:

- If increase the age of prisoners by 1 year then the self-reported general health status will decrease by 0.017.
- If increase the score of self-reported mental health status, then the self-reported general health status will increase by 0.536.
- If prisoners are smokers, then the self-reported general health status will decrease by 0.283.
- If increase the score of nutrition conditions during detention then the self-reported general health status will increase by 0.148.
- If increase the score of cleanliness in communal areas and in cell, then the self-reported general health status will increase by 0.160.
- If increase the score of general satisfaction on detentions conditions, then the self-reported general health status will increase by 0.168.

	Unstandardized Coefficients		Sig.	95% Confidence Interval for B	
Variables	**B**	**Std. Error**	**Lower Bound**	**Upper Bound**	
Constant	**2.14**	**0.233**	**0**	**0.682**	**2.598**
Age	-0.017	0.004	0	-0.024	-0.01
Self-reported mental health status	0.536	0.04	0	0.457	0.616
Smoking	-0.283	0.098	0.004	-0.475	-0.092
Nutrition conditions during detention	0.148	0.051	0.004	0.049	0.248
Cleanliness in communal areas and in cell	0.16	0.048	0.001	-0.255	-0.065
Overall satisfaction on detention conditions	0.168	0.065	0.01	0.04	0.297

Table 3: Female prisoners' self-reported general health.

	Unstandardized Coefficients		Sig.	95% Confidence Interval for B	
Variables	**B**	**Std. Error**	**Lower Bound**	**Upper Bound**	
Constant	1.487	0.306	0	0.885	2.089
Age	0.009	0.003	0.007	0.003	0.016
Current self-reported general health status	0.506	0.039	0	0.429	0.584
Feelings of anxiety. sadness or discomfort	-0.344	0.043	0	-0.429	-0.259
Access to health services	0.145	0.044	0.001	0.058	0.232
Accommodation conditions during detention	0.113	0.062	0.071	-0.01	0.235
Nutrition conditions during detention	0.145	0.055	0.008	-0.252	-0.037
Cleanliness in sanitary areas	0.094	0.045	0.036	0.006	0.182

Table 4: Female prisoners' self-reported mental health status.

Also a linear model was performed in order to determine the factors which affect the self-reported mental health status (Table 4).

The model showed that:

- If increase the age of prisoners by 1 year then the self-reported mental health status will decrease by 0.009.
- If increase the score of current self-reported general health status, then the self-reported mental health status will increase by 0.506.
- If increase the feelings of sadness, anxiety or discomfort, then the self-reported mental health status will decrease by 0.344.

- If prisoners have access to health services, then the self-reported mental health status will increase by 0.145.
- If increase the score of accommodation conditions during detention, then the self-reported mental health status will increase by 0.113.
- If increase the score of nutrition conditions, then the self-reported mental health status will increase by 0.145.
- If increase the score of cleanliness in sanitary areas, then the self-reported mental health status will increase by 0.094.

Discussion

To the best of our knowledge the studies attempting to assess the impact of incarceration on female prisoners' self-reported health status are limited in Greece. Three studies have been carried out assessing inmates' health status only in the female prison of Attica [39-41].

The present study focuses on the whole female prisoners' population in Greece. Our results revealed that approximately 3 out of 10 inmates rated their general health status as poor compared to that before incarceration, while more than two-thirds reported that their health status worsened during detention. The vast majority expressed negative feelings which affect their everyday habits. Nearly half of the participants reported that the access to health services and the quality of provided healthcare in prison did not meet their needs. With regards to detention conditions, one out of two of the respondents was not satisfied with the accommodation, the nutrition, the cleanliness of the facilities and the whole prison environment. Also, our results revealed that inmates' satisfaction on the detention conditions and on the access to and quality of healthcare seem to influence their self-reported general and mental health status.

Most of our findings are consistent with the international literature. In Greece and other European countries, the common reasons of female imprisonment are drug-trafficking, financial reasons and theft/robbery, while the violent crimes and murders are observed more frequently in the male prison population or in women incarcerated in USA [11,31,35,46-54].

Prisoners' poor health status as well as a high prevalence of mental disorders and mental health deprivation have been reported in various studies [3,5,8,55-59]. Furthermore, it is confirmed that prisoners report a deterioration of their health status during their detention [3,30,60-62]. The age constitutes an important factor. Older inmates report a lower level of general health compared to younger prison population [3,14,63-65]. On the contrary, younger prisoners report lower self-reported mental health status in contrast to older inmates [66]. Literature review with regard to the age-related data is consistent with our findings where it has been found that female prisoners' self-reported general and mental health status is affected by the age.

Prisoners tend to use health services more frequently than the general population [14,67]. Our study findings regarding female prisoners' views and opinions on the access to and quality of health services also seem to be consistent with other studies reporting that inmates are provided a low level of health care during incarceration, since they do not have a direct equivalent access to health services in the community and they cannot choose their health providers, compared to the general population, [13,30,32,37,59,68-71].

With regard to risk factors, two thirds of the participants said that they were using tobacco during their incarceration. Almost the same and higher rates of smokers have been reported in other Greek and international surveys [33,34,36,38,72-77]. According to the study results, women increased their smoking habits by 20.8% during their detention period, while in previous surveys conducted in two Greek male prisons the relevant increase rates were higher (37.7% and 43.4% respectively) [33,34].

Dissatisfaction with the detention conditions was also reported in a Greek study focused on male prisoners as well as in the international literature [61,78,79]. However, the results of a survey in a male prison in Crete were different as two out of three respondents stated that the detention conditions were good or tolerated [32]. In addition, in a Scottish Prison survey the majority of prisoners expressed positive views about prison cleanliness and was generally satisfied with the provided nutrition [44,77].

There are numerous strengths in our study. The most important is that our findings can be generalizable to the country since they come from both female prisons existing in Greece, focusing on the whole female prisoners' population. Moreover, the questionnaire and was completed during face to face interviews without the presence of the prison's social workers. Consequently, prisoners could not misreport their physical and mental health status in an attempt to avoid being stigmatized or to avoid the risk of being deprived of certain privileges such as being allowed to work in prison or being allowed to leave the prison on temporary license [36].

The lack of a standardized questionnaire for assessing prisoners' health status, access to and quality of health services as well as detention conditions might be a potential limitation; however, the tool developed for data collection was based on international literature review, it was tested on a convenience sample and also it has been already used in other two published studies [40,41].

Conclusions

The findings suggest that female imprisonment is associated with deterioration of self-reported health status. Restrictions on the access to health services and bad incarceration conditions are aggravating factors. Our findings should be used for decision making purposes in order to prevent the effects of incarceration on prisoners' health and to introduce more effective interventions aiming at meeting their health needs, improving everyday life in prison and also life after release.

Acknowledgements

We would like to thank the Ministry of Justice and the Directorates of the detention centers for allowing us to conduct this study and providing us with useful information and data. We would also like to express our sincere thanks to prison staff for the cooperation, support and valuable advice. Finally, we thank all the female prisoners who accepted to participate in this study.

References

1. Walmsley R (2016) World Prison Population List, 11th ed. Institute for criminal policy research, Birkbeck, University of London, London.
2. Walmsley R (2015) World female imprisonment List, 3rd ed. Institute for criminal policy research, Birkbeck, University of London, London.
3. Nobile CG, Flotta D, Nicotera G, Pileggi C, Angelillo IF (2011) Self-reported health status and access to health services in a sample of prisoners in Italy. BMC Public Health 11: 529.

4. Galea S, Vlahov D (2002) Social determinants and the health of drug users: Socioeconomic status, homelessness, and incarceration. Public Health Rep 117: S135-S145.
5. Butler T, Kariminia A, Levy M, Murphy M (2004) The self-reported health status of prisoners in New South Wales. Aust N Z J Public Health 28: 344-350.
6. Kunst AE, Bos V, Lahelma E, Bartley M, Lissau I, et al. (2005) Trends in socioeconomic inequalities in self-assessed health in 10 European countries. Int J Epidemiol 34: 295-305.
7. Greenberg GA, Rosenheck RA (2008) Jail incarceration, homelessness, and mental health: A national study. Psychiatr Serv 59: 170-177.
8. Conklin TJ, Lincoln T, Tuthill RW (2000) Self-reported health and prior health behaviours of newly admitted correctional inmates. Am J Public Health 90(12): 1939-1941.
9. Van den Bergh BJ, Gatherer A, Møller LF (2009) Women's health in prison: Urgent need for improvement in gender equity and social justice. Bull World Health Organ 87: 406.
10. Fazel S, Baillargeon J (2011) The health of prisoners. Lancet 377: 956-965.
11. Marshall T, Simpson S, Stevens A (2000) Health care in prisons: A health care needs assessment. University of Birmingham, Birmingham.
12. Walmsley R (2009) World prison population list, 8th ed. International Centre for Prison Studies, London.
13. World Health Organization (WHO) (2013) Good governance for prison health in the 21st century: A policy brief on the organization of prison health. WHO Regional Office for Europe, Copenhagen.
14. Lindquist CH, Lindquist CA (1999) Health behind bars: Utilization and evaluation of medical care among jail inmates. J Community Health 24: 285-303.
15. Clow B, Pederson A, Haworth-Brockman M, Bernier J (2009) Rising to the challenge: Sex and gender based analysis for health planning, policy and research in Canada. Atlantic Centre of Excellence for Women's Health, Halifax, NS.
16. Moschetti K, Stadelmann P. (2015) Disease profiles of detainees in the Canton of Vaud in Switzerland: Gender and age differences in substance abuse, mental health and chronic health conditions. BMC Public Health 15: 872.
17. Mooney M, Hannon F, Barry M, Friel S, Kelleher C (2002) Perceived quality of life and mental health status of Irish female prisoners. Ir Med J 95: 241-243.
18. Gunter TD (2004) Incarcerated women and depression: A primer for the primary care provider. J Am Med Womens Assoc 59: 107-112.
19. Plugge E, Fitzpatrick R (2005) Assessing the health of women in prison: A study from the United Kingdom. Health Care Women Int 26: 62-68.
20. Young M, Waters B, Falconer T, O'Rourke P (2005) Opportunities for health promotion in the Queensland women's prison system. Aust N Z J Public Health 29: 324-327.
21. Harris F, Hek G, Condon L (2007) Health needs of prisoners in England and Wales: The implications for prison healthcare of gender, age and ethnicity. Health Soc Care Community 15: 56-66.
22. World Health Organization (WHO) (2009) Women's health in prison: Correcting gender inequity in prison health. WHO Regional Office for Europe, Copenhagen.
23. Van den Bergh BJ, Gatherer A, Fraser A, Moller L (2011) Imprisonment and women's health: Concerns about gender sensitivity, human rights and public health. Bull World Health Organ 89: 689-694.
24. Fazel S, Bains P, Doll H (2006) Substance abuse and dependence in prisoners: A systematic review. Addiction 101: 181-191.
25. Hawton K, Linsell L, Adeniji T, Sariaslan A, Fazel S (2014) Self-harm in prisons in England and Wales: An epidemiological study of prevalence, risk factors, clustering, and subsequent suicide. Lancet 383: 1147-1154.
26. Harlow CW (1999) Prior abuse reported by inmates and probationers. Bureau of Justice Statistics, Washington, DC.
27. Corston B (2007) A report of a review of women with particular vulnerabilities in the criminal justice system. Home Office, London.
28. Social Exclusion Task Force (2009) Short study on women offenders. Cabinet Office, London.
29. Prison Reform Trust (2012) Women in prison. Prison Reform Trust, London.
30. Bernier J, MacLellan K (2011) Health status and health services use of female and male prisoners in provincial jail. Atlantic centre of excellence for women's health, Halifax, NS.
31. Fotiadou M, Livaditis M, Manou I, Kaniotou E, Xenitidis K (2006) Prevalence of mental disorders and deliberate self-harm in Greek male prisoners. Int J Law Psychiatry 29: 68-73.
32. Dandoulaki M, Kosteri V, Milaki V (2008) The psychology of prisoners. The case of prison in New Alikarnasos. Thesis, Technological Educational Institute of Crete, Heraklion, Greece.
33. Papadodima SA, Sakelliadis EI, Sergentanis TN, Giotakos O, Sergentanis IN, et al. (2010) Smoking in prison: A hierarchical approach at the crossroad of personality and childhood events. Eur J Public Health 20: 470-474.
34. Makris E, Gourgoulianis KI, Hatzoglou C (2012) Prisoners and cigarettes or 'imprisoned in cigarettes'? What helps prisoners quit smoking? BMC Public Health 12: 508.
35. Babasikas KD (2013) Inmates in greek prisons and their behavior: The role of institutional, psychological and spatial environment. Doctoral thesis, Aristotle University of Thessaloniki, Thessaloniki, Greece.
36. Togas C, Raikou M, Niakas D (2014) An assessment of health related quality of life in a male prison population in Greece associations with health related characteristics and characteristics of detention. BioMed Res Int p: 274804.
37. Athanasopoulou P (2016) Provision of nursing care to prisoners. Thesis, Western Greece University of Applied Sciences, Patra, Greece.
38. Bania EG, Daniil Z, Hatzoglou C, Alexopoulos EC, Mitsiki E, et al. (2016) COPD characteristics and socioeconomic burden in Hellenic correctional institutions. Int J Chron Obstruct Pulmon Dis 11: 341-349.
39. Vasilopoulou V, Vezyraki D, Chatzaki M (2008) Study of mental health in Greek and immigrant prisoners in detention of Korydallos. E-Thesis: Institutional Repository, Heraklion, Greece.
40. Geitona M, Milioni SO (2016) Health status and access to health services of female prisoners in Greece: A cross-sectional survey. BMC Health Serv Res 16: 243.
41. Geitona M, Milioni SO (2016) Female prisoners' views and satisfaction on incarceration conditions: Findings of a cross-sectional survey in Greece. J Psychol Psychother 6: 284.
42. Douglas N, Plugge E (2006) Health needs assessment for young women in young offender institutions. Youth Justice Board for England and Wales, London.
43. Brooker C, Fox C, Callinan C (2009) Health needs assessment of short sentence prisoners. University of Lincoln, Lincoln.
44. Carnie J, Broderick R (2011) Prison survey 2011. Scottish Prison Service, Falkirk.
45. Rea LM, Parker RA (2005) Designing and conducting survey research: A comprehensive guide, 3rd ed. San Francisco: Jossey-Bass. A Wiley Imprint pp: 30-32.
46. Fickenscher A, Lapidus J, Walker P, Becker T (2001) Women behind bars: Health needs of inmates in a county jail. Public Health Rep 116: 191-196.
47. Parke R, Clarke-Stewart A (2002) Effects of parental incarceration on young children. Urban Institute, Washington, DC.
48. Maguire K, Pastore AL (2003) Sourcebook of Criminal Justice Statistics-2002. Bureau of Justice Statistics, Washington, DC.
49. Taylor R (2004) Women in prison and children of imprisoned mothers: Preliminary research paper. Quaker United Nations Office, Geneva.
50. Bloom B, Owen B, Covington S (2005) Gender-responsive strategies for women offenders: A summary of research, practice, and guiding principles for women offenders. National Institute of Corrections, Washington, DC.

51. Quaker Council for European Affairs (QCEA) (2007) Women in Prison: A review of the conditions in member states of the council of Europe: Executive summary. Quaker Council for European Affairs, Bruxelles.
52. Aebi MF, Delgrande N (2010) Council of Europe Annual Penal Statistics. SPACE I: Survey 2008. Council of Europe, Strasbourg.
53. Harner HM, Riley S (2013) The impact of incarceration on women's mental health: Responses from women in a maximum-security prison. Qual Health Res 23: 26-42.
54. Prison Reform Trust (2016) Bromley briefings prison factfile. Prison Reform Trust, London.
55. Fazel S, Danesh J (2002) Serious mental disorder in 23000 prisoners: A systematic review of 62 surveys. Lancet 359: 545-550.
56. Andersen HS (2004) Mental health in prison populations. A review-with special emphasis on a study of Danish prisoners on remand. Acta Psychiatr Scand Suppl 424: 5-59.
57. Watson R, Stimpson A, Hostick T (2004) Prison health care: A review of the literature. Int J Nurs Stud 41: 119-128.
58. Clarke JG, Hebert MR, Rosengard C, Rose JS, DaSilva KM, et al. (2006) Reproductive health care and family planning needs among incarcerated women. Am J Public Health 96: 834-839.
59. Plugge E, Douglas N, Fitzpatrick R (2006) The health of women in prison study findings. University of Oxford, Oxford.
60. Robert D, Frigon S, Belize S (2007) Women, the embodiment of health and carceral space. Int J Prison Health 3: 176-188.
61. Douglas N, Plugge E, Fitzpatrick R (2009) The impact of imprisonment on health: What do women prisoners say? J Epidemiol Community Health 63: 749-754.
62. Proctor J (2009) The impact imprisonment has on women's health and health care from the perspective of female inmates in Kansas. Women Crim Justice 19: 1-36.
63. Colsher PL, Wallace RB, Loeffelholz PL, Sales M (1992) Health status of older male prisoners: A comprehensive survey. Am J Public Health 82: 881-884.
64. Fazel S, Hope T, O'Donnell I, Piper M, Jacoby R (2001) Health of elderly male prisoners: Worse than the general population, worse than younger prisoners. Age Ageing 30: 403-407.
65. Butler T, Belcher JM, Champion U, Kenny D, Allerton M, et al. (2008) The physical health status of young Australian offenders. Aust N Z J Public Health 32: 73-80.
66. Marshall T, Simpson S, Stevens A (2001) Use of health services by prison inmates: Comparisons with the community. J Epidemiol Community Health 55: 364-365.
67. James D, Glaze L (2006) Mental health problems of prison and jail inmates. Bureau of justice statistics, Washington, DC.
68. Feron JM, Paulus D, Tonglet R, Lorant V, Pestiaux D (2005) Substantial use of primary health care by prisoners: Epidemiological description and possible explanations. J Epidemiol Community Health 59: 651-655.
69. Lee J, Vlahov D, Freudenberg N (2006) Primary care and health insurance among women released from New York City jails. J Health Care Poor Underserved 17: 200-217.
70. Bjørngaard JH, Rustad AB, Kjelsberg E (2009) The prisoner as patient: A health services satisfaction survey. BMC Health Serv Res 9: 176.
71. Sarpong AA, Otupiri E, Yeboah-Awudzi K, Osei-Yeboah J, Berchie GO, et al. (2015) An assessment of female prisoners' perception of the accessibility of quality healthcare: A survey in the Kumasi Central Prisons, Ghana. Ann Med Health Sci Res 5: 179-184.
72. Cropsey K, Eldridge GD, Ladner T (2004) Smoking among female prisoners: An ignored public health epidemic. Addict Behav 29: 425-431.
73. Belcher JM, Butler T, Richmond RL, Wodak AD, Wilhelm K (2006) Smoking and its correlates in an Australian prisoner population. Drug Alcohol Rev 25: 343-348.
74. Sieminska A, Jassem E, Konopa K (2006) Prisoners' attitudes towards cigarette smoking and smoking cessation: A questionnaire study in Poland. BMC Public Health 6: 181.
75. Nijhawan AE, Salloway R, Nunn AS, Poshkus M, Clarke JG (2010) Preventive healthcare for underserved women: Results of a prison survey. J Womens Health 19: 17-22.
76. Qadir M, Murad R, Qadir A, Mubeen SM (2014) Prisoners in Karachi: A health and nutritional perspective. Annals Abbasi Shaheed Hospital & Karachi Medical & Dental College 19: 67-72.
77. Carnie J, Broderick R (2015) Prison Survey 2015. Scottish Prison Service Falkirk.
78. Singh KVP (2010) Human rights of prisoners: A case study of central jail Amristar. Thesis, Guru Nanak Dev University, Amritsar, India.
79. Cheliotis L (2012) Suffering at the hands of the state: Conditions of imprisonment and prisoner health in contemporary Greece. Eur J of Criminol 9: 3-22.

Prevalence of Dysmenorrhea and its Effects on School Performance: A Cross-sectional Study

Derseh BT[1*], Afessa N[2], Temesgen M[2], Semayat YW[2], Kassaye M[2], Sieru S[2], Gizachew S[2] and Ketsela K[2]

[1]*Department of Public Health, Institute of Medicine and Health Sciences, College of Health Sciences, Debre Berhan University, Ethiopia*

[2]*Department of Nursing, Institute of Medicine and Health Sciences, College of Health Sciences Debre Berhan University, Ethiopia*

[*]**Corresponding author:** Derseh BT, Department of Public Health, Institute of Medicine and Health Sciences, College of Health Sciences, Debre Berhan University, Ethiopia, E-mail: minastariku@gmail.com

Abstract

Introduction: Dysmenorrhea is a painful menstrual cramp of uterine origin. It is the most common gynecologic complaints in adolescence and young women among university female students. Major symptoms including pain, adverse effect on daily life and school performance, causing recurrent short-term school absenteeism among female adolescents. Therefore, this study aimed to estimate the prevalence of dysmenorrhea and its effect on school performance.

Methodology: Cross-sectional study was conducted in Debre Berhan University, which is one of public higher institutions in Ethiopia. Cluster sampling technique was used to enroll 307 students. Data were collected using a self-administered questionnaire which was designed for this research. The questionnaire was anonymously completed by each participant who were consented to participate in the study. Data was cleaned, coded and entered into statistical product for service solution (SPSS V.16) for analysis. Pearson's Chi-square test was used to determine linear relationship between dependent and independent categorical variables. Bivariabe and multivariable logistic regression was executed to determine the effect of dysmenorrhea on school performance.

Results: The age of the respondent ranges from 18-29 with a mean and standard deviation of 20.35 ± 1.55. Most of the participants 249 (84.4%) were in the age category of 18 to 21. Concerning the age of menarche, the average was 15.1 ± 1.79 years. Regarding painful menses, 197 (66.8%) of students were suffering from dysmenorrhea. Out of dysmenorric students, 119 (60.4%) of them reported that their school performance was affected attributed to the pain and this was explained by loss of concentration and class absenteeism. Pearson Chi-square test revealed that severity of pain among dysmenorric students had effect on their academic performances (X^2df=2=25.1, $p<0.001$). The result also showed that statistical significance evidence was found among severity of pain and class absentees (X^2df=2=15, $p<0.001$); loss of concentration in class (X^2df=2=12.85, $p<0.05$) and lack of focus on exam (X^2df=2=7.4, $p<0.05$). Moreover, students who are suffering from dysmenorrhea were 8 times more likely their educational performance had been affected than those students who had no dysmenorrhea (AOR=8.013, 95%CI: 3.41, 17.305). It also had psychological effect on students (AOR=2.52, 95%CI: 1.135, 5.595).

Conclusion and Recommendation: Primary dysmenorrhea is a common problem among female students of Debre Berhan University and brought a number of physical and emotional symptoms. As a result the condition affected their school performance and limited their daily class activities. Therefore, to combat these effect students most probably expected to change their lifestyle particularly regular physical exercise. Moreover, awareness should be brought to school authority and teachers about dysmenorrhea to provide psychological and academic support to affected students.

Keywords: Absenteeism; Dysmenorrhea; Effect; Menarche; School performance

Introduction

Menstruation is a normal physiological process that occurs approximately once a month in women of reproductive age as a result of the breakdown of the endometrial tissue. But dysmenorrhea refers to the occurrence of painful menstrual cramps of uterine origin. It is the most common gynecologic complaints in adolescence and young women, occurring in 60% to 93% of school girls and young women [1-5].

Major symptoms, including pain, adversely affect daily life and school performance, causing recurrent short-term school absenteeism among female adolescents [6]. Previous epidemiologic investigations have reported the magnitudes of dysmenorrhea ranged from 43% to 91% in school girls [1-7]. There are a limited number of studies conducted on university female students with the problem of dysmenorrhea in Ethiopia. Likewise, as far as our knowledge is concerned such study is the first to deal with dysmenorrhea and academic performance in our study area. However, some studies reported different prevalence; for instance, at Bahir Dar University the prevalence of dysmenorrhea and premenstrual syndrome were 85.1% and 72.8%, respectively [8].

Likewise, the prevalence of premenstrual syndrome (PMS) at Mekelle University college of Health Science reported as 34% [9]. At the same time studies out of the country reported prevalence rate of dysmenorrhea. In Indian nursing college, situated in campus of largest tertiary care hospital in central and south Gujarat, the reported prevalence was 45% [10].

In Egypt, it was reported a highest prevalence rate of dysmenorrhea (94.4%) with (49.0%) for mild pain, 34.4% for moderate pain and 16.6% for severe pain [11]. In Japanese high school students the prevalence reported was 72.8% [12]; findings from Mansoura University-Egypt, showed relatively high prevalence of dysmenorrhea, that was 78.8% among technical secondary schools girls [13].

The prevalence of dysmenorrhea among Hong Kong University student reported was 80% (95%CI; 75, 85%) [14]. Study conducted in Iraq revealed that the frequency of dysmenorrhea was estimated to be 85.31% [15]; likewise, a cross-sectional study carried among female students aged 18 to 27 years in Isfahan University of Medical Sciences-Iran, the prevalence was 89.1% [16]. Study conducted in Parakou high school showed that the prevalence of primary dysmenorrhea was 78.35% with 95% CI [74.07-82.11%].

It was mild in 33.3% of the cases; moderate in 37.8% and severe in 28.8% [17]. Similarly, cross-sectional study conducted on 356 female medical students at Mohiuddin Islamic University, Mirpur Azad Kashmir revealed a prevalence of 56% [18]. In other studies among Turkish and Serbian students, prevalence of dysmenorrhea was found to be 72.7% and 29.9%, respectively [19,20].

Different researchers argue that female university students had experienced less academic performance and other negative effects as a result of dysmenorrhea. The most common effects were class absenteeism as reported in [9,12,13,17,21-24], unable to concentrate on their classes or study [13,14,17,18], had bad relationships with their families/friends [13,14,18], unable to do homework [17] and missed exam [24].

So far we have seen the prevalence and effects of dysmenorrhea on school performance in different university students. The gap identified was that previous studies pay little attention on the need for strategy design at university level to compensate lost classes and improve poor performance attributed to dysmenorrhea. Therefore, this study aimed to estimate the prevalence of dysmenorrhea and its effect on school performance and seek appropriate strategy as a remedy.

Materials and Methods

Study area

Debre Berhan University is one of the thirteen new universities in Ethiopia which was established in 2007 G.C and located in Amhara Region, North Showa Zone, in Debre Berhan Town 130 km, away from Addis Abeba. Currently, the total number of regular students is estimated to be 10, 258. From this 6444 are males and 3714 are females.

Study design and period

Institution based cross-sectional study design was carried out to assess the prevalence of dysmenorrhea, its effect on academic performance among female students from March 1-7, 2016 G.C.

Sample size

The sample size for this particular study was determined by using single population proportion formula, considering 95% confidence level, 5% of marginal error (0.05), prevalence of dysmenorrhea (p=0.85) at Bahir Dar University [8]. Multiplying the result by 1.5 to minimize the sampling error that arises from cluster sampling technique and taking 10% non-response rate, the total sample size required was 307 undergraduate students.

Data collection and operational definitions

Data were collected using a self-administered questionnaire which was designed for this research. The questionnaire was anonymously completed by each participant who consented to participate in the study. Before actual data collection, pretest was performed on 30 female students to check the soundness of data collection tool and to determine the time of data collection. Then, the students were asked to provide information about their socio demographic and gynecologic or obstetric information. Women who reported that they had experienced menstrual pain completed additional questions regarding the characteristics of pain and influence of pain on their ability to perform everyday activities including academic performance and class absenteeism, if any. The period between the first day of menstruation and the day immediately prior to the next menstruation was defined as the menstrual cycle.

Menstrual cycles were considered to be regular if ranged between 21 to 35 days. A family history of dysmenorrhea was defined as positive if a student's first degree relative (mother or sister) had a history of dysmenorrhea. Mild pain during menses refers to painful menses but not inhibits normal activity (class activities), Moderate pain refers daily activity affected and required analgesics which give relief and severe pain refer activity clearly inhibited and poor effect of analgesics.

Data management and analysis

Data was cleaned, coded and entered in to statistical package for service solution (SPSS V.16) for analysis. Descriptive statistics, such as frequency, percentage, mean, standard deviation, tables and graphs were used to describe study population. Pearson's Chi-square test was used to determine the relationship between dependent and independent categorical variables. The differences were considered significant if probability of null hypothesis was less than 0.05. To determine the potential influence of dysmenorrhea on academic and psychology of female students, binary logistic regression was used to calculate crude and adjusted odds ratios with adjustments for covariates.

Ethical Consideration

The study was approved by the Ethical Committee of the Institute of Medicine and Health Sciences, Debre Berhan University. The rationale of the study was explained to the students. Confidentiality of information was maintained by omitting any personal identifier from the questionnaires and collected data were kept safe to avoid disclosure to third party except principal investigators.

Results

Out of 307 self-administered distributed questionnaires, 295 female students returned the questionnaires after completing the required information, giving a response rate of 96.1%. The respondent's age ranges from 18-29 with a mean (±SD) of 20.35 ± 1.55. Most of the participants, 249 (84.4%) were in the age category of 18 to 21. Concerning the age of menarche, the average was 15.1 ± 1.79 years. Almost half, 146 (49.5%), of the respondents age of menarche were in age group of 12-15 years. Regarding the regularity of menstrual cycle, students reported that 252 (85.4%) of them had regular menstrual cycle (Table 1).

Variables		Frequency	Percentage
Age of the students (in years)	18 to 21	249	84.40%
	21 to 25	42	14.20%
	25+	4	1.40%
	Mean ± standard deviation	20.35 ± 1.55	
Age at first menarche (in years)	<12	25	8.50%
	12 to 15	146	49.50%
	15+	124	42.00%
	Mean ± standard deviation	15.1 ± 1.79	
Duration of menstrual flow (in days)	<3	132	44.75%
	3 to 7	163	55.25%
	Mean ± standard deviation	4.16 ± 1.425	
Amount of flow (pad/days)	≤3 pads (little)	270	91.50%
	4 to 7 pads (moderate)	25	8.50%
Menstrual cycle	Regular	252	85.40%
	Irregular	43	14.60%
Habit of physical exercise	Yes	85	28.81%
	No	210	71.19%

Table 1: Socio-demographic and menstrual characteristics of female students, DBU, Ethiopia, 2016.

Prevalence of dysmenorrhea and its severity

According to this study, 197 (66.8%) of the students reported that they were suffering from primary dysmenorrhea. We asked and classified students having menstrual pain that hindered with daily activities and required medication during each menstrual period and reported severe pain in 34 (17.26%), moderate pain in 81 (41.11%) and mild pain in 82 (41.63%). The location of this pain varies with students and mostly it was reported in lower abdomen (142/197; 72.1%) followed by abdominal pain that extends to thighs (20.8%), back pain in 38 (19.3%) and pack pain extending to anus in 11 (5.6%). Regarding symptoms associated with dysmenorrhea the most common symptoms reported were stomach cramp in 176 (89%), backache in 73 (37%), mood change in 58 (29%), fatigue present in 104 (52.8%), diarrhea present in 8 (4.0%) and headache present in 47 (23.8%) (Table 2).

Variables	Frequency	Percentage
Presence of dysmenorrhea		
Yes	197	66.80%
No	98	33.20%
Severity of dysmenorrhea		
Mild	82	41.63%
Moderate	81	41.11%
Severe	34	17.26%
Symptoms associated with pain		
Stomach cramp	176	89.00%
Backache	73	37.00%
Mood changes	58	29.00%
Fatigue	104	52.80%
Diarrhea	8	4.00%
Headache	47	23.80%
Nausea	32	16.24%
Edema	7	3.60%

Table 2: Prevalence, severity and symptoms of dysmenorrhea among female students, DBU, Ethiopia, 2016.

Effects of dysmenorrhea

As indicated in Table 3 below, Pearson Chi-square test were performed to determine the relationship between dysmenorrhea and its effect on school performance. The test revealed that severity of pain among dysmenorric students had effect on their academic performances (X^2df=2=25.1, p<0.001). The result also showed that there were high statistical significance between severity of pain and class absenteeism, loss of concentration in class and lack of focus on exam (p<0.05) (Table 3). Likewise, pain during menses affected student's psychology, it is also statistically significant under bivariate logistic regression [COR=6.002; 95%CI (3.018, 11.94)] (Table 4).

Characteristics	Severity of Dysmenorrhea						x^2	df	P-value
	Mild		Moderate		Severe				
	Count	Percent	Count	Percent	Count	Percent			
Effect on Education									
Yes	34	17.25%	53	26.90%	31	15.73%			
No	47	23.85%	28	14.21%	4	2.06%	25.1	2	<0.001*
Class absentee									
Yes	9	7.62%	30	25.42%	23	19.49%			
No	25	21.18%	23	19.49%	8	6.80%	15	2	<0.001*
Lost Concentration									
Yes	27	22.88%	30	25.42%	11	9.32%			
No	7	5.93%	23	19.49%	20	16.96%	12.85	2	0.002*
Decreased class input									
Yes	12	10.17%	22	18.64%	6	5.10%			
No	22	18.64%	31	26.27%	25	21.18%	4.33	2	0.115
Lack of focus on exam									
Yes	15	12.71%	12	10.17%	5	4.25%			
No	19	16.10%	41	34.74%	26	22.03%	7.4	2	0.025*
Unable to answer exam									
Yes	6	5.08%	6	5.08%	5	4.25%			
No	28	23.72%	47	39.83%	26	22.04%	0.773	2	0.679
Effect on psychology									
Yes	31	15.73%	35	17.76%	19	9.64%			
No	51	25.88%	46	23.35%	15	7.67%	3.2	2	0.202
Effect on relationships									
Yes	9	10.89%	8	9.41%	5	5.88%			
No	22	25.88%	27	31.76%	14	16.47%	0.329	2	0.848
Mood change									
Yes	15	17.64%	12	14.12%	5	5.88%			
No	16	18.82%	23	27.06%	14	16.47%	0.273	2	0.255
Note: X^2=chi square; df=degree of freedom; P<0.05 indicates statistical significance (*)									

Table 3: Association between severity of dysmenorrhea and its effects on education among female students, DBU, Ethiopia, 2016.

Bivariable and multi-variable analysis

Premenstrual symptom was an important indicator for the presence of dysmenorrhea. It was found that those respondents who had PMS were 3.259 times more likely to have dysmenorrhea compared to those who do not experienced PMS (AOR=3.259, 95%CI: 1.783, 5.954). According to the analysis, dysmenorrhea has negative effect on student's academic performance and their psychology. These can be supported by our findings that students who had primary dysmenorrhea were 8.013 times more likely their educational performance affected than those female students who had no dysmenorrhea (AOR=8.013, 95%CI: 3.41, 17.305). Similarly, dysmenorrhea also had a psychological effect twice as those who do not have the pain (AOR=2.52, 95%CI: 1.135, 5.595) (Table 4).

Variables	Presence of Dysmenorrhea No. (%)		COR (95% CI)	AOR (95% CI)
	Yes	No		
Family History				
Yes	115 (38.98)	44 (14.92)	1.721 (1.056, 2.805)*	1.077 (0.59, 1.965)
No	82 (27.79)	54 (18.31)	1	1
Duration of menses flow in days				
Less than 3 day	80 (21.12)	52 (17.63)	1.653 (1.015, 2.694)*	1.265 (0.702, 2.278)
3 to 7 days	117 (39.66)	52 (17.63)	1	1
Premenstrual Symptoms				
Yes	143 (48.47)	37 (12.54)	4.366 (2.61, 7.304)*	3.259 (1.783, 5.954)*
No	54 (18.31)	61 (20.68)	1	1
Effect on School Performance				
Yes	118 (40.00)	79 (26.78)	13.144 (6.44, 26.82)*	8.013 (3.71, 17.305)*
No	10 (03.39)	88 (29.83)	1	1
Psychological Effect				
Yes	85 (28.81)	11 (03.73)	6.002 (3.018, 11.94)*	2.52 (1.135, 5.595)*
No	112 (37.97)	87 (29.49)	1	1

Table 4: Bivariate and multivariate analysis of dysmenorrhea and effects on education among female students, DBU, Ethiopia, 2016.

Discussion

The prevalence of dysmenorrhea among female students is 66.8%, which is higher compared with studies conducted in different parts of the world. This figure is relatively higher than prevalence reported by Shah et al. [10], Yasir et al. [18] and Pejcic et al. [20]. In contrasts, the prevalence was relatively lower in studies conducted by Teshome et al. [8], El-Hameed et al. [11], Mohamed et al. [13], Chia et al. [14], Khodakarami et al. [15], Habibi et al. [16] and Sidi et al. [17]. The possible reasons for the discrepancy among the estimates could be the difference in the life style of study subjects, the difference in use of selected age group, difference in perception of pain during menstruation, the absence of universally accepted technique of defining dysmenorrhea, a probable disparity in the methods of data collection, study definitions of dysmenorrhea and pain. But our study was consistent with studies done in Japanese Female Junior High School Students and other studies as mentioned by Kazama et al. [12], Unsal et al. [19], Kumbhar et al. [23] and Charu et al. [25].

In our study, subjects suffering from dysmenorrhea (n=197) presented with the following symptoms like stomach cramp, mood change, backache, headache, fatigue, and vomiting/diarrhea were reported. Such symptoms were the major reasons for difficulty in concentration during class time (34.5%), absenteeism (32%), less participation in school activities (20%), lack of focus on exam (16.5%) and inability to answer the correct response during exam (8.6%). Based on these findings, one can learn that painful menses in our study setting is an important health problem in university female students and has a negative effect on their academic performance. The Chi-square analysis also showed that dysmenorrhea is responsible for significant absenteeism from class (X^2=15; df=2; p=0.001), loss of concentration (X^2=12.85; df=2; p=0.02), lack of focus on exam (X^2=7.4; df=2; p=0.025). Different studies agree with our study findings [9,12-14,17,18,21-24]. The negative effect of dysmenorrhea comes at its peak when it brings about missed exams and absenteeism.

Limitation of the Study

Since the study design was cross-sectional, temporal relations could not be established between dysmenorrhea and its effect on academic performance. In addition there could be a memory decay that leads to recall bias and over-reporting of the condition because students were asked for conditions within the last years prior to the study.

Conclusion and Recommendation

Primary dysmenorrhea was a common problem among female students and brought a number of physical and emotional symptoms. As a result it affected female students' school performance and limited their daily school activities. Therefore, strategies should be designed for early detection of the problems and management through change in students' life style like promoting regular physical exercises. Performing regular physical exercise reduced primary dysmenorrhea symptoms as mentioned by Noorbakhsh Mahvash et al. [26]. Thus, because of high potential benefits of physical exercise in reducing the negative effects of primary dysmenorrhea symptoms, university students should be recommended to take part in regular physical activity programs. Moreover, school authorities and teachers should be aware of the problems of dysmenorrhea to provide psychological and academic support through tutorial class to affected group of students. Alongside, health professionals who are working in the university's student clinic should design health education program to mobilize university community to change students' life style.

Authors' Contribution

BTD comprehended the idea, designed the study, conducted analyses, interpreted and prepared the manuscript; all the others conducted, analyzed, interpreted the result, read and approved the final manuscript.

Competing Interests

We, the authors, declare that we have no competing interests.

Acknowledgment

We would like to appreciate all students who were volunteer and willing to give us their time to offer all relevant information to this investigation. Our deepest gratefulness also goes to Debre Berhan University and Debre Berhan Health Science College for their support.

References

1. Maybin JA, Critchley HO (2011) Progesterone: A pivotal hormone at menstruation. Ann N Y Acad Sci 1221: 88- 97.
2. Berbic M, Ng CH, Fraser IS (2014) Inflammation and endometrial bleeding. Climacteric 17: 47-53.
3. Hillard PJA (2006) Dysmenorrhea: consultation with the specialist. Pediatr Rev 27: 64-71.
4. Calis KA, Popat V, Dang DK, Kalantaridou SN (2016) Dysmenorrhea. eMed Gynecol Obstet p: 253812.
5. Proctor ML, Murphy PA, Pattison HM, Suckling J, Farquhar CM (2007) Behavioral interventions for primary and secondary dysmenorrhea. Cochrane database Syst Rev 3: CD002248.
6. Harel Z (2008) Dysmenorrhea in adolescents. Ann NY Acad Sci 1135: 185-195.
7. Sultan C, Gaspari L, Paris F (2012) Adolescent dysmenorrhea. Endocr Dev 22: 171-180.
8. Shiferaw MT, Wubshet M, Tegabu D (2014) Menstrual problems and associated factors among students of Bahir Dar University, Amhara National Regional State, Ethiopia: A cross-sectional survey. Pan Afr Med J 17: 246.
9. Tolossa FW, Bekele ML (2014) Prevalence, impacts and medical managements of premenstrual syndrome among female students: Cross-sectional study in college of health sciences, Mekelle University, Mekelle, Northern Ethiopia. BMC women's health 14: 1.
10. Shah M, Monga A, Patel S, Shah M, Bakshi H (2013) A study of prevalence of primary dysmenorrhea in young students-A cross-sectional study. Health line 4: 30-34.
11. El-Hameed NA, Mohamed MS, Ahmed NH, Ahmed ER (2011) Assessment of dysmenorrhea and menstrual hygiene practices among adolescent girls in some nursing schools at EL-Minia Governorate, Egypt. J Am Sci 7: 223.
12. Kazama M, Maruyama K, Nakamura K (2015) Prevalence of dysmenorrhea and its correlating lifestyle factors in japanese female junior high school students. Tohoku J Exp Med 236: 107-113.
13. Mohamed HE, Mansour SE (2013) The effect of dysmenorrhea on quality of life of technical secondary schools girls. Med J Cairo Univ 81: 83-90.
14. Chia CF, JHY Lai, PK Cheung, LT Kwong, FPM Lau, et al. (2013) Dysmenorrhoea among Hong Kong university students: Prevalence, impact, and management. Hong Kong. Med J 19: 3.
15. Khodakarami B, Masoumi SZ, Faradmal J, Nazari M, Saadati M, et al. (2015) The severity of dysmenorrhea and its relationship with body mass index among female adolescents in Hamadan, Iran. J Midwifery Reprod Health 3: 444-450.
16. Habibi N, Huang MSL, Gan WY, Zulida R, Safavi SM (2015) Prevalence of primary dysmenorrhea and factors associated with its intensity among undergraduate students: A cross-sectional study. Am Society Pain Management Nurs 16: 855-861.
17. Sidi I, Hounkpatin B, Obossou AAA, Salifou K, Vodouhe M, et al. (2016) Primary dysmenorrhea in the schools of Parakou: Prevalence, Impact and Therapeutic Approach. Gynecol Obstet 6: 376.
18. Yasir S, Kant B, Farooq MD (2014) Frequency of dysmenorrhoea, its impact and management strategies adopted by medical students. J Ayub Med Coll Abbottabad 26: 349-352.
19. Unsal A, Ayranci U, Tozun M, Arslan G, Calik E (2010) Prevalence of dysmenorrhea and its effect on quality of life among a group of female university students. Ups J Med Sci 115: 138-145.
20. Pejcic A, Jankovic S (2016) Risk factors for dysmenorrhea among young adult female university students. Ann Ist Super Sanita 52: 98-103.
21. Shete JS, Warbhe P, Padmini D (2012) Class absenteeism among female medical students: A study reflecting its association with common menstrual disorders. Int J Recent Scientific Res 6: 5307-5309.
22. Singh A, Kiran D, Singh H, Nel B, Singh P, Tiwari P (2008) Prevalence and severity of dysmenorrhea: a problem related to menstruation, among first and second year female medical students. Indian J Physiol Pharmacol 52: 389-397.
23. Kumbhar SK, Reddy M, Sujana B, Reddy R, Bhargavi K, et al. (2011) Prevalence of dysmenorrhea among adolescent girls (14-19 yrs.) of Kadapa district and its impact on quality of life: A cross sectional Study. Natl J Community Med 2: 265-268.
24. Kakoma JB, Gasana GK, Nkurunzinza J, Ngirinshuti JP (2010) Dysmenorrhea and other menstrual characteristics in Rwandan female students at National University of Rwanda and Nyanza school girls. Rwanda Medical Journal 68: 3.
25. Charu S, Amita R, Sujoy R, Thomas GA (2012) Menstrual characteristics' and 'Prevalence and effect of dysmenorrhea' on quality of life of medical students. IJCRIMPH 4: 4.
26. Mahvash N, Eidy A, Mehdi K, Zahra MT, Mani M (2012) The effect of physical activity on primary dysmenorrhea of female university students. World Applied Sciences Journal 17: 1246-1252.

Permissions

All chapters in this book were first published in JWHC, by OMICS International; hereby published with permission under the Creative Commons Attribution License or equivalent. Every chapter published in this book has been scrutinized by our experts. Their significance has been extensively debated. The topics covered herein carry significant findings which will fuel the growth of the discipline. They may even be implemented as practical applications or may be referred to as a beginning point for another development.

The contributors of this book come from diverse backgrounds, making this book a truly international effort. This book will bring forth new frontiers with its revolutionizing research information and detailed analysis of the nascent developments around the world.

We would like to thank all the contributing authors for lending their expertise to make the book truly unique. They have played a crucial role in the development of this book. Without their invaluable contributions this book wouldn't have been possible. They have made vital efforts to compile up to date information on the varied aspects of this subject to make this book a valuable addition to the collection of many professionals and students.

This book was conceptualized with the vision of imparting up-to-date information and advanced data in this field. To ensure the same, a matchless editorial board was set up. Every individual on the board went through rigorous rounds of assessment to prove their worth. After which they invested a large part of their time researching and compiling the most relevant data for our readers.

The editorial board has been involved in producing this book since its inception. They have spent rigorous hours researching and exploring the diverse topics which have resulted in the successful publishing of this book. They have passed on their knowledge of decades through this book. To expedite this challenging task, the publisher supported the team at every step. A small team of assistant editors was also appointed to further simplify the editing procedure and attain best results for the readers.

Apart from the editorial board, the designing team has also invested a significant amount of their time in understanding the subject and creating the most relevant covers. They scrutinized every image to scout for the most suitable representation of the subject and create an appropriate cover for the book.

The publishing team has been an ardent support to the editorial, designing and production team. Their endless efforts to recruit the best for this project, has resulted in the accomplishment of this book. They are a veteran in the field of academics and their pool of knowledge is as vast as their experience in printing. Their expertise and guidance has proved useful at every step. Their uncompromising quality standards have made this book an exceptional effort. Their encouragement from time to time has been an inspiration for everyone.

The publisher and the editorial board hope that this book will prove to be a valuable piece of knowledge for researchers, students, practitioners and scholars across the globe.

List of Contributors

Francis Olayemi Adebayo, Olatunde Onafowokan and Nathaniel Adewole
Department of Obstetrics and Gynecology, University of Abuja Teaching Hospital, Abuja-FCT, Nigeria

Sanjay Jayawant Rode
Department of Economics, S.K. Somaiya College, Mumbai University, India

Duko B, Tadesse B, Gebre M and Teshome T
Faculty of Health Sciences, College of Medicine and Health Sciences, Hawassa University, Ethiopia

Solomon Gebre
Mearg General Hospital, Emergency Surgical Department, Dansha, West Tigray, Ethiopia

Ataklti Negasi
Mygaba Primary Health Unit, Emergency Surgical Department, Mygaba, West Tigray, Ethiopia

Assefa Hailu
Freweyni Primary Hospital, Emergency Surgical Department, Freweyni, Eastern Tigray, Ethiopia

Fageeh WMK
Department of Obstetrics and Gynecology, Faculty of Medicine, King Abdulaziz University Hospital, Kingdom of Saudi Arabia

Currie J
Health and Physical Education, University of Technology Sydney, Australia

August S Bassani, Daniel Banov and Maria Carvalho
Professional Compounding Centers of America (PCCA), Houston, TX, USA

Massaldjieva R Ivanova, Desislava Bakova, Maria Semerdjieva, Bianka Torniova, Boris Tilov and Ekaterina Raikova
Department of Health Care Management, Medical University of Plovdiv, Bulgaria

Krishnavelh Kathleen Nadasen
Department of Anthropology and Sociology, University of the Western Cape, Bellville, South Africa

Muhammad Basheer Yahya and Tepanata Pumpaibool
Department of Clinical Pharmacy and Pharmaceutical Care, Faculty of Pharmaceutical Sciences, Gombe State University, Gombe, Nigeria

Pranti Dutta
Department of Biosciences and Bioengineering, Indian Institute of Technology, Guwahati, India

Bodhisattva Sengupta
Department of Humanities and Social Sciences, Indian Institute of Technology, Guwahati, India

Nasser Saeed Al-Qahtani
Department of Family and Community Medicine, College of Medicine, Najran University, KSA, Saudi Arabia

Lisa B Phipps and Kristopher J Pickens
Office of Learning Innovation and Student Success and Institute for Women's Health, Virginia Commonwealth University, Virginia, USA

Allison Sepulveda
Institute for Women's Health, Virginia Commonwealth University, Virginia, USA

Nicole Karjane
Department of Obstetrics and Gynecology, Virginia Commonwealth University, Virginia, USA

Donna Miles
Carolina Population Center, University of North Carolina at Chapel Hill, North Carolina, USA

Susan Kornstein
Department of Psychiatry, Institute for Women's Health, Virginia Commonwealth University, Virginia, USA

Dace S Svikis
Department of Psychology, Psychiatry, Obstetrics and Gynecology, Virginia Commonwealth University, Virginia, USA

Khan NM, Rampat S and Sannassee L
Faculty of Social Sciences and Humanities, University of Mauritius, Moka, Mauritius

Teklehaymanot AN, Niguse D and Tesfay A
Department of Population and Family Health, College of Health Sciences, Jimma University, Ethiopia

Asrat Meleko Mara, Mengistu Ayenew, Haile Haftu and Binyam Aregay
Department of Public Health, Mizan-Tepi University, Mizan Aman, Ethiopia

Jose Luis Turabian, Minier-Rodriguez LE, Moreno-Ruiz S, Rodriguez-Almonte FE, Cucho-Jove R and Villarin-Castro A
Specialists in Family and Community Medicine, Health Center Santa Maria de Benquerencia, Toledo, Spain

Neto JB
Department of Aesthetic Vaginal Surgery, Centro Clínico Mãe de Deus, Brazil

Van der Pligt P, Ball K, Hesketh KD, Teychenne M, Crawford D and Campbell K
Institute for Physical Activity and Nutrition (IPAN), School of Exercise and Nutrition Sciences, Deakin University, Geelong, Australia

Dodd J
The University of Adelaide, School of Paediatrics and Reproductive Health, Robinson Research Institute, Adelaide, South Australia, Australia
Department of Perinatal Medicine, The Women's and Children's Hospital, Women's and Babies Division, North Adelaide, South Australia, Australia

Mohammed Feyisso and Alebachew Girma
Department of Public Health, College of Health Sciences and Medicine, Dilla University, Dilla, Ethiopia

Hamid Yimam
Department of Public Health, College of Health Sciences and Medicine, Mizan Tepi University, Mizan, Ethiopia

Sileshi Hailu
Department of Anesthesia, College of Health Sciences and Medicine, Dilla University, Dilla, Ethiopia

Lemma E
Public Health Expert at Fantale District, Oromia Regional State, Fantale, Ethiopia

Husein G
Department of Public Health, College of Health Science, Arsi University, Assela, Ethiopia

Yitagesu Sintayehu and Kasiye Shiferaw
Department of Midwifery, College of Health and Medical Sciences, Haramaya University, Ethiopia

Birhanu Hordofa
Department of Nursing and midwifery, College of Health and Medical Sciences, Addis Ababa University, Ethiopia

Andrade Martin C, Fernandes Alvares R, Reis Nascimento T, Waldemar Paranaiba SS, Karen da Silva Morais T and Carvalho Santos D
Physical Therapist, Studio-100 Pilates, Brasilia, Brazil

Himani Sharma, Singh SK and Shobhit Srivastava
Department of Mathematical Demography and Statistics, International Institute for Population Sciences, Mumbai, Maharashtra, India

Salifou K, Obossou AAA, Noudamadjo A, Houkponou F, Sidi R and Vodounhe M
Department of Mother and Child, Faculty of Medicine, University of Parakou, Bénin

Perrin XR and Alihonou E
Department of Mother and Child, Faculty of Health Sciences of Cotonou, University of Abomey-Calavi, Bénin

Jay Lincoln
Master in Public Health, School of Public Health and Primary Care, Fiji National University, Fiji Islands

Masoud Mohammadnezhad
Associate Professor in Public Health, School of Public Health and Primary Care, Fiji National University, Fiji Islands

Sabiha Khan
Lecturer in statistics, School of Public Health and Primary Care, Fiji National University, Fiji Islands

Merga Dheresa, Nega Assefa, Bizatu Mingiste and Yadeta Dessie
Department of Health and Medical Sciences, Haramaya University, Harar, Ethiopia

Yemane Berhane and Alelmayhu Worku
Addis Continental Institutes of Public Health, Addis Ababa, Ethiopia

Takele Gezahegn Demie, Tufa Kolola Huluka and Helen G Libanos
Department of Public Health, College of Health Sciences, Debre Berhan University, Debre Berhan, Ethiopia

Tigist Demissew
Department of Surgical, College of Health Sciences, Debre Berhan University, Debre Berhan, Ethiopia

Derara Workineh
Dawe Serer District Health Office, Bale Zone, Oromia Regional State, Ethiopia

Mastewal Arefaynie Temesgen
Public Health Department, College of Medicine and Health Sciences, Wollo University, Ethiopia

Sidra Manzoor
Department of Molecular Biology and Biotechnology, University of Veterinary and Animal Sciences, Lahore, Pakistan

Mubashar Aziz
Department of Pathobiology, Faculty of Veterinary Sciences, Bahauddin Zakariya University, Multan, Pakistan

Ahsan Sattar Sheikh
Institute of Food Science and Nutrition, Bahauddin Zakariya University, Multan, Pakistan

Bagnan-Tonato JA, Lokossou MSHS, Ogoudjobi OM, Tognifode V, Aboubacar M, Adisso S, Ali ARORS, Lokossou A and Perrin RX
Department of Mother and Child, Faculty of Health Sciences of Cotonou, University of Abomey-Calavi, Bénin

Obossou AAA
Department of Mother and Child, Faculty of Medicine, University of Parakou, Bénin

Maysoon Sharief, Dhamya Salih Alharoon and Hutham Tariq Mohammed
Department of Gynecology and Obstetrics, College of Medicine, University of Basrah, Basrah Health Directorate, Basrah, Iraq

Haile Anchebi T
Department of public Health, College of Health Sciences, Adama General Hospital and Medical College, Adama, Ethiopia

Zeleke Shiferaw B
Department of Nursing, Wolkite University, College of Medicine and Health Sciences, Wolkite, Ethiopia

Olana Fite R
Department of Nursing, College of Medicine and Health sciences, Woliata Sodo University, Woliata Sodo, Ethiopia

Garoma Abeya S
Department of Social and Population Health, Adama Hospital Medical College, Adama, Ethiopia

Abay Woday
Department of Public Health, College of Medical and Health Science, Samara University, Ethiopia

Yonatan Menber, Fuad Yimam and Negesse Melese
Department of Public Health, College of Health Science, Alkan University, Ethiopia

Samuel Dagne
Department of Public Health, College of Health Science, Woldia University, Ethiopia

Takeshi Hasuda
Department of Obstetrics and Gynecology, Jikei Hospital, Kumamoto, Japan

Atsushi Ueda and Chang-Nian Wei
Department of Public Health, Faculty of Life Sciences, Kumamoto University, Kumamoto, Japan

Sara Lee and Rina Lazebnik
Department of Pediatrics, University Hospitals Cleveland Medical Center, Cleveland, Ohio, USA

Noam Lazebnik
Department of Obstetrics and Gynecology, University Hospitals Cleveland Medical Center, Cleveland, Ohio, USA

Krystel Tossone
Begun Center for Violence Prevention Research and Education, Case Western Reserve University, Cleveland, Ohio, USA

Matthew Bauer
School of Medicine, Case Western Reserve University, Cleveland, Ohio, USA

Stella-Olga Milioni and Mary Geitona
Department of Social and Educational Policy, University of Peloponnese, Damaskinou and Kolokotroni Str, 20100, Corinth, Greece

Derseh BT
Department of Public Health, Institute of Medicine and Health Sciences, College of Health Sciences, Debre Berhan University, Ethiopia

Afessa N, Temesgen M, Semayat YW, Kassaye M, Sieru S, Gizachew S and Ketsela K
Department of Nursing, Institute of Medicine and Health Sciences, College of Health Sciences Debre Berhan University, Ethiopia

Index